FUNDAMENTALS OF ESTHETIC IMPLANT DENTISTRY

FUNDAMENTALS OF ESTHETIC IMPLANT DENTISTRY

Abd El Salam El Askary

Blackwell
Munksgaard

Fundamentals of Esthetic Implant Dentistry

Authorized reprint by Wiley India Pvt. Ltd., 4435-36/7, Ansari Road, Daryaganj, New Delhi – 110002.

Wiley also publishes its books in a variety of electronic formats. Some content that appears in print may not be available in electronic books. For more information about Wiley products, visit our website at: www.wiley.com.

Reprint: 2014

Printed in India

ISBN: 978-0-8138-1448-3

I dedicate this work to the one who teacheth by the pen, Teacheth man that which he knew not.

Contents

List of Contributors

Main author:

Abd El Salam El Askary, B.D.S
39 Abdelsalam aref. St.
Elbostan
Alexandria, Egypt
E-mail: askary@dataxpres.com.eg
Phone: +2 012 214 8642
Fax: +2 03 5850770

Co-authors:

Chapter 7
Hom-Lay Wang, D.D.S., M.S.D.
Professor and Director of Graduate Periodontics
Department of Periodontics and Oral Medicine
University of Michigan School of Dentistry
1011 North University Avenue
Ann Arbor, Michigan 48109-1078, USA
Phone: 734-763-3383
Fax: 734-936-0374
E-mail: homlay@umich.edu

Rodrigo F. Neiva, D.D.S.
Clinical Assistant Professor
Department of Periodontics and Oral Medicine
University of Michicgan School of Dentistry
Ann Arbor, Michigan 48109-1078, USA

Chapter 9
Dr. Dritan Turhani
AKH-General Hospital of Vienna
Department of Cranio-Maxillofacial and Oral Surgery
Waehringer Guertel 18-20
1090 Vienna, Austria
E-mail: dritan.turhani@gmail.com

Elisabeth Stein, Martina Weinβenböck, and Rolf Ewers also contributed

Chapter 10
Dr. Peter Gehrke
Bismarck str.27
67059 Ludwigshafen
Germany
Phone: 49 62 21 68124456
Fax: +49 621 68124469
Email: Dr-gehrke@dr-dhom.de

Chapter 11
Stephen J. Chu, DMD, MSD, CDT, MDT
150 East 58th Street, Suite 3200
New York, New York 10155
Phone: 212-752-7937
Fax: 212-980-9647
E-mail1: schu@csdny.com
E-mail2: schudmd@aol.com

Foreword

Osseointegration is no longer a possibility but rather a given in implant dentistry today. However, with this predictability that we have come to expect, has also come a shift into concerns that at one time were not even thought about. Today, the concept of beauty and esthetics are also equally as important as the pure function of mastication. In fact, in some cases with high smile lines, it is more important than just function and will in fact determine the treatment plan of choice.

This textbook is a wonderful accumulation of the thoughts and work of Dr. El Askary and other professionals from around the world. I want to congratulate Dr. El Askary for his dedication to this project, which is considered to be an ongoing work in progress over his outstanding career. His involvement with esthetics and implant dentistry is as intense as anyone's in this field, and his dedication and pursuit of excellence is to be commended.

This textbook has many wonderful chapters for both the specialist as well as the novice in this field. It is presented in a clear meaningful way that all clinicians can relate to easily. Many of the latest concepts have been put into this work, some of which have not been seen in print before. It is also wonderful to see the fact that facial esthetics and smile analysis has been integrated into the evaluation of the patient. This is something that dentists often forget about, and Dr. El Askary has made sure to emphasize the face and mouth as part of the stage that is set up for the teeth and intraoral tissues.

In addition, the chapters on modern diagnostic methods, perioplastic surgery, socket preservation, papilla regeneration, and bone reconstruction are all beautifully illustrated and documented. The scientific community and those involved in esthetic treatment of their patients will have a sense of fulfillment after viewing this text. It will be a reference text that will guide them to improve their performance and to help solve the clinical dilemmas that they face daily.

Congratulations again to Dr. El Askary, whose dedication and pursuit of excellence is to be applauded.

Dennis Tarnow
Professor and Chairman
Department of Periodontology and Implant Dentistry
New York University College of Dentistry

Preface

In the name of God, the Beneficent, and the Merciful.

Implant dentistry today focuses more on the patient's overall appearance than ever before, contributing not only to enhanced social interaction but also to self-confidence and self-esteem. As a result, esthetic implantology procedures are expected to become a more integral part of modern dentistry, encompassing quality of life along with routine functional establishment. Bennett and Weyant (1993) caution, however, that overall improvement in oral and facial esthetics may improve the patient's social ease, but it may not alter others' perceptions of his or her honesty, virtue, helpfulness, potency, or general emotional adjustment.

Implant dentistry offers a unique opportunity for collaboration and interaction among clinicians. This is witnessed by the numerous study groups and specialty conferences held on an almost weekly basis around the world. The growth of implant therapy has influenced almost every aspect of dentistry, from manufacturing implant components to marketing and financing strategies that further promote implant therapy.

These in turn lead to new loading concepts, versatile restorative options, challenging implant designs, minimally invasive surgical approaches, and new esthetic therapies. As a result, we can now use dental implants under more accurate surgical and biomechanical protocols, thus achieving outstanding treatment success rates. Simply put, we have entered an era of clinical predictability.

Applying clinical periodontal plastic surgery procedures to modern implant dentistry has enabled us to achieve, preserve, and maintain the natural peri-implant soft and hard tissue contours. Therefore, we should extend our gratitude to the forerunners of periodontal plastic surgery and the champions of modern esthetic implantology who inspired us with their exceptional dedication and innovation. Thanks should also go to pioneers such as Tarnow, Misch, Lazara, Bragger, Belser, Buser, Potashnick, Hurzeler, Belser, H. Salama, M. Salama, Bengazi, Moy, Spears, Garber, Semion, Chiche, Wöhrle, Saadoun, Grunder, Bitchacho, Magne, Jovanovich, Kan, Allen, Zitzmann, Simion, and many others who have made valuable scientific and clinical advancements in implant dentistry, and whose contributions have personally benefited me greatly. It is my firm belief that esthetic implant dentistry should be rooted in the understanding that we as clinicians do not create esthetics anew, but imitate the esthetics created by God. Therefore, we value our work according to our ability to imitate Nature, not our ability to create artifice.

This book presents a comprehensive overview of modern esthetic implant dentistry, with particular emphasis on achieving beauty through the close study of related facial details and the importance of smile analysis in any esthetic dentistry treatment plan. All aspects of esthetic implant therapy have been carefully presented in a manner which, hopefully, is both reader friendly and clinically applicable.

Chapter 1 defines beauty in particular and general terms, highlights the value of esthetics to both patients and clinicians, demonstrates how to achieve conceptual thinking when performing an esthetic treatment, and discusses the clinician-patient relationship during esthetic implant therapy. Chapter 2 covers the merits of any successful practice by applying the optimal diagnostic tools and features the most up-to-date assessment techniques in diagnosis and planning. Chapter 3 is intended as a solid grounding in the relationship of facial esthetics to the intraoral clinical picture. It urges clinicians to place a greater emphasis on studying the facial features and linking them to the intraoral condition before starting treatment to achieve an optimal and appropriate outcome.

Chapter 4 discusses accurate 3D implant positioning within the alveolar ridge and relates the optimal implant position to achieving a healthy biological emergence profile and healthy contours. It also highlights the impact of modern implant designs on the treatment outcome. Chapter 5 provides comprehensive insights on the most up-to-date peri-implant soft tissue procedures and techniques for achieving optimal esthetics. It starts with the basics of performing atraumatic soft tissue handling and concludes with soft tissue closure and maintenance.

Chapter 6 presents the immediate implant placement in both flapless and flapped surgical protocols. Methods of using natural teeth as provisional restorations in immediate implant cases are detailed in this chapter. Chapter 7 explains the optimal preservation methods of the socket environment for allowing predictable implant placement. It also offers clinical solutions for each socket condition.

Chapter 8 assists the reader in understanding the behavior and nature of the interimplant papilla. The difference in the papillae between natural teeth and implants is thoroughly explained, as is the predictability of most available methods of interimplant papilla regeneration. This chapter also discusses future clinical advancements trials in this field.

Chapter 9 predicts future trends in bone grafting by applying genetic engineering methods to present-day implant dentistry and outlines the best grafting methods to offer highly predictable results. Chapter 10 defines the prosthodontic procedures used to achieve esthetically pleasing implant-supported restorations, covers most implantology-related advanced prosthetic and therapeutic techniques made to obtain natural contours and biological harmony with implant-supported restorations, and draws attention to novel methods used to assist the clinician in achieving predictable esthetics.

Chapter 11 highlights the importance of shade matching in esthetic implant dentistry and details the roles of color and light in achieving successful esthetic restorative outcomes. Chapter 12 shows the clinical consequences of mishandling implants in the esthetic zone. It extensively portrays the major complications that can occur during the course of treatment and provides suggestions for solving complications resulting from positioning errors, soft and hard tissue grafting errors, or prosthetic errors.

I hope this book will offer readers the professional success and satisfaction that I have enjoyed. I also hope that, as so many have given their time and advice freely to me, I might be able to reciprocate this valuable gift and offer my own expertise and in turn help with the advancement of this specialty.

Reference

Bennett ME, Weyant R J. 1993. Letter to the editor. J Dent Res 72:850.

Acknowledgments

> Say. Surely my prayer and my sacrifice and my life and my death are [all] for Allah, the Lord of the worlds. (006.162 Al-Anaam, The Holy Koran)

With this statement, I started working on this project, which I want to dedicate to the gracious Creator of Earth and Heaven. I truly thank him for giving me the power and vision to make this contribution to the world of esthetic implant dentistry.

I am delighted and honored just to think that I might be a part of the communication between the East, West, and the rest of the world, because I believe that science has no borders, no territory, and no nationality. It has been transmitted and alternated from culture to culture and from civilization to civilization throughout the ages.

I thank the readers who purchased my first book, *Reconstructive Aesthetic Implant Surgery*, especially those who purchased it before it went to the printer—what unique support! Thanks also to my fellow dentists and colleagues worldwide who purchased my previous book. The outstanding number of copies sold contributed positively to the decision to undertake this current project.

I express my profound appreciation for the remarkable educator who guided me with great and selfless dedication—Dr. Roland M. Meffert of San Antonio, Texas—who taught me the ABCs and mindset of oral implantology, and put the smile of a father on top of his great teaching skills. Thank you, Dad. Other inspiring mentors who I thank are Dr. Kenneth Judy and Dr. Karl Misch, co-chairmen of the International Congress of Oral Implantologists (ICOI), who gave me—and still give me—tremendous support in my career. I thank Dr. Sherif Abulnaga of Cairo, who taught me many things in life, Dr. Magid Amin, Dr. Griffin of Boston, who inspired me with his marvelous surgical skills in the early stages of my career, and Dr. Perel of Providence, and his wife Jane. I also thank the executive staff of the ICOI, represented by its dynamic director Craig Johnson.

Thanks go to Dr. Dennis Tarnow of New York just for being himself! He has been of great assistance to me and many others; he never ignored anyone's request. The higher he goes (chairman of two departments in the New York University College of Dentistry), the more humble and down-to-earth he gets. Thank you, Dennis, for your support and for the great Foreword that you contributed to this book. Dr. Sang-Choon Cho has also been of great assistance to me. He never let me down when I asked him to provide me with any literature that I needed for this project. Thank you, Dr. Cho.

I must thank my friends and colleagues who contributed to this book—your efforts and contributions have added great value. I also deeply thank the laboratory technicians who complemented my work and provided original work for this project: Walter Lummer, my master technician, and Hassan al Hakeem.

I thank the Zimmer Dental family who offered unlimited support. I can only recall a few of them now: Tom Shea, the president, Brian Marshall, Alexander Ochsner, Michael Studer, and former staff members Celine Cendras-Maret and Russ Bonafede. A word of appreciation also goes to Mike Werner from Zimmer Dental, who spared no effort in helping to provide me with any requested scientific material.

Supportive colleagues must be thanked here: Drs. El Ibrashi K. (may God rest his soul in peace), Sameh Labib, El Sharkawy H. Khaled Zekry, Amr Abdelazeem, Tarek Abdelsamad, Mohammad Ashour, Sherif Effat, Khaled Abdelghaffar, Hesham Nasr of New Orleans, Professor Mohammad Sharawy of Georgia, Mohammad Abdel Maksoud of Florida, Nabeel Barakat of Lebanon, Abbas Zaher of Alexandria, Mona Elsannea of Kuwait, and Professor Abdullah el Shemary of Riyadh.

Friends whom I thank for just being themselves are Rosa and Mario of Italy, Amgad Salwa of Cairo, and Mona and Moaazam of Boston. They really loved me from the bottom of their hearts. My true friend Ahmad Bakry and his wife Amal of Alexandria, my friend the great Egyptian actress Yousra, my dear friend Tannaz of Los Angeles, my close friends Sherif Elsebaay and Walid Yousry—thanks to all of you for your patience and support. I enjoyed your companionship very much. I

also acknowledge my very sincere friends Dr. Duke Aldridge of Oregon, Dr. Ed Hobbs from Dallas, and Dr. Jerry Burd from Beaumont.

I give a special word of gratitude and remembrance to Dr. Bassant Elraffa, who used to share my dreams, even those that seemed unachievable. She listened to me with care and undivided attention at all times and added her input to my ideas. She was an honest, great person. Unfortunately she passed away last year, after battling illness. I ask the almighty Allah to rest her soul in peace. I also want to thank my dear friend and teacher Dr. Sameer Mostafa who passed away recently. I won't forget your support and encouragement.

I cannot and would not forget some people who helped me with the first book. I salute the manager of my past project, Mrs. Lynn Bishop, for her patience and support, as well as the chief editor, Ms. Bonnie Harman, for her guidance and corrections. Both of them spent many hours editing my poor English and my grammar mistakes. Thank you for your kindness.

Thanks to the graphics team that assisted me in this current project, under the command of the talented graphic designer Iman Ahmad of Alexandria. She is a young woman from the heart of Egypt who has shown great professional talent and ethical spirit. Thank you for your great artwork. Another word of thanks goes to Dr. Ahamad el Attar who taught me the basics of graphics and audiovisual presentations. My gratitude also goes to Salwa Abdelsattar, who greatly assisted with the word processing of this project.

My family support is always immense, and I thank my mother, father, and brother Hesham and his wife Lina who focused their prayers toward asking Allah to assist me in my work. Thank you for being there for me and thank you for your endurance and patience. To my wife Mahy, thank you for your unlimited and unconditional love. Your patience and care have brought a new dimension to my life; may Allah reward you for your genuine feelings.

I also specially thank my former and present executive team and staff: Enjy Mohammad, my former secretary who helped much in this project, and Iman Abdelsattar, my present secretary. Mr. Saied Atiea, Hoyda and Ebtesam; Drs. Ahamad Shawkat, Sherif Hayaty, Motaaz Fatahallah, Mohamad Monier, Dalia John, Ziad Rabie, Maha el Kabany, and Tarek Nasr; without your assistance, I would not have been able to complete this project.

Finally, a word of gratitude goes to the current Blackwell senior staff who I have come to know closely. I acknowledge the high moral attitude as well as subtle professionalism of Sophia Joyce, who has been of great assistance on this project. I thank Caroline Connelly in England for her genuinely professional attitude. I also thank Erica Judisch, the editorial assistant of this book, for her professional assistance and patience, as well as Erin Magnani, the associate project manager at Blackwell Publishing, and Peggy Hazelwood, the copyeditor for this project.

About the Author

Abd El Salam El Askary graduated from Alexandria Dental School, University of Alexandria, Egypt in 1986. He obtained his postgraduate training in many reputable international institutions in Europe and in the United States of America. Dr. El Askary is an international lecturer and pioneer in the field of esthetic implant dentistry.

Dr. El Askary is a former associate clinical professor at the University of Florida, Jacksonville, and a visiting lecturer in the continuing education center at the University of New York.

He currently maintains a private practice limited to periodontics, implantology, and oral reconstruction in Alexandria, and Cairo, Egypt.

He is currently the President of the Arabic Society of Oral Implantology, Cairo, Egypt; a member, fellow, and the vice president of the International Congress of Oral Implantologists (ICOI) for Egypt; a board member of the Egyptian Scientific Society for Dental Implantologists; and a fellow of the International Academy for Dental Facial Esthetics.

FUNDAMENTALS OF ESTHETIC IMPLANT DENTISTRY

Chapter 1

Introduction

Abd El Salam El Askary

Adornment and Beautification

Beautification and adornment are mutually inclusive terms that involve cosmetics, clothing, jewelry, body piercing, tattooing, and so forth. They are fueled by our subconscious drive to look attractive and feel good about ourselves. We also enjoy the attention we get from others when they notice our attractiveness (Boucher 1965), which explains the contemporary high demand for cosmetics by all classes of society.

Our inherited ancient cosmetic practices have inspired and contributed to current cosmetic practices. Evidence points to cosmetic use dating back 5,000 to 6,000 years. Although Nefertiti's name means "the beauty has come," even she did not rely on her natural looks alone (Kunzig 1999). Her darkened eyebrows and boldly outlined eyes are as popular today as they were in the pharaonic times. Tattooing the whole body with blue pigments was a common practice in the late thirteenth century. Famous rock star Billy Idol's distinctive spike hairdo can be traced back to the end of the Iron Age (1000 BC to 50 BC), when Celts and Gauls used to wash their hair with limewater—a white, chalky substance—to create striking white spikes of hair. The hair curlers used by women today are actually an ancient beauty ritual practiced by men and women alike. One of the earliest examples of hair curling is seen in Venus of Willendorf, a mummy from to the Paleolithic Age (Faure 1923).

Archeological evidence suggests that prehistoric people contrived their own techniques for preparing cosmetic pigments. As many as 17 different colors were reported to have been created from a few primary sources: lead, chalk, or gypsum (for white); charcoal (for black); and manganese ores (for shades of red, orange, and yellow). These pigments were blended with greasy substances to give them the right consistency for painting on bodies.

For ancient Egyptians, life was not as important as the afterlife, and their desire to look appealing extended beyond the grave. The large quantities of perfume and makeup found buried with the dead prove that these were indispensable funerary gifts (Kunzig 1999).

So far, no one has found a sample of ancient Egyptian lipstick. However, the Louvre Museum in Paris indicated that Nefertiti had perhaps attempted painting her lips. Surprisingly, both men and women of the upper classes used ground ant's eggs to paint their eyelids. The dye from henna plants was used to color hair and fingernails and to adorn the palms and soles of feet. To freshen their breath ancient Egyptians chewed on natron, a naturally occurring sodium carbonate (Cosmetice 2000). Ancient chemists synthesized the black or gray makeup, referred to as *mesdemet* by the ancient Egyptians, that later acquired the name *kohl* from Arabs (Breuer 1965).

Scents constituted a large percentage of Egypt's exports at one time. Raw essences were bought from neighboring Mediterranean countries and used to make perfumes, creams, and lotions, which were later exported. Beauty inventions of the pharaohs spread so far that women from the Roman Empire began to rely on cosmetics brought from Egypt and other parts of the region.

Records show that the Sumerians, Babylonians, and Hebrews employed these compounds as much as the Egyptians did for ceremonial, medicinal, and ornamental purposes. Locally, however, their use was most often confined to mummification rituals. According to researchers, the apparent beauty of royal women in ancient times was essentially found in their ability to use natural resources to enhance their appearance (Breuer 1965). They believed that makeup was only an adjuvant to one's own natural beauty.

Cosmetics and Esthetics

The term *cosmetic* refers to substances and procedures that are used to enhance features or correct defects in appearance. Cosmetics are the preparations used to change the appearance or enhance the beauty of the face, skin, or hair. The intraoral cosmetic surgical procedures with minimal invasive incisions were inspired by the cosmetic surgeries for the face. They are linked with regard to factors such as the fragility of the oral tissues and the muscular movements of the facial muscles. See Figures 1.1A–E and 1.2A–F.

The term *esthetics* is different from cosmetic in that it signifies "natural beauty"—a quality that comes from within. It can be defined as the science of beauty that is applied in nature and in art. While beauty is generally described as "a pleasurable psychological reaction to a visual stimulus," the word *art* is derived from the Latin *ars*, meaning "skill" (Encyclopedia of Word Art 1959). For artwork to be valued as good, it must be satisfactory to the senses, and that is referred to in the visual arts as "the relationships among colors, lines, and masses in space" (Gombrich 1978). Cosmetic dentistry was defined by Philips (1996) as an elective procedure aimed at altering the existing natural or unnatural periodontium to a configuration perceived by the patient to enhance the appearance, while esthetic dentistry is a rehabilitative procedure that corrects a functional problem using techniques that will be less

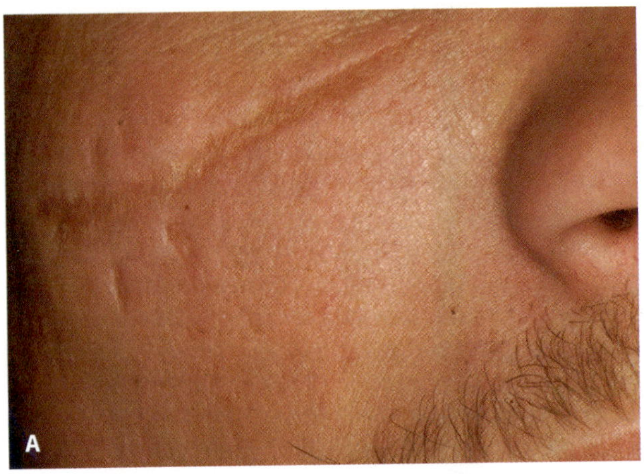

Figure 1.1A. Scar tissue of the face.

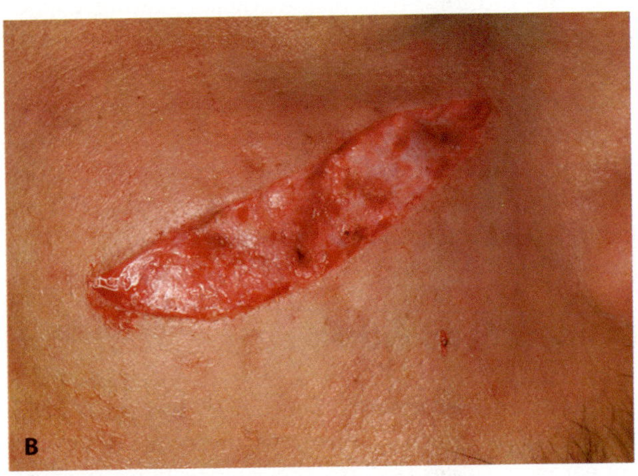

Figure 1.1B. Excision of the scar tissue.

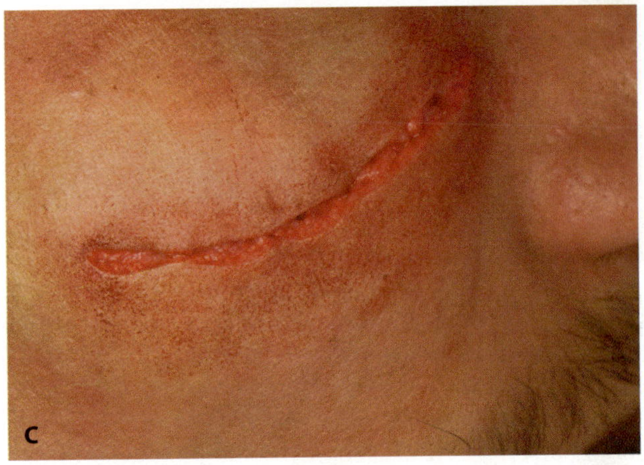

Figure 1.1C. Primary wound closure.

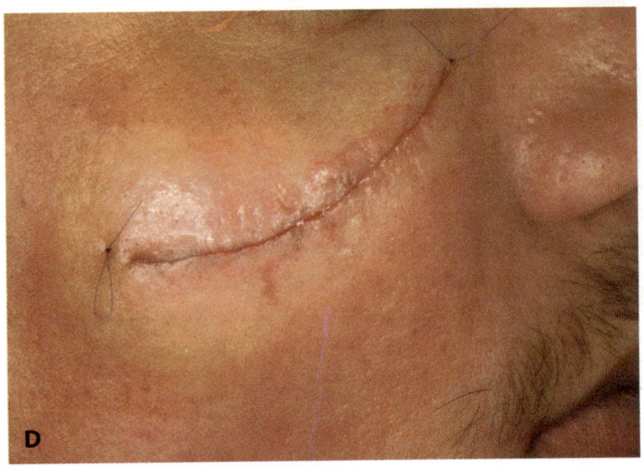

Figure 1.1D. Final wound closure.

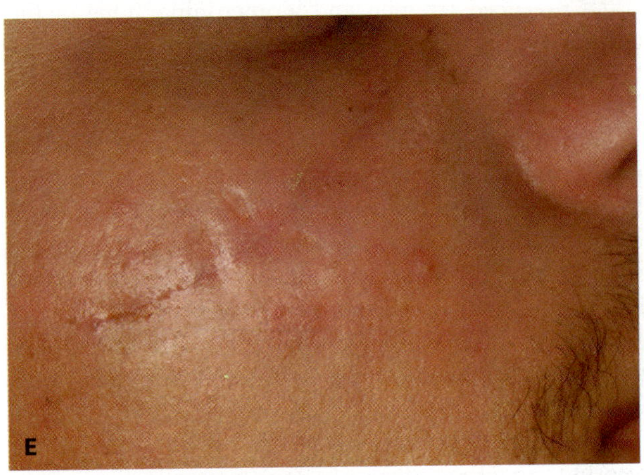

Figure 1.1E. One month posthealing.

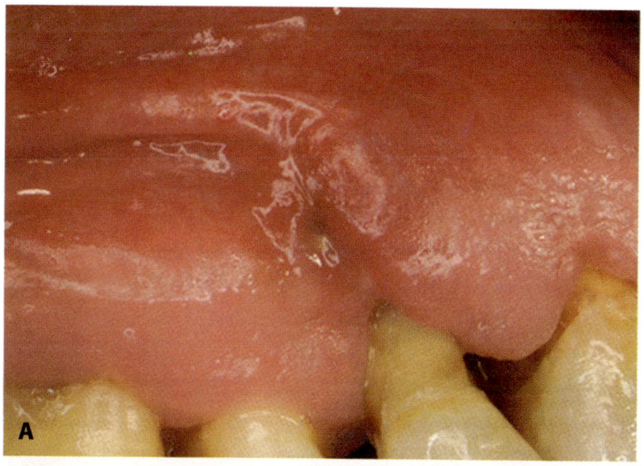

Figure 1.2A. Intraoral scar tissue and gingival recession of the first premolar that necessitates correction.

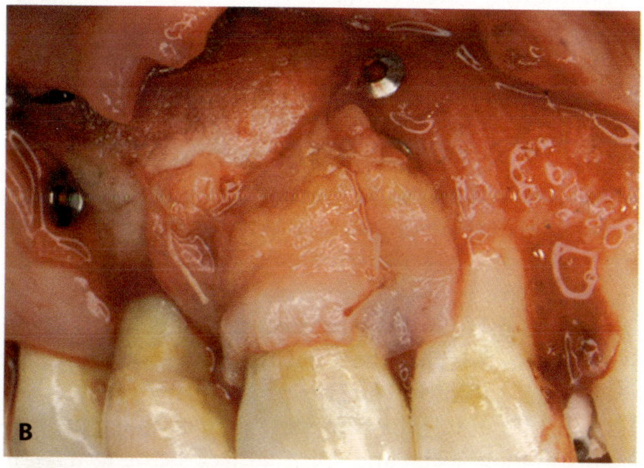

Figure 1.2B. Mucoperiosteal flap reflection and connective tissue graft stabilization.

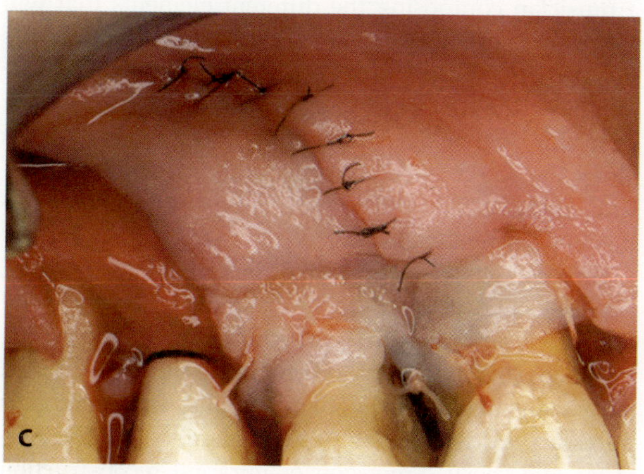

Figure 1.2C. Lateral sliding flap in combination with coronal repositioning of the entire flap.

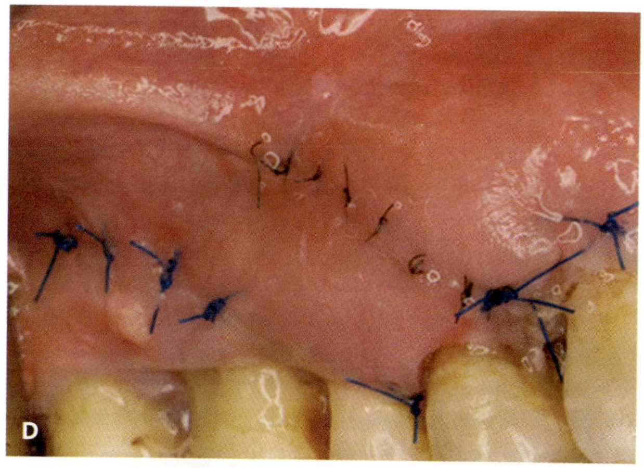

Figure 1.2D. One week postoperative healing.

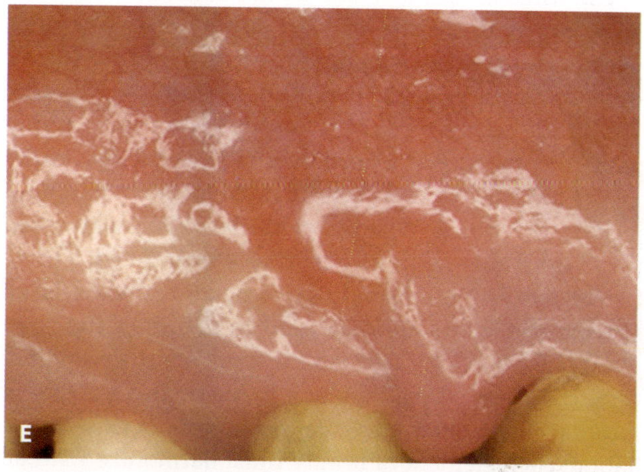

Figure 1.2E. Two months postoperative result that shows complete elimination of the scar tissue and improvement of the gingival recession.

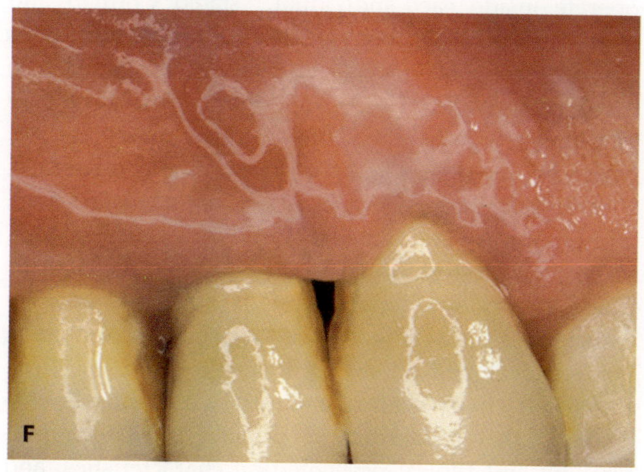

Figure 1.2F. Six months postrestorative, showing total soft tissue healing and maturation.

apparent in the remaining natural periodontium and/or associated tissues.

People usually interpret beauty differently; each individual defines it according to his own concept. In his Vision of the Prophet, Kahlil Gibran manipulated magnificent pieces of poetry and prose to express his view of natural beauty: "Beauty is that which attracts your soul, and that which loves to give and not to receive" (Gibran 1980).

Dante also viewed art as a natural imitation: "Art, as far as it is able, follows nature, as a pupil imitates his master." Leonardo da Vinci's famous Mona Lisa, the enigmatic woman whose identity remains a mystery to this day, reveals his perspective on beauty (Corson 1972). In the Mona Lisa, da Vinci demonstrates that the secret to this woman's natural and everlasting beauty is simply the mysterious smile on her face, which could be interpreted as either angelic or quite devilish (Gunn 1973). Most artists have one thing in common: they use their talent to imitate the real beauty they find in a certain thing, such as nature or the beauty of a face or soul. In this way, Peter Paul Rubens expressed his true feelings toward his beloved, Susanna Fourment, by imitating her beauty in "a portrait of my love" (Gunn 1973).

Art has always been instrumental in the imitation of beauty or nature. When Honore de Balzac was asked what art is, his reply was "nature concentrated." Thus, artists derive their inspiration from nature and of us; all artistic endeavors are compared to nature as the standard of excellence. Likewise, the work of artists and, not less, clinicians, should attempt to maintain a balance of proportions in their work. Perfection cannot exist in isolation; each element of beauty must harmonize with all other related elements to create the whole. For example, a face cannot be called beautiful unless all facial features are in harmony.

"Facial forms are a reflection of vital forces which operate inside each individual," stated Corman and Nouveau (1981). Throughout the centuries, numerous attempts have been made to relate facial features to moral qualities (Eco U. 1993) and the concept that it may be possible to judge the nature of a man on the basis of his body structure is found in the writings of Aristotle, Cicero, Quintilian, Seneca, Galeno, Campanella, Darwin, and Lombroso, and hinted at in physiognomic science. From the oldest physiognomy, we proceed to scientific physiognomy, in which analysis is not based on easy associations (beauty, goodness, wickedness, ugliness), but is developed according to more subtle markers. Rufenacht (1992) dealt abundantly with "morphopsychology," that is, the study of correlations between morphology and typical psychological characteristics, and evaluated the dynamic and evolutionary factors that determine them (environment, psyche).

Harmony and Esthetics

Each time I look at the facial details of my patients while they are smiling, I am amazed at the perfection. They are fabricated with high precision and perfection; the harmony between the facial structures that we overlook most of the time is worthy of watching. When you look deeper at the human face, notice that the lips act as a curtain that reveals the dentition beneath when an emotional reaction takes place. Watch the muscular activity of the mouth when mastication occurs. The food bolus management inside the mouth, along with the saliva acting as a lubricant, works for years and years with no technical problems. Note the effect of a very tiny structure called the interproximal papilla when it complements the overall shape of the dentition. These observations inspired many scientists to record their findings on the harmony of the human creation.

I dedicated much of my work to the area of regenerating the interimplant papilla and have used several techniques to achieve this goal. As is the case with facial harmony, intraoral esthetic harmony can be achieved by paying attention to the fine details of the natural teeth. Therefore, the term *esthetic implantology* seeks harmony in all details to simulate the natural teeth's appearance and achieve the desired overall beauty—a major concern for many patients seeking esthetic rehabilitation therapy. In other words, beauty in today's dentistry does not differ widely from the concepts of general art. Experience has shown that most patients not only appreciate the functional improvements provided by prosthodontic rehabilitation, but also note remarkable improvements in their social and spiritual well-being as a result of the changes in their appearance.

The philosophy of beauty and beautification is so wide ranging it has attracted people of all kinds: artists, musicians, clinicians, and even the common man. Like a musician composing the different elements that will orchestrate his music, a successful clinician integrates the elements of treatment for a particular patient before executing the treatment plan. The success of an esthetic procedure can be determined only when the eye moves along the object to be corrected and perceives its cohesion and harmony with all the other relevant esthetic elements (Copper 1980).

Any esthetic restoration requires imaginative skills, superior clinical talents, and the comprehension of all facial relationships that make treatment successful. While logic is important to composing a treatment plan and analyzing the available elements, imagination is necessary for composing the treatment vision. Furthermore, the social dimension of intraoral reconstruction should not be underestimated. For example, natural teeth are not mere white physical structures, they have social attributes that are vital to one's self-image, social interaction, and physical attractiveness. This consideration has led to the understanding of the importance and the value of esthetic oral rehabilitation.

Esthetic Implant Therapy

Carlsson and others (1967) found that esthetics is a determining factor for complete denture success. Both the patient's and observer's concept of the esthetic result have been found to be highly significant (Waliszewski 2005). Several authors have found further evidence that esthetics is the predominant factor in complete denture success (Vallittu et al. 1996, Brewer 1970, Hirsch et al. 1972). Liefer and others (1962) reported they had statistically fewer adjustment appointments and a greater number of satisfied patients when all esthetic decisions were made by the patient. This implies that when the esthetic result was successful, the dentures were more successful overall, a finding echoed by Vig (1961). A survey by Vallittu and others (1996) found that patients wearing removable dentures considered the appearance to be the most important asset of the teeth.

Brewer (1970) demonstrated through a limited clinical trial that denture patients almost exclusively chose the more esthetic denture over the more comfortable or functional denture. Despite the fact that solutions to functional and comfort-related problems are available, successfully restoring the appearance of an edentulous patient remains problematic. Early literature projected the importance of esthetics. White (1872) introduced what is probably the most original esthetic concept when he described his theory of correspondence and harmony. He highlighted the relationship among age, gender, and appearance; the proper tooth-to-face size proportion; and color harmony between face and teeth (White 1884).

Esthetic implant therapy is an advanced treatment modality in today's field of implantology, aiming to achieve an ideal esthetic and functional treatment outcome within the alveolar ridge or the edentulous spaces. Esthetic implant therapy has become an integral part of modern implant dentistry, because it complements the overall results of oral implantology. Significant advances have been introduced recently, including novel techniques to develop or regenerate implant recipient sites by stimulating both hard and soft tissues and to reproduce healthy peri-implant tissue contours that resist mechanical forces and masticatory trauma.

Despite the advances and the success seen in many clinicians' practices, there is insufficient scientific support regarding the overall success and longevity of esthetic implant therapeutical techniques in well-controlled, long-term studies. The advances in esthetic implant therapy and soft tissue and hard tissue regeneration are more the author's observations than standard protocols that are used in clinicians' daily practices.

Therefore, a standard surgical and prosthetic protocol for esthetic implant therapy is mandatory. Esthetic implant therapy demands evidence-based publications, and fewer case reports, to establish a standard of care for every clinician. All efforts should be made to standardize methodologies for every clinical situation, and then test those procedures against evidence-based protocols.

Past advances resulted from patients' unwillingness to accept dental restoration with metallic margins or unmatched. These challenges, some of which have been extremely difficult to address, have benefited from original plastic periodontal surgical techniques that are now used routinely to correct various soft tissue defects such as gingival recession, mucogingival defects, and imbalanced gingival contours.

While these traditional periodontal plastic surgery techniques for natural teeth have been helpful, their usefulness for dental implants is limited in terms of timing and predictability. As a result of these continuous adaptations, new classifications of hard and soft tissue defects have been developed to describe each patient's clinical situation and improve communication among the dental team.

"Reconstructive esthetic implant therapy" has been suggested as a term to describe the different intraoral procedures and their clinical implications. This classification should be continually updated by setting a standard protocol for detailing certain procedures, defining new terms, and confirming the evidence behind clinical concepts. This in turn will help esthetic implantology emerge as a distinct specialty of implantology, which will continue to develop and expand, along with functional implantology (Kazor et al. 2004).

Over the past 35 years dental implantology has proven to be a predictable method for restoring function in the oral cavity (Adell et al. 1981, Engquist et al. 1988, Schnitman et al. 1988). The late 1980s and early 1990s witnessed the expansion of dental implants to include treatment of partially edentulous patients with fixed, implant-supported restorations. These new clinical applications include the treatment of missing anterior single dentition, which has a documented success rate in excess of 90% (Schmitt and Zarb 1993, Engquist et al. 1995, Anderson et al. 1995, Ekfeldt et al. 1994). As awareness of this treatment has increased, restoration of missing maxillary anterior single teeth with implant-supported restorations is quickly becoming the preferred treatment modality, despite the fact that it remains one of the most esthetically difficult and challenging of all implant restorations.

Clinicians' efforts to improve the esthetic dimension of dental implants and achieve restorations that mimic the appearance of natural teeth have played a significant role in raising the awareness of and popularity about dental implants. Successfully achieving an esthetic implant-supported restoration that mimics the natural tooth appearance requires very meticulous treatment procedures. The process involves detailed presurgical planning, optimal three-dimensional implant placement, meticulous soft tissue management, the use of predictable bone grafting techniques when required, and skillful use of various prosthetic components. Many researchers have dedicated their efforts to improving and developing techniques that help achieve predictable, esthetic results with dental implants. Some have laid out the fundamentals of presurgical planning (Jansen and Weisgold 1995), and others (Spielman 1996, Parel and Sullivan 1989) have set guidelines for achieving a natural-looking final restoration with esthetic implant positioning.

Soft tissue sculpture (Bichacho and Landsberg 1994), the use of connective tissue grafts (Khoury and Happe 2000) and free gingival grafts (Miller 1982), improvement of soft tissue contours (Lazara 1993), the use of enhanced conservative new mucoperiosteal flap designs (Nemcovsky et al. 2000), and methods to improve soft tissue topography at the time of second-stage surgery (Sharf and Tarnow 1992) were all invented to benefit esthetic outcomes. Many techniques have been introduced to achieve an adequate height and width of the alveolar bone to obtain an optimal natural emergence profile (Pikos 2000, Simion et al. 1994). Jovanovic (2000) defined the term *esthetic bone grafting* as the regeneration of the lost osseous structure to its original biological dimensions, not only to serve functionally, but also esthetically.

Restoring a single missing tooth with an implant-supported prosthesis can be a difficult task, but not as difficult as restoring multiple adjacent missing teeth in the esthetic zone (El Askary 2000). When only a single tooth is to be restored, the establishment of the peri-implant papillae and surrounding tissues is highly predictable (Petrungaro et al. 1999). However, in the case of multiple implant placements, the interimplant papilla is unpredictable. Some authors (Beagle 1992, Shapiro 1985, Jemt 1997, Hurzeler and Dietmar 1996) have suggested soft tissue surgical interventions as a solution for this problem, while others (El Askary 2000, Salama et al. 1995) have used hard tissue reconstructive procedures. Tarnow and others (1992) and Salama and others (1998) have proposed helpful tools for predicting the inter- and peri-implant papillae with classifications that have assisted in the assessment of various clinical papillary conditions.

Clinicians are urged to preserve the peri-implant soft tissue architecture during any plastic surgical procedures that attempt to regenerate the interimplant papilla. Misch (1997) stated that esthetic enhancement techniques are very often accomplished at the expense of sulcular health because some of the clinical procedures can be invasive to peri-implant tissues. Therefore, esthetic surgical procedures should focus on preserving the surrounding tissues and being less invasive in nature.

The Predictability of Esthetic Implant Therapy

Esthetic implant therapy should not be a separate treatment discipline, but rather an integral part of all other treatment modalities (Sorensen 1997). Function should complement esthetics and vice versa, because the final objective of esthetic implant dentistry is a perfect prosthetic outcome that simulates the natural tooth appearance. See Figure 1.3. Many simple principles of

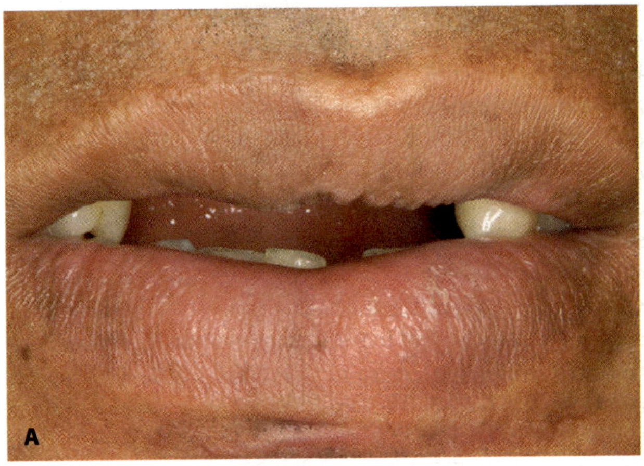

Figure 1.3A. Lost anterior teeth due to a car accident.

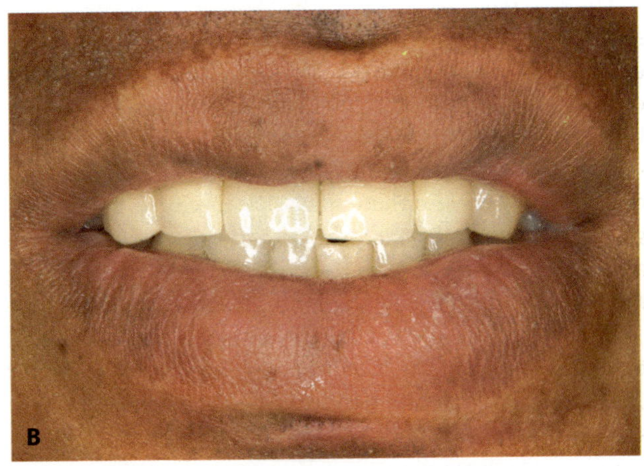

Figure 1.3B. The oral condition postimplant therapy.

prosthetic design that have been routinely used for decades can be applied to anterior dental esthetics to create harmony while maintaining natural beauty, and can turn an average case into an ideal one (Golub-Evans 1994). The goal of esthetic implant therapy is to complement any given treatment plan, because the treatment planning for an esthetic case will slightly differ from that for a functional case.

The delivery of a state-of-the-art implant-supported prosthesis enriches the implantology practice, not vice versa, and solves clinical issues and mysteries such as the interimplant papilla. This surely will make a great impact on modern implant therapy. Recently an interesting study by Belser and others (2004) evaluated the esthetic implant therapy literature about from 1997 to 2003 regarding outcomes of implant restorations in the anterior maxilla to formulate consensus statements about esthetics in implant dentistry. Articles without a scientifically proven basis were excluded. The treatment outcome of implant therapy for maxillary anterior single tooth replacement was evaluated prospectively. The study reported that stable long-term results (both esthetic and clinical) can be achieved with anterior single-implant crowns in spite of the fact that clinical parameters for measurement did not exist in many articles. The success rate in the anterior maxilla or the esthetic zone was almost the same as in the other locations in the oral cavity. In the case of anterior single tooth replacement in sites without tissue deficiencies, predictable treatment outcomes, including esthetics, can be achieved because of tissue support provided by adjacent teeth interproximally. The replacement of multiple adjacent missing teeth in the anterior maxilla with fixed implant restorations is poorly documented. Therefore, restoring lost esthetics is unpredictable, particularly regarding the interimplant papilla.

The study also stated that the literature was inconclusive regarding the routine implementation of many esthetic procedures such as flapless surgery and immediate implant placement with or without immediate loading/restoration in the anterior maxilla. However, most of these studies do not include well-defined esthetic parameters. The need for a universal index or global scoring system is essential for future evaluations, and would subsequently help to standardize clinical evaluations and findings.

Another study by Belser and others (2004) evaluated the clinical procedures regarding esthetics in implant dentistry. It discussed three aspects: (1) outcome analysis of implant restorations located in the anterior maxilla, (2) anatomical and surgical considerations of implant therapy in the anterior maxilla, and (3) practical prosthodontic procedures related to anterior maxillary fixed implant restorations. The evaluation concluded that most of these studies do not include well-defined esthetic parameters. The success rate of dental implants placed and restored in the esthetic zone has a success rate that is similar to that reported for other segments of the jaws. Single anterior tooth replacement therapy revealed that predictable treatment outcomes, including esthetics, can be achieved routinely. The research stated that implant therapy in the anterior maxilla is considered an advanced or complex procedure and requires comprehensive preoperative planning and precise surgical execution based on a restoration-driven approach. Patient selection should be approached with caution when it comes to esthetic implant therapy, because esthetic results are less consistent in smokers and systemically involved patients.

The study recommended optimal implant size and morphology selection favoring soft tissue health and integrity, and noted that optimal three-dimensional (3D) implant positioning is essential for any esthetic treatment results in an implant shoulder located in an ideal position, allowing for an esthetic implant restoration with stable, long-term peri-implant tissue support. Finally, the study objectively defined the esthetic zone as any dento-alveolar segment that is visible upon full smile. Subjectively, the esthetic zone can be defined as any dento-alveolar area of esthetic importance to the patient.

Clinician–Patient Relationship

The patient's satisfaction with the esthetic outcome of implant therapy is considered a cornerstone of implant therapy. Therefore, treatment plans should focus on the patients' satisfaction. One of the principal criteria of appraisal is the level of the patient's expectations. Patients with realistic expectations will be more easily satisfied than those with unrealistic expectations. Rittersma and others (1980) reported that 20% to 40% of patients who had undergone orthognathic surgery had not been sufficiently informed about the psychological risks (depression) and physical consequences (pain, dysesthesia) that arise postsurgery. On the other hand, patients who were duly informed and aware that immediately after the operation they may experience personal inconvenience for a short time easily overcame these effects. Women showed a higher degree of neurosis and a less favorable perception of their body image (Kiyak et al. 1981), and it was also noticed that unmarried patients did not increase their social and recreational activities with their friends of the opposite sex after surgical correction of their facial deformities (Lam et al. 1983).

In general, satisfaction is reduced if the patient feels that the esthetic improvement obtained is less than his expectations; therefore, an accurate appraisal of the patient's psychological profile at the time of treatment planning is mandatory. There must be no discrepancy between the patient's own perception of his body image and the esthetic appraisal of the clinician. Solid communication between the patient and the clinician is certainly fundamental. This allows the patient to obtain complete information about the relationship between the cost of treatment, its benefits, and its risks. Good communication also allows the clinician to identify any pre-existing psychological disorders as well as whether the patient's motives for undergoing surgery are real and whether the patient's expectations are realistic or unrealistic.

Patient satisfaction with various types of implant-supported prostheses has been evaluated. De Bruyn et al. (1997) evaluated the importance of patient satisfaction in a study consisting of 61 implant patients that had undergone implant therapy. The study emphasized esthetics, phonetics, comfort with eating, and the overall satisfaction with the treatment. Most of the patients experienced their implant restorations as "natural" teeth and stated that they would undergo the treatment again or recommend it to others. Another study (Levi et al. 2003) assessed 78 patients using a self-reported satisfaction survey regarding maxillary anterior dental implant treatments in terms of implant position, restoration shape, overall appearance, effect on speech, and chewing capacity; these factors were considered treatment variables. These results also indicated the importance of overall satisfaction with patient acceptance of the dental implant treatment modality.

The nature of the clinician–patient relationship is somewhat critical and requires special emphasis at the beginning of treatment. The relationship with a patient who seeks rehabilitative esthetic work often starts with a recommendation from a former patient or a colleague. Patients usually do not have clear preconceived notions about oral reconstructive surgeries. A trained office receptionist can recognize determine the patient's desires, goals, and expectations.

Patient's expectations are considered to be the first valuable piece of information collected prior to clinical examination; many patients were disappointed with their clinicians because they ultimately felt that their expectations, although unrealistic, were not fulfilled. Finances are another important issue. Clinicians should fully explain the possibilities of exceeding the stated costs; some major reconstructive cases require additional corrective surgeries. All possible risks and treatment complications should be addressed and explained prior to treatment, not only for financial reasons but also so patients know what to expect in terms of discomfort. Studies show that patients tend to better accept any postoperative complications such as swelling, bruising, etc., if they are previously notified.

It is important to determine patients' oral habits before beginning treatment. Smoking and parafunction can influence the success of implant therapy. Special care should be given to apprehensive and anxious patients. Generally, pretreatment apprehension is a result of the faulty information that the patients gathered from other sources. The dental staff's attitude toward the patient is also a natural concern—the staff should communicate with the patient in quiet, reassuring tones, addressing the patient by name while avoiding inappropriate personal terms.

The start of treatment should never be rushed. It does not improve patient acceptance. On the contrary, it can sometimes cause anger, hesitation, and despair.

Operating rooms are notoriously (and wrongly) cold; instead, a comfortable temperature should be maintained, with a relaxing atmosphere that has minimizes the show of medical devices or surgical instruments as much as possible. Sophisticated patients require more postoperative assurance than other patients; they want to be able to reach the clinician and any of the staff at any time to have their inquiries or complaints answered. In most cases, they want to be reassured that they are improving and that they are on the right treatment track.

Many factors can influence patient satisfaction with dental implants, including age, gender, occupational status, and socioeconomic class. However, the literature lacks valid studies of the relationship between satisfaction and personality profiles. In general, fixed prostheses and removable over-dentures retained by dental implants enhance patient satisfaction. However, determining which prosthodontic protocol has a better impact on the quality of life and overall satisfaction is still considered to be a controversial issue. Satisfaction and quality of life assessments are among the most critical factors that govern such success. As most of the related studies showed, dental implants provided promising and predictable results regarding patient satisfaction and various aspects of life assessment.

Any treatment complications, both foreseen or unforeseen, should be communicated to the patient along with a plan for resolution. It has been proven that the vast majority of the patients welcome and admire truthfulness and straightforward statements. Repetition of the answers and reassurance are valuable psychological aids to patients.

In the case of uncontrolled treatment complications, consultation with another clinician can be a valuable tool, because the patient is usually reassured that everything possible is being done to solve the problem. Almost invariably, the patient returns to her original clinician with her confidence restored. If the request for a consultation comes from the patient, it should be welcomed as a way of obtaining needed help and showing sincere concern for the patient's welfare.

When a new patient who left his original treating office seeks your assistance, contacting the patient's original clinician in the presence of the patient (with the patient's permission) can help him feel that all efforts are being made. This approach has shown to be more efficient than hiding words and speaking philosophically. Note that it is the clinician's responsibility to accept this patient if all parties agree.

References

Adell, R., U. Lekholm, and B. Rocker. 1981. A 15 year study of osseointegrated implants in the treatment of the edentulous jaw. *Int J Oral Surg* (10), pp. 387–416.

Anderson, B., P. Odman, A.M. Lidvall, et al. 1995. Single tooth restoration supported by osseointegrated implants: Results and experience from a prospective study after 2 to 3 years. *Int J Oral Maxillofac Implants* (10), pp. 702–711.

Beagle, J.R. 1992. Surgical reconstruction of the interdental papilla: Case report. *Int J Periodontics Restorative Dent* (12), pp. 145–151.

Belser, U., D. Buser, and F. Higginbottom. 2004. Consensus Statements and Recommended Clinical Procedures Regarding Esthetics in Implant Dentistry. *Int J Oral Maxillofac Implants*, 19, pp. 873–874.

Belser, U., B. Schmid, F. Higginbottom, et al. 2004. Outcome Analysis of Implant Restorations Located in the Anterior Maxilla: A Review of the Recent Literature. *Int J Oral Maxillofac Implants*, 19, pp. 30–42.

Bichacho, N., and C.J. Landsberg. 1994. A modified surgical prosthetic approach for an optimal single implant-supported crown, part I: The cervical contouring concept. *Pract Periodont Aesthet Dent* (6), pp. 35–41.

Boucher, F. 1965. *20,000 Years of Fashion: The History of Costume and Personal Adornment*. New York: Harry N. Abrams, Inc., Publishers; Contini, Mila.

Breuer, M. 1965. *Cosmetic Science. 2 vols. 1978–1980. Fashions from Ancient Egypt to the Present Day.* London.

Brewer, A. 1970. Selection of denture teeth for esthetics and function. *J Prosthet Dent*; 23, pp. 368–373.

Carlsson, G.E., A. Otterland, A. Wennstrom, et al. 1967. Patient factors in appreciation of complete dentures. *J Prosthet Dent*; 17, pp. 322–328.

Copper, D.F. 1980. Interrelationships between the visual art, science and technology. *Leonardo*, (13), pp. 29–33.

Corman, K., and M. Nouveau. 1981. *Detnorpho-pscologie* Paris: Stock P1us.

Corson, R. 1972. *Fashions in Makeup*. London: Peter Owen.

Cosmetice. 2000. Microsoft® Encarta® Online Encyclopedia.

De Bruyn, H., B. Collaert, U. Linden, et al. 1997. Patient's opinion and treatment outcome of fixed rehabilitation on Branemark implants. A 3-year follow-up study in private dental practices. *Clin Oral Implants Res.*, 8(4), pp. 265–271.

Eco, U. 1993. Il linguaggio del volto. In: Lavater, J.C. *Della fisiognomica*. Milano: Ed Associati.

Ekfeldt, A., G. Carlsson, and G. Borgesson. 1994. Clinical evaluation of single tooth restorations supported by osseointegrated Implants. A retrospective study. *Int J Oral Maxillofac Implants* (9), pp. 179–183.

El Askary, A.S. 2000. Interimplant papilla reconstruction by means of a titanium guide. *Implant Dent* (9), pp. 85–89.

Encyclopedia of Word Art. 1959. Vol. 15 McGraw-Hill, p. 68.

Engquist, B., T. Bergendal, T. Kallus, et al. 1988. A retrospective multi-center evaluation of osseointegrated implants supporting over dentures. *Int J Oral Maxillofac Implants* (3), pp. 129–134.

Engquist, B., H. Nilson, and P. Astrand 1995. Single tooth replacement by osseointegrated Branemark implants: A retrospective study of 82 implants. *Clin Oral Implant Res* (6), pp. 238–245.

Faure, E. 1923. *History of Art*. Vol. 3, Renaissance Art. New York: History and Brothers Publishers.

Gibran, K., 1980. *Visions of the Prophet*.

Golub-Evans, J. 1994. Unity and variety; essential ingredients of a smile design. *Curr Opin Cosmet Dent*, pp. 1–5.

Gombrich, E. 1978. *The Story of Art*, 13th ed. London: Phaidon Press.

Gunn, F. 1973. *The Artificial Face: A History of Cosmetics*. London: Trinity Press.

Hirsch, B., B. Levin, and N. Tiber. 1972. Effects of patient involvement and esthetic preference on denture acceptance. *J Prosthet Dent*, 28, pp. 127–32.

Hurzeler, M.B., and W. Dietmar. 1996. Peri-implant tissue management: Optimal timing for an aesthetic result. *Pract Periodont Aesthet Dent* (8), pp. 857–869.

Jansen, C., and A. Weisgold. 1995. Presurgical treatment planning for the anterior single tooth implant restoration. *Compendium* (16), pp. 746–762.

Jemt, T. 1997. Regeneration of gingival papillae after single implant treatment, *Int J Periodontics Restorative Dent* 17, pp. 327–333.

Jovanovic, S.A. 1997. Bone rehabilitation to achieve optimal aesthetics. *Pract Periodont Aesthet Dent*, (9), pp. 41–52.

Kazor, C.E., K. Al-Shammari, D.P. Sarment, et al. 2004. Implant plastic surgery: a review and rationale. *J Oral Implantol*. 30(4), pp. 240–254.

Khoury, F., and A. Happe. 2000. The palatal subepithelial connective tissue flap method for soft tissue management to cover maxillary defects: A clinical report. *Int J Oral Maxillofac Implants* (15), pp. 415–418.

Kiyak, H.A., T. Hohl, P. Sherrick, R.A. West, R.W. McNeill, and F. Bucher. 1981. Sex differences in motives for and outcomes of orthognathic surgery. *J Oral Surg*, 39, pp. 757–764.

Kunzig, R. 1999. *Style of the Nile*. September.

Lam, T., H.A. Kiyak, T. Hohl, R.A. West, and R.W. McNeill. 1983. Recreational and social activities of orthognathic surgery patients. *Am J Orthod*, 83, pp. 143–152.

Lazara, R.J. 1993. Managing the soft tissue margin: The key to implant aesthetics. *Pract Periodont Aesthet Dent* (5), pp. 81–87.

Lefer, L., M.A. Pleasure, and L. Rosenthal. 1962. A psychiatric approach to the denture patient. *J Psychosom Res*; 6, pp. 199–207.

Levi, A., W.J. Psoter, J.R. Agar, S.T. Reisine, and T.D. Taylor. 2003. Patient self-reported satisfaction with maxillary anterior dental implant treatment. *Int J Oral Maxillofac Implants*, 18, pp. 113–120.

Miller, P.D. 1982. Root coverage using a free soft tissue autograft following citric acid application. Part I: Technique. *Int J Periodont Rest Dent* (2), pp. 65–70.

Misch, E.C. 1999. Single tooth implant. In: Misch, C.E., ed. *Contemporary Implant Dentistry*. St. Louis: Mosby, pp. 397–428.

Nemcovsky, C.E., O. Moses, and Z. Artzi. 2000. Rotated palatal flap in immediate implant procedures. *Clin Oral Implant Res* (11), pp. 83–90.

Parel, S.M., and D.Y. Sullivan. 1989. *Aesthetics and Osseointegration*. Dallas, TX: Taylor Publishing Co., 11.

Petrungaro, P.S., M.D. Smilanich, and N.W. Windmiller. 1999. The formation of proper interdental architecture for single tooth implants. *Contemp Esthet Rest*, (3), pp. 14–22.

Philips, E.D. 1996. The anatomy of a smile. *Oral Health* (86), pp. 7–9, 11–3.

Pikos, M.A. 2000. Block autografts for localized ridge augmentation: Part II. The posterior mandible. *Implant Dent* (9), pp. 67–75.

Rittersma, J., A.F. Casparie, and E. Reerink. 1980. Patient information and patient preparation in orthognathic surgery: a medical audit study. *J Oral Maxillofac Surg*, 8, pp. 206–209.

Rufenacht, C.R. 1992. *Principi di estetica*. Milano: Scienza e Tecnica Dentistica Edizioni Internazionali.

Salama, H., M.A. Salama, D. Garber, and P. Adar. 1995. Developing optimal peri-implant papilla within the esthetic zone: Guided soft tissue augmentation, *J Esthet Dent* (7), pp. 125–129.

Salama, H., M. Salama, D. Garber, and P. Adar. 1998. The interproximal height of bone. A guidepost to predictable esthetic strategies and soft tissue contours in anterior tooth replacement. *Pract Periodont Aesthet Dent* (10), pp. 1131–1141.

Schmitt, A., and G.A. Zarb. 1993. The longitudinal clinical effectiveness of osseointegrated dental implants for single tooth replacement, *Int J Prosthodont* (6), pp. 187–202.

Schnitman, P.A., J.E. Rubenstein, P.S. Whole, et al. 1988. Implants for partial edentulism. *J Dent Educ* (52), pp. 725–736.

Shapiro, A. 1985. Regeneration of the interdental papillae using periodic curettage. *Int J Periodontics Restorative Dent* (5), pp. 27–33.

Sharf, D.R., and D.P. Tarnow. 1992. Modified roll technique for localized alveolar ridge augmentation. *Int J Periodontics Restorative Dent* (12), pp. 415–425.

Simion, M., P. Trisi, and A. Piatelli. 1994. Vertical ridge augmentation using a membrane technique associated with osseointegrated implants. *Int J Periodont Rest Dent* (14), pp. 497–511.

Sorensen, J.A. 1997. Aesthetics at what cost? *Pract Periodont Aesthet Dent* (9), pp. 969–970.

Spielman, H.P. 1996. Influence of the implant position on the aesthetics of the restoration. *Pract Periodont Aesthet Dent* (8), pp. 897–904.

Tarnow, D., A. Magner, and P. Fletcher. 1992. The effect of the distance from the contact point to the crest of the bone on the presence or absence of the interproximal dental papilla. *J Peridontol* (63), pp. 995–996.

Vallittu, P.K., A.S.J. Vallittu, and V.P. Lassila. 1996. Dental aesthetics: a survey of attitudes in different groups of patients. *J Dent*, 24, pp. 335–338.

Vig, R.G. 1961. The denture look. *J Prosthet Dent*, pp. 9–15.

Waliszewski, M. 2005. Restoring dentate appearance: A literature review for modern complete denture esthetics. *J Prosthet Dent*, 93, pp. 386–394.

White, J.W. 1872. Aesthetic dentistry. *Dental Cosmos*, 14, pp. 144–145.

White, J.W. 1884. Temperament in relation to the teeth. Dental Cosmos, 26, pp. 113–120.

Chapter 2

Diagnostic Considerations for Esthetic Implant Therapy

Abd El Salam El Askary

Oral implantology is the fastest-growing science within dentistry; it offers safe, effective, and predictable results for patients with complete or partial edentulism. It also offers a permanent long-term functional and esthetic solution to many clinical circumstances that lacked solutions prior to the routine use of implant therapy.

Successful dental implantology always starts with optimal treatment planning. When esthetics are a major concern the treatment plan should consider whether the patient is appropriate for such a procedure, as well as the particular procedure itself, the materials that are needed, the proper timing of the procedure, and the treatment duration for the entire plan. Considering these basic elements strengthens the treatment plan and offers predictability, which improves the chances of long-term success on both the functional and esthetic levels.

Treatment planning may involve several specialties, including periodontics, prosthodontics, and orthodontics. Any treatment plan should include the least risky procedures in terms of success rate and longevity, because it is no longer appropriate to consider a high-risk procedure when a more predictable alternative such as dental implant is available. The value of higher risk endodontic or periodontal procedures to save teeth for prosthodontic abutments is sometimes questionable because dental implants are a more predictable alternative. For example, procedures such as root amputation or tooth hemisection, which have a five-year failure rate of 30% to 50%, are less appealing options than dental implants, which have a better success rate and are less risky (Langer et al. 1981, Buhler 1988, Green 1986).

Treatment that includes long-span fixed partial dentures and multiple splinted teeth should be carefully compared to the implant alternative. Additionally, endodontic procedures such as apicoectomies or retrofills should be carefully considered, not only because of the limited benefit and lower success rate, but also because of the possibility of compromising a potential implant site in terms of infection and soft and hard tissue loss. Also, periodontal procedures such as crown lengthening should be considered because bone volume may be reduced, which might compromise both the hard and soft tissue for a future implant site (Curtis et al. 2002).

Successful preplanning of implant therapy shortens the treatment time, ensures predictable results, and allows for easier implication of the preset treatment protocol. Presurgical planning in major esthetic cases is unlike that in simple functional cases. Planning for esthetic cases requires more time and a different diagnostic perspective; it should include additional factors such as smile patterns and lip size, etc. This textbook focuses on planning for predictable esthetics; therefore it deals with soft tissue health and biotypes more than loading and functional concerns.

Accurate and precise planning includes detecting any existing clinical difficulties prior to the treatment and viewing or foreseeing the final result before the treatment is started. This requires imagination, creativity, and farsightedness on the part of the clinician, but surely helps the dentist determine what is needed to restore the missing dentition and/or its supporting structures if dental implants are to be considered.

Gathering and analyzing all available information and every available diagnostic tool will determine whether the therapy is a modern or obsolete clinical tool. Modern technology has offered a wide selection of modern diagnostic tools that vary from digital imaging to computer-aided design/computer-aided manufacturing (CAD/CAM) machines, surgical microscopes, computer-guided surgical templates, laser technology, computer software simulation, and a wide array of bone-grafting materials and implant designs. In addition, there are revolutionary new loading dental implant concepts. Today's new loading concepts are being used predictably and routinely to greatly reduce treatment time.

Tissue preservation also is in the spotlight in many modern implantology treatments. This is the result of a better understanding of the bone's response after tooth extraction and its reaction to loading and nonloading. The better understanding of tissue biotypes has led to an understanding of the possible reaction of the hard and soft tissue surrounding dental implants. Therefore, tissue preservation concepts have become a routine clinical application in any treatment plan that concerns both esthetics and function.

This thinking has led to the use of strategic tooth extraction as a way to preserve adequate tissues for dental implants. Tooth removal procedures must be carefully planned to preserve as much of the soft and hard tissues as possible, not only to create the best esthetic result but also to ensure the most functional and long-lasting results. It is now uncommon to remove an anterior tooth without considering preserving the surrounding alveolar ridge regardless of whether the missing tooth will be restored by a fixed partial denture or an implant-supported restoration. The prognosis of this approach is of course highly influenced by the clinician's skills to preserve and regenerate soft and hard tissue in preparation for dental implants (Curtis et al. 2002).

Guided bone regeneration is a highly predictable treatment option that improves bone topography. This provides better whiteness than the biological guided tissue membranes, and the introduction of the devices to obtain the plasma-derived growth factors enhance the outcome of the regenerative therapy on both soft and hard tissue levels.

Radiographic, modern diagnostic evaluation tools are considered to be the logical stepping stones to ensuring a successful treatment. Besides radiographs, old photographs or slides provided by the patient are fairly important components of the treatment plan. The photographs can offer a glimpse of what the original teeth looked like before the tooth or teeth were lost. In some cases, the patient may want to duplicate what they previously looked like; in others, they may wish to hide a deformity or abnormality that they used to have. Learning the patient's desires and expectations by using old, original pictures as a reference can be very helpful in anterior oral rehabilitations. This pretreatment appraisal influences not only treatment modality selection but also treatment timing, sequence, and prognosis.

Generally speaking, when patients seek implant therapy, they don't have a complete and full knowledge about the treatment sequence and nature of the procedure. This may be because there is a lack of public awareness about this new type of treatment, or because the general dentist did not offer them this treatment modality until all of the other treatment options had expired. Therefore, gathering information about the patient's knowledge of the treatment in general, as well as their expectations, becomes another important factor in the treatment plan.

The clinician must be prudent and visualize what is feasible and realistic based on the existing clinical condition. It is the patient's right to be made aware not only of the prognosis of dental implant therapy but also of all other available treatment alternatives that apply to the their condition. The patient must be informed about the benefits, risks, and potential complications involved in the selected treatment plan. The clinician must inform the patient prior to initiating treatment about how realistic their expectations are, as well as the time frame that is expected to accomplish the task. It is the absolute right of the patient to be acquainted with the treatment prognosis and possibilities. The patient must be informed of any possible discomfort, pain, or temporary compromise in function that they might experience. Furthermore, a patient seeking implant replacement therapy requires reassurance that the selected treatment plan will be successful at the end of the treatment. Consequently, it is only humane for the clinician to try to minimize the time of the actual treatment.

Making a study cast is extremely valuable in completing the remaining diagnostics; much information can be gathered from the cast alone. A well-prepared diagnostic study cast sheds light on fundamental aspects of the oral cavity's topographic status and its associated clinical conditions, including the type of occlusion; the number, shape, and condition of the remaining dentition; the remaining interdental and interarch space that is available for tooth replacement; the remaining alveolar bone and its topography; and the detection of any existing pathological lesions or parafunctional habits. The diagnostic information obtained prior to the initiation of treatment can provide valuable information for planning the surgical and restorative phases of treatment. These data can also be used to help select the position, size, type, and design of the future implants; determine the need for any grafting or bone augmentation procedures; determine the surgical approach; position the implant in the alveolar ridge; select the prosthetic components; and determine the type of future restoration.

Most implant therapy patients have lost their teeth directly or indirectly as a result of poor oral hygiene. Evaluating the patient's oral hygiene practice before implant therapy can provide clues on the prognosis of the implants after therapy. However, the relationship between dental plaque and implant failure is not yet totally confirmed. In generalized terms, maintaining soft tissue health around the abutment is imperative to ensuring the long-term survival of the implant-supported prosthesis. A patient's ability and willingness to practice meticulous oral hygiene influences both the consideration of placement of osseointegrated fixtures and the type of prosthesis to be made afterwards. If a patient is insufficiently motivated to assure a reasonable degree of oral hygiene, perhaps a tissue-integrated prosthesis might not be their best treatment option.

Patients with poor oral hygiene must be notified of the potential danger that neglected hygiene has on the fixture survival and the likely need to remove a fixed prosthesis from time to time to adequately clean the prosthesis and abutments. The need for this service may increase the long-term added cost for many patients. Furthermore, special consideration should be given to patients with physical handicaps who are likely unable to practice acceptable oral hygiene. Although a nurse or spouse may be willing to assist in this regard, that approach is seldom as desirable as personal oral hygiene. For those patients, it may be much more practical to choose a treatment approach that excludes dental implant therapy.

In addition to the diagnostic factors that should be considered, several technical factors must also be discussed with the working team. These include the type of prosthesis to be used, access for clinical care, design of the fixtures, and interarch space limitations. Prior to implant fixture installation, the number, position, and angulation of fixtures should be determined and translated to the surgical template. The accuracy of the fixture positioning is another influential aspect of the overall success of implant therapy. Although placing the greatest number of the longest possible fixtures gives the greatest surface area of integration, placing the dental implant fixtures in the esthetic zone may take another route, according to several critical esthetic factors such as the presence of the interimplant papilla.

The type of the abutment used also might influence the angulation of the fixture position itself. The abutment can be screw-retained or cement-retained. This requires attention to the value of a precisely fabricated surgical template. The level of the occlusal plane and the type of prosthesis to be used should be recorded before surgical placement of fixtures. Preoperative articulation of the diagnostic casts must use a technique that permits this evaluation, and a wax trial denture must be prepared to determine optimal placement. In case of reduced intermaxillary space, the options include resective osseous therapy, orthodontic intrusion, bite raise, and so on.

Matching tooth color is obviously essential to the overall final result. The optimal arrangement of the various esthetic elements to proper proportion or relation according to known principles becomes necessary. The ultimate goal of any treatment plan is to achieve a pleasing composition in the smile that matches the intraoral prosthetic reconstruction (Goldstein and Goldstein 1988).

Communication between dentist and dental technician is another key to the treatment's success, because there is nothing more frustrating for the clinician and the technician than to have to modify or remake a prosthesis (Winter 1990). The clinician should determine the general tooth shape, shade arrangement, and alignment, then transfer it on the prescription form to the technician. This valuable information is determined clinically and cannot be second-guessed in the laboratory. Intraoral photographs and full-face or profile pictures can help give an improved perspective on the depth and shape of the teeth but not the shade. They are, however, invaluable for assessing shade distribution and special color effects (Shelby 1977).

Achieving successful long-term function of dental implant restorations on a routine bases requires a solid foundation of diagnosis, treatment planning, and case preparation. Implant success thus requires a personalized approach, based on the functional, esthetic, and psychological needs of the implant candidate. Hence, diagnosis and treatment planning are necessary for safe integrated implant therapy.

Medical Evaluation

A complete medical and dental history provides insight into the patient's current state of health. Patients are urged to reveal any ongoing or previous medical treatment and/or any medications they are taking as well as any influencing habits. This highlights contraindications or important areas of concern for dental implant therapy (Malamed 1995, Sabes et al. 1970). The medical evaluation can also provide useful information on the potential prognosis of implant treatment (Halstead 1982, Misch 1982, Little and Falace 1993). Areas of medical risks (Wakley and Baylink 1988) associated with dental implant placement can be evaluated through a detailed medical history or physical and laboratory examination. Furthermore, clinicians should approach medically compromised patients with caution and be aware that patients who are seen frequently could already be contraindicated to receiving implant therapy. If any suspicious symptoms exist, the patient should be referred to their physician to follow the condition and deliver a clear report. Following this protocol could prevent possible complications during the course of treatment. In some cases, treatment may need to be postponed.

Renal disease is a major concern to dental implant therapy. First, it should be carefully evaluated through the medical history (Wakley and Baylink 1988), because epinephrine and norepinephrine are naturally produced in the medulla of the kidney and are responsible for regulation of blood pressure, myocardial contraction, and excitability. Glucocorticoids from the cortex are responsible for regulation of carbohydrates, fat, and protein metabolism. Hypofunction of the adrenal gland may lead to Addison's disease, which is manifested by weight loss, hypotension, and nausea with or without vomiting. Oral manifestation is hyperpigmentation of lips and gingiva. The hyperfunction causes Cushing's syndrome, manifested by moon face, hypertension, and decreased collagen production—patients suffer from poor wound healing, osteoporosis, and increased risk of infection. Normal creatinine levels are 0.7–1.5 mg/100 mL. The disturbance may indicate kidney dysfunction and warrants further investigation; ignoring the disturbance may lead to osteoporosis and decreased bone healing. Patients who have any chronic renal problems should receive additional steroids prescribed by an experienced physician.

Blood dyscrasias such as anemia, leukemia, bleeding/clotting disorders, etc. also affect dental implants. The symptoms of mild anemia are fatigue, anxiety, and sleeplessness. Chronic anemia is characterized by shortening of breath, abdominal pain, bone pain, tingling of the extremities, muscular weakness, headache, fainting, change in heart rhythm, and nausea. Oral symptoms of anemia include a sore, painful, smooth reddish tongue, loss of taste sensation, and paresthesia of oral tissues. Anemia may lead to further complications such as impaired bone maturation and development; a faint large trabecular pattern of bone may even appear radiographically, which indicates a 25% to 40% loss of trabecular bone pattern.

Decreased bone density affects initial placement and may influence the initial amount of mature lamellar bone forming at the interface of osseointegrated implants. Preoperative and postoperative antibiotics should be administered and hygiene appointments should be scheduled more frequently and the anemic condition should be corrected.

The blood leukocytic disorders entail leukocytosis, which is a result of leukemia, neoplasm, acute hemorrhage, and/or diseases associated with acute inflammation, necrosis, or leukopenia, which may accompany certain infections (e.g., hepatitis) or bone marrow damage (from irradiation therapy). Both conditions may cause complications that compromise the success of dental implant therapy, because infection, edema, and bleeding can be common due to thrombocytopenia. A more conservative treatment plan should be formed when leukocytic disorders are present.

Vitamin D level is another factor to be considered in implant therapy. Vitamin D, which is synthesized in the liver, skin, kidney, intestine, and parathyroid gland, helps to increase the absorption of calcium and phosphate from the intestine and kidney. Deficiency of vitamin D is called *osteomalacia*. Oral effects of osteomalacia include a decrease in trabecular bone, indistinct lamina dura, and an increased tendency for chronic periodontal disease.

Hyperparathyroidism also has distinctive oral consequences such as loss of lamina dura, loosening of the teeth, and an altered trabecular bone pattern (ground glass appearance). Central and peripheral giant cell tumors may develop. Implants are relatively contraindicated in such cases of hyperparathyroidism. Patients with severely compromised immune systems and severe gastrointestinal diseases (e.g., hepatitis, malabsorption, etc.) should also be excluded from dental implant installation.

Patients with progressive musculoskeletal diseases (e.g., osteoporosis, osteopetrosis, and Osteitis deformas [Paget's disease]) due to increased osteoblastic activity are usually marked by increased serum alkaline phosphates and calcium levels. Bony enlargements can be palpated and appear radiographically as cotton or wool shapes. These patients are predisposed to osteosarcoma and in these cases dental implants are totally contraindicated.

Osteoporosis is a common oral bone disease that influences implant placement. The problem arises from the imbalance between the rate of bone resorption and formation, with emphasis on resorption. The cortical plates become thinner, the trabecular bone pattern is more discrete, and advanced demineralization occurs. Osteoporosis affects women twice as often as men, especially after menopause. It does not constitute an absolute contraindication for dental implants, but it influences the treatment path. Precautions should include estrogen therapy intake, dietary calcium intake, and progressive bone loading. Implant designs should be greater in width and coated with hydroxyapatite to increase bone contact (Wakley and Baylink 1988).

Some situations preclude the success of implant therapy because they compromise the body's health either generally or locally. Pregnancy, persistent oral infections, AIDS, neurologic disorders (e.g., stroke, palsy, mental retardation, etc.) that may render a patient incapable of maintaining adequate oral hygiene on a daily basis, and malignancies are examples of such contraindicating situations for dental implant therapy (Smiler 1987).

Relative contraindications to dental implant therapy are conditions that are debilitating to the body's immune system. Although they do not directly pose a potential threat to dental implant survival, these contraindications will eventually cause the implants to fail in the host body. These relative contraindications include prolonged corticosteroid or immunosuppressive drug therapy, chemotherapy, or collagen diseases (Smiler 1987).

Smoking is increasingly cited in the literature as a risk factor in soft tissue healing (Rees et al. 1984), periodontal health (Bergström and Preber 1994, Grossi et al. 1997), and implant therapy. Modern science has shown that smoking poses a potential increased risk to the long- and short-term success of dental implants (Bain and Moy 1993, Gorman et al. 1994, De Bruyn and Collaert 1994, Bain 1996).

A recent study (Persson et al. 2003) that evaluated the soft tissue response to smoking stated that tobacco smoking has considerable negative effects on the outcome of periodontal treatment. This may be related to an altered neutrophill activity in terms of elastase and/or matrix metalloproteinase-8 (MMP-8), as well as protease inhibitor alpha-1-antitrypsin (a-1-AT) and alpha-2-macroglobulin (a-2-MG) activities. The study included 15 smoking and 15 nonsmoking patients with moderate to severe periodontitis who received surgical treatment. Clinical examinations and collection of gingival crevicular fluid (GCF) were conducted prior to surgery and one and five weeks following treatment. The elastase activity was measured with a chromogenic low-molecular substrate and the levels of a-1-AT, a-2-MG, and MMP-8 with enzyme-linked immunosorbent assay. Results showed unaltered levels of a-1-AT, a-2-MG, and MMP-8 in smokers following surgery. In nonsmokers, the levels of a-1-AT and a-2-MG increased, whereas MMP-8 levels decreased. The levels of elastase remained in both smokers and nonsmokers.

The results indicated that in the presence of smoking, the levels of a-1-AT, a-2-MG, and MMP-8 remained unaltered during the recovery period following surgical treatment. This is interpreted as a possible interference of smoking with the treatment response and may, in part, explain the clinical evidence of poor treatment outcome in patients who smoke. These findings support clinicians who exclude smokers from periodontal and implantology treatment until they follow a strict cessation protocol.

Another study (Henemyre et al. 2003) determined the effect of physiologically relevant nicotine levels on porcine osteoclast function as measured by resorption of calcium phosphate. The study used pure nicotine that was diluted in a medium to the following concentrations: 0.03 μm, 0.15 μm, 0.30 μm, 0.60 μm, and 1.50 μm. Porcine osteoclasts were seeded onto calcium phosphate multitest slides and incubated at 37°C with half media changes every 24 hours. Cells received 0, 0.15, 0.30, 0.60, and 1.50 μm nicotine, or 25 nm parathyroid hormone (PTH). Osteoclast resorption was quantified by measuring the resorbed surface area of the calcium phosphate substrate.

The study showed an increase in osteoclasts in a linear relationship to the increasing nicotine concentrations; however, no correlation was found between osteoclast number and the amount of resorption. It was concluded that nicotine appears to stimulate osteoclast differentiations and resorption of calcium phosphate, which is the major component of bone. Nicotine-modulated osteoclast stimulation may, in part, explain the increased rapidity of periodontal bone loss and refractory disease incidence in smokers.

Allergies are yet another source of concern. It is important to identify allergies that could dictate the use or avoidance of certain drugs of other substances in dental implant therapy. Due to its high passivity and biocompatibility, no allergies to titanium or titanium alloy have been reported in the dental literature (Latta et al. 1993, Bezzon 1993). However, allergies to dentures were reported (Hansen and West 1997) and such restorative base metals as chromium cobalt (Henemyre et al. 2003, Hansen and West 1997), nickel (Bezzon 1993, Hansen and West 1997), and palladium-copper-gold alloys (Fielding and Hild 1993) have appeared in research abstracts.

Patients with artificial joints may develop bacteremia due to implant surgery, which can cause hematogenous seeding at the joint implants. It was hypothesized that bacteria may seed the prosthesis and cause infection due to dental procedures. Preoperative antibiotic coverage is highly indicated.

The salivary glands and ducts must be inspected for unobstructed asymptomatic salivary flow that might cause lack of lubrication to any oral prosthesis and may mandate a change in the proposed prosthodontic plan.

Liver function should be assessed because liver cirrhosis reduces synthesis of clotting factors, abnormal synthesis of fibrinogen and clotting proteins, vitamin K deficiency, enhanced fibrinolytic activity, and quantitative and qualitative platelet deficiency. The liver's ability to detoxify drugs is another factor in implant therapy. Bilirubin altered range (total 0.7 mg/100 mL) indicates liver disease, which affects tissue healing, drug pharmacokinetics, and the patient's long-term overall health. In minor procedures, postoperative control of bleeding should be controlled by using bovine collagen and additional sutures. Advanced surgical procedures require hospitalization to control hemorrhage.

A history of osteomyelitis or irradiation therapy in the region of the proposed implant receptor site should be well investigated; the relationship between dental implant failure and irradiation therapy is not quite clear. Irradiation for the treatment of oral cancer does not seem to reduce the survival rate of implants as compared to those placed in the nonirradiated jaws. The main problem with irradiated patients is decreased salivary flow (xerostomia) (Jisaander et al. 1997), the liability for infection due to the decrease in blood supply, and the possibility of osteoradionecrosis (Marx and Johnson 1987).

Radiation complications begin when the dose exceeds 64 Gy (Murray et al. 1980). Some authors stated that the maxilla is more prone to failure with dental implants after irradiation therapy (Jisaander et al. 1997). The waiting period between the end of radiation therapy and implant placement varies. Some authors suggest three to six months (King et al. 1979). Others suggest six months (El Askary et al. 1999a) because that much time is needed for fibrosis to begin in the irradiated tissues as a result of reduced cell reproducibility and progressive ischemia. Although it seems the failure rate of dental implants after oral radiotherapy is minimal (Keller 1997), a longer healing period and hyperbaric oxygen (HBO) therapy, especially in the maxilla, are recommended to improve the healing capacity, avoid soft tissue ulceration, and reduce fibrous tissue formation (Jisaander et al. 1997).

Endocrine systemic diseases (e.g., uncontrolled diabetes, hyperthyroidism, pituitary/adrenal disorders, etc.) should be approached with caution because 75% of patients with diabetes mellitus exhibit increased alveolar bone loss and inflammatory gingival changes that might negatively affect osseointegration (Proceedings of the 1996 World Workshop in Periodontics 1996). Hypoglycemia is the most serious complication for diabetic patients during any dental procedure. It occurs as a result of excessive insulin levels or hypoglycemic drugs or inadequate food intake. Hypoglycemia signs and symptoms include weakness, nervousness, tremors, palpitations, and/or sweating. In the worst cases, confusion and agitation can lead to seizures, or even coma.

Diabetes mellitus does not directly affect the success of dental implants. A consensus expressed that the placement of implants in patients with metabolically controlled diabetes mellitus does not result in a greater risk of failure than in the general population (Proceedings of the 1996 World Workshop in Periodontics 1996), but a group study stated that diabetic patients experience more infection in clean wounds than nondiabetics (Goodson and Hunt 1979). The increased risk of infection is probably due to thinning and fragility of the blood vessels, which alters the blood supply. Therefore, the current surgical opinion is that patients with well-controlled diabetes (below 250 mg/dL) probably do not encounter inordinate operative risks, whereas patients with poorly controlled diabetes or those who are at high risk (more than 250 mg/dL) may frequently experience wound healing failure (Smith et al. 1992). Poorly controlled diabetic patients present more difficult management problems, and postponing the surgery is recommended until better control is achieved (Smith et al. 1992).

Alcohol consumption is detrimental to the success of dental implantology procedures (Sampson et al. 1996, Spencer et al. 1986) because it contributes negatively to osteoporosis and osteopenia. This is supported by studies that suggested that alcohol intake leads to a negative bone balance effect and progressive bone loss (Lindholm et al. 1991). This in turn may lead to insufficient bone volume for application of dental implants. A study (Bombonato et al. 2004) that evaluated the possible effect of alcoholic beverages on reparative bone formation around hydroxyapatite tricalcium phosphate implants inside the alveolar socket in rats confirmed that a significant delay in reparative bone formation was detected in the alveolus of alcoholic rats by a histometric differential point counting method.

It is also imperative that the clinician take all steps to detect early signs of an undiagnosed disease (Marx and Johnson 1987). Bidigital palpation of the lips; buccal mucosa; hard and soft palates; oral pharynx; and submental, submandibular, and cervical lymph nodes should be made to assess the presence of any masses (Smith et al. 1989). By gently grasping and lifting the tongue forward, upward, and laterally, the floor of the mouth and the tongue can also be examined (Smith et al 1989). Recording the patient's vital signs (pulse, blood pressure, respiratory rate, and temperature) can be important in assessing the patient's present overall health. Other medical tests and/or consultations with the patient's physician may be necessary when compromised medical conditions exist or are suspected. It is important to note that the literature suggests evaluating medically compromised implant candidates on a patient-by-patient basis, because compromised medical status alone is not necessarily indicative of implant failure (El Askary et al. 1999a, 1999b).

Finally, in addition to evaluating the patient's physical conditions, his psychological ability to commit to long-term treatment and maintenance programs also must be assessed. For example, phobic or highly anxious individuals may have low pain thresholds and refuse follow-up visits. On the other hand, patients whose dental complaints stem from somatization disorders will probably not be satisfied with the results of implant therapy (Melamed 1989). People afflicted with acute psychiatric or psychological disorder may contraindicate for dental implant therapy (Wakley and Baylink 1988). These disorders may be subdivided into the following disorders:

(a) Inability to understand information, follow instructions, or make reasonable decisions (e.g., psychotic syndromes, severe neurotic conditions, or character disorders, etc.)
(b) Impaired memory or motor coordination necessary for routine oral hygiene (e.g., cerebral lesion syndromes, presenile dementia, etc.)
(c) Chronic, severe drug addiction (because of a high propensity for poor motivation, inadequate nutrition, and lack of compliance with oral hygiene regimen) (Smith et al. 1989)

As always, it is best to select candidates whose level of understanding and cooperation is superior, for that guarantees a successful end result.

Study Cast

The study cast, which assists in developing and executing the treatment plan, is perhaps the most valuable tool in case planning (See Figure 2.1) (Misch 1999a). The fact that the patient can only be examined for a limited time per visit emphasizes the value of the cast because it provides an almost exact replica of the oral condition at the time the impression is made and it remains for any evaluation request at any time after the patient has been

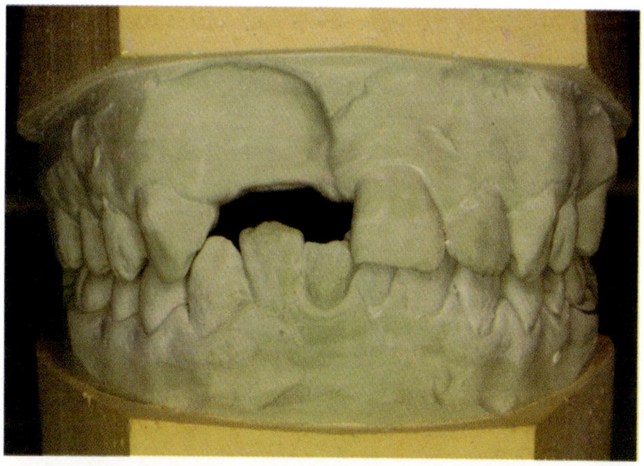

Figure 2.1. Study casts mounted on a simple hinge articulator showing a missing maxillary right central incisor.

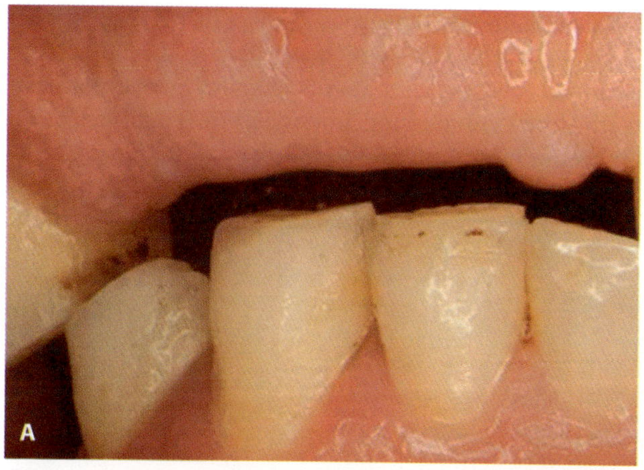

Figure 2.2A. Decreased interarch space that does not allow the stacking of the implant restorative components.

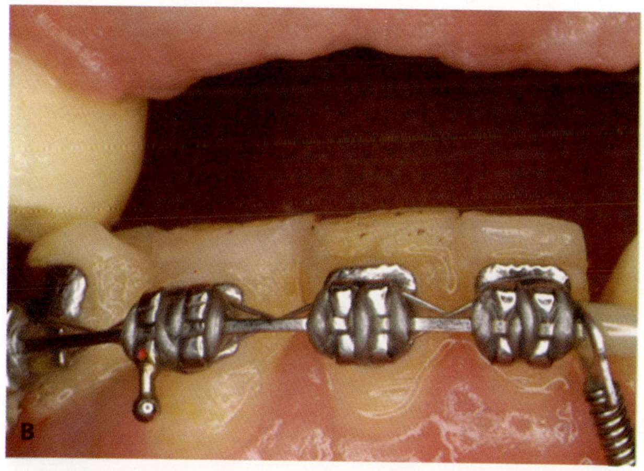

Figure 2.2B. Creating an improved interarch space via using orthodontic teeth intrusion.

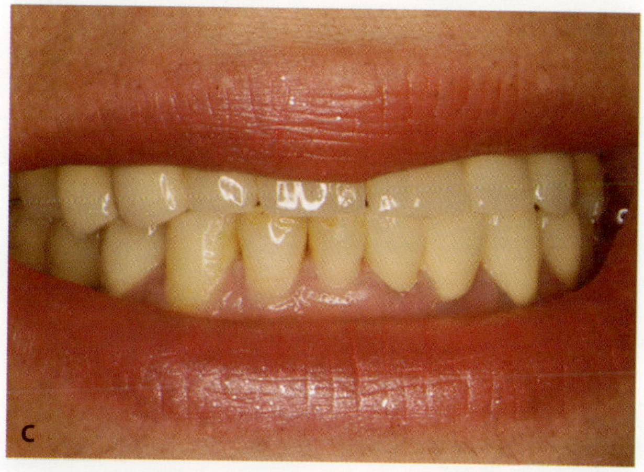

Figure 2.2C. Case finally restored.

dismissed. Therefore, transferring the patient's intraoral condition to a dental cast becomes a vital prerequisite to presurgical planning by enabling the clinician to comprehend the treatment elements required to satisfy all of the esthetic and functional demands in the proposed treatment plan (Jovanovic 1997).

The master study cast may be duplicated two or three times for various clinical applications. One duplicate may be used in fabricating the surgical template, another in constructing a provisional restoration for the patient, and another may be retained and preserved as a record for any future demand or for the comparison between the treatment progress.

While study casts have a number of advantages, they are especially helpful in providing information that is measurable and verifiable. They also help determine the interarch space and sulcus depth. These measurements are necessary to calculate the future crown-implant ratio, the need to perform a bone-grafting procedure, the type of implant used, the type of the final abutment, the type of the prosthetic design, and the extent of the final restoration.

The evaluation of the interarch space is best done on the study cast, and not in the patient's mouth, because the palatal and lingual sides of the teeth can be clearly visualized. The interarch space can be divided in to three distinctive categories—optimal, diminished, or excessive. Every category requires a different clinical approach, and many factors, including the amount of available osseous support, the tissue biotype, and the nature of the opposing arch, influence the treatment of a deficient interarch space. In cases where the interarch space should be improved for implant therapy, the treatment should focus on the functional adaptation to this new position with the aid of the provisional restorations (See Figures 2.2A–C and 2.3A–J) (Dawson 1974).

A proper occlusal recording should provide a precise reference for accurate articulation of the dental casts.

Silicone materials offer ease of dispensing and simplicity over traditional wax materials. It should not be assumed that when patients possess intact posterior teeth along with missing anterior teeth, it is sufficient for an accurate occlusal relation of the casts. Missing anterior teeth result in loss of anterior stop and frequently lead to several possible intercuspations of the casts in the laboratory. In this case, a silicone record is most often all that is necessary to accurately tripodize the casts for an accurate relation (Breeding and Dixon 1992).

Not only can missing teeth size and number be detected on the study cast, but also the available restora-

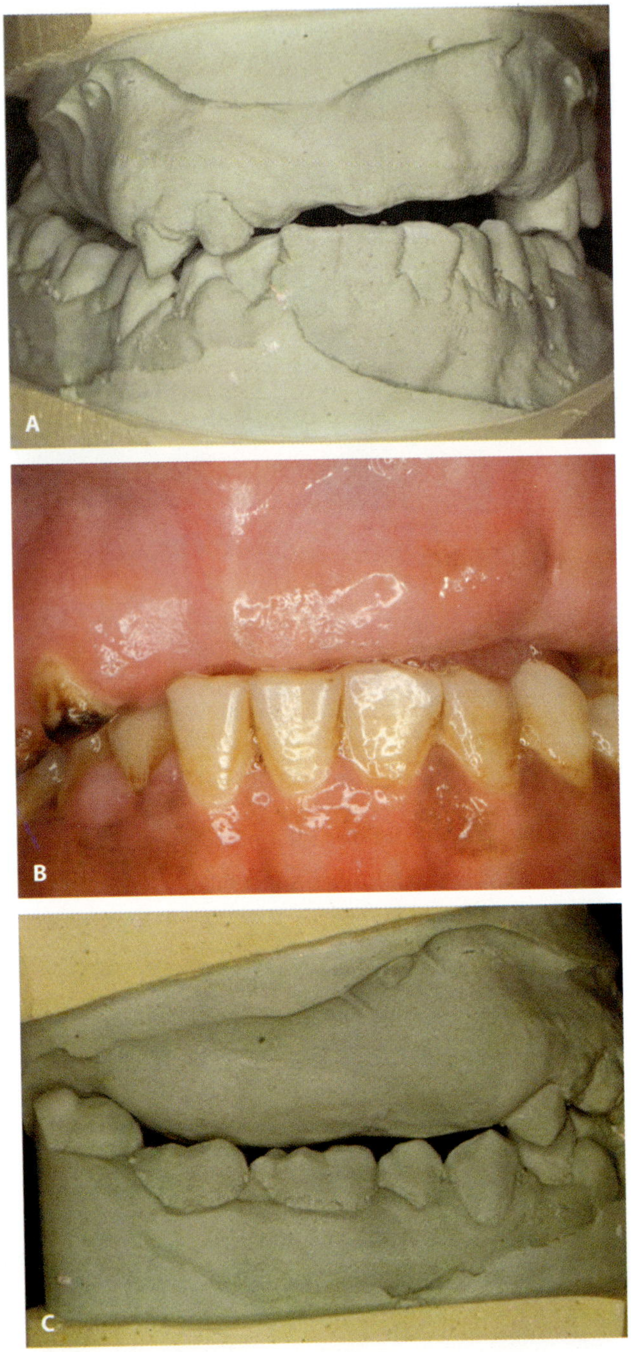

Figure 2.3A, B, C. Different views for an intraoral condition and a study cast showing severely diminished interarch space that limits implant placement and restoration.

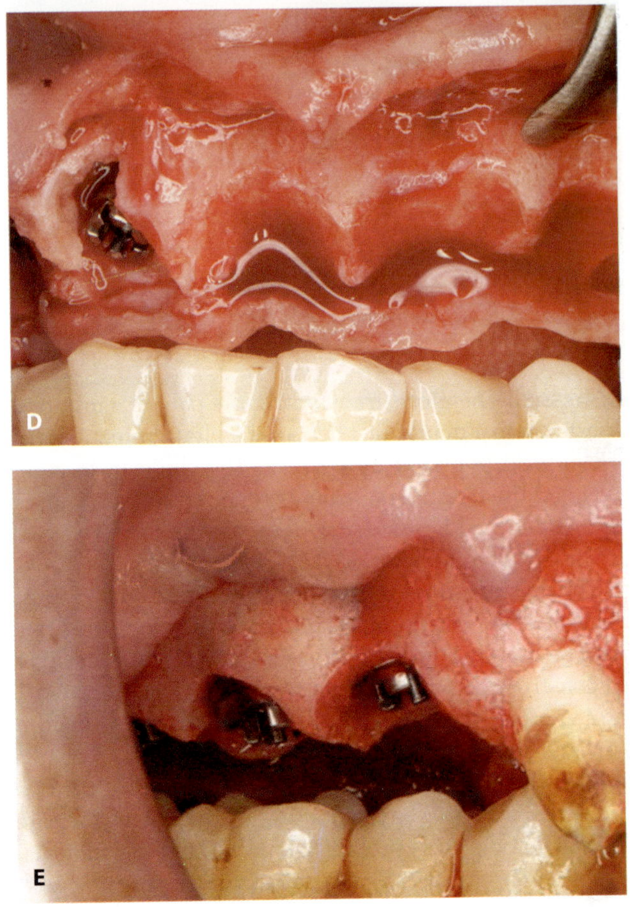

Figure 2.3D, E. Ressective osseous therapy (osteoplasty) is performed to create an interarch space. This decision was made due to the ample bone height.

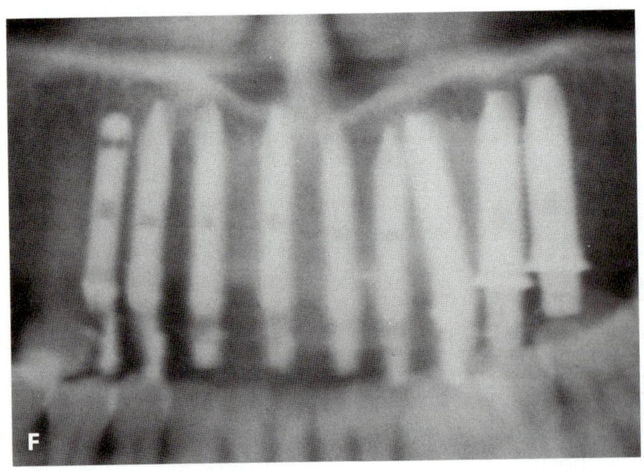

Figure 2.3F. A radiographic view showing implants in place, not the improved width and height of the implants used after bone resection.

tive space in terms of mesiodistal and buccolingual dimensions. Therefore, it is helpful in deciding on the number of the future implants to be used. In areas where function is of prime importance, as in replacing missing posterior dentition, a maximum number of implants should be used to assist in better loading. This provides a larger surface area of support, because loads are magnified as they move farther posteriorly in the oral cavity.

On the other hand, in areas where esthetics are desirable and biting forces are less damaging, it is preferable to reduce the number of implants used (without compromising the function). This is sometimes called the *pontic enhancement method* or *pontic development technique*, and is shown in Figures 2.4A–C. This technique can

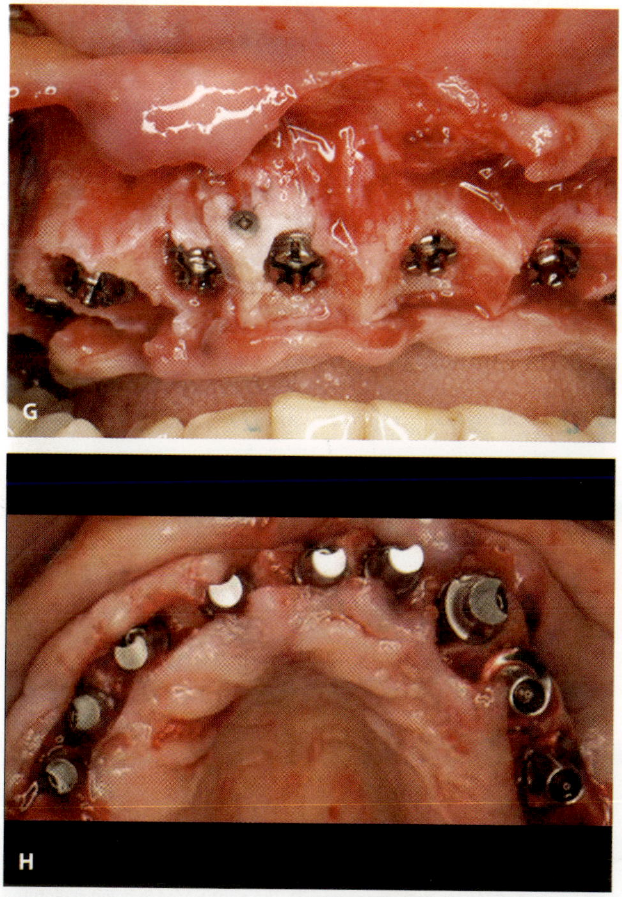

Figure 2.3G, H. Implants in place and abutments connected for immediate functional loading.

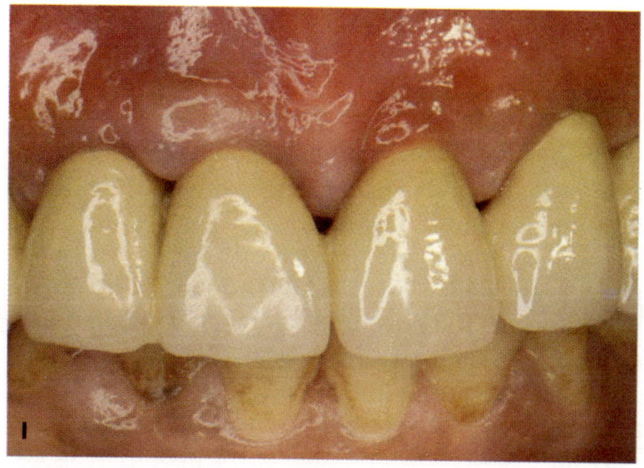

Figure 2.3I. Intraoral picture of the case restored.

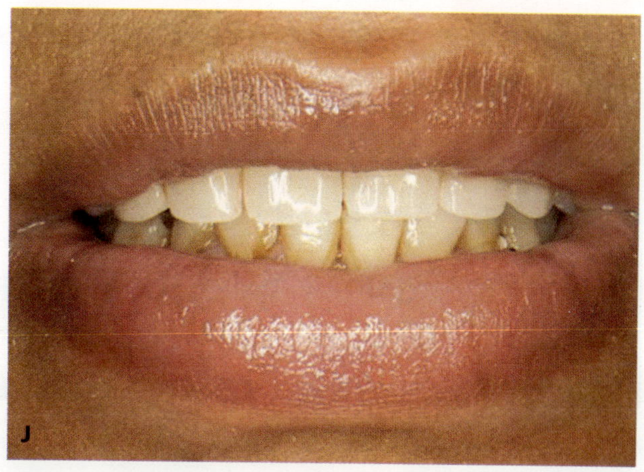

Figure 2.3J. Extraoral view showing the overall patient improvement.

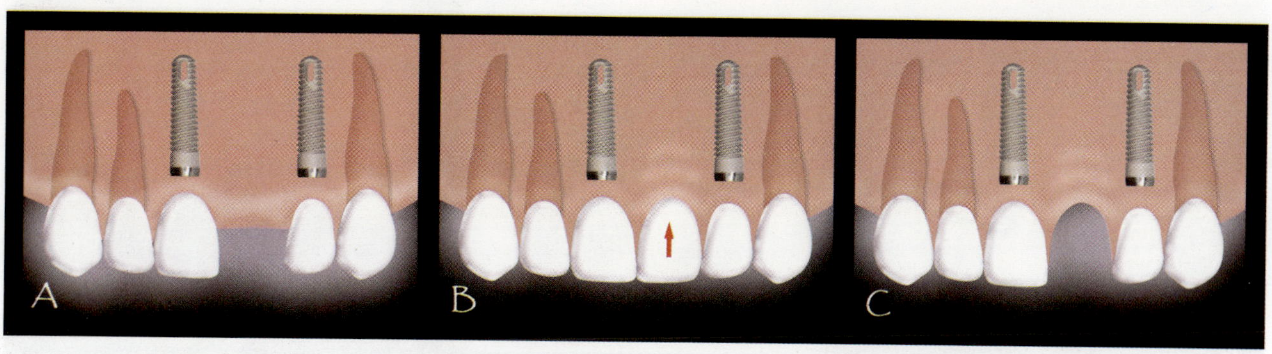

Figure 2.4A, B, C. Illustrations showing the use of a reduced number of implants to enable enhanced peri-implant soft tissue architecture via the pontic development method. In 2.4B, note the effect of the pressure of the pontic at the red arrow.

strikingly improve the esthetic outcome by enhancing and stimulating the peri-implant soft tissue architecture. To duplicate the appearance of natural dentition esthetics in the esthetic zone, a provisional fixed prosthesis supported by dental implants is used to simulate the natural gingival architecture. The goal is to turn the flat osseous and gingival contours into natural soft tissue contours that simulate the interdental papillae-like shape (See Figures 2.5A–G). This is achieved via the ovate pontic in both the interim and definitive fixed prostheses to support facial and inter-proximal soft tissues (Kinsel and Lamb 2002.) The technique entails the use of gingivoplasty to the edentulous ridge at the sites of the ovate pontic while a coordinated modification is made on the diagnostic cast.

The goal is to create gingival embrasures and interdental papillae that replicate those found surrounding natural teeth. The pressure from the underlying pontic of the fixed prosthesis affects the alveolar ridge. When a removable prosthesis is used, the patient is instructed to wear the transitional prosthesis full time, with removal only for oral hygiene procedures. The pontic site development method can allow the clinician to obtain a natural emergence profile as well as papillary-like architecture (Spear 1999). Caution must be exercised when using pontic site development methods. Shorter implants, which are not clinically predictable are bio-

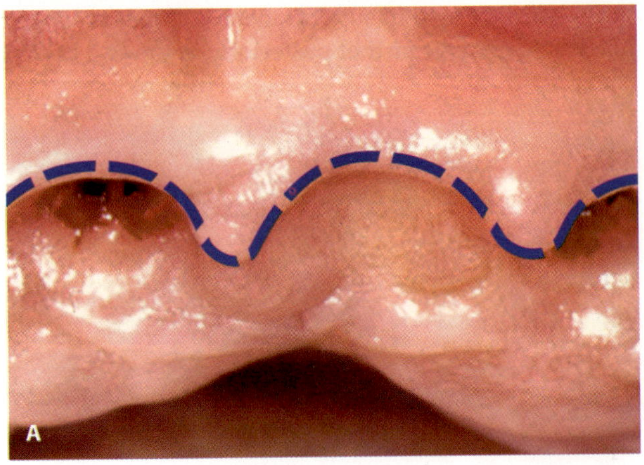

Figure 2.5A. An intraoral view showing the use of two implants to support a three-unit fixed bridge. The blue interrupted line shows the resultant gingival architecture.

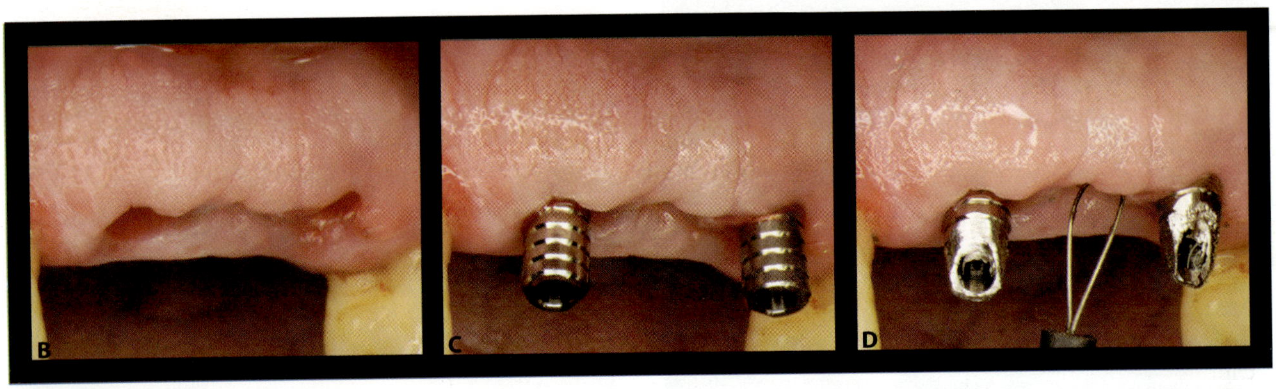

Figure 2.5. **B.** Preopertative view of a case that is indicated for pontic development method. **C.** Abutments connected. **D.** The pontic area is being sculptured using electrosurgery.

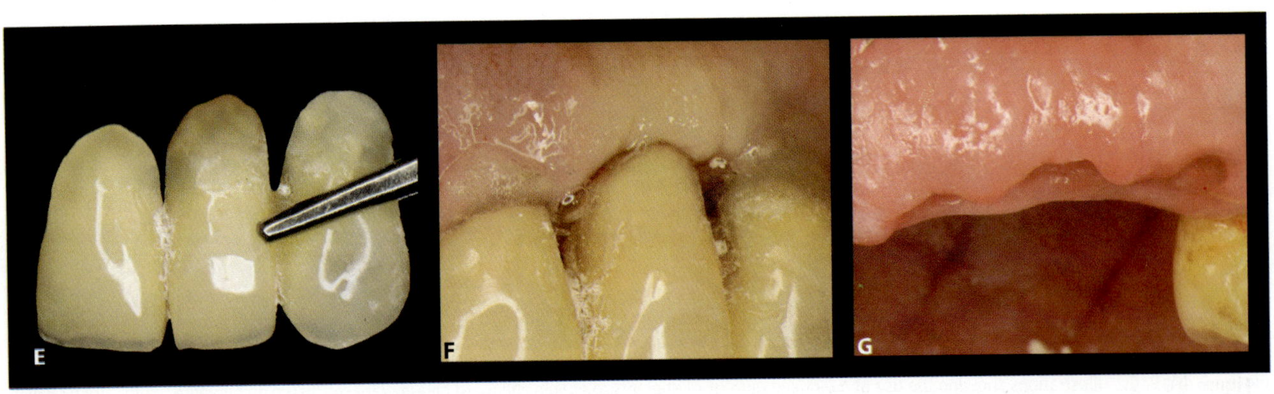

Figure 2.5. **E.** A provisional bridge is fabricated that conforms to the new pontic outline. **F.** The provisional bridge is in place. Note the effect on the pontic area. **G.** The pontic effect on the soft tissue. Note the natural gingival architecture starts to develop.

mechanically doomed. Therefore, longer and surface-enhanced implants are recommended to provide a better implant–bone contact that can maintain the biting forces and offer long-term success.

A study that was designed to examine the clinical and histological characteristics of the human alveolar ridge mucosa adjacent to an ovate pontic–designed restoration used 12 patients requiring maxillary fixed partial dentures (either implant- or tooth-supported) with a pontic site in the premolar or molar region (Zitzmann et al. 2002). Twelve patients, four men and eight women, with a mean age of 54 years (range, 36 to 66 years) were studied. The pontics had an ovate design and were adapted to the underlying mucosa with tight but non-compressive contact. After 12 months, soft tissue biopsy specimens about 3×3 mm in size were obtained from the ridge mucosa in contact with the pontic (test site) and from an adjacent uncovered masticatory mucosal area (control site). Histometrically, the thickness of the epithelium and the keratin layer and the height of the connective tissue papillae were measured. Morphometrically, the composition of the connective tissue of the specimens was analyzed.

The results indicated that only three pontic sites showed clinical signs of mild inflammatory reaction at 12 months, whereas the other test sites and all control sites appeared healthy with larger tissue fractions of inflammatory cells found in pontic sites than in control areas in the zone immediately subjacent to the epithelium. The adequate adaptation of the ovate pontic to the alveolar ridge mucosa with daily hygiene practice of the area underneath the pontic did not cause substantial changes with regard to the height of the epithelium and the rete pegs. The epithelium in the pontic site was always identified as keratinized, but the keratin layer itself was thinner than in the reference area. The keratin layer contributes to the protection of the masticatory mucosa against mechanical and/or microbial insult. The enhanced volume of inflammatory cells in the subepithelial zone of pontic sites, as compared with control sites, may in part be explained by this thinner keratin layer. The authors suggested that hyperpressure resulted in a thinner epithelium with shorter rete pegs when compared with the adjacent uncovered mucosa. The results of this study suggested that long-term mucosal health can be maintained with an ovate pontic design, provided that the infrapontic area is carefully adapted and regularly cleaned (See Figures 2.6A–C and 2.7A–B).

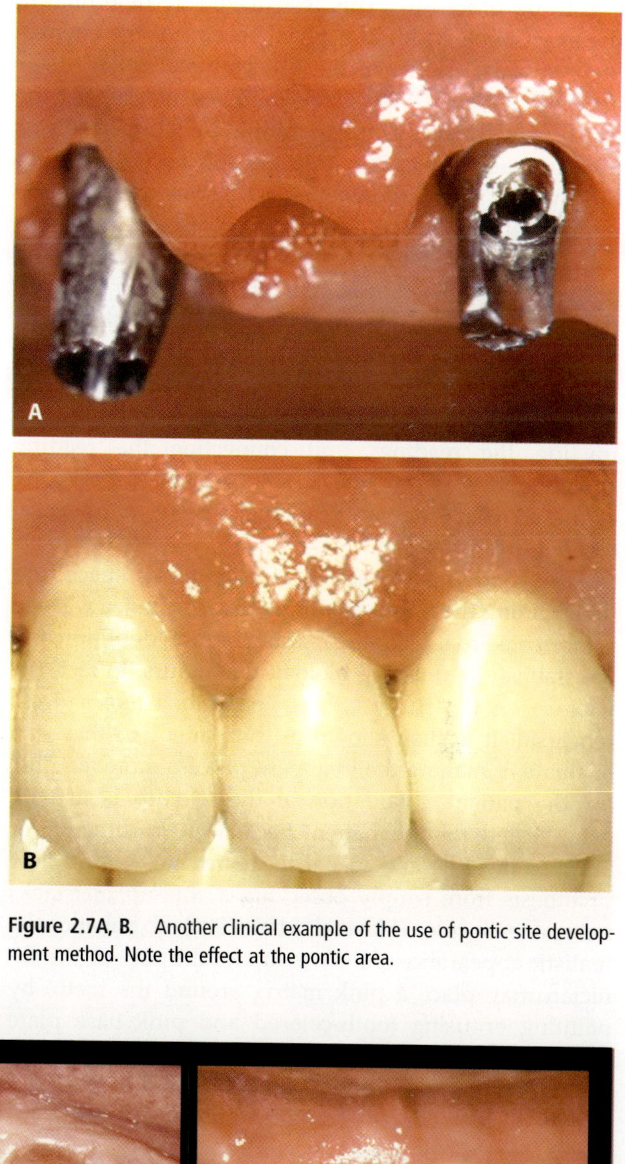

Figure 2.7A, B. Another clinical example of the use of pontic site development method. Note the effect at the pontic area.

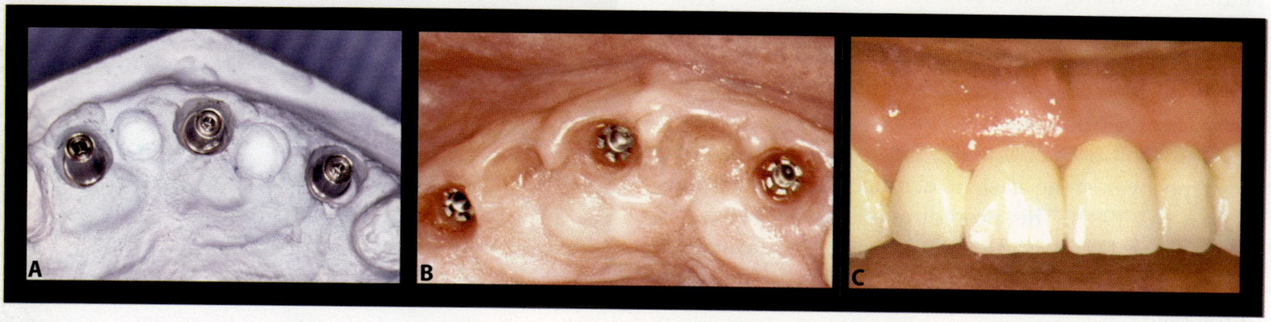

Figure 2.6. **A.** Master cast showing the use of three implants to restore five missing anterior teeth. Note the sculpture of the pontic area. **B.** Final clinical result after pontic development technique. Note the formed papillary-like architecture. **C.** Final restoration cemented in place restoring the natural emergence and papillary architecture.

Precise radiographic images can be a useful aid in detecting clinical information, but, sometimes it can add cost and more exposure to radiation. A specially prepared study cast can occasionally give a valuable indication of the nature of available osseous support as well as soft tissue thickness. In addition, it can be used to assess the amount of available bone and precisely determine whether the available bone is sufficient for housing an implant fixture or whether the area requires a grafting procedure. This is achieved by determining the exact bone width at a given section of the edentulous alveolar ridge using a technique called *ridge mapping* (Wilson 1989). This involves measuring the mucosal thickness by inserting a thin puncture needle or a tissue gauge or caliper into the soft tissue investing the alveolar ridge following a vertical line drawn in the middle of the edentulous area of interest. A thin vacuum-formed template can be used to index the probing sites. The measurement is then repeated at two or three locations along the vertical line both facially and lingually. The collected depth readings are then transferred onto the corresponding locations on the sectioned study cast at the same vertical line. By subtracting the readings and connecting the reading spots together in one line, it will form the topography of the alveolar ridge and the thickness of the mucosa. (See Figures 2.8A–B).

After studying the available edentulous space and determining the number of implants required, a wax-up is fabricated to replace the missing natural dentition and re-establish the missing biological contours. In fact, the wax-up on the study cast is very much like a dress rehearsal. It is then shown to the patient so they can evaluate it, making the treatment process more tangible for the patient. Evaluation of the wax-up is usually complicated for the patient because it is difficult for them to imagine and visualize themselves with a new prosthesis from simply observing a wax-up that lacks natural teeth color (Marizola et al. 2000). To enhance the realistic appearance of the wax-up for the patient, the clinician may place a pink matrix around the teeth, by painting or using tooth-colored and pink base plate wax, to simulate gingival appearance (Roge and Preston 1987). Sometimes adding a lip impression to the pink matrix on the study cast will provide a 3-D vision for the patient (Rifkin and Materdomini 1993). Natural tooth and soft tissue color also improve the perspective of shape over stone cast or acrylic resin restorations (Ganz et al. 1989). This procedure allows the patient to be an integral part of the treatment plan, and it makes the patient feel somewhat responsible for the outcome of the plan.

After the patient approves the wax-up, the locations of the future implants are then marked on the cast. The diagnostic wax-up incorporates the planned modifications, and the provisional restorations are then constructed from this waxing. The waxing may be tested and modified intraorally if necessary. Computerized imaging may replace diagnostic waxing or complement it, according to the clinical situation (See Figures 2.9A–B). A surgical template is then constructed on the study cast according to the marking of the future implant locations that had been determined earlier. This procedure transfers the planned first stage of surgery onto the surgical site.

A vast array of variable devices are available to assist in transferring the data from the planned study cast to the oral cavity. The clinician should select the correct tool for executing the treatment plan.

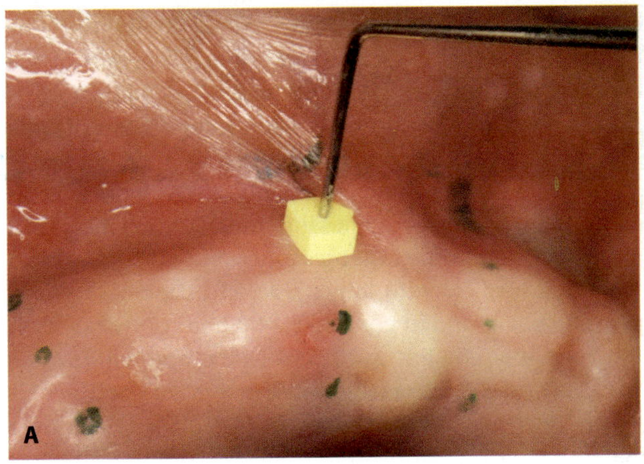

Figure 2.8A. Three pin markings labially and three pin markings palatally are made. A needle punching the soft tissue to mark the place to record the soft tissue depth is shown.

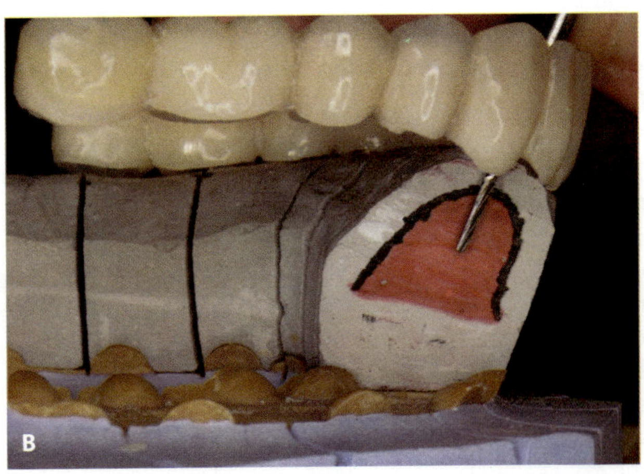

Figure 2.8B. A sectioned model showing the actual thickness of bone after tracing the collected data; the dark blue color represents the bone thickness.

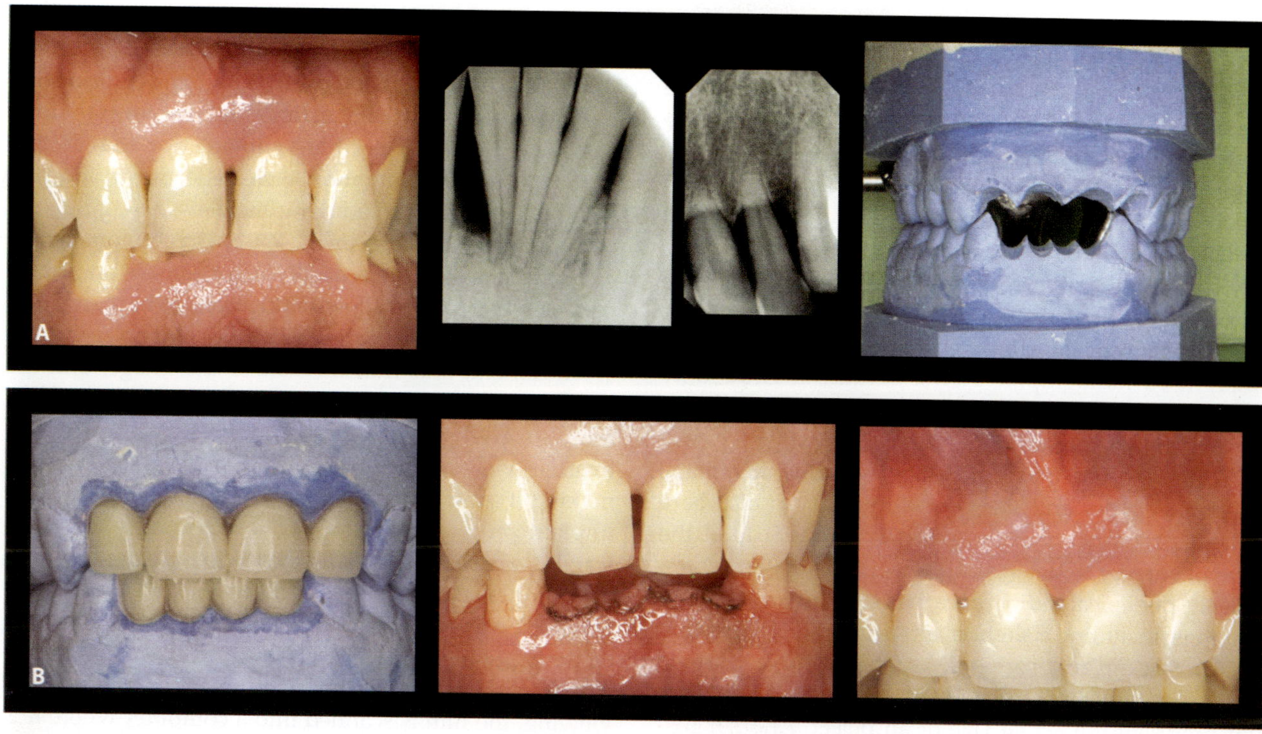

Figure 2.9A, B. A surgical template and a wax-up for missing teeth, showing the replication of the missing tissue contours.

Diagnostic Radiography

The accurate assessment of the topography of the alveolar process is an absolute necessity prior to implant therapy. It allows precise implant positioning, determines any alveolar bone deficiency, and determines the position of the future implant and the need to carry out any grafting procedures. The contiguous structures adjacent to the site of interest and soft tissue profile can also be evaluated. The oral mucosa hides the actual dimensions of the underlying osseous structure, which makes it invisible and undetectable; therefore the recognition of the shape and the volume of the remaining alveolar bone becomes very important to the treatment (Misch 1999a, Wood and Lee 1994).

Various available radiographic views can help assess the quantity, quality, and inclination of the residual alveolar ridge. Such related anatomical details as the nasal floor, maxillary sinus, and anterior mental looping may also be identified. Any pathology or bone disease related to the working site may be detected and dealt with before treatment commences. Preoperative radiographs may be helpful for postoperative comparisons and reviews of treatment progress with the patient. In the event of future medicolegal problems, radiographs are used as evidence of the patient's situation at present and both pre- and postoperatively.

In addition to accurately determining bone dimensions and density (Gher and Richardson 1995), the available technical advancements in radiography have helped improve case design and treatment planning, thus improving the predictability of clinical results (Garg and Vicari 1995). This, in turn, helps the dental team select the proper implant size and design, surface texture and angulation, and surgical technique to be used for implant placement. Overall, this information helps the clinician visualize hidden elements and build the treatment plan.

Today's digital technology has enabled us to view the underlying bone structure like never before, and to gain an exact picture of the underlying bone topography. There are numerous radiological techniques and views available, and each has its own merits and drawbacks. The clinician should be able to select the most suitable radiographic method for each patient according to several factors, such as the patient's age, health condition, and financial status, as well as the possibility of re-exposure to X-ray radiation, availability of modern equipment, magnification errors, data required from a specific view, and value of the procedure to be carried out. Because sophisticated modern radiography, such as digital scans, is not an absolute routine prerequisite for every case, at times basic and simple radiographic methods will suffice.

Periapical and panoramic views are the most commonly used views in daily dental patient care. They offer only a two-dimensional imagery, providing an idea of bone volume and density (Garg and Vicari 1995). This view can be helpful in evaluating the condition of the periodontium to assess the location of the roots relative to the neighboring anatomical structures and/or a particular future implant receptor site. Periapical and panoramic X-ray views are cost effective, because most dental offices offer at least one of these radiographic devices. The devices are easy to use and involve minimal additional expense for the patient.

The periapical view ranks number one among the routinely used radiographic views. Because it is the only available method for routine, accurate monitoring of crestal bone levels around previously restored dental implants, the periapical view has a unique advantage over other types and views of X-rays. It can also be a valuable reference that the clinician can refer to at the time of surgery to determine the depth of drilling. Conversely, periapical radiography has some inherent shortcomings, including a slight magnification of images that is inconsistent and varies according to the technique used. Consequently, an image in a periapical film does not represent the actual size of an object. Another disadvantage is the small size of the film, which restricts the viewed area and thus limits its clinical applications.

Digital radiography has taken periapical views to a new level, enabling the practitioner to execute the treatment plan with ease and predictability. It provides accurate information regarding the site of interest. The best advancement in digital radiography is that it reduces 90% of the radiation exposure for the patient and subsequently reduces the scattered radiation levels. Digital radiography also enhances communication with patients, provides easy storage and retrieval, enables simplified electronic claims, simplifies dental staff consultation, perfects duplication, and eliminates film development chemicals and their subsequent disposal. The regular film is replaced with a sensor that is connected to a computer, where the image can be viewed instantaneously (Farman and Farman 1999).

The radiation reduction benefits both the clinician and the patient, because digitalization allows several views to be taken in a shorter time without fear of radiation hazard. It is also thought to be cost effective in comparison with the regular radiographic views.

Two types of platform of sensors are commercially available: metal oxide semiconductor sensors and phosphorus sensors. Both allow radiographs to be stored digitally with a time and date stamp; allow for enlargement, enhancement, and transmission of the image; and are good for patient education. Two types of digital viewing are also available: direct and indirect. Direct viewing involves viewing the image within seconds of exposure, making it a timely application for both endodontic and implant procedures. However, direct images are rigid, fragile, and expensive. Indirect viewing uses a scanner as an intermediate step between capturing and viewing the image. The sensor cannot be re-exposed until it is scanned, or the original image is lost. However, these images are less fragile, and they can be somewhat flexible. After viewing, the film is scanned into a computer where it is then available for viewing, saving to a hard drive, or transmitting electronically (See Figures 2.10A–D).

The digital radiography image can be enhanced and modified into many forms, and the clinician can make direct measurements on the screen that are accurate at the time of the surgery. A new digital radiography that is now available is the VisualiX® eHD (Gendex-KaVo, Milan, Italy). It is a digital sensor based on charge coupled device (CCD) technology that ensures a high quality image. The pixel size has been reduced to 19.5 microns, providing a theoretical resolution of roughly 26 μmeter. It is designed with a cesium iodide scintillator, grown vertically on a carbon layer. The vertical growth process generates a columnar microstructure, which drives light directly on the CCD surface, reducing loss

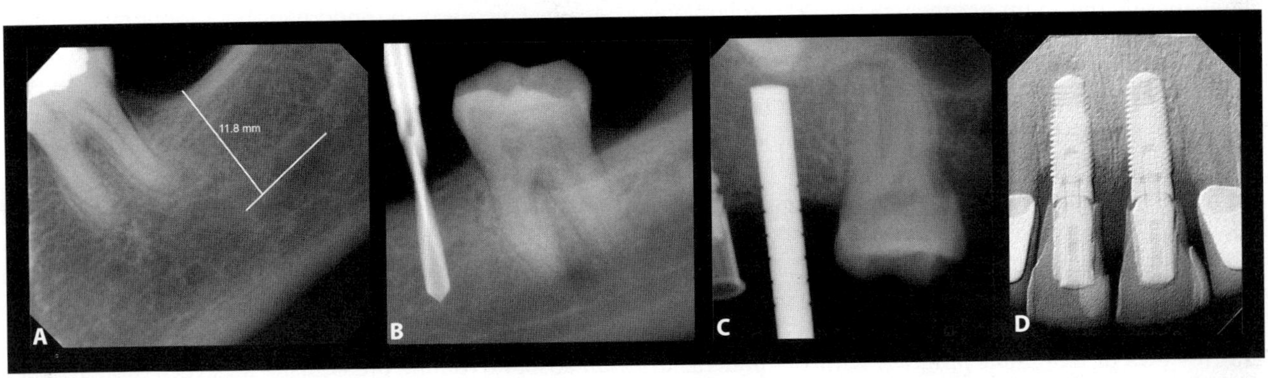

Figure 2.10. **A.** Digital periapical radiographic views showing direct measurement of the bone height. **B.** Digital periapical radiographic views showing the detection of the drilling depth. **C.** Digital periapical radiographic views showing the relationship to the anatomical vital structure. **D.** A 3D view of the periapical digital radiograph.

and providing an unsurpassed image quality. In addition, the VisualiX® eHD unique "auto-trigger" function eliminates the need to manually activate the sensor before the exposure. The sensor automatically recognizes the presence of the X-ray emission and passes the image to the personal computer. The sensor has a special drop-like shape, smooth edges, and round corners, which follows the anatomical shape of the oral cavity, thus simplifying sensor positioning and maximizing patient comfort (See Figure 2.11).

The occlusal view is another radiographic intraoral view. It has very limited applications in today's implantology because of superimposition of anatomical structures and the fact that the change in the X-ray tube angulation can lead to distortion in most of the images and difficulties in accessing the posterior regions of the oral cavity (Reddy and Wang 1999). The most popular panoramic view is also the most commonly used diagnostic tool in dental implantology, although it is limited to two-dimensional viewing; thus it fails to show the width of the object. It has lower resolution (especially in the anterior zone) than intraoral radiographs, which provide magnified images up to 15–22%. Hence, it is difficult to calculate the exact bone height, or mesiodistal distance, without performing a mathematical calculation to eliminate the magnification error.

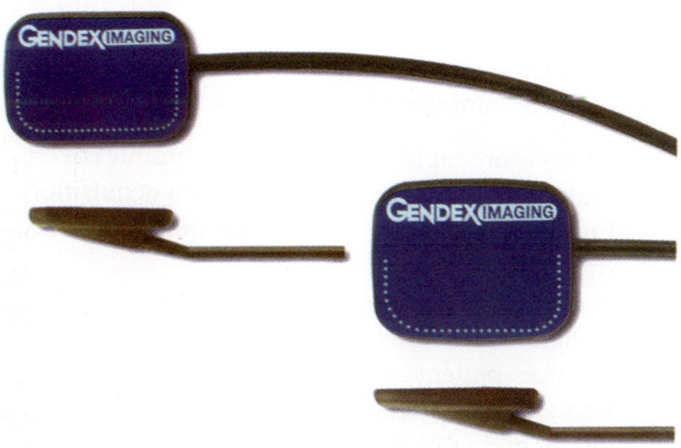

Figure 2.11. VisualiX® eHD digital Xray sensor (Gendex, KaVo, Milan, Italy). Note the smooth margins and rounded corners that offer maximum patient comfort.

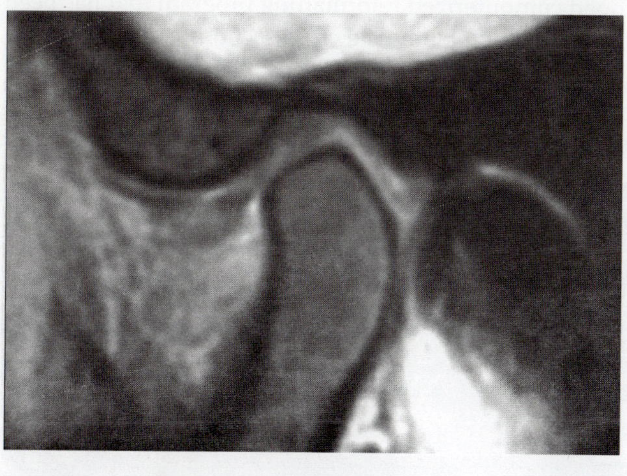

Figure 2.12. Magnetic resonance view of the TMJ.

With today's technology, specifically the digital imaging technology, panoramic views have overcome their inherent shortcomings (See Figure 2.12). The digital version of panoramic systems may be represented in the most updated machine, the Orthoralix 8500 (Gendex-KaVo, Milan, Italy). This is an example of modern, basic, digital panoramic radiography and features up to four microprocessor computer-controlled motors that provide superior mechanical performance, giving the rotating arm the freedom of motion needed to accurately follow the patient's morphology. The multimotorized rotation allows the X-ray generator to rotate and relocate itself in the horizontal plane, thus permitting the best focal imaging and allowing for optimal reproduction of the entire dento-maxillo-facial region.

The Orthoralix 9200 (Gendex–KaVo, Milan, Italy) has been recently introduced. It offers real-time acquisition for the panoramic images using a linear tomographic technique that offers three transverse cross sections of the upper and lower jaw at 7-mm intervals. It offers a choice of two focal layers of either 3 mm or 6 mm and the possibility to show the right or left dental arch on the same film. Maximum precision is also obtained in patient positioning by using an efficient triple light beam system, thus the intervention of the operator is highly reduced. The device features the Transcan (transversal tomographic system) and temporomandibular joint (TMJ) programs. It also features automatic exposure control (AEC) system mode, which makes the correct choice of technical factors easier, and features automatic profile recognition (APR), making real-time corrections to ensure optimum balance between contrast and image resolution. Artifact suppression and lack of redundant shadows from the spinal cord are evident. Lateral views are obtained of the TMJ where the major condylar axis is produced for an accurate examination of the base and section of each joint. The system also features several cephalometric views: latero-lateral(LL), antero-posterior(AP), and submento-vertex (SV). The tomographic slice on a relatively ample cross section at the maxillary sinuses in posteroanterior view is also available, in which the image layer position can be determined by the clinician (See Figure 2.13).

Lateral cephalometric radiographs are usually only used in dental implantology to assess the anterior maxilla and mandible in terms of angulation and lateral osseous and dental topography. The trajectory and angulation of the residual alveolar ridge are required.

Therefore, cephalographs provide information regarding the angulation of the implants to be placed. They are, however, limited in their application in dental implantology to completely edentulous patients.

Computerized tomography (CT) has benefited dental implants immensely. Specifically, CT offers the following advantages of digital radiography in general: produces sharp images, eliminates the need for film processing, uses a lower dose of radiation, presents precise measurements directly without magnification, and provides a digital image that can be stored on the computer for future comparisons (Reddy and Wang 1999). CT is based on a software program that constructs a 3-D model. It creates clear tomographic sections for the alveolar bone and differentiates between soft and hard tissues clearly as never before. It reformats the image data to create a tangential and cross-sectional tomographic image of the future implant site and precisely verifies the bone quality. The 3-D model is computed using several radiographic views from specific angles (James et al. 1991). Because of its ability to provide a complete 3-D image, CT provides a highly sophisticated format for precisely defining jaw structure and locating critical anatomical structures (See Figures 2.14A–D) (Misch 1999a, Dula et al. 2001, Reddy et al. 1994, Potter et al. 1997, Scaf et al. 1997).

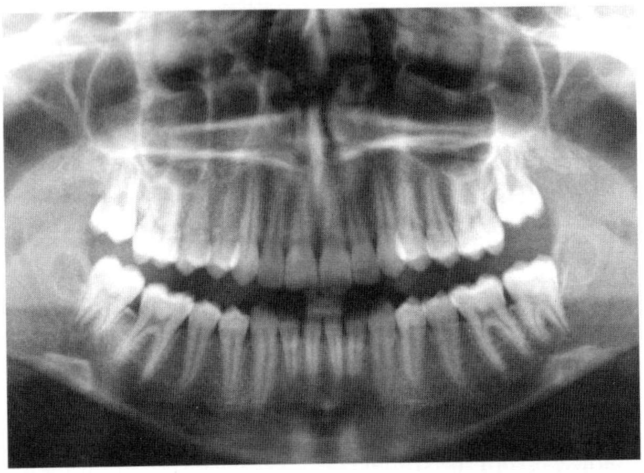

Figure 2.13. Panoramic view showing all the dentition and related anatomical landmarks.

The ability to plan oral rehabilitation using computerized axial tomography (CAT) data by incorporating measurements that define bone volume and density with the planned dental restoration represents the cutting edge of imaging and treatment planning. Special dental processing software programs that are capable of reformatting CATs into more useful image orientations provide panoramic and cross-sectional images in addition to 3-D images. Software (SIM/Plant, Columbia Scientific, Columbia, Maryland, USA) allows the CATs to interact with CT scan data on a personal computer. The interactions within the program provide implant, prosthetic, and bone augmentation simulations and fabrication of a surgical guide. The software assists the planning of surgical prosthetic methods (i.e., the abutment component of the restoration can be coordinated ahead of time on the planned implant). Bone density can also be determined with Hounsfield equipment. Knowledge of the density of the proposed implant site can be helpful in customizing the time between implant placement and implant loading.

Recently, the multislice helical CT was introduced; it has several advantages over the classic conventional CT:

1. Offers more rapid and extended anatomic coverage
2. Reduces patient motion during data acquisition
3. Provides increased z-axis resolution of reconstructed data
4. Is capable of acquiring 0.5-mm slices
5. Is eight times faster at providing thick tissue slices
6. Reduces patient breath-holding time
7. Reduces partial volume effect
8. Offers higher contrast
9. Offers decreased image noise
10. Offers less waiting for tube cooling

Dentascan (MPDI, Torrance, CA) is a specially developed computerized reformatting program that has been developed to obtain true cross-sections of the mandible and maxilla for patients being considered for dental implant surgery. It generates a referenced cross-sectional

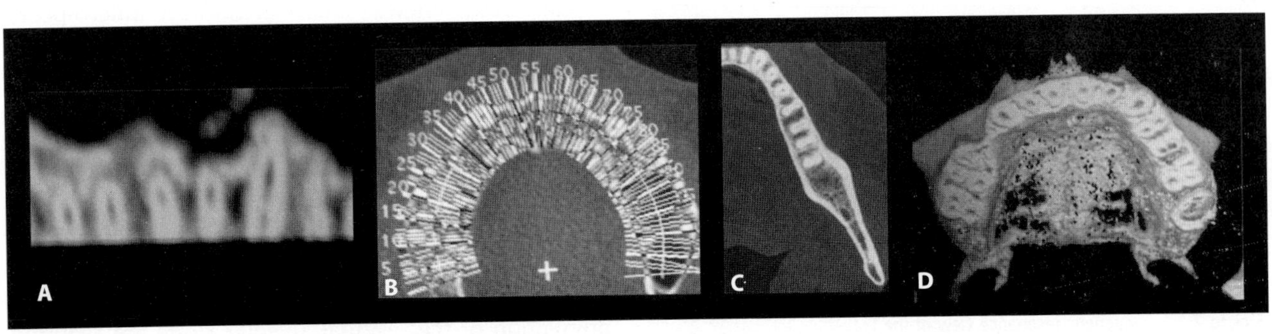

Figure 2.14A, B, C, D. Different views of a computerized tomography (CT) of the maxilla and mandible.

and tangential panoramic image of the alveolar bone along with 3-D images of the arch. It consists of a software modification of the CT data to produce images specifically helpful for preoperative assessment of the alveolar bone before implant placement. The program also provides serial slices through the alveolar ridge at specific intervals. The surgeon is then able to visualize the alveolar bone in a 3-D image and measure the size of the ridge directly from the scan. Regular axial scans are obtained at 1 mm continuously through either the maxilla or mandible. Using the axial scan through the roots of the teeth, the curvature of the alveolar ridge is drawn on the computer screen. Then a software program produces sequential oblique cross-sections every 2 mm or 3 mm around the entire curvature of the alveolar ridge. Each of the cross sections is sequentially numbered and matched to tick marks on the axial views. Finally, five panoramic views are obtained, and the oblique views are keyed to the panoramic scans as well. The CT scans are photographed in true life-size format with vertical scale in millimeters; this method has its drawbacks in terms of cost and processing time (Schartz et al. 1989).

Magnetic resonance imaging (MRI) is a relatively new technology that employs a noninvasive strong magnet field and radio waves to allow clinicians to examine and diagnose many different parts of the body. MRIs may be used to appraise the existing alveolar bone, especially for use with dental implants. It is a useful scanning method that may be used in the TMJ areas or in areas where CT software programs are not available, or with patients who do not desire or cannot be exposed to further radiation. It should be noted, however, that these types of images have not attained popularity in dental implantology (Zabalegui et al. 1990).

Digital subtraction radiography (DSR) is the most versatile and sensitive method for measuring bone loss. It can detect both bone height and changes in bone mass surrounding dental implants. DSR addresses the limitations in detecting postoperative changes that are present in other radiographic modalities. By eliminating information that has not changed, DSR allows the clinician's eye to focus on actual changes that have occurred between the recording of two images (Garg and Vicari 1995, Reddy and Wang 1999).

Recently, Voxgram (Voxel, Park City, UT, USA) was introduced as an exciting tool in medical imaging. The images record and display the data from regular CT and magnetic resonance (MR) scans. A single life-sized Voxgram image provides an enhanced display of the patient's imaging data. It directly overcomes the physician's difficulty in mentally assimilating vast quantities of visual information. Voxgram images display patient anatomy and pathology as transparent 3-D "sculptures of light" projected toward the observer in real 3-D space. These images provide a uniquely accurate perspective of patient anatomy, which increases the clinician's understanding, saves time, and improves clinical outcomes. It allows surgeons to interactively place implants and measuring devices directly into the hologram, as if navigating within the actual patient's anatomy. This "X-ray vision" allows clinicians to select and plan the best surgical approach, and to be safer, faster, more precise, and more confident during diagnosis and therapy planning, in the operating room, and during follow-up (See Figure 2.15).

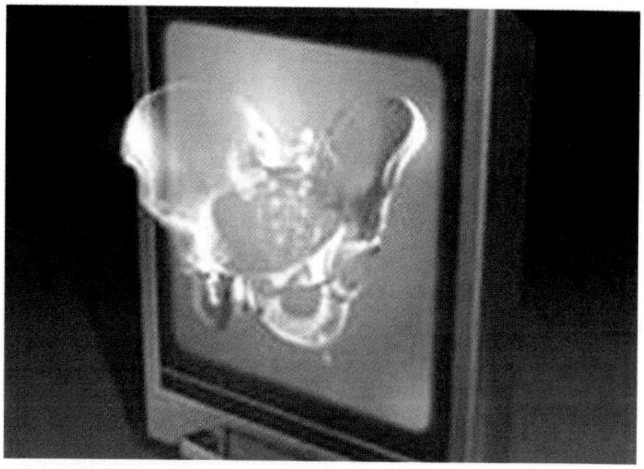

Figure 2.15. Voxel hologram image.

Selecting the most suitable radiographic view for presurgical planning stage requires rational decision and sound judgment. Sophisticated and expensive radiographic procedures sometimes may not be helpful in detecting the various parameters needed to make a precise diagnosis; sometimes the regular, readily available radiographic techniques may be sufficient.

Osseous Site Management

Healthy osseous structure of the alveolar ridge maintains the esthetic soft tissue appearance around natural dentition and provides a framework for peri-implant soft tissue contours. Alveolar bone deficiency due to postextraction bone resorption can result in functional and esthetic problems that require augmenting procedures to reestablish the missing original dimension. The advent of novel osseous regenerative therapy has significantly increased the functional and esthetic potential of dental implants by restoring alveolar ridge defects to their original dimensions, which allows for optimal implant placement and, in turn, increases the credibility of dental implant therapy as a unique treatment alternative.

An optimized osseous structure allows both optimal implant positioning as well as successful final implant-supported restoration, but it is not frequently performed in an optimal osseous volume due to many factors, including postextraction bone resorption and trauma.

Correction of osseous deficiencies allows not only ideal implant placement but it also creates more natural soft tissue profiles, influencing crown anatomy and emergence, and consequently complementing the overall esthetics. Hence, bone enhancement therapies may be a prerequisite for successful implant dentistry (See Figures 2.16A–B and 2.17A–B) (Wilson 1989).

Osseous housing for any future implant site is the main supporting structure that keeps the implant functioning and surviving on a long-term basis (Misch 1999b, Misch 1999c, Holmes and Loftus 1997), thus the importance of healthy and sufficient bone volume becomes a great value to implant therapy. Therefore, emphasis should be placed on inserting an implant in an optimal osseous foundation when a predictable, successful esthetic and functional outcome is to be achieved. Achieving an optimal esthetic implant restoration requires a thorough and meticulous anatomic site analysis of the alveolar ridge anatomy. The analysis must assess many factors: bone width, height, and density, and the presence or absence of bone atrophy.

The severity of the alveolar bone deficit determines the optimal grafting approach. Depending on the extent and morphology of the bone defect, a staged or a non-staged approach can be undertaken. The treatment of the bone defect depends on the proper identification of the type of the osseous deficit itself. A horizontal defect is unlike a vertical one, in terms of clinical management and prognosis. A complex defect that combines vertical and horizontal defects probably will require a different treatment approach; therefore, the type of the tissue deficit and its dimension must be addressed and managed carefully throughout the course of treatment.

Unfortunately, the behavior of the alveolar bone post-tooth extraction complicates the routine implant installation procedures, due to the reduced bone volume and the approximation from the anatomical landmarks that might limit the optimized implant placement. It has been reported that the alveolar bone loses almost 30% of its size within two years following tooth extraction (Lam 1967). Both the maxilla and mandible have distinctive resorption patterns that affect both the width and height of the alveolar bone (Parkinson 1978, Pietrokovski et al.

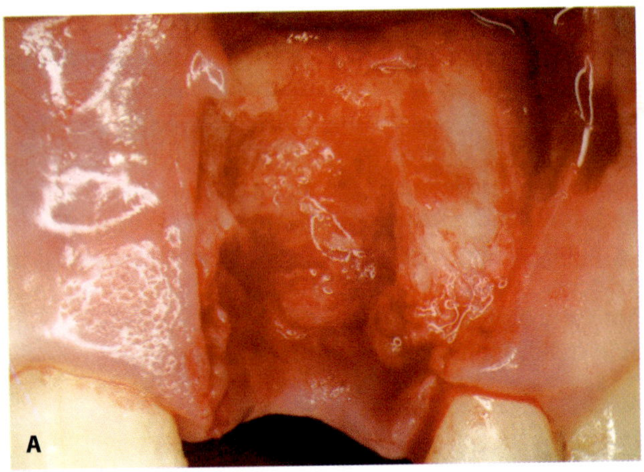

Figure 2.16A. Vertical osseous defect.

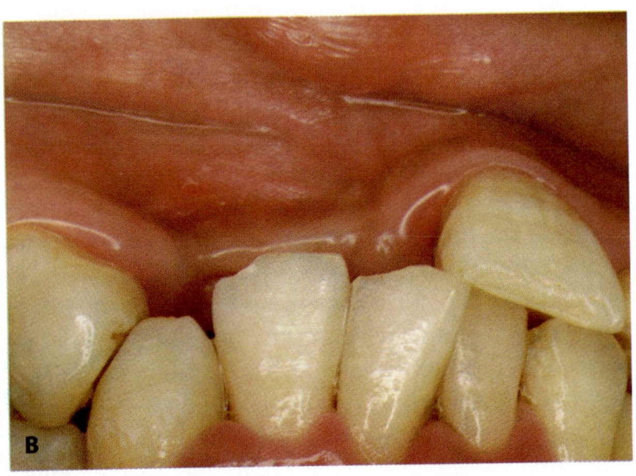

Figure 2.16B. Horizontal osseous defect.

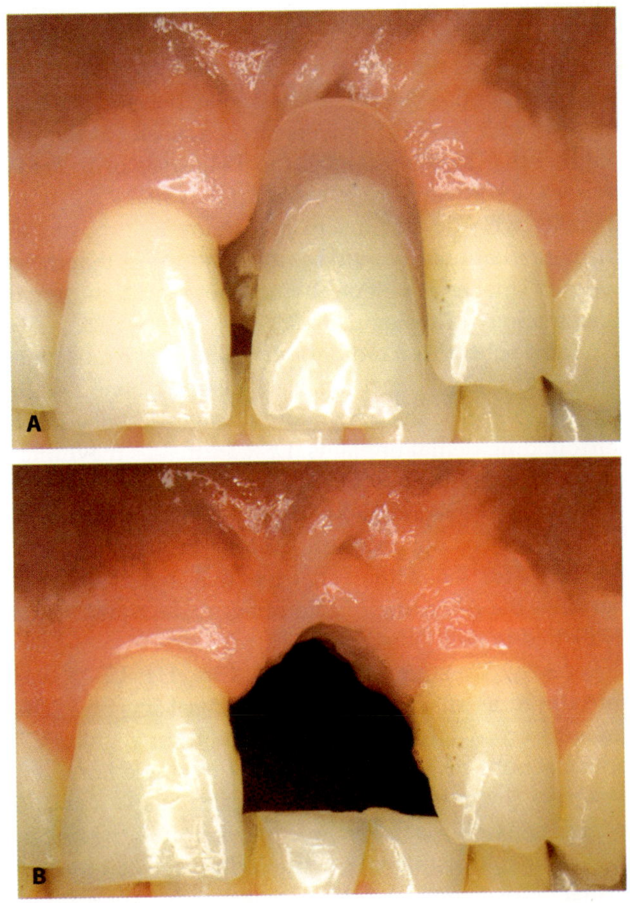

Figure 2.17A, B. Improperly designed prosthesis due to poor osseous defect management.

1967) and negatively affect the overall prognosis of the implant-supported prosthesis. The anterior mandible (the intermental foramina), where the best bone volume can be found, may not necessarily be the best quality for fixture placement. In the posterior mandible there is often insufficient bone height over the inferior alveolar canal. In the maxilla, the pyramid of bone between the medial wall of the antrum and the lateral wall of the nose is frequently the best available bone volume for placement of implant fixtures, while in the posterior maxilla, there is often insufficient bone over the antrum posteriorly and over the nasal fossa anteriorly.

Bone resorption patterns also vary according to location. The maxilla resorbs superiorly and medially while the mandible resorbs inferiorly and laterally. Fixtures placed in these resorbed jaws will be more palatal in the maxilla and more lateral in the mandible than the original position of the natural teeth, thus negatively affecting the overall prognosis. A reverse buccolingual relationship may also occur posteriorly, becoming particularly evident in long-term partially edentulous patients or those with natural teeth in the opposing arch. The position of the artificial teeth in the completed prosthesis must be determined before fixture placement. Fixtures placed too far labially or buccally may result in a prosthesis that is unacceptable esthetically and functionally.

The need for quantitative and qualitative parameters of the available osseous structure is important; it can help the practitioner precisely determine the specific bone category of each particular condition. This, in turn, enables the clinician to select the appropriate treatment protocol. Subsequently, a surgical technique can be chosen to provide an optimal treatment prognosis with maximum predictability from either an esthetic or functional aspect. Misch (1999b) has classified the available alveolar bone volume into four distinct divisions:

- Division A (abundant bone): Alveolar bone width is more than 5 mm, height greater than 10–13 mm, mesiodistal length greater than 7 mm, and the load's angulation does not exceed 30 degrees between the occlusal plan and the implant body. In addition, the crown-implant body ratio is less than 1. This type of bone is optimal for hosting an implant with a diameter between 4 and 5 mm.
- Division B (barely sufficient bone): A slight to moderate atrophy has occurred, leading to a decrease in the width of the available bone at the expense of only the facial cortical bone. The height remains stable at a minimum of 10 mm. The remaining available bone width varies between 3 mm and 5 mm and is thus able to accommodate an implant of 4 mm maximum width. The load's angulation may not exceed 20 degrees. Treatment options presented for this type are osteoplasty, bone augmentation, or the use of narrower diameter root form dental implants.
- Division C (compromised bone): Moderate to advanced atrophy is present, with the width less than 2.5 mm, height less than 10 mm, load angulation greater than 30 degrees, and crown-implant body ratio equal to or greater than 1. The posterior maxillary and mandibular regions demonstrate this type of alveolar bone more than the anterior segments.
- Division D (deficient bone): This type demonstrates severe atrophy, accompanied by basal bone loss. Therefore, the use of autogenous bone grafts is strongly recommended to augment the deficient alveolar bone. This kind of bone usually results in complications related to soft tissue management, grafting, and early implant failure.

Adequate bone requires no augmentation and is greater than 5 mm in width, 10 mm to 13 mm in height, and 7 mm in length (Misch 1990). Barely sufficient bone is 2.5 mm to 5 mm in width, greater than 10 mm to 13 mm in height, greater than 12 mm in length, and can be modified with osteoplasty or augmentation of the hard or soft tissues, depending on the nature of the defect (B-w). Compromised bone necessitates osteoplasty and some form of hard or soft tissue augmentation depending on the extent of the defect in height (less than 10 mm, C-h) or width (less than 2.5 mm, C-w). Deficient bone requires substantial hard tissue augmentation from extra oral sites and is generally not amenable to implant rehabilitation. Salama and Salama (1993) have introduced another classification that considers the available bone according to the socket condition that will host the future implant fixture. This classification can be helpful when an immediate implant placement is the treatment of choice, because the condition of the alveolar socket might influence the treatment plan.

Lekholm and Zarb (1985) classified the residual jaw shape into five categories or types ranging from A to E, with decreasing amounts of bone remaining. In type A residual ridges, there has been little residual ridge resorption, intermaxillary space is minimal, and fabrication of the prosthesis may be compromised accordingly. Type B and C residual ridges are found with moderate to advanced resorption and are usually ideal for placement of osseointegrated fixtures and fabrication of the prosthesis. Type D and E residual ridges have advanced resorption and may require onlay bone grafts in advance of or in conjunction with fixture placement, especially in the maxilla.

Buser and others (2004) recently published a classification system for implant patients (SAC). In the SAC classification system, the "S" represents simple, "A" represents advanced, and "C" represents complex treatment procedures. The system highlights the different clinical conditions that often present in the anterior maxilla and the frequent need for bone augmentation procedures. The classification states the treatment protocol according to the clinical condition either in sites without osseous defects or in sites that has osseous defects.

Accurate detection of bone density, either via radiographic views, computing, or location during surgery, is an important factor in determining the optimal implant surface to be used. In 1988, Misch (1999a, 1999b) introduced four bone density groups based on macroscopic cortical and trabecular bone characteristics. The regions of the jaws with similar densities were often consistent. Suggested implant design, surgical protocol, treatment plans, and loading time spans have been described for each bone density type. The macroscopic description of the Misch bone density classification of D1 bone is primarily dense cortical bone. D2 bone has dense-to-thick porous cortical bone on the crest and within coarse trabecular bone. D3 has a thinner porous cortical crest and fine trabecular bone. D4 bone has almost no crestal cortical bone. The fine trabecular bone comprises almost all of the total volume of bone next to the implant. A very soft bone, with incomplete mineralization, may be considered D5 bone. This usually describes immature bone.

Poor bone density can be dealt with locally or systemically. The systemic methods entail the administration of bisphosphonates that may favor the bone deposition rate more than the bone resorption rate. Clinicians also prescribe an oral dose of bisphosphonates for patients at risk for osteoporosis to help delay the onset of the disease by slowing the natural progression of bone tissue destruction or to reduce its complications. Bisphosphonates inhibit bone resorption, and thus bone renewal, by suppressing the recruitment and activity of osteoclasts, thus shortening their life span.

However, recently the effects of the bisphosphonates have been linked to the osteonecrosis of the jaws. Health professionals should be aware of a strong drug precaution regarding osteonecrosis of the jaw (ONJ) that has been observed in cancer patients who underwent invasive dental procedures such as dental implants or tooth extractions while receiving treatment with intravenous bisphosphonates. ONJ can cause severe, irreversible, and often debilitating damage to the jaw. The two intravenous bisphosphonates that were mentioned in the precautions are marketed under the trade names Aredia and Zometa (Novartis Farma, USA). Orally administered bisphosphonates are not the subject of the drug precautions. However, the Food and Drug Administration (FDA) noted that there have been anecdotal reports of ONJ in association with oral bisphosphonates administered for osteoporosis.

Recently three bisphosphonates, Pamidronate (Aredia, Novartis Pharmaceuticals, East Haven, NJ, USA), Zoledronate (Zometa, Novartis Pharmaceuticals), and Alendronate (Fosamax, Merck Co., West Point, VA), have been investigated by Marx and others (2005). The study, which involved 119 total cases of bisphosphonate-related bone exposure, investigated the link between the drugs and painful refractory bones. Thirty-two of 119 patients (26%) received Aredia, 48 (40.3%) received Zometa, 36 (30.2%) received Aredia—later changed to Zometa, and three (2.5%) received Fosamax. The mean induction time for clinical bone exposure and symptoms was 14.3 months for those who received Aredia, 12.1 months for those who received both, 9.4 months for those who received Zometa, and three years for those who received Fosamax. Sixty-two (52.1%) were treated for multiple myeloma, 50 (42%) for metastatic breast cancer, four (3.4%) for metastatic prostate cancer, and three (2.5%) for osteoporosis. The number of subjects who presented findings in addition to exposed bone were 37 (31.1%) asymptomatic, 82 (68.9%) with pain, 28 (23.5%) with mobile teeth, and 21 (17.6%) with nonhealing fistulas. Eighty-one (68.1%) bone exposures occurred in the mandible alone, 33 (27.7%) in the maxilla, and five (4.2%) occurred in both jaws.

The study concluded that complete prevention of this complication in not currently possible. However, pretherapy dental care reduces this incidence, and nonsurgical dental procedures can prevent new case development. For those who present with painful exposed bone, effective control to a pain-free state without resolution of the exposed bone is 90.1% effective using a regimen of antibiotics along with 0.12% chlorohexidine antiseptic by mouth.

The local methods entail using surgical bone condensation methods and/or using hydroxyapatite- (HA) coated implants. Many treatment modalities for bone volume density are available today, as are several modalities to preserve the available osseous structure from undergoing resorption. One method is placing dental implants immediately. This offers several advantages: preventing bone resorption, maintaining alveolar crest width and height, reducing the complexity of the surgical procedures, reducing treatment time, and offering enhanced esthetic results. The implant is seated in the exact natural tooth angulation and aligned optimally with the adjacent teeth.

Osseous defects generally can be divided into three categories according to the severity and location of the defect: vertically, horizontally, or a combination. The corrective methods can be performed along with implant installation or prior to implant installation to correct vertical bone defects along with an implant installation. Autogenous bone chips can correct the defect if it is less than 2 mm in depth, but if there is more than a 2 mm defect, a veneer graft or what might be called an *onlay graft* can be used predictably.

Autogenous bone grafting in any reconstructive procedure is considered to be the gold standard of all bone grafting procedures, because it provides proteins such as bone-enhancing substrates, minerals, and vital bone cells to the recipient site, which enhances the overall success of the grafting procedure and results in high success rates. In a study that evaluated 63 patients with inadequate topography of the edentulous ridge and who were treated with mandibular ramus body grafts after four months of osseous healing, 187 implants were placed in the grafted sites (Bedrossian 2000). The study concluded that the mandibular ramus body grafts remained viable regardless of the age or the extent of alveolar resorption in the patients. The ease of harvesting this graft in the office setting, its long-term resistance to resorption, and minimal postoperative morbidity makes the method reliable for horizontal alveolar augmentation.

The technique entails a papillae-sparing incision on both sides, exposing the buccal alveolar bone 3 mm to 5 mm apical to the mucogingival junction. The length and height of the recipient site are measured to ascertain the size of graft needed. A buccal vestibular incision is made to expose the mandibular ramus. A 1 mm to 1.2 mm fissure bur in a straight rotary instrument is recommended for outlining the osteotomy. The initial cut is made antero-posteriorly, followed by proximal and distal vertical cuts. The depth of bur penetration is limited to the buccal cortical plate. Upon completion of the cortical osteotomy, the harvest site is outlined by the blood in the cancellous portion of the bone. Five-mm thin, curved and straight osteotomes are used to separate the graft. Therefore, an absolute determination of the out-fracture pattern must be made prior to removal of the bone from the oral cavity. The atraumatic exposure of the lateral aspect of the inferior alveolar canal, exposing the nerve, does not result in neuropraxia, while the dissection of the inferior alveolar nerve trapped in the grafted bone may lead to paresthesia. The monocortical graft is adapted to the recipient site, ensuring intimate contact between the medial portion of the graft and the buccal plate. Perforation of the recipient site with a small bur to allow for revascularization of the graft is recommended.

Fixation of the bone graft to the recipient site is accomplished using self-tapping titanium mini-screws. Initial stabilization of the graft is crucial. Absolute immobilization is necessary for the complete healing of the bone graft without a fibrous component. At least two screws should be placed to eliminate micro-movement and rotation of the graft during the healing phase. Irregularities at the peripheral aspect, as well as the medial side of the graft, can be filled with any bone grafting particulated material prior to soft tissue closure. An optimal soft tissue closure of the recipient site is absolutely essential. However, the use of other areas inside the oral cavity as donor sites can give predictable results as well, and they offer less frequency of postoperative complications at the donor site area, such as the chin (See Figures 2.18A–S).

The surgical entry to access and harvest a block graft in the mandible should provide the best and allow better access with no possibility for postoperative sloughing or root injury. The preparation of the donor site influences the fate of the bone grafting procedure.

To assess the influence of bed preparation on the incorporation of autogenous bone grafts in mandibles, six dogs with three different types of receptor beds were studied. The three receptor beds were cortical, perforated, and decorticated. After 45 and 90 days, the animals were sacrificed and block sections of grafted and adjacent bone were removed. The specimens were prepared and stained with hematoxylin and eosin and Masson's trichromic. The autogenous bone grafts were integrated with the receptor bed, mainly in the perforated and decorticated groups because no connective tissue intervened in the cortical beds.

The size of the graft itself should be stable with perforated receptor sites (See Figure 2.19) (De Carvalho et al. 2000). Autogenous bone grafts are highly osteogenic and, in theory, best fulfill the requirements for bone regeneration. However, they possess some important practical shortcomings: (1) harvesting the graft requires an additional surgery, which increases the patient postoperative inconvenience; (2) another osseous defect at the donor site is created, which presents an extra risk of infection and/or morbidity; (3) extensive graft resorption can be expected, especially with iliac grafts, but less with mandibular grafts (because they are from the same embryonic origin as the recipient site); (4) only limited amounts of graft material can be harvested from the intraoral donor sites; and (5) the possibility of apical root injury (in chin grafts) or sensory nerve damage exists.

These shortcomings have led to the development and use of other readily available grafts (allografts, xenografts, and alloplasts) that can be used routinely and safely in the dental office. The use of the cortico-cancellous allograft bone blocks might offer some advantages, because harvesting of the graft from the donor site is eliminated and the patient's acceptance toward this treatment modality is better than the intraoral autogenous graft. However, allograft bone blocks are not yet solidly supported by the literature, in spite of the promising clinical success they show (See Figures 2.20A–S and 2.21A–P).

Bone interpositioning grafting techniques, which allow osseous site dilatation, may be clinically reliable when used in conjunction with the allografts or autografts harvested from the illium or any other places. The method entails the splitting of the deficient alveolar ridge and then, after osseous dilatation occurs, introducing autogenous bone in the split space. This method maintains a blood supply to both sides of the bone graft and it might not require screw retention; however, it requires an

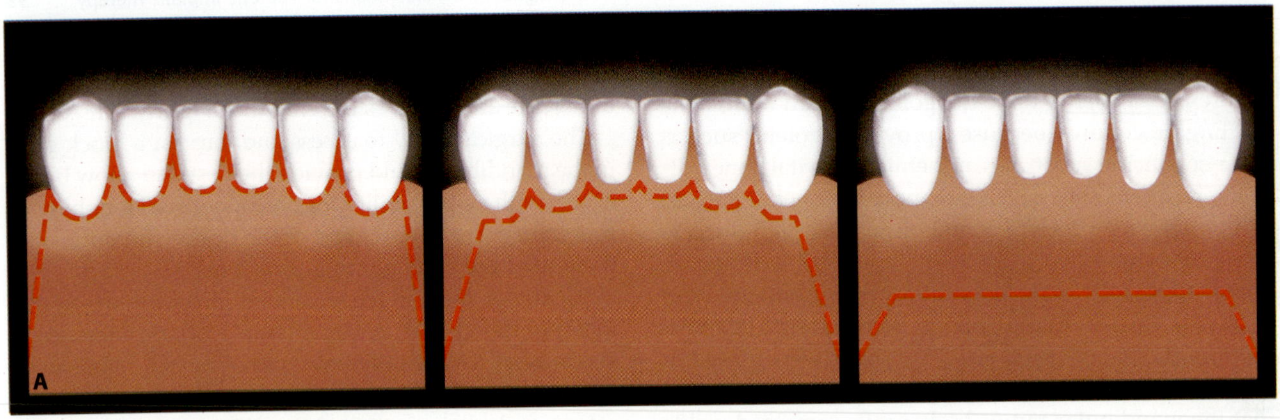

Figure 2.18A. Different incision designs for harvesting chin grafts (Marginal, Midbuccal, Vestibular).

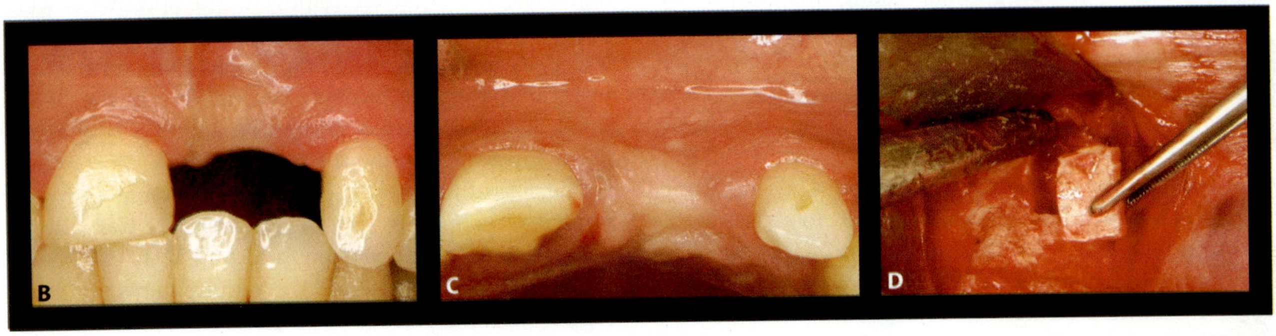

Figure 2.18. B, C. Two different intraoral views of horizontal osseous defect. D. Harvesting corticocancellous graft from the chin area.

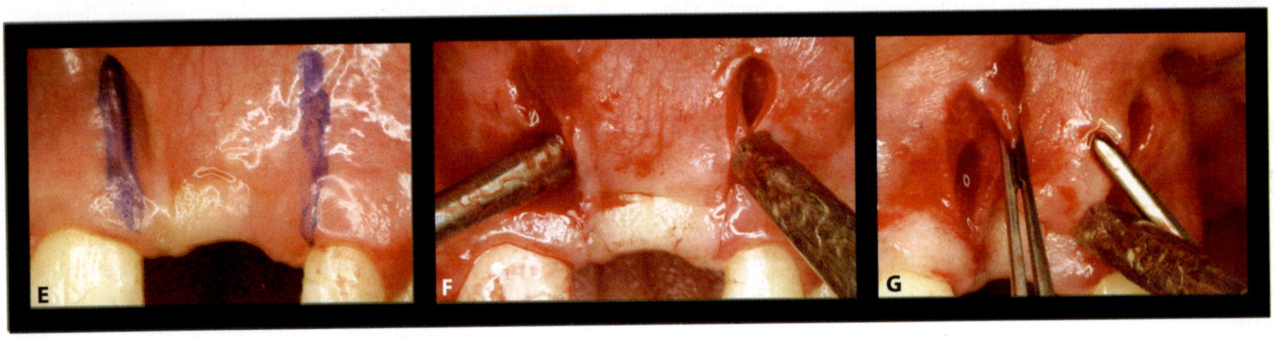

Figure 2.18. E. Incision line marked on the mucosa. Two vertical incisions with no crestal incision are allowed to allow for tunneling method. F. The start of dissecting the tunnel via periosteal elevator. G. Complete mobility of the tunnel.

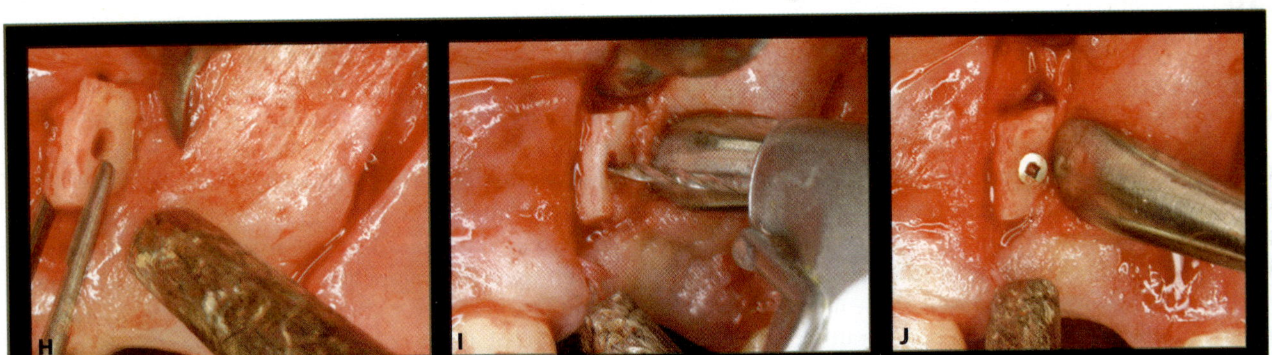

Figure 2.18. H. The graft is being introduced to the tunnel after being perforated for screw stabilization. I. The drilling procedure in the osseous bed. J. The mesial end of the graft is being stabilized with the screw.

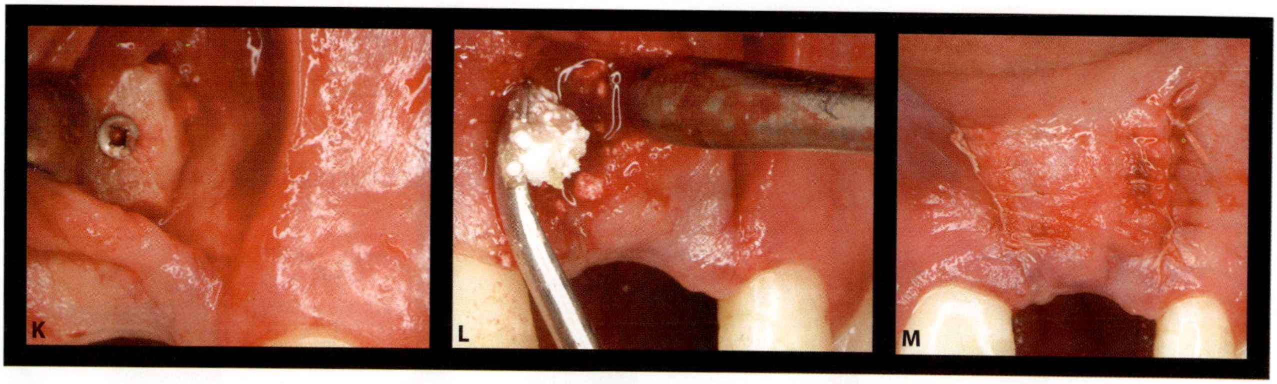

Figure 2.18. **K.** The distal end of the graft is being stabilized. **L.** The voids are being filled with particulated bone graft. **M.** The flap is sutured and closed with no tension.

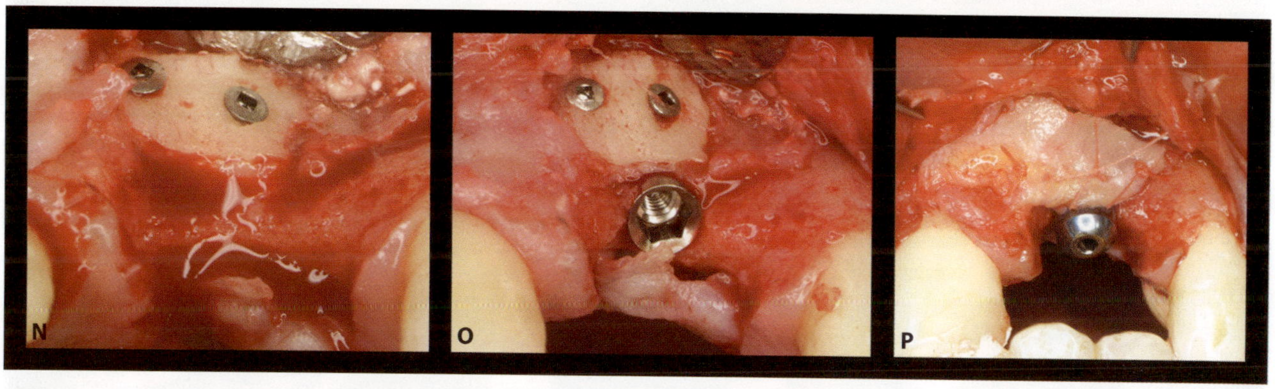

Figure 2.18. **N.** Implant installation surgery showing the amount of bone augmented. **O.** TSV implant (Zimmer Dental, Carlsbad, CA, USA) was installed. **P.** Connective tissue graft is used to profile the soft tissues.

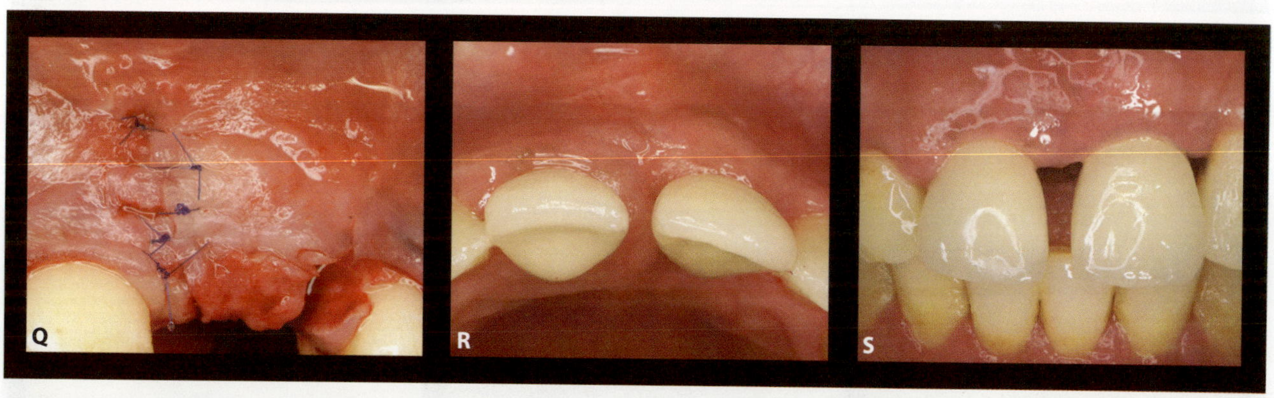

Figure 2.18. **Q.** Soft tissue closure is attempted. **R.** Incisal view postrestorative showing remarkable improvement of the labial profile. **S.** Frontal view of the case postrestorative.

optimal soft tissue closure. The preferable soft tissue closure method is the connective tissue pedicle from the palate, which does not disturb the keratinized tissue continuity in the maxilla (See Figures 2.22A–R).

Revolutionary methods of bone grafting that offer more predictable results and are less invasive will soon be introduced. Tissue engineering techniques typically entail seeding of progenitor cells on a scaffold, which mimics the tissue surrounding cells. Cells are then cultured *in vitro* so that they can proliferate and produce the phenotype of the tissue they are replacing. A number of available technologies have enhanced the feasibility of tissue engineering, including the development of matrices, which are porous, absorbable scaffolds that mimic the environment surrounding cells in the body.

Another development is the advancement of cell culture techniques that allow proliferation of cells in culture that retain their pheno-type. The availability

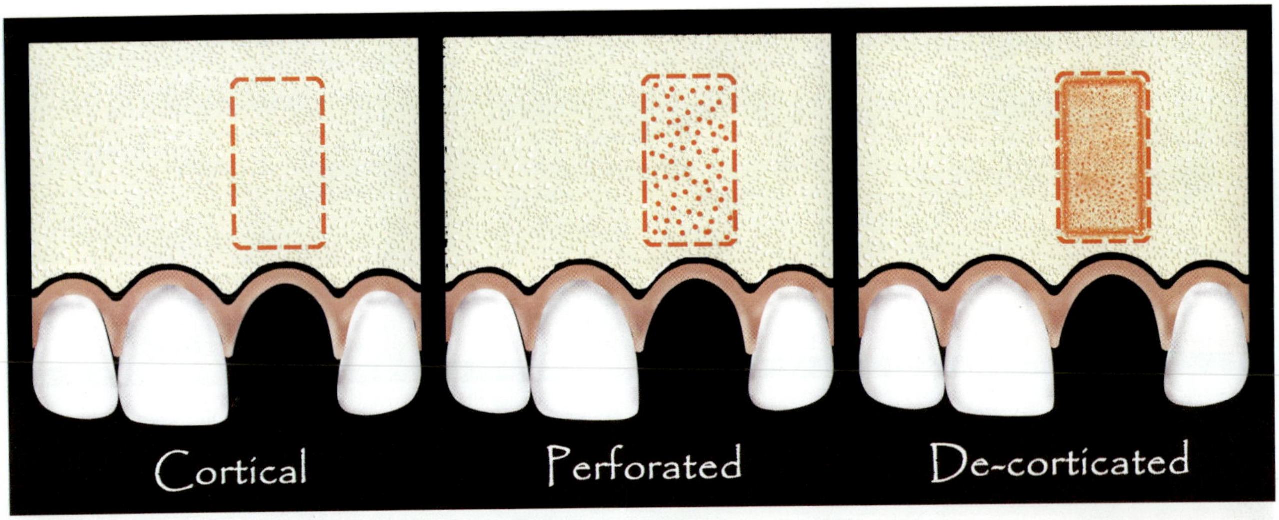

Figure 2.19. Different types of receptor bed sites: cortical, perforated, and decorticated.

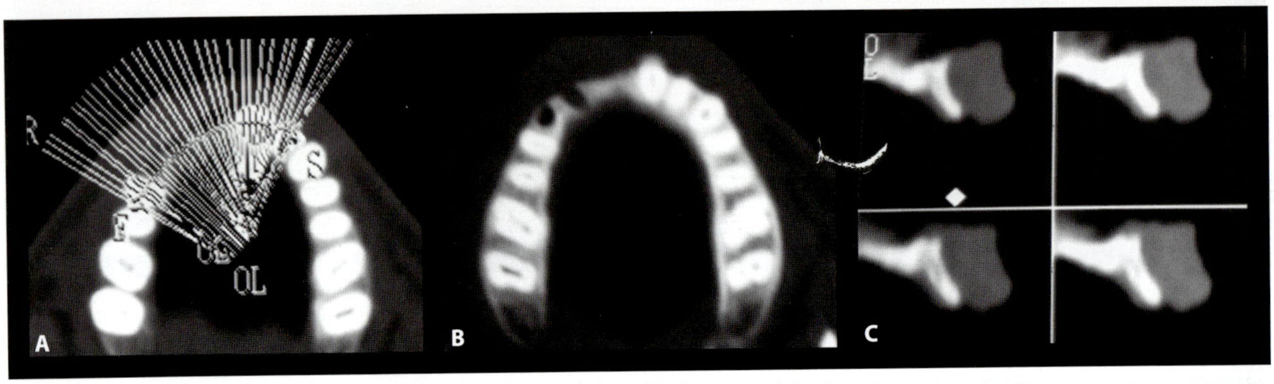

Figure 2.20. **A.** CT scan showing a defective osseous site. **B, C.** Horizontal and axial CT scan images showing the amount of osseous defect.

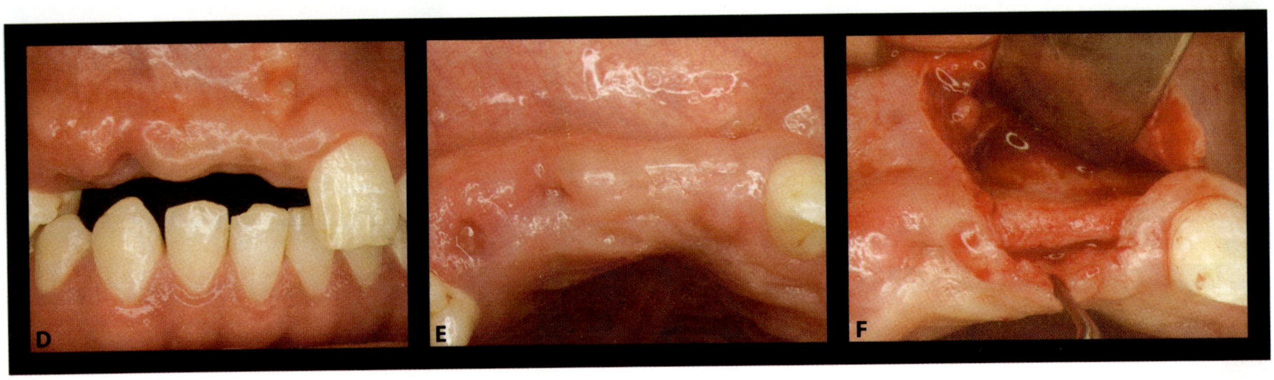

Figure 2.20. **D.** Facial view for the missing anterior teeth that shows the amount of bone loss. **E.** Incisal view of the osseous defect. **F.** The mucoperiosteal flap reflected showing severe horizontal osseous defect.

of genetically engineered growth factors is another important advancement, because growth factors are essential for regulating regeneration (Chai and Slavkin 2003). Recombinant growth factors, such as bone morphogenetic protein-2 and osteogenic protein-1, are currently in clinical use in orthopedic surgery. However, these growth factors have been used experimentally for oral reconstructive surgery.

A more recent development is the application of gene therapy to provide sustained release of these growth factors in the local environment. This is a therapeutic modality involving transfer of a specific DNA fragment

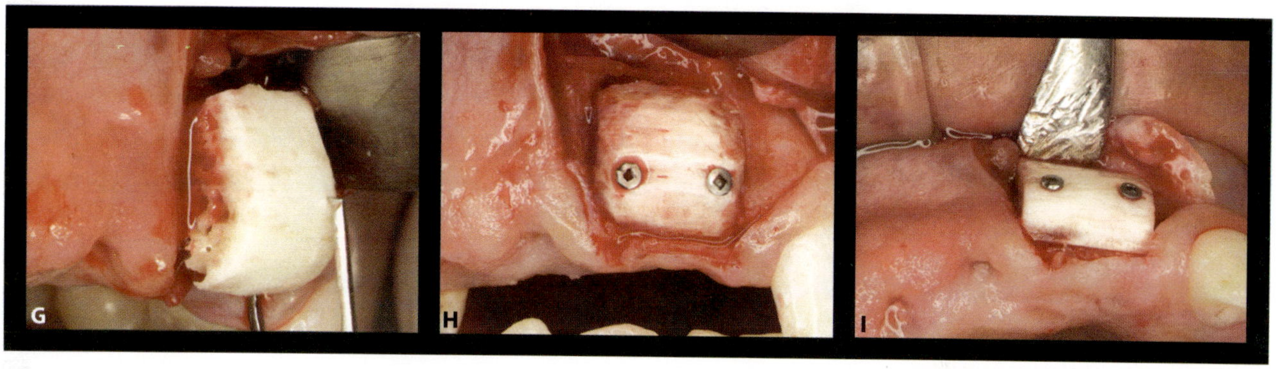

Figure 2.20. G. Allograft corticocancellous block is being fitted to the site. H. Facial view showing the block is stabilized to the osseous bed via two titanium screws. I. Incisal view showing the block is stabilized to the osseous bed.

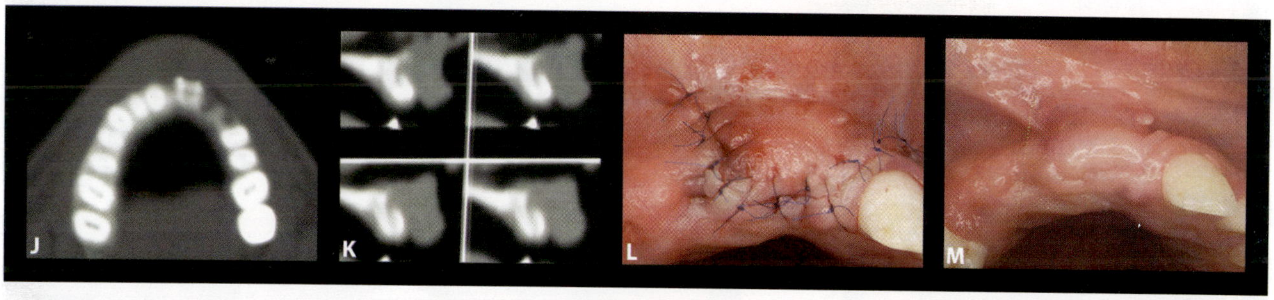

Figure 2.20. J, K. CT horizontal and axial views showing the osseous topography improvement. L. The area sutured. M. An incisal view of postgrafting tissue profile improvement.

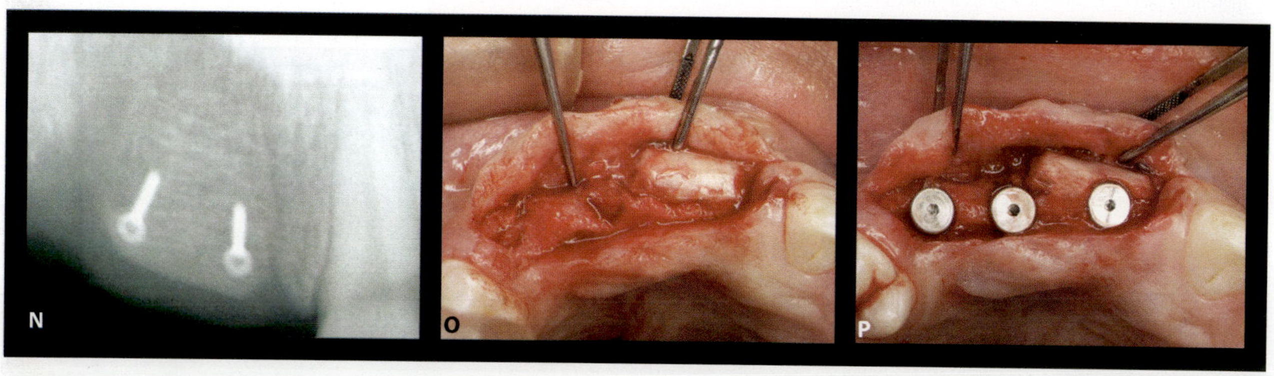

Figure 2.20. N. Radiographic view showing the block in place 5 months postgrafting. O. Surgical reentry for implant placement showing the amount of bone regenerated. P. Three implants placed.

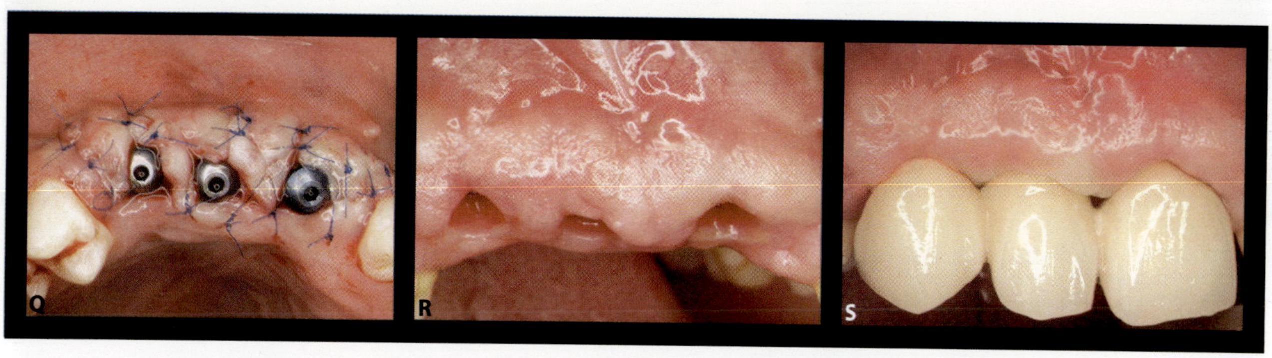

Figure 2.20. Q. Healing abutments connected and the flap sutured. R. Three weeks post soft tissue healing. S. Case finally restored.

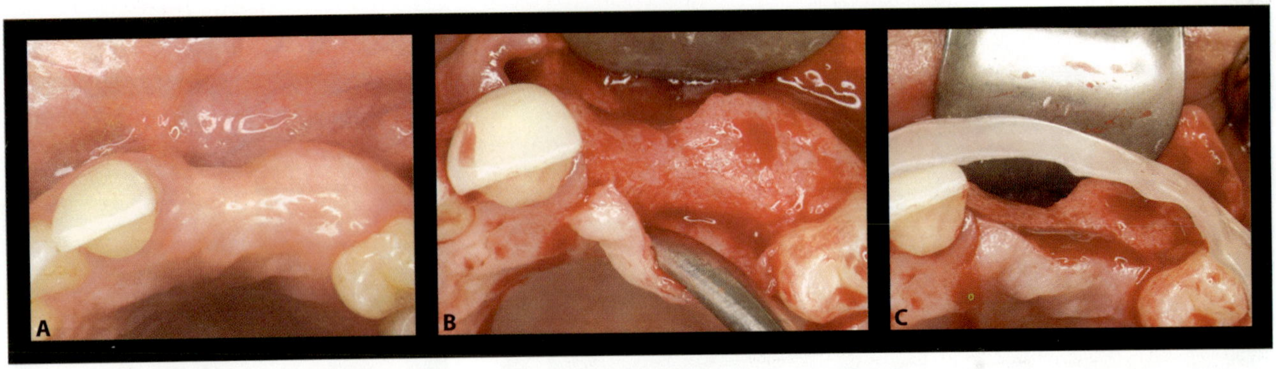

Figure 2.21. **A.** A moderate-sized horizontal osseous defect. **B.** The mucoperiosteal flap reflected and the bone defect assessed. **C.** The surgical template in place to assess the size of the osseous defect.

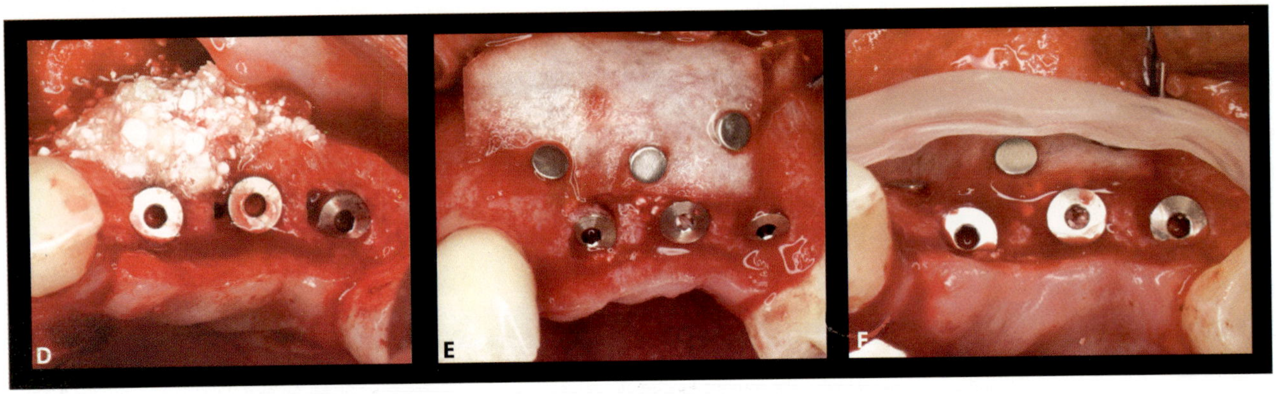

Figure 2.21. **D.** Implants were placed and the defect was filled with allograft bone substitute (Puros Allograft, Zimmer Dental, Carlsbad, CA, USA). **E.** A BioMend membrane is placed to cover the graft (Zimmer Dental, Carlsbad, CA, USA). **F.** The graft size is being rechecked.

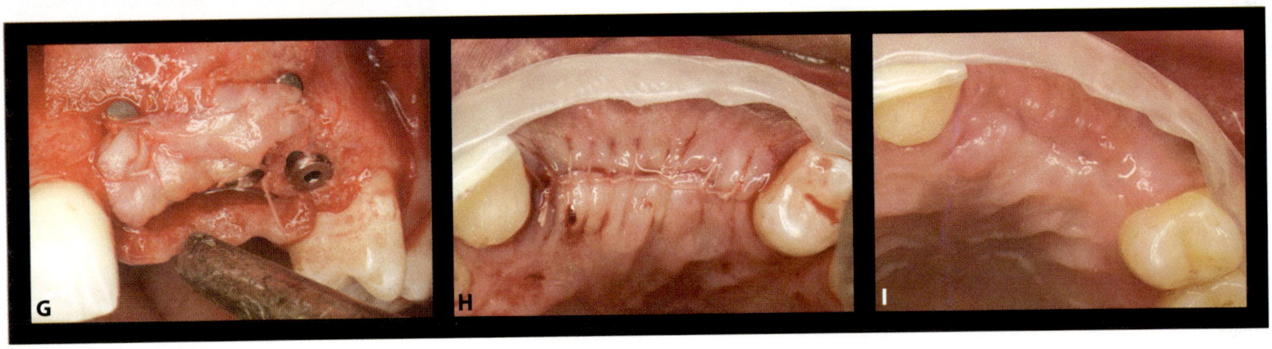

Figure 2.21. **G.** Connective tissue graft is placed on top to allow for an enhanced soft tissue profile. **H.** The flap closure achieved. **I.** Two weeks posthealing clinical picture.

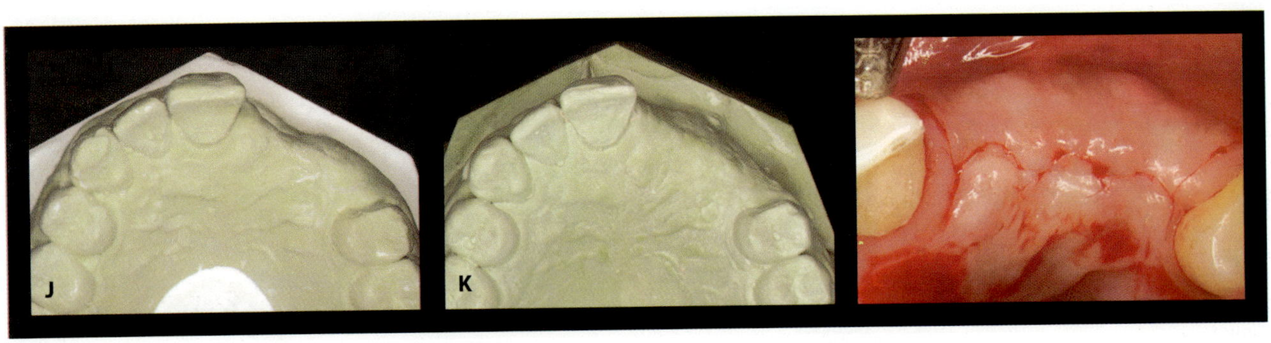

Figure 2.21. **J, K.** Pre- and postoperative bone grafting result on the study cast. **L.** Second-stage surgery incision.

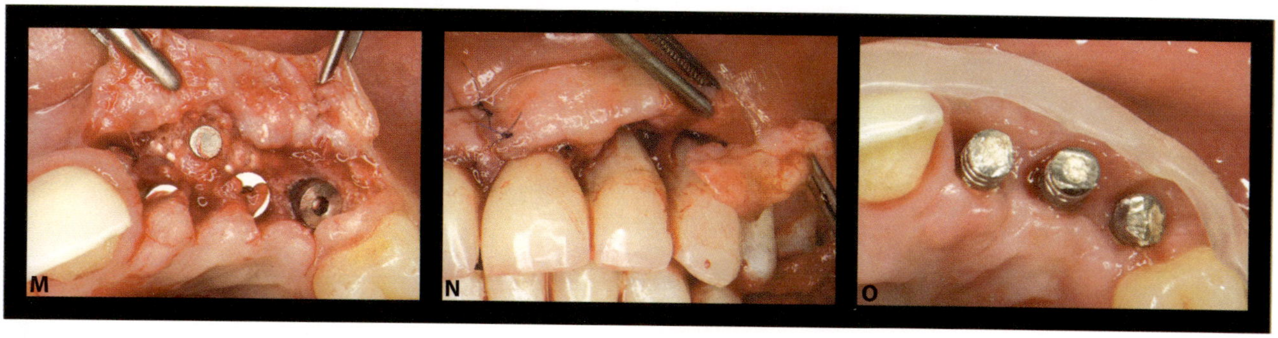

Figure 2.21. **M.** Regenerated bone at the time of the second-stage surgery. **N.** Adding a subepithelial connective tissue graft to enhance the profile and to act against tissue remodeling. **O.** Improved soft tissue topography according to the surgical template.

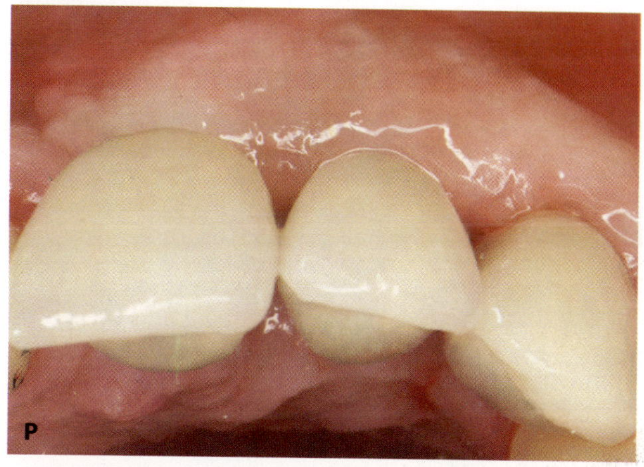

Figure 2.21. **P.** Incisal view of the final prosthesis showing optimized bone topography.

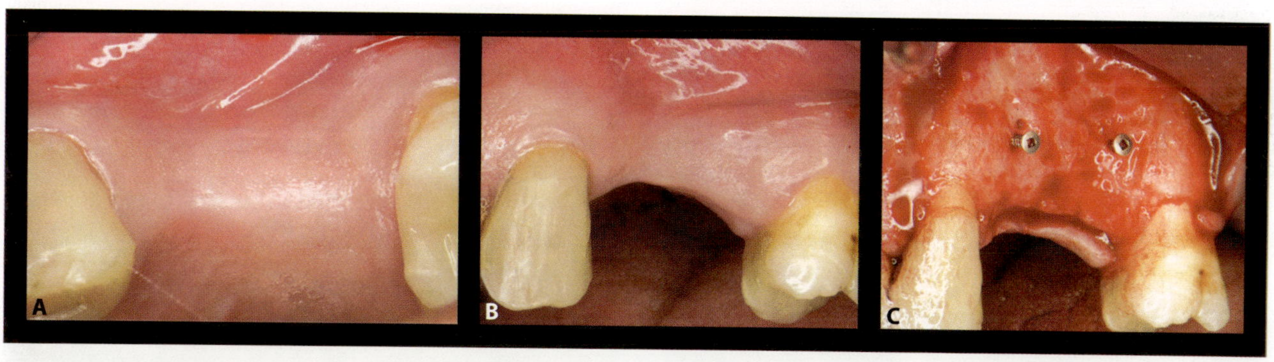

Figure 2.22. **A.** Preoperative occlusal view for postextraction 3D bone resorption. **B.** Preoperative labial view of the defect. **C.** The flap is reflected and two screws are placed as tenting pods.

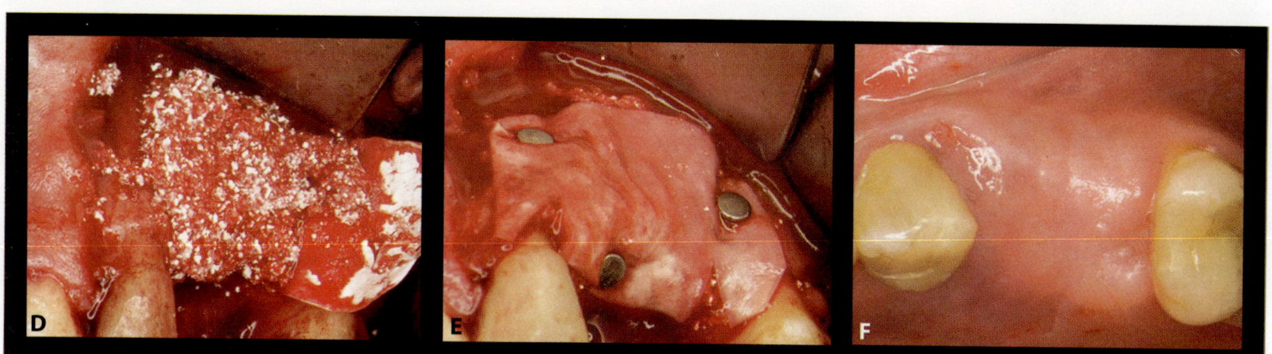

Figure 2.22. **D.** The area is filled with porous allograft (Zimmer Dental, Carlsbad, CA, USA). **E.** The area covered with resorbable collagen membrane. **F.** Post-grafting view showing the enhanced alveolar ridge profile.

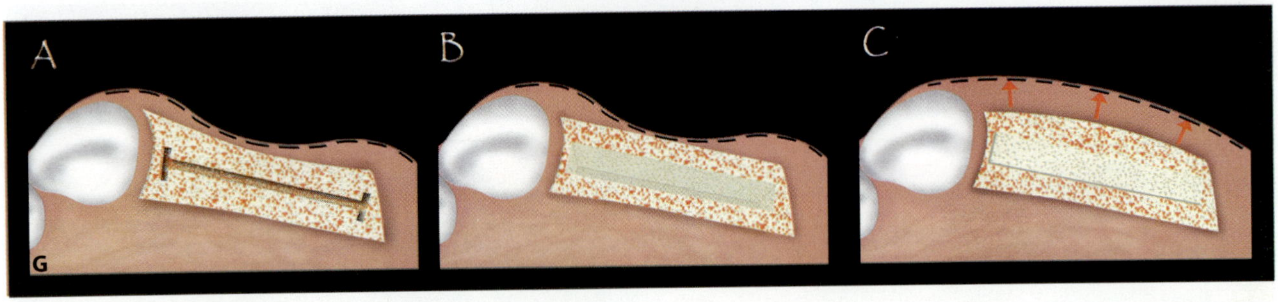

Figure 2.22G. An illustration showing the bone interpositioning grafting technique.

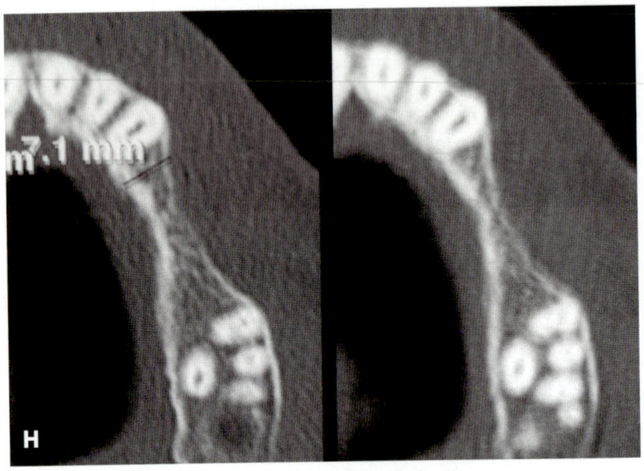

Figure 2.22H. CT radiographic view showing a remarkable alveolar ridge deficiency.

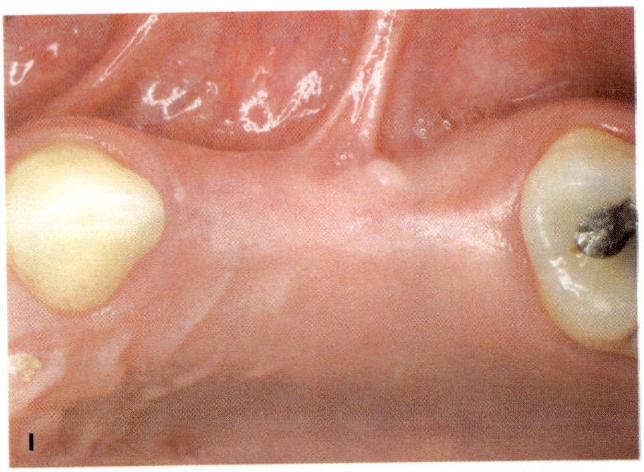

Figure 2.22I. Preoperative clinical view of the osseous defect.

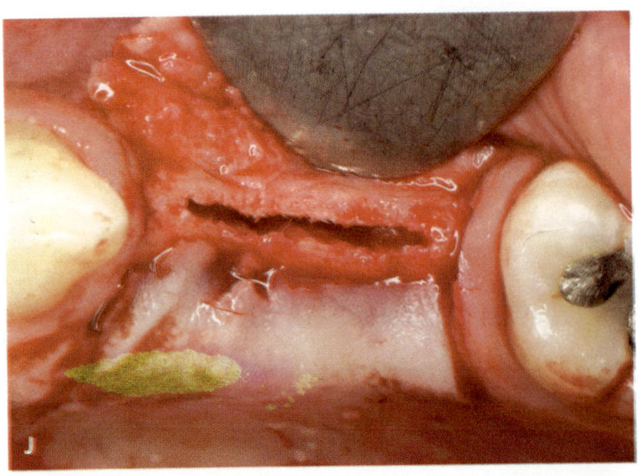

Figure 2.22J. Intra-surgical view showing the maxillary bone initial splitting.

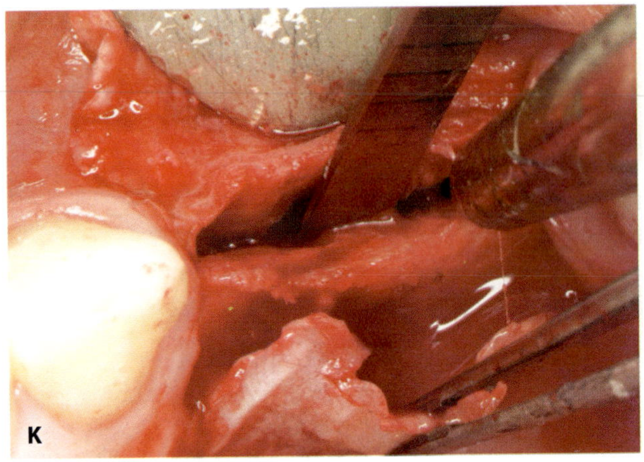

Figure 2.22K. Osseous site dilation using osteotomes and bone splitters.

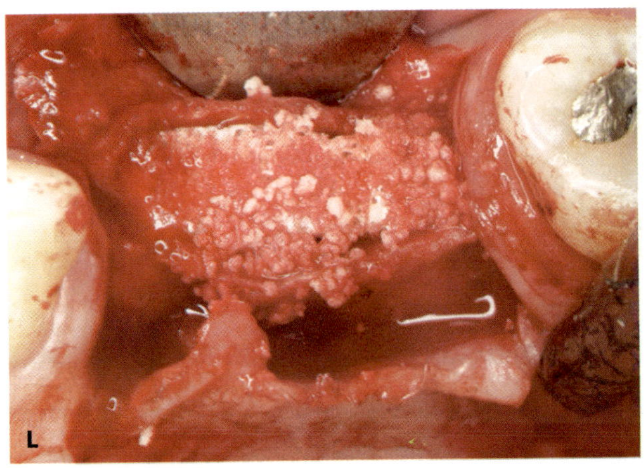

Figure 2.22L. The allograftis fully seated in place, receiving its blood supply from both sides.

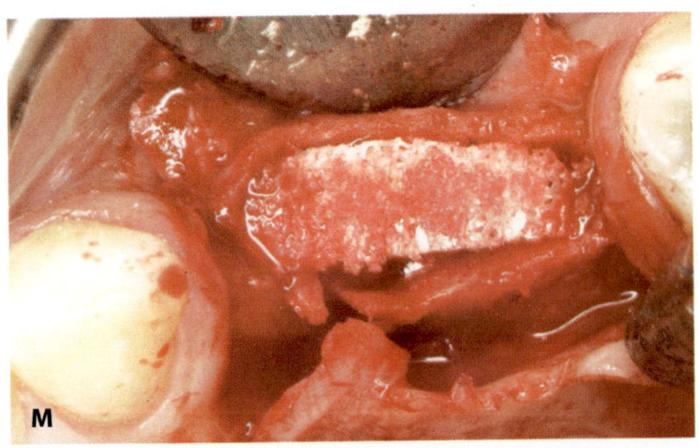

Figure 2.22M. The voids are filled with particulated bone graft material.

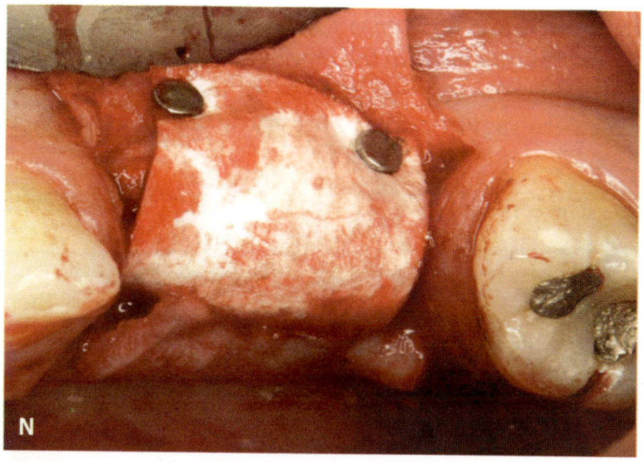

Figure 2.22N. BioMend membrane (Zimmer Dental, Carlsbad, CA, USA) is placed on top and stabilized with tacks.

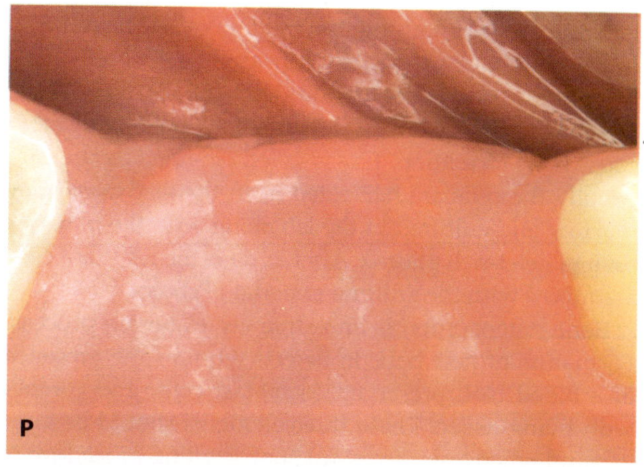

Figure 2.22P. The final tissue healing showing a remarkable improvement in the tissue buccal contour.

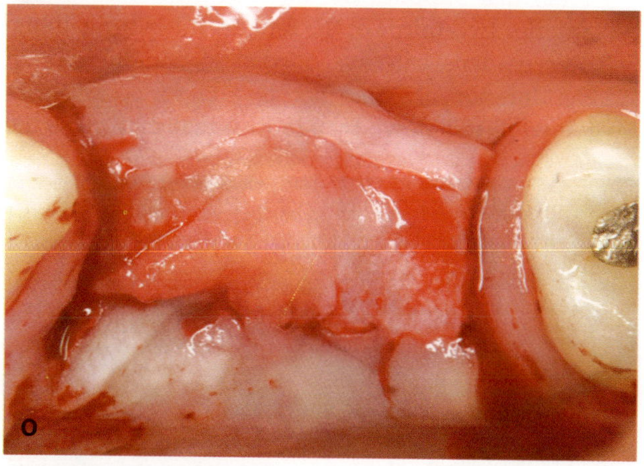

Figure 2.22O. Soft tissue approximation using connective pedicle. Note the tension-free approximation.

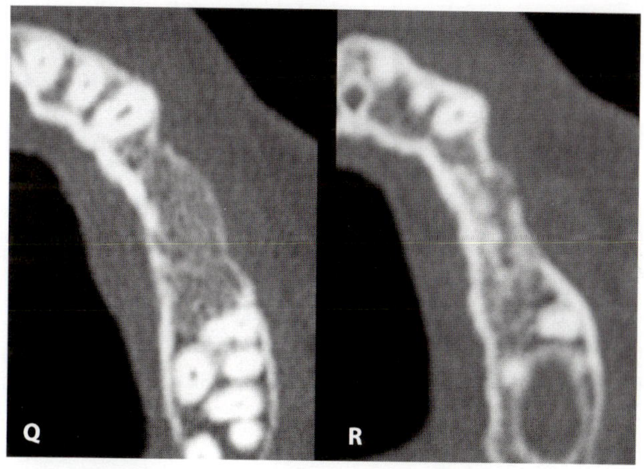

Figure 2.22Q, R. Two different CT radiographic pictures showing the improvement of the buccal bone contour.

to target cells. The application of this technology in bone regeneration is to induce a sustained release of growth factors necessary for bone regeneration (Jin et al. 2004). The DNA may either be introduced into cells directly in the patient, or the DNA may be inserted into target cells outside the patient first (*ex vivo* gene therapy), followed by transfer of cells carrying the DNA into the patient. DNA can be inserted into cells by the aid of viruses or other nonviral means such as liposomes (lipid spheres).

A laboratory breakthrough has occurred on the implant surface characteristics that have been shown to modify cell behavior and regulate integrin expression and resulting integrin-mediated cellular activity that are essential components for tissue healing and homeostasis. A study that evaluated the influence of titanium surface roughness on integrin expression and cell morphology has used human gingival fibroblasts cultured on smooth (polished) and rough (sand-blasted acid-etched) titanium surfaces and a cell culture plastic (control) surface (Oates et al. 2005). A total ribonucleic acid (RNA) was isolated from experimental and control cells, and levels of integrin subunit messenger RNA (mRNA) were assessed by reverse transcription-polymerase chain reaction. The products were analyzed by polyacrylamide gel electrophoresis, confirmed via DNA sequencing, and quantified using computer-assisted densitometry. The expression of the integrin subunits was analyzed at the protein level using flow cytometry.

The results demonstrate the presence of multiple integrin subunits in human gingival fibroblasts grown in contact with titanium implant surfaces and show that titanium surface roughness alters cellular morphology but appears to have limited effects on integrin expression. The study provides insight into the complicated cellular and molecular events occurring at the implant surface that may be critical to optimizing the soft tissue interactions with the soft tissue-implant interface. The future of intraoral bone grafting seems very promising. Currently work is proceeding to allow the stromal stem cells to be cultured in the laboratory to expand an autogenous osteoblast lineage in a four-week period (Ueda et al. 2005). These cells, when injected into bone defects, will predictably cause bone formation. This is called *cell-based therapy* and usually the cells are harvested from the iliac crest bone marrow and cultured in the lab along with the patient's own platelet-rich plasma. After 28 days the resultant cells are mixed with the grafting material of choice.

Bone regeneration is an extremely elaborate process. Formation of new bone in defects requires the presence of a blood clot, preserved osteoblast cells, and contact with living tissue. These three elements should be kept in mind when any successful bone grafting procedure is to be achieved.

The optimization of the remaining osseous topography is considered to be an important factor to the long-term success of dental implant supported prostheses on both the functional or esthetic levels. Today's practitioner has a wide array of grafting materials available that can be used in several clinical applications. The use of these materials has widened the scope and expectations for implant surgery tremendously. Research and clinical experience have shown that certain materials are better suited for specific applications than others and that some are much easier to handle than others. Keeping this in mind, the clinician must give priority to thorough presurgical planning and considering the least invasive procedures to attain the most predictable results.

Anatomical Considerations

Before beginning any implant surgery, one should be fully aware of the anatomical landmarks that are related to the site of the surgery. Complete awareness of the anatomical landmarks could rescue the patient from postsurgical complications as a result of an anatomical structure injury. The anatomical structures related to the jaws include arteries, venus plexuses, nerves, muscle attachments, and air spaces.

The mandibular anatomical structures that should be well identified include some important muscles such as the mylohyoid muscle, which constitutes the mouth floor. It originates from the medial aspect of the mandible and inserts mainly into the hyoid bone. The genioglossus muscle originates from the mandibular genial tubercles and inserts anteriorly in the dorsum of the tongue and posteriorly in the hyoid bone. The buccenator muscle, which forms the sides of the cheek's body along with the buccal pad of fat, originates from the alveolar bone of the mandible and maxilla posteriorly and is fused along with the fibers of the orbicularis oris muscle. Lateral and medial pterygoid, masseter, and temporalis muscles also have a great role in mastication and the opening and closing mechanisms of the mouth (Sharawy 1990).

The important nerves that are of interest to the clinician performing implant therapy in the mandible are (See Figures 2.23 and 2.24):

- The inferior alveolar nerve (n. alveolaris inferior) is the largest branch of the mandibular nerve. It descends along with the inferior alveolar artery, at first beneath the pterygoideus externus, and then between the sphenomandibular ligament and the ramus of the mandible to the mandibular foramen. It then passes forward in the mandibular canal, beneath the teeth, as far as the mental foramen, and then divides into the mental and incisive nerves.
- The lingual nerve (n. lingualis) is a branch of the mandibular nerve in infratemporal fossa (DuBrul 1982) that supplies the mucous membrane of the anterior two-thirds of the tongue. It lies beneath the pterygoideus externus, medial to and in front of the inferior alveolar nerve, and is occasionally joined to this nerve by a branch that may cross the

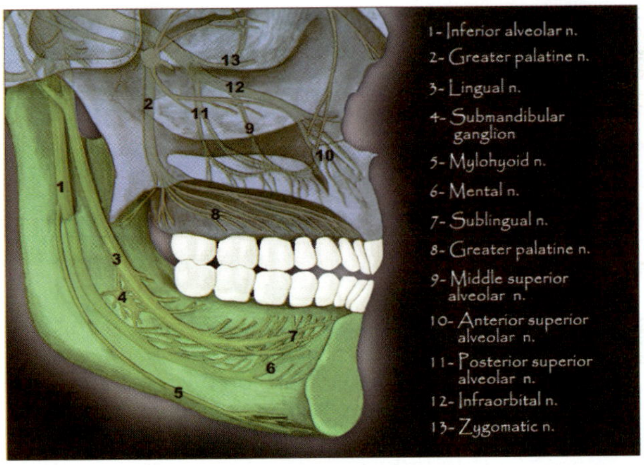

Figure 2.23. Innervation of the mandible and maxilla.

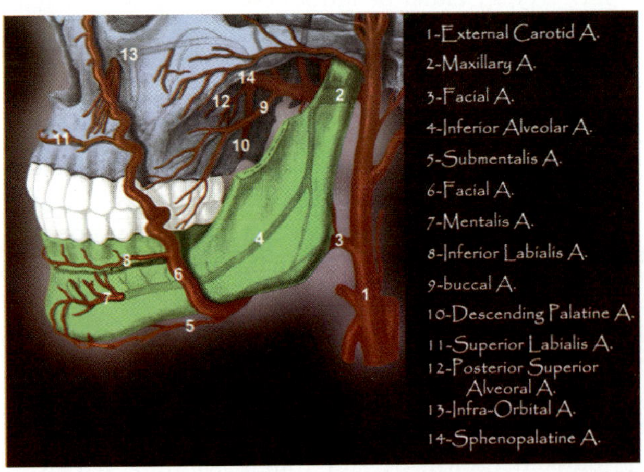

Figure 2.24. Arterial supply of the mandible and maxilla.

internal maxillary artery, which can be easily injured when working closely opposite to the second and third mandibular molars. It passes downward and forward between the ramus of the mandible and medial pterygoid muscle. It enters the oral cavity above the posterior edge of the mylohyoid muscle close to its origin at the third molar area.

- The masseteric nerve (n. massetericus) passes laterally, above the pterygoideus externus, in front of the temporomandibular articulation, and behind the tendon of the temporalis muscle. It crosses the mandibular notch with the masseteric artery to the deep surface of the masseter muscle, in which it ramifies nearly as far as its anterior border. It gives a filament to the temporomandibular joint.
- The buccinator nerve (n. buccinatorus, long buccal nerve) passes forward between the two heads of the pterygoideus externus, and downward beneath or through the lower part of the temporalis. It emerges from under the anterior border of the masseter, ramifies on the surface of the buccinator, and unites with the buccal branches of the facial nerve. It supplies a branch to the pterygoideus externus during its passage through that muscle, and may give off the anterior deep temporal nerve (Perlnt 1949).
- The mylohyoid nerve (n. mylohyoideus) is derived from the inferior alveolar nerve just before it enters the mandibular foramen. It descends in a groove on the deep surface of the ramus of the mandible, and reaches the under surface of the mylohyoid muscle and supplies the anterior belly of the digastricus.
- The m ental nerve (n. mentalis) emerges at the mental foramen and divides beneath the triangularis muscle into three branches: one descends to the skin of the chin and two ascend to the skin and mucous membrane of the lower lip. These branches communicate freely with the facial nerve (Williams and Warwick 1980).

The salivary glands are important structures related to the mandible. The parotid gland lies just anterior to the ear. The superficial lobe lies over the ramus of the mandible, and the gland curves around behind the mandible to form the deep lobe. The gland lies within the superficial fascia of the neck and is completely invested in this connective tissue. The parotid duct leaves the anterior border of the gland to pass over the buccinator muscle and pierce the cheek opposite the second upper molar tooth. The duct may have some associated accessory glandular tissue. The submandibular gland lies just under the middle of the body of the mandible. The gland lies on the outer surface of the omohyoid muscle and curves around the free border of that muscle posteriorly to lie in the floor of the mouth. The duct runs along the floor of the mouth to open on the floor on either side of the frenulum of the tongue. The superficial part of the gland is closely related to the facial artery before it passes upward over the mandible. The sublingual salivary glands lie below the tongue and open through several ducts into the floor of the mouth (See Figure 2.25).

The arterial supply of the mandible includes important arteries such as the lingual artery. It arches superanteriorly, about 5 mm superior to the tip of the greater horn of the hyoid bone, and then passes deep to the hypoglossal nerve, the stylohyoid muscle, and the posterior belly of digastricus muscle. At the anterior border of this muscle, it turns superiorly and ends by becoming the deep lingual artery. The facial artery, which has a strong link to the mandible, passes superiorly under the cover of the digastricus and stylohyoid muscles and the angle of the mandible. It loops anteriorly and enters a deep groove in the submandibular gland. The facial artery hooks around the inferior border of the mandible and enters the face. Here the pulsation of this artery can be felt (anterior to the masseter muscle).

While the major venous drainage of the mandible mainly involves only two major veins, the external jugular vein and the pterygoid plexus of veins that corresponds to all branches of the maxillary artery drain into the pterygoid plexus of veins situated between the temporalis and lateral pterygoid muscles. Because the plexus communicates with the cavernous sinus through the inferior ophthalmic vein, any orodental infection can spread from the deep facial and alveolar regions to the cavernous sinus, where infection can be fatal.

The maxilla has close muscle attachments to the buccinator, levator anguli oris muscles (caninus). The maxilla has several important anatomical structures. The most important maxillary anatomical structure to dental implantology is probably the maxillary sinus. The adult maxillary sinus is pyramidal-like in shape and has a

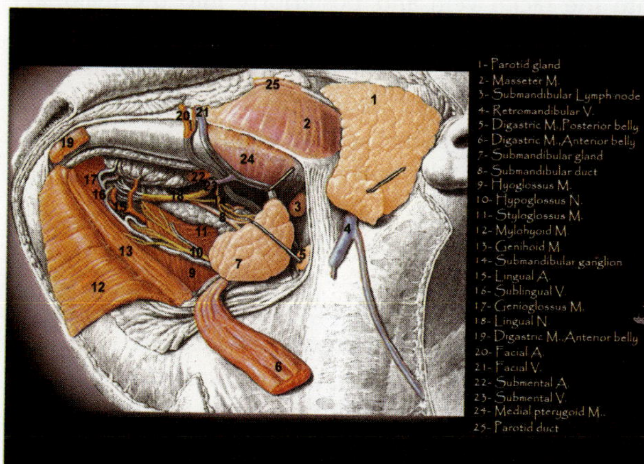

Figure 2.25. The anatomy of the floor of the mouth.

volume of approximately 15 mL (34 × 33 × 23 mm). The base of the pyramid is the nasal wall with the peak pointing toward the zygomatic process. The anterior wall has the infraorbital foramen located at the midsuperior portion, with the infraorbital nerve running over the roof of the sinus and exiting through the foramen. The thinnest portion of the anterior wall is just above the canine tooth—the canine fossa. The roof is formed by the orbital floor and transected by the course of the infraorbital nerve. Behind the posterior wall are the pterygomaxillary fossa, the internal maxillary artery, sphenopalatine ganglion, the vidian canal, the greater palatine nerve, and the foramen rotundum. The floor, as discussed above, varies in its level. From birth to age nine, the floor of the sinus is above that of the nasal cavity. At age nine, the floor is generally at the level of the nasal floor. The greater palatine nerve and the branches of the infraorbital nerve are responsible for the innervations of the maxillary sinus. The sinus arterial supply is from the infraorbital, lateral branches of the sphenopalatine, greater palatine, and the alveolar arteries.

The posterior superior lateral nasal artery is relatively close to the sphenopalatine artery and may anastomose with the facial or other nasal arteries. It can course intraosseously in the medial wall of the sinus. This effect presents the theoretical potential for a significant bleeding complication during lateral approach sinus elevation surgery. Given that the posterior lateral nasal artery or its branches can be intraosseous, it may be possible to sever this artery or a branch during elevation of the sinus lining at the medial posterior wall by vigorous curettage of the thin bone. Bleeding from this artery may be controlled with electrosurgery or an endoscopic ligation of the artery or the sphenopalatine artery. Endoscopic ligation by an appropriately trained surgeon may be indicated. Elevation of the head can decrease nasal blood flow. In-office electrocautery may be the most effective method of controlling the bleeding of a small arteriole (Flanagan 2005).

Venous drainage of the maxillary sinus runs anteriorly into the facial vein and posteriorly into the maxillary vein and jugular veins. The innervation of the maxilla involves the maxillary nerve and its branches, the meningeal and ganglionic branches, the zygomatic nerves, and the superior alveolar nerves, which are divided into the following:

1. The posterior superior alveolar nerve arises from the maxillary nerve while it is still in the pterygopalatine fossa. It passes along the posterolateral surface of the maxilla, the region associated with the infratemporal fossa. It then passes into the bone and supplies the maxillary sinus. It divides into several small branches that are intermingled and attached to each other to form the superior dental plexus. It supplies the molar teeth and the adjacent gums and cheek.
2. The middle superior alveolar nerve arises from the infraorbital nerve and runs downward and forward in the lateral wall of the maxillary sinus. It terminates as several small branches that communicate with the dental plexus. It supplies the premolars in the maxilla. Sometimes this nerve is absent.
3. The anterior superior alveolar nerve arises from the lateral aspect of the infraorbital nerve in the canal and descends in its own canal in the anterior wall of the maxillary sinus. It divides into several branches that supply the incisor and canine teeth. It takes part in formation of the dental plexus and also gives a small nasal branch that supplies part of the lateral wall of the nasal cavity below the entrance of the maxillary sinus. The infraorbital nerve is the continuation of the main trunk of the maxillary division. It exits the orbit through the infraorbital foramen.

The greater palatine nerve enters the oral cavity through the greater palatine foramen. It runs forward in grooves in the inferior surface of the hard palate together with its artery and vein to supply palatal mucosa up to incisor teeth. As the maxilla atrophies, it shifts to the palate and crest of the ridge. The nasopalatine nerve enters the oral cavity through the nasopalatine canal and exits through the incisive foramen. It must be anaesthetized before elevation of the mucosa of the floor of the nose for subnasal grafts or implants that engage the nasal floor. The maxilla gets its arterial supply mainly from the branches of the third part of the maxillary artery. These arterial branches are:

1. The posterior superior alveolar artery descends downward and forward giving numerous branches that enter through the posterolateral aspect of the maxilla to become intraosseous branches that supply the molar and premolar teeth. Other branches supply gingival of teeth.
2. The infraorbital artery passes forward through the inferior orbital fissure and appears at the face at the infraorbital foramen, and through the infraorbital canal to form (a) the anterior superior alveolar artery that supplies the anterior maxillary teeth and mucous membrane of maxilla and (b) the middle superior alveolar artery, which is usually absent. Both anterior and posterior alveolar arteries join to form the arterial loop.
3. The greater palatine artery descends from the greater palatine canal and opens on the side of the hard palate in the greater palatine foramen. As it descends, it forms the lesser palatine arteries, which supply the soft palate, that exit from the lesser palatine foramina. The soft palate is also supplied by the ascending pharyngeal artery from the facial artery and palatine branches of the ascending pharyngeal artery. Part of the mucoperiosteum of

the anterior maxilla is supplied by the superior labial artery, which is a branch of the facial artery. The venous drainage of the maxilla drains in to the retromandibular vein and the pterygoid venous plexus.

Peri-implant Soft Tissue Optimization

Establishing healthy esthetic gingival appearance around dental implant-supported restorations requires a meticulous assessment of any gingival or periodontal defects, and subsequently has the capacity for restoring any existing defect. Esthetic gingival and periodontal defects can be addressed during the preoperative clinical examination of implant candidates.

Examples of gingival and periodontal defects or discrepancies prior to implant therapy are plenty, including loss of attachment levels, loss of the keratinized mucosa, asymmetrical or unbalanced adjacent gingival contours, localized reduction of tissue volume, absent or blunting of the interproximal papillae, and all known types of gingival recession. The unoptimized soft tissue quality or quantity may arise due to many factors, including aggressive tooth brushing (Flanagan 2005), smoking habits (Robertson et al. 1990), plaque accumulation (Kennedy et al. 1985), and tissue injuries due to trauma. If any of these previous factors exist at the time of clinical evaluation, the factors should be eliminated and corrected prior to selecting any clinical approach for dental implant therapy.

Esthetics in the anterior region relies heavily on the very existence of healthy keratinized gingival margins. This fact applies to both natural dentition and implant-supported restorations (Berglundh and Lindhe 1996); it also facilitates long-term maintenance of implant-supported restorations. This should be established during the clinical examination at the presurgical stage. The gingival form and color should also be evaluated along the course of the presurgical phase.

It is valuable to detect the gingival hyperpigmentation, because it can be detrimental to the overall treatment result. Oral pigmentation is most commonly physiologic in nature; however, nonphysiologic pigmentations may be encountered. Physiologic pigmentation results primarily from melanin produced by melanocytes present with the stratum basale of the oral epithelium and is typically more generalized than its nonphysiologic counterparts. The etiology of these pigmentations may be hereditary, due to pregnancy, or medication-induced. Nonphysiologic pigmentations may be pathologic or nonpathologic. Examples of localized pathologic pigmented lesions include hemangiomas, Kaposi's sarcoma, and melanoma, among others. Pathologic pigmented lesions may also be generalized when associated with systemic conditions such as Addison's disease, PeutzJeghers syndrome, neurofibromatosis, or heavy metal ingestion. Localized, nonphysiologic pigmentations are typically due to implanted material within the oral mucosa resulting in a clinically evident discoloration. The exogenous pigments may include carbon, iron dust, metallic silver (amalgam tattoos), or graphite (Phillips and John 2005).

The existence of pigmented gingival tissues warrants exercising care to avoid scar tissue formation, which would contribute negatively to the esthetic result, especially in high smile line patients. The continuity of the keratinized band should be preserved using less invasive therapeutic techniques, such as flapless surgical entries (See Figure 2.26A). Gingival components that contribute to an esthetically pleasing implant-supported restoration are the marginal radicular form, the interdental tissues status, and the color and texture of healthy keratinized tissues (Tarnow and Eskow 1995a).

The original width of attached gingiva in the maxillary anterior area can vary widely from approximately 2 mm to 8 mm. The labiolingual dimension of gingival tissue is approximately 1.5 mm at the base of the gingival sulcus (Goaslind et al. 1977). The literature makes no conclusions about the amount of soft tissue that is needed to achieve predictable implant esthetics and function; some states that neither the absence of inflamed soft tissue nor a specific amount of keratinized mucosa is required to ensure a successful osseointegration (Adell et al. 1981). On the contrary, some authors have confirmed that the absence of a keratinized mucosa might jeopardize implant survival (Cox and Zarb 1987, Zarb and Schmitt 1990). In addition, some authors have stated that a minimum of 2 mm of keratinized tissue width is needed to achieve optimal health of the tissues surrounding natural dentition (Lang and Lǫ 1972, Dorfman et al. 1980) while others have suggested that

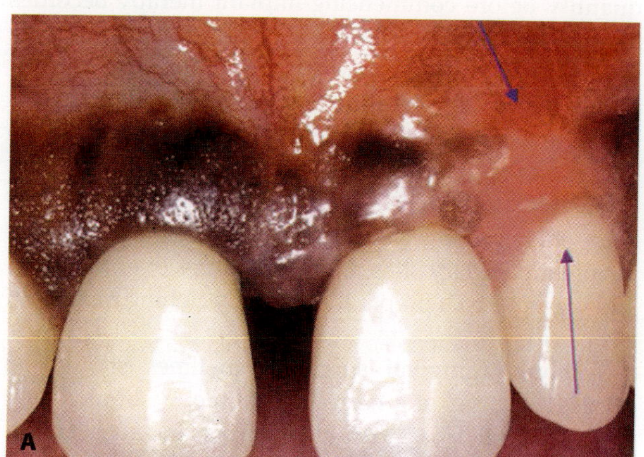

Figure 2.26A. An intraoral view showing scar tissue opposite to the upper left lateral incisor that leads to discontinuity of the keratinized band in pigmented gingiva.

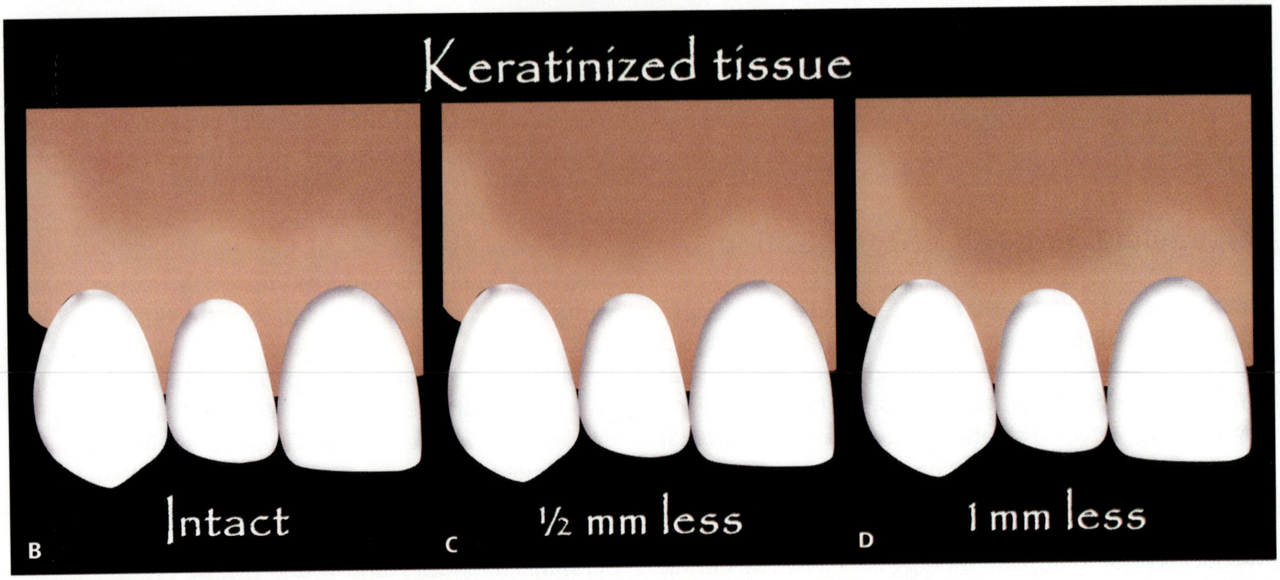

Figure 2.26B, C, D. The clinical assessment parameters for the available keratinized tissues.

less than 1 mm of keratinized tissue can be adequate, provided the bacterial plaque is well controlled (See Figures 2.26B–D) (Stetler and Bissada 1987).

Generally and logically speaking, the presence of a sufficient band of keratinized mucosa will surely improve the esthetic outcome of the definitive implant-supported restoration. The presence of the keratinized band can also minimize postoperative gingival recession, endure the trauma of brushing, resist muscle pull, and reduce the probability of soft tissue dehiscence above implant fixtures. Because soft tissues have the tendency to recede almost 1 mm after surgical and restorative implant procedures (Bengazi et al. 1996), a sufficient amount of healthy keratinized gingival tissue band should exist prior to implant placement for compensation. Therefore, optimizing the soft tissue quality and quantity before commencing implant therapy becomes a vital prerequisite.

Diagnosing the type and the reason for intraoral soft tissue defects, as well as setting the proper treatment, is valuable to implantology success. One of the methods to enhance the soft tissue condition is the free gingival graft or onlay graft because it offers great predictability. It has been enhanced by using thicker grafts, butt joints on recipient papillary sites, mattress sutures over the graft, and vigorous root preparation, and by etching roots with citric acid.

Vestibular gingival surgery sometimes should be selected in cases of a narrow vestibule; vestibuloplasty is probably the best treatment option for such conditions. Care must be exercised not to displace the tissue to its original position due to the action of the related muscles. Recently, connective tissue grafts have attained great popularity in implant dentistry. This offers fair improvement of deficient soft tissue volume and profile. Apical and coronal repositioning surgeries either used alone or in combination with other surgeries offer great clinical predictability whenever the biological width is preserved at its normal known limits.

There is a strong relationship between periodontal disease and implant dentistry. The development or pre-existence of any periodontopathic condition can disrupt the clinician's ability to recreate long-term successful implant therapy. This is especially critical in the maxillary anterior region, where the soft tissue is complex and its relationship to the implant restoration and adjacent dentition often determines the implant's success. This also influences the treatment planning to a great extent. Any existing periodontal condition should be well assessed, diagnosed, and treated prior to implant therapy.

A study by Gouvoussis and others (1995) suggested that transmission of periodontopathic organisms from periodontitis sites to implant sites in the same mouth is likely. It calls to the clinician's attention the potential of cross infection from periodontitis sites to implant sites. This was confirmed by the results of cross-sectional microbiologic studies of failing implant sites. The data suggested similar microbial profiles between these sites and those of periodontitis pockets (Becker et al. 1990). This study offered a strong link between a periodontally involved patient and dental implant failure, which is evidenced with the findings that there is an increase of the gram negative anaerobic flora with high levels of spirochetes associated with failing implants (Rosenberg et al. 1991). These studies support the concept that microbiota associated with stable and failing implants are similar to the microbiota of periodontally healthy and diseased teeth, respectively.

In an interesting confirmation of the previous conclusion, Sanz and others (1991) reported elevated levels of polymorphonuclear neutrophils (PMN) associated with disease progression around dental implants, and Kao and others (1995) found gingival crevicular fluid IL-1B levels of diseased implants to be elevated threefold as compared to clinically healthy sites. These findings are similar to those of a study that evaluated periodontal degeneration around natural teeth that is caused by the inflammatory mediators such as PGE_2, IL-1B, and possibly IL-6 produced by the chronic inflammatory cells of the periodontal tissues and that initiate pathways that stimulate osteoclastic bone resorption, which indicates the similarity in the inflammatory response (Genco 1992). These studies all indicate that the need for a clinical protocol that includes the elimination of periodontal disease prior to implant placement is mandatory.

Soft Tissue Biocharacterization and Influence

The composition and structure of the periodontium influence the implant prognosis from the esthetic and functional aspects. Distinguishing and identifying the periodontal biotypes is critical to the treatment plan and the proper selection of the surgical approach. Identifying the patient biotype not only influences the surgical technique but also the fate of the implantology procedure.

Healthy human periodontium is comprised of radicular cementum, periodontal ligament, gingival bone, and investing alveolar bone (Glickman 1972). It can also be divided into the gingival unit and the attachment apparatus. The gingival unit consists of the free gingival, attached gingival, and alveolar mucosa. This gingival unit has a lining epithelium of either masticatory mucosa, which is thick keratinized epithelium with a dense collagenous connective tissue corium, or lining mucosa, which is thin, nonkeratinized epithelium with a loose connective tissue corium containing elastic fibers. Masticatory mucosa is found in the free and attached gingival, hard palate, and dorsum of the tongue, and lining mucosa is found everywhere else in the oral cavity. Briefly, the free gingiva is that part of the gingiva located above the base of the gingival sulcus. It usually measures less than 3 mm in height. The alveolar mucosa is reddish in color because of the thin nature of the epithelium overlying the vascular corium.

The attachment apparatus consists of the alveolar bone, cementum of the tooth, and the collagen fiber attachment. The alveolar bone mainly consists of an outer compact bone with inner trabecular bone, the compact bone, which lines the alveolar socket and acts as the attachment for collagen fibers that are incorporated into the compact bone. The bone is known as *bundle bone*. The cementum, which invests the root structure of the tooth, acts as the origin of the collagen fibers of the principal groups in the periodontal ligament. The principal fiber group is made up of collagen fibers running from the cementum of the root and does not insert in the bone. The dentogingival group runs from the cementum into the free gingival. The dentoperiosteal group runs from the cementum apically, over the alveolar crest of bone to the mucoperiosteum of the attached gingival. The circular fibers are not attached in cementum; they run in the free gingival around the tooth in a circular manner and the transseptal group, which runs from the cementum over the alveolar crest bone to the cementum of the adjacent tooth. These groups of fibers are immensely important to esthetics because they are the main structures that are responsible for the shape and the position of the interdental papilla. They only benefit natural teeth, and not dental implants, because dental implants do not possess an insertion place for the fibers as in the case with natural root cementum.

The periodontal fiber group is also made up of collagen fibers. They are also called the *dentoalveolar group* because they insert in the alveolar bone. They are composed of alveolar crestal fibers that run from the supraalveolar cementum down to the alveolar crest. Horizontal fibers run straight across from cementum to the alveolar bone, and the oblique fibers (largest group) run from the cementum, apically, from the root to the bone. All of these biological elements maintain the periodontium in a state of harmony, making it a unique creation.

The natural morphology of the healthy periodontium is characterized by a rise and fall of the marginal gingiva following the underlying alveolar crest contour both facially and proximally. Two distinctive periodontal patterns are present in the oral cavity: the thin scalloped biotype and the thick flat biotype. The thick flat type is more prevalent, constituting almost 85% of the population; the thin scalloped biotype composes 15% of the population (Ochsenbein and Ross 1973, Weisgold 1977, Olson and Lindhe 1991). Each type has distinctive morphological characteristics.

Recognizing and distinguishing these basic types is essential in selecting the implant size, implant type, and surgical approach, and in predicting the overall prognosis that will result in biological harmony between the dental implants and the existing dentogingival structures. The thick flat biotype is characterized by adequate amounts of masticatory mucosa. It is dense and fibrous in nature with minimal height difference between the highest and lowest points on the proximal and facial aspects of the marginal gingival; therefore, it is called flat. Larger-sized teeth that are most likely square characterize this type of periodontium. This bulkiness of the tooth shape results in a broader, more apically positioned contact area, a cervical convexity that has greater prominence, and an embrasure that is completely filled with the interdental papilla. The root dimensions are broader mesiodistally, almost equal to the width of the crown at the cervix, which causes a diminution in the amount of bone interproximally. The typical reaction of this tissue biotype to trauma such as tooth preparation, impression making, endodontic abscess, cracked tooth, or failing endodontic treatment is inflammation and apical migration of the junctional epithelium with a resultant pocket formation.

With thick flat tissue biotype, marginal inflammation is described in its acute form as marginal redness or magenta-cyanotic in appearance. With chronic inflammation, marginal gingivitis is present with gingiva coloration ranging from red to magenta. The gingiva may range from a normal shape to a boggy, enlarged shape. As inflammation persists, periodontal pocketing tends to occur. In regions with a relatively thick bulk of bone, the pocket formation occurs in conjunction with infrabony defects (See Figure 2.27). The thick flat tissue type is ideal for placing dental implants and restoring it with high esthetic predictability. Here the gingival and osseous scalloping is normally parallel to the cementoenamel junction (CEJ) (Gargiulo et al. 1961). The minimal undulation of the CEJ between adjacent teeth, which predictably follows the natural contour of the alveolar crest, makes the gingival tissues more stable. Consequently, this type of periodontium is less likely to exhibit soft tissue shrinkage postoperatively (See Figures 2.28A–B) (Gargiulo et al. 1961).

The thin scalloped biotype of periodontium exhibits its own distinctive features. These include thin, friable gingiva with a narrow band of attached masticatory mucosa, and a thin facial bone that usually exhibits dehiscence and fenestration, as shown in Figure 2.29. The tooth crown shape usually exhibits a triangular or thin cylindrical form, and the contact areas are smaller and located in a further incisal location. The cervical convexity is less prominent than that of the thick biotype. The interdental

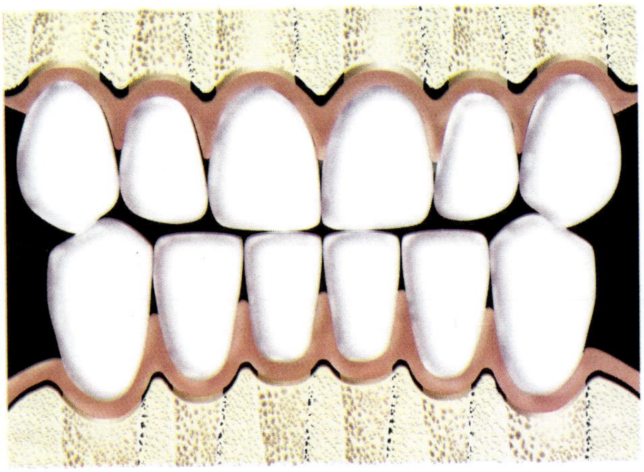

Figure 2.27. An illustration showing the thick flat tissue biotype features.

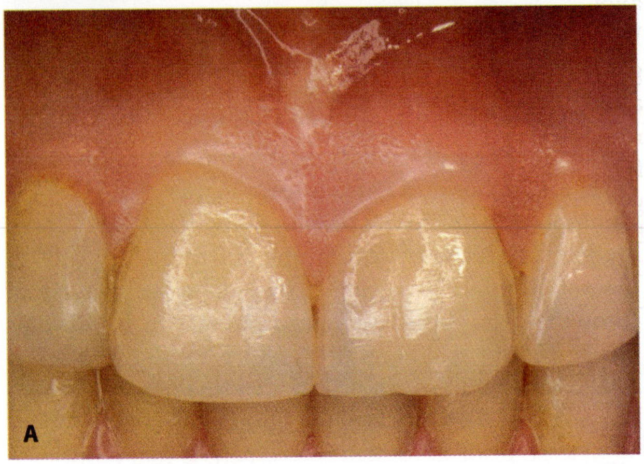

Figure 2.28A. Intraoral view showing a clinical picture of thick flat tissue biotype. Note the square shape of the crown and the width of the keratinized tissue band.

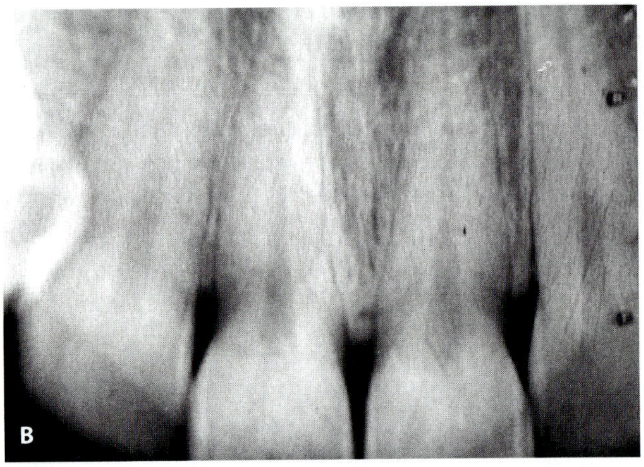

Figure 2.28B. Periapical view showing the morphological characters of the thick flat tissue biotype. Note the reduced interradicular bone thickness.

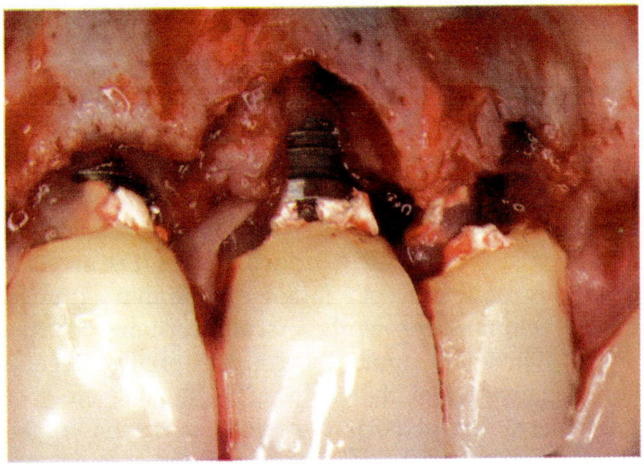

Figure 2.29. Typical thick flat tissue reaction to insult by pocket formation.

papilla is thin and long but does not fill the embrasure space completely, resulting in a scalloped appearance (Jansen and Weisgold 1995). Additionally, this biotype possesses a root that is narrow with an attenuated taper, allowing for an increased amount of interradicular bone. When inflicted with trauma, this tissue type undergoes gingival recession both facially and interproximally. Both acute and chronic inflammation will result in gingival recession. There are no pockets or infrabony defects that form because the thin bony plate resorbs in advance of the gingival recession. There is at least 0.5 mm to 0.8 mm of bone loss (Reynolds and Bowers 1996, Wilderman et al. 1970). Subsequently the thin labial plate recedes apically, and the soft tissue will follow the bone, causing recession. The extent of this recession is difficult to predict due to the varying thickness of the labial plate of bone among patients, as shown in Figure 2.30.

Placing dental implants in the esthetic zone becomes a critical task with this particular tissue biotype because it is difficult to achieve symmetrical soft tissue contours, probably due to the proximity of the implant to the natural tooth periodontium next to it, and the reduced amount of masticatory mucosa (Esposito et al. 1993). The resultant recession and bone resorption leave a flat profile between the roots, with marginal exposure of the restoration and subsequent partial loss of the interproximal papilla (Tarnow et al. 1992). Ridge preservation procedures must be carried out for any planned tooth extractions in this tissue biotype. Flapless implant installation are optimal for this type of bone, provided an intact labial plate of bone is present (See Figures 2.31A–B, 2.32A–B, and 2.33). However, a mixture of thick and thin tissue types in the same patient can be detected. Areas of thin labial plate are commonly associated with the canine eminencies, the mesial roots of maxillary first molars, and mandibular incisors. These areas tend to have thin gingiva as well. In such cases, these can be

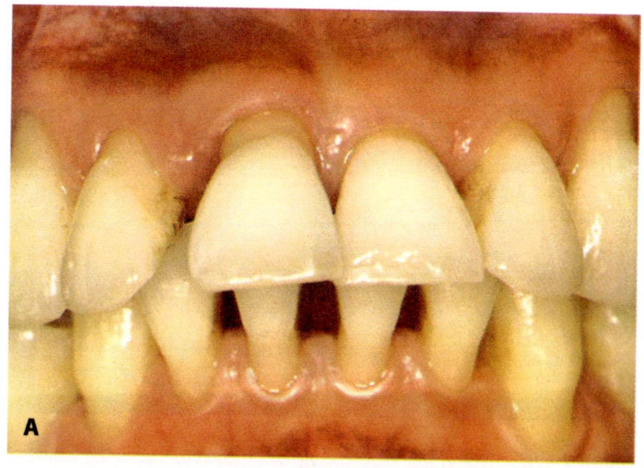

Figure 2.31A. Clinical picture of the thin scalloped tissue biotype. Note the reduced crown width and the apically located interdental papillae.

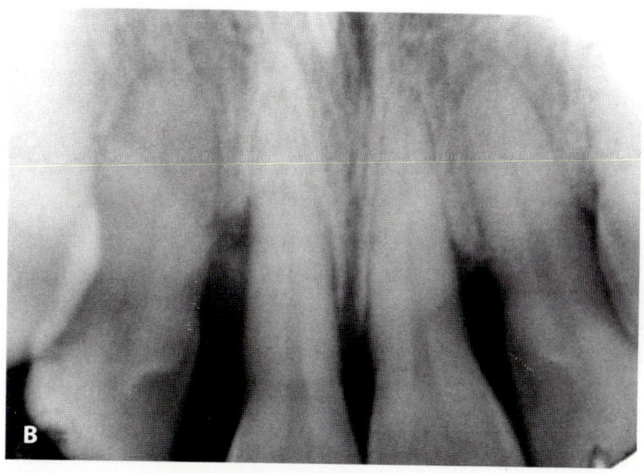

Figure 2.31B. A periapical radiographic view showing thin scalloped tissue biotype. Note the spacing between the roots.

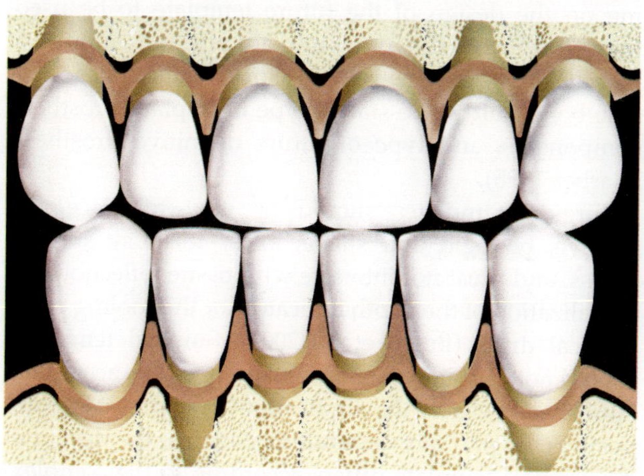

Figure 2.30. An illustration showing the clinical features of the thin scalloped tissue biotype.

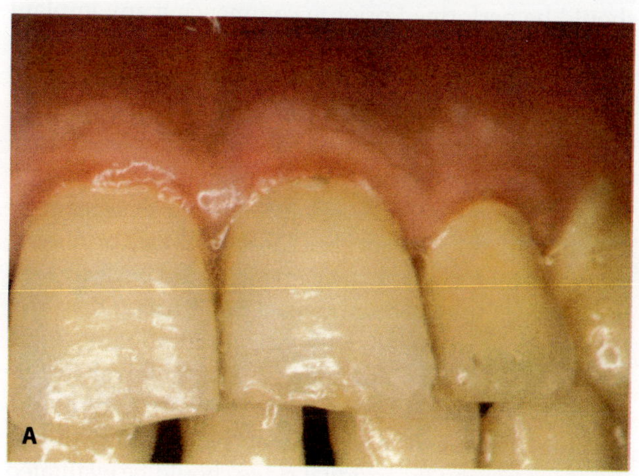

Figure 2.32A. Clinical picture of the thin scalloped tissue biotype of the upper front teeth.

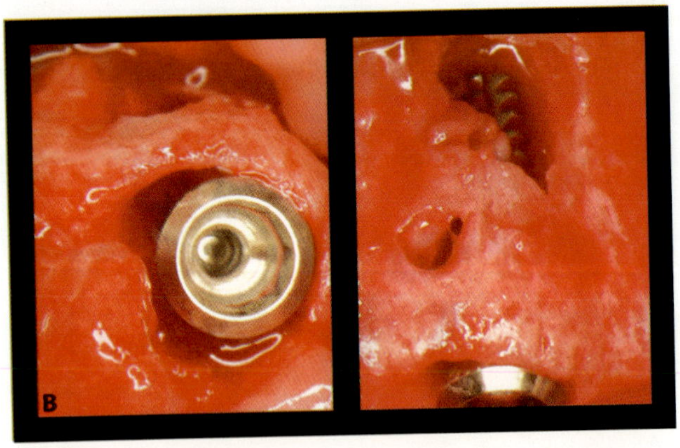

Figure 2.32B. Typical thin scalloped tissue reaction to trauma by fenestration and thinning.

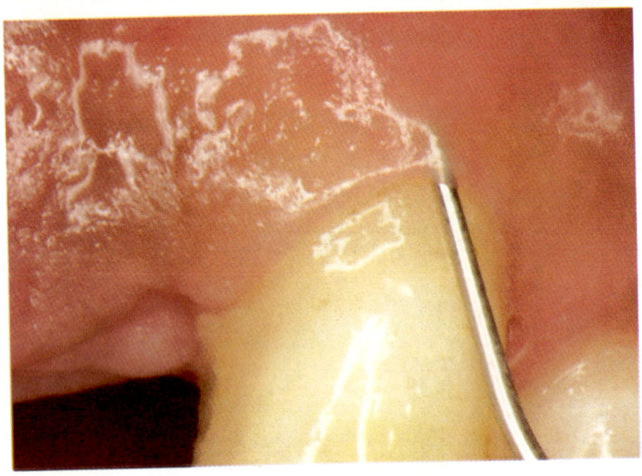

Figure 2.33. The explorer can be seen through the gingiva in a typical thin scalloped biotype.

called thick, thin, or mixed thick-thin gingiva (Reynolds and Bowers 1996, Wilderman et al. 1970).

The qualitative assesment of the periodontium is of great value. A proper appraisal of the periodontium should be performed prior to commencing any implant therapy in the esthetic zone. The clinician should be able to predict the response of the periodontal apparatus to restorative margins, inflammation, and regular trauma.

A tissue-integrated prosthesis must be placed in a healthy tissue environment. Any primary or secondary disease process must be resolved before placement of dental implants. Any localized inflammatory or fibrous processes that require management should be dealt with in advance. Inflammation caused by ill-fitting dentures can often be resolved with tissue-conditioning techniques prior to implant surgery. Any gingival hyperplastic tissues should be excised if they are a result of a reactive process. The degree of redundancy of the mucosa covering the residual ridge should be evaluated before fixture placement, if there has been significant resorption of the bone without a corresponding atrophy of the overlying mucosa. A mobile soft tissue ridge crest may be present and should be excised prior to surgery. Muscle pull in conjunction with alveolar mucosa such as that found in the front mandibular area should be considered for repositioning. Recent advances in periodontal surgery have made it possible not only to reposition or regenerate tissues to meet esthetic demands, but also to change the tissue quality of the restorative environment for more predictable treatment outcomes.

Soft tissue handling before implant placement increases the predictability of a satisfying treatment outcome. These procedures are indispensable in critical esthetic regions, but they unfortunately necessitate additional surgical procedures and increased cost to the patient (Kazor et al. 2004).

Fabricating Optimal Surgical Guides

Using an accurately fabricated surgical template ensures a predictable esthetic implant-supported restoration. The template is also another key determining factor to the optimal implant position in a 3-D fashion, because the precise implant placement complements esthetics and function, clear patient phonetics, and easier oral hygiene. Thus, transfer of the information regarding the predetermined position and angulation for the implant fixture from the study cast onto the surgical site becomes mandatory to allow a prosthetic driven implant placement protocol. A precisely fabricated surgical template or guide has an active role in executing the treatment plan at the first stage of surgery; it assists in the maintenance of a healthy natural biological space between the implant and the neighboring roots. In addition, it assists in keeping the recommended distance between implant fixtures themselves.

Factors must be taken into consideration before deciding on the design of the future template to be used; these encompass the future implant position, number of implants to be used, existing occlusion, amount of available bone, soft tissue status, type of implant prosthetic components, and type of future definitive prosthesis (Garber 1995).

Surgical templates should be easy to place and remove, be rigid and stable, allow for easy surgical access, and must not interfere with tissue reflection and visualization of the depth indicators or the cooling of the surgical drills (Buser et al. 2004). Surgical templates should not be rough or sharp. They should be accurately fabricated to ensure the duplication of the preset implant position. In partially edentulous patients, the design of the surgical template differs according to the complexity of the case. In partially edentulous cases, where the edentulous area is bounded by remaining dentition, the template does not need to be extended antroposteriorly more than two teeth on each side of the edentulous space and can be trimmed accordingly (Cowan 1990). It can only be fabricated, however, after completion of the wax trial denture. The guide must be developed so that the fixtures are placed in proposed tooth positions, not in proposed embrasure positions. The failure to do so could lead to an outcome that is unacceptable esthetically and phonetically. The prosthesis must be fabricated in a manner similar to a fixed partial denture.

The simplest surgical template is fabricated from a clear resin duplicate of the diagnostic wax-up. It has guiding grooves or cutouts at the location of the potential implant sites. These are usually fabricated according to the original position of the missing dentition. The exact amount of hard and soft tissue that should be regenerated to provide a healthy biological contour will be automatically identified after the template construction (Palacci 2001). The template is placed on the working cast, and drill holes of 3 mm diameter are prepared through the cingula of the anterior teeth and/or on the center of the occlusal surfaces of posterior teeth. These guide holes will be used to guide the pilot drill in the bone. An alternative device can be fabricated in the opposing arch that indicates fixture position when the mandible is closed to the proper vertical dimension. It can be fabricated in an edentulous or dentulous opposing arch and should include a vertical stop at the proper vertical dimension. The vertical stop must be located in an area where the mucoperiosteum will not be raised for fixture placement (See Figures 2.34A–B and 2.35).

Most of the fabricated surgical templates are limited to two planes, excluding the apicoincisal plane of the implant (Touati 1997a). Because of the greater accuracy of the surgical template fabrication, more precise implant positioning is obtained. A 3-D positioning surgical template could also be constructed to indicate the distance required to countersink the implant, which makes the third dimension achievable, and adds to the buccolingual and the mesiodistal dimensions. The best way to indicate these positions is to fabricate a complete diagnostic wax-up that features the soft tissue margin position, facial surface, and embrasure form of the proposed restoration. Working backward from this wax-up generates a template that will place the implant in a position that will support the planned restoration (Jansen and Weisgold 1995, Tarnow and Eskow 1995b).

The surgical template can also be a partial denture with indented markings on the acrylic teeth indicating the site of the future implants (with palatal or lingual relief) (Engelman et al. 1988, Shepherd 1996). The transparent and the partial denture replica surgical templates lack precise implant positioning because the template does not provide any control for the buccolingual movement of the drill nor the apicocoronal movement. Any

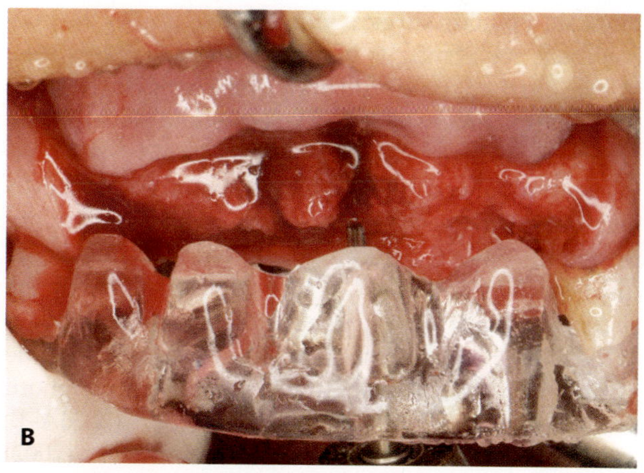

Figure 2.34B. The basic transparent template.

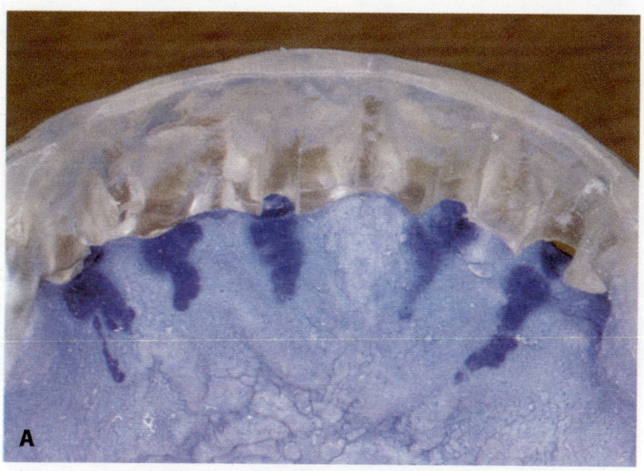

Figure 2.34A. The commonly used surgical template that has guiding grooves lacks axial movement control of the drill.

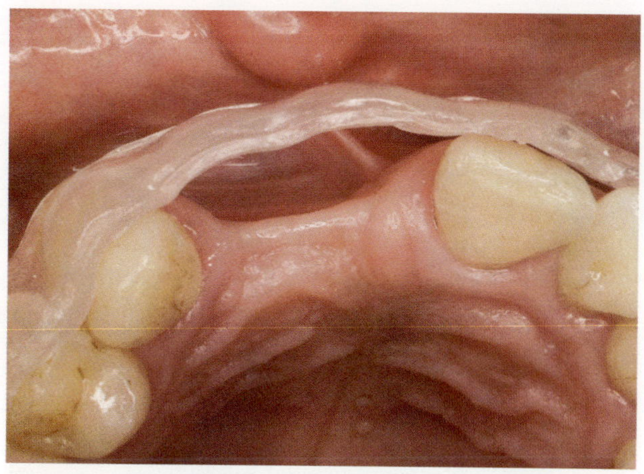

Figure 2.35. An acrylic template that shows the amount of bone to be regenerated to regain the original contours.

deviation in the direction of the drilling angulation will subsequently alter the planned implant position.

A panoramic radiograph can be taken with the surgical template in place to help determine the best location and angulation of implants relative to the proposed prosthesis; radiopaque ball bearings of a known diameter are luted into the template and appear suspended over potential implant placement sites on the radiograph. By dividing the actual diameter of the ball bearing by the diameter of its image on the radiograph, the distortion factor of the panoramic image can be calculated for each proposed implant location (Garg and Vicari 1995). The actual height of the residual ridge can then be calculated by multiplying the distortion factor by the distance from the crest of the ridge to any anatomical landmark. This procedure assists in the selection of an accurate implant length.

After radiographic assessment is made, the ball bearings are removed and the template is perforated and sterilized for use during the implant surgery (Garg and Vicari 1995). The preferred and most popular method to fabricate a precise surgical template that guides the buccolingual positioning is by integrating a stainless steel sleeve into the acrylic resin body of the template over the drill hole (Kennedy et al. 1998, Becker and Kaiser 2000). This type of template permits exact implant positioning with more accurate parallelism because the sleeves help maintain parallel holes throughout the drilling procedure. They also prevent the acrylic resin from being distorted or chipped off at the surgical site (from the sharp frictional rotation of the surgical drill with the sides of the template). Presence of the sleeves provides a stable position for the drill and fixed angulation throughout the drilling procedure, as shown in Figures 2.36A–B, 2.37A–B, and 2.38A–B. Cehreli and others (2002) described how to make impressions of both arches to fabricate an accurate stainless steel surgical template.

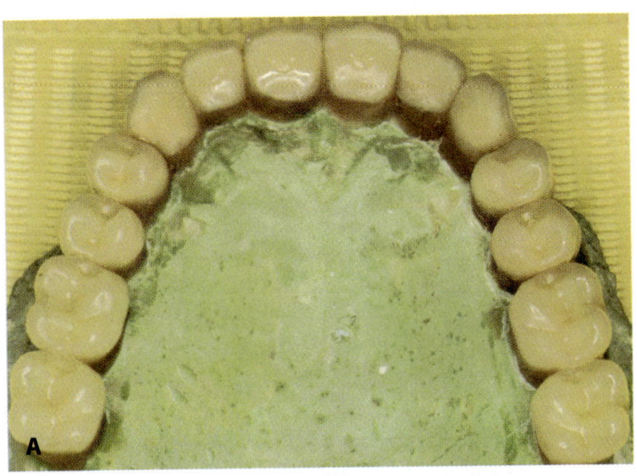

Figure 2.36A. Wax-up of a missing right central incisor.

Next, casts are poured in type III dental stone (Moldano; Bayer, Leverrusen, Germany). Complete maxillomandibular records and mount casts in a semiadjustable articulator (Model 8500; Whip Mix Corp,

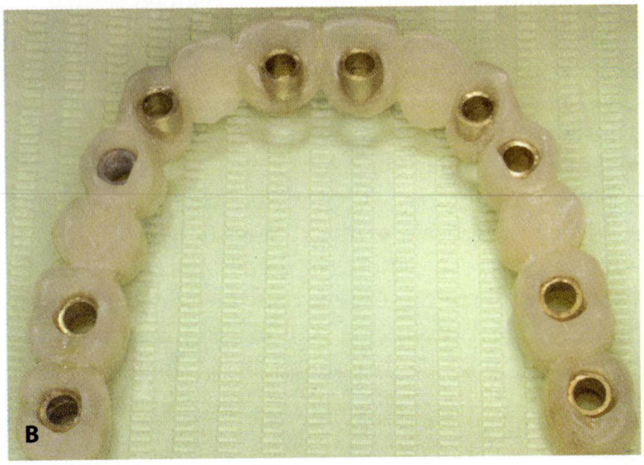

Figure 2.36B. The metal sleeve attached to the acrylic frame.

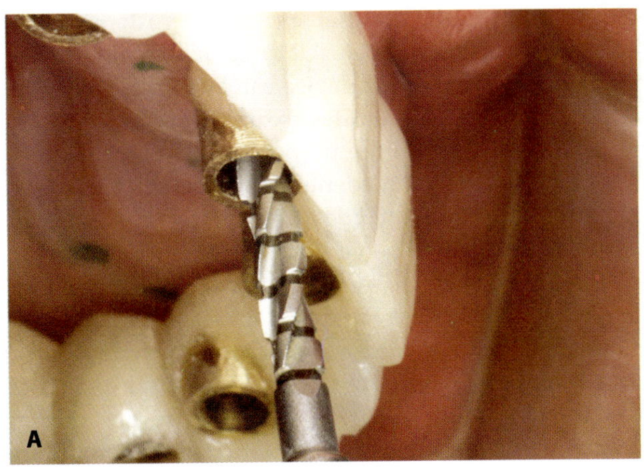

Figure 2.37A. The surgical template framework in place.

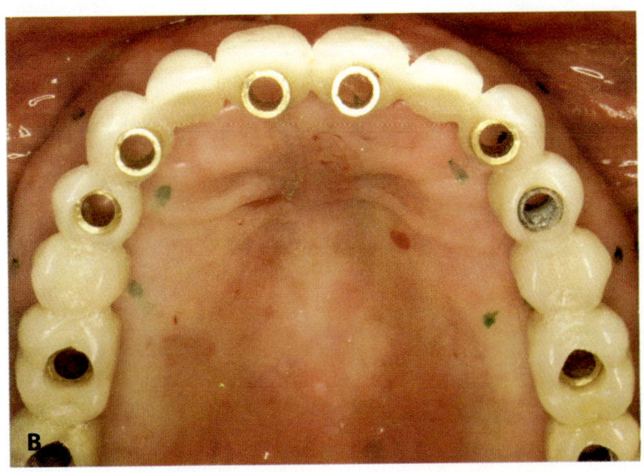

Figure 2.37B. The stainless steel sleeves are attached to the acrylic template for accurate implant positioning.

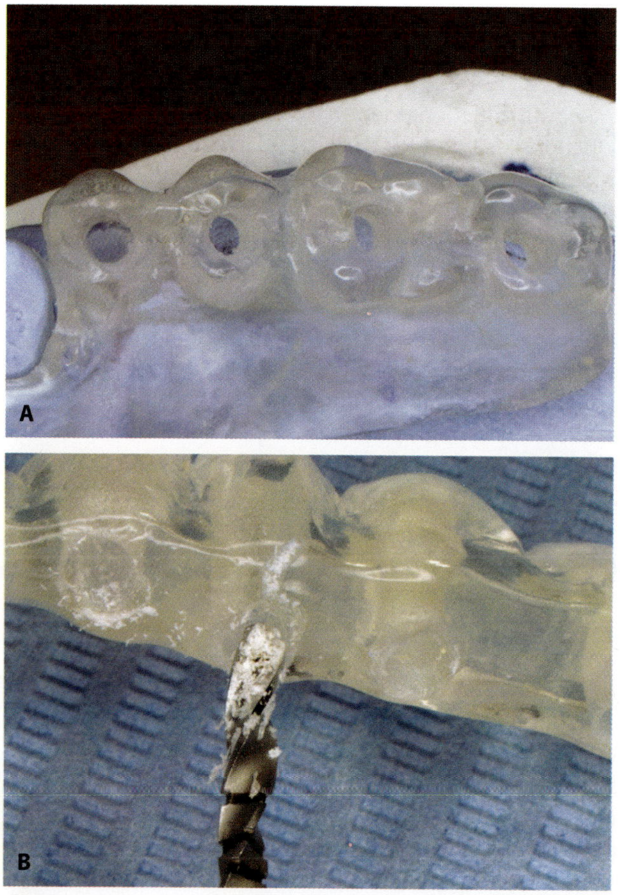

Figure 2.38A, B. The effect of the drilling on the pure acrylic resin template, showing the flaking of the resin into the wound area.

Louisville, KY, USA) then determine the dental implant recipient sites and complete an appropriate setting of artificial teeth. To do this, make a single-mix of condensation silicone (Coltene/Whaledent, Mahwah, NJ, USA) impression to the artificial teeth. Upon setting, remove the impression and the denture teeth from the cast. Eliminate wax with hot water, and coat the cast with a tinfoil substitute. Flow a mix of autopolymerized methyl methacrylate resin (Orthocryl 2000; Dentaurum, Ispringen, Germany) into the impression in the space previously occupied by the artificial teeth. Reinsert the cast into the impression, secure it with an elastic band, and place the assembly into a pressure pot for polymerization. Upon polymerization, remove the resin guide from the cast. Finish and polish the guide. Place the cast and the acrylic resin guide as an assembly onto a surveying table. Tilt the table to determine the desired angulation of the proposed dental implants. For each implant site, prepare a pinhole, 1 mm in diameter, at the anticipated central axis of the implant in the acrylic resin guide. When the pins are secured in each hole, double check the optimal angulation both on the cast and the CT by placing the guide in the patient's mouth and obtain two-dimensional (2-D) CT images. Measure the dimensions and angulation of the available bone and determine the appropriate location and angulation of the implants. The difference between the angulations of the bone and the pin is the required change in the tilt of the surveying table.

For each implant site, the absolute vertical alignment of a pin presents the original situation. When the pin is initially incorporated into the guide, the mesiodistal angulation of the pins is determined according to the angle of the tooth neighboring the edentulous ridge. Remove the portion of the guide where the stainless steel surgical guides will be incorporated. Secure a 2-mm surgical twist drill of the desired system to be used to the surveyor as an analyzing rod, and pass the drill through the assembled prefabricated stainless steel surgical guides. The height of the stainless tubes used is 4 mm, and the inner diameter of each tube has 0.1-mm machining tolerance to allow surgical drills to pass through easily. The guides for 2 mm and 3 mm drills also have collars that extend horizontally and rest on the consecutive guide. Secure the internally stacked guides to the surgical guide with acrylic resin.

A dual-purpose template is yet another precise surgical form that maintains a correct labiolingual position of dental implants (Cenrell and Sahin 2000). The objective of this type of template is to fabricate a surgical guide that offers critical information about the location and angulation of the implant, as well as the position and angulation of the anticipated abutment relative to the predesigned superastructure with computed tomographic evaluation. Modification of the device for surgical procedures is accomplished thereafter. During CT imaging, radiopaque markers are incorporated into the radiographic template to provide proper guidance in determining the location and the axis of the implant and the future abutment. Relevant data should be transferred to the working cast through the markers, which dictate accurate reorientation of the surveying table for guiding channel preparation. An effective radiopaque marker should stay in place during the modification procedures.

Conversion of the radiographic template to a surgical aid should facilitate correct placement of the implants with the desired path of insertion, which is correlated with the data obtained from a 2-D scan image. The surgical guide should rest firmly on anatomical structures and provide the clinician with ease in site preparation and accurate visualization of the implant sites (Verdi and Morgano 1993). Recently, the terms *computer-guided surgery* and *computer-milled surgical templates* have been introduced to complete the vast array of the assisting devices to implant therapy (Klein and Abrams 2001).

The computer-milled surgical template (Compu-surge Template, Implant Logic Systems, Cedarhurst, New York, USA) provides a connection between the CT scan and the surgical template. It uses reformatted CT data in combination with a 3-D simulation of the implant position to produce a computer-milled surgical template. The simulated implant position is created via SIM/Plant software (SIM/Plant, Columbia Scientific, Columbia, Maryland, USA). The 3-D coordinates of the simulated implant position are transferred to a five-axis computer-controlled milling machine that creates an appliance with the SIM/Plant plan. Drill guide components are then installed in the milled surgical template to direct the drilling procedure. The novel guide template plays an active role in the drilling procedure to achieve optimal esthetic results. This guide template is best used when placing multiple adjacent implants (Minoretti et al. 2000). It is fabricated from the wax-up on the diagnostic cast.

Precise determination of the implant angulation is obtained by providing a guide sleeve on the 0.8 mm Kirschner wires within the template. The template is placed in position over the intact mucosa surface. The template guides the Kirschner wires to pierce through the mucosa into the bone. The wires are attached to a special insert using a dental coupling fitted into the dental hand piece. The insert facilitates easy insertion of the wires into the bone. The wires are then trimmed 5 mm to 7 mm above the bone level, and incisions are made to connect the wires to each other or to the adjacent natural tooth. After the insertion of the wires, the implant osteotomies are prepared with a trephine drill guided over the wires alone or over wires combined with a special guidance cylinder fitting the trephine drill, as shown in Figures 2.36A and 2.36B.

This method may alleviate some of the problems common to conventional template techniques, in which the template directly guides the drill. With this method, the guiding wires allow for precise implant positioning in the alveolar ridge. This type of template may also help to improve the security during the surgical procedure. It reduces the danger of plastic or metal debris of the guiding sleeve or template being introduced into the wound, and it causes no obstruction in sight or movement of the template when raising the mucoperiosteal flap (See Figures 2.39A–C).

A multifunctional template has been introduced that functions as the following: (1) a radiographic implant positioning guide, (2) an accurate bone sounding guide, and (3) a surgical guide and an aid in flap reflection and a pick-up impression tray. Drilling slots of the template allow drill placement from a buccal direction to allow better visualization. It can be used for patients with limited mouth opening, and to facilitate the flow of coolant from hand pieces with external irrigation systems. Transgingival bone sounding allows mapping of the bony topography of an implant site. The resultant readings are accurate, reproducible measurements that allow the resulting image to be analyzed with confidence. The design of this template allows the clinician to accurately read the probe depth, even after probing multiple sites, due to the thickness of the material and its ability to shield blood and maintain visualization of the probe. This, in turn, improves accuracy of recording and reduction of measurement errors (Quinlan et al. 1998).

In another attempt to fabricate a surgical template that offers great accuracy and optimal 3-D positioning of the implant, a technique has been introduced that uses, along with its newly designed set of drills, a radiographic stent with a vertical orientation pin to the occlusal plane positioned in the central fossa of each pontic tooth (Weinberg and Kruger 1998). A CT scan is then obtained with the stent in place. The panoramic image provides the anteroposterior implant inclination, while the cross-sectional image provides the buccolingual implant inclination which was to be replicated by the surgical guide. Thus, the precise locations of each implant with a true vertical reference are superimposed onto the corresponding reformatted images. Preoperative panoramic and CT images are reproduced by an in-office Polaroid camera (or 35-mm prints). The vertical

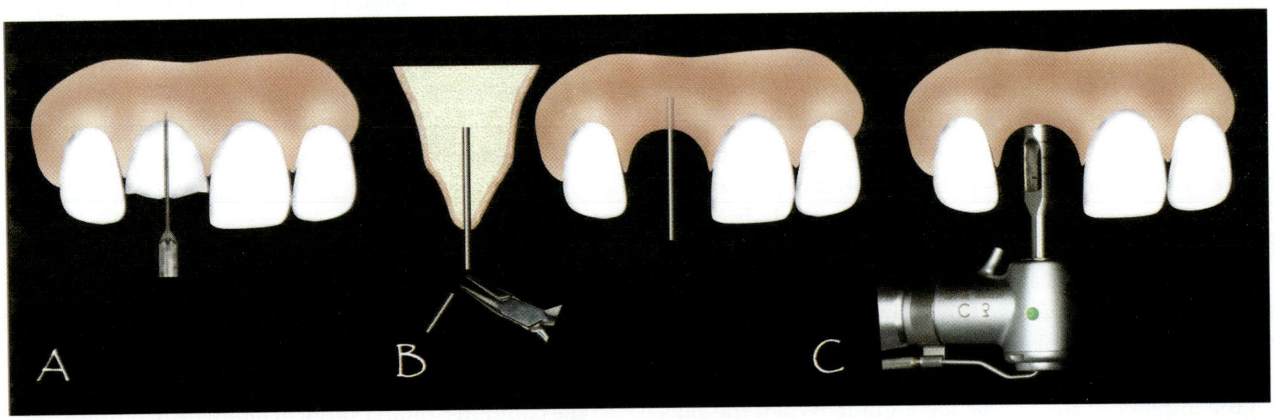

Figure 2.39. **A.** The Kirschner wire being introduced through the mucosa. **B.** The wire trimmed off. **C.** The remaining Kirschner wire is the guide for the trephine drill. Note that in using the novel guide, the pilot drill is replaced with a small-diameter trephine drill.

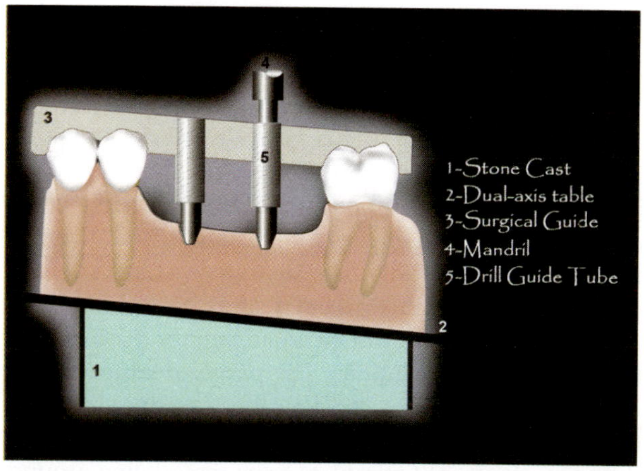

Figure 2.40. A three-dimensional (3D) positioning device.

orientation pin images provide a true vertical reference line that is drawn on each picture, indicating the osteotomy starting point. A line is drawn on the Polaroid print through the starting point and along the optimum implant orientation selected. The angle between the true vertical line of reference and the optimum implant orientation is measured and recorded. A dual-axis table is used to facilitate the reproduction of the individual buccolingual and mesiodistal inclinations of each implant. Surgical drill guide tubes are positioned within the surgical guide. This type of template offers a greater predictability in terms of apicocoronal and labiolingual positioning (See Figure 2.40).

The common surgical templates possess some technical difficulties such as difficulty in guiding the drills in the correct position and angulation in the ridge, poor visibility, problems with cooling during the drilling procedure, and difficulty in reliably positioning the template in completely edentulous arches after the reflection of the soft tissues. Furthermore, the templates often guide only the pilot drilling, and a misalignment of subsequent drills may still result.

Modern Provisionalization in Esthetic Implantology

Implant-supported restorations for partially and fully edentulous patients have been a well-accepted and predictable treatment modality. However, restoring function and esthetics during the healing period remains a difficult clinical task. A critical stage in tooth replacement in the esthetic zone is in the interim between implant insertion and surgical uncovering at the second-stage surgery, because a healing period ranging from a few months to one year might be required to achieve fully integrated dental implants in their osseous housing. The number of implants used, the condition of the alveolar bone, the location of the implants, and the type of implant design are all factors in the length of the osseointegration waiting period.

During this time, many patients experience apprehension about losing their social image or daily function routine, which can translate into fear or rejection of dental implant therapy. Therefore, clinicians should provide a stable, functional, and esthetic provisional restoration to the patients during this critical period (El Askary and Shawkat 2003).

For years, provisionalization was viewed as a thoughtless type of treatment procedure that sought only a rapid, feasible, inexpensive method to obtain disposable crowns and bridges (Shavell 1979). This thinking implied that provisional restorations should not be perfected, because they would not serve in the patient's mouth for a long period. Today, with the wide application of dental implants as a routine tooth replacement therapy, the role of provisional prostheses has changed dramatically. Patients might have stayed edentulous for long times before implant therapy, especially those who were "esthetically conscious" tended to ask the usual question ("Will I stay toothless till dental implants integrate?") because it becomes embarrassing when the patient is seen in public without teeth or with a temporary tooth that is obviously artificial (Goldstein 1997). This question was encountered because after patients selected the dental implants as a treatment option they also started to get ready for a new social and esthetic era in their lives. The provisional prostheses should be designed to sustain or improve the quality of life for patients undergoing implant therapy (Balshi and Garver 1986).

As the word *provisional* suggests, provisionalization involves something that is used temporarily or for a short period of time, until the permanent service is rendered. Its application to dental treatment is no exception. When fabricating a provisional prosthesis, several factors should be considered:

1. The provisional restoration should not interfere with primary wound closure.
2. The provisional restoration should provide the patient with harmonious occlusion.
3. The provisional prosthesis should restore esthetics and phonetics.
4. The provisional prosthesis should protect the underlying gingival tissues (i.e., maintain the dentogingival unit health).
5. The provisional prosthesis should not exert any direct biting loads to the underlying implants, in case a delayed method of loading is selected.

A properly fabricated provisional restoration can be an important source of biomechanical information. It can be a valuable aid in determining the final tooth position, exact tooth shade, and occlusal scheme of the definitive prosthesis. Moreover, it can reveal some new additional touches for improved esthetics and patient comfort (Balshi and Garver 1986). After the second-stage surgery, a provisional restoration can help to guide healing of the soft tissues around dental implants to develop the emergence profile until it reaches the original anatomical dimensions. This can minimize the need for further soft tissue manipulation (Biggs 1996). Therefore, the interim prosthesis might act as a reference in designing the final prosthesis (Soballe et al. 1990).

The type of provisional prosthesis should be determined by the dental team during the presurgical planning phase. When considering a provisional prosthesis for a patient who will receive an implant-supported restoration, the available options are plentiful. These include an existing prosthesis that the patient already uses or a removable partial denture, a resin-bonded bridge, or the modified socket seal template technique, which includes temporary implants and the use of the socket seal methods (natural teeth provisionalization).

Using or Modifying an Existing Prosthesis

When the patient seeks implant therapy to replace an existing prosthesis because it does not function properly, the old prosthesis can be used as a temporary solution. When the patient is presented with an old bridge, the following steps should be followed: an overall impression is made with the failed bridge in place before attempting to remove it. An indirect or direct provisional bridge is then created and cemented in place after the old bridge is removed. Or, when the old bridge has already been removed from its place, it can be temporarily cemented after relieving pontic areas that touch the soft tissue, as shown in Figure 2.41.

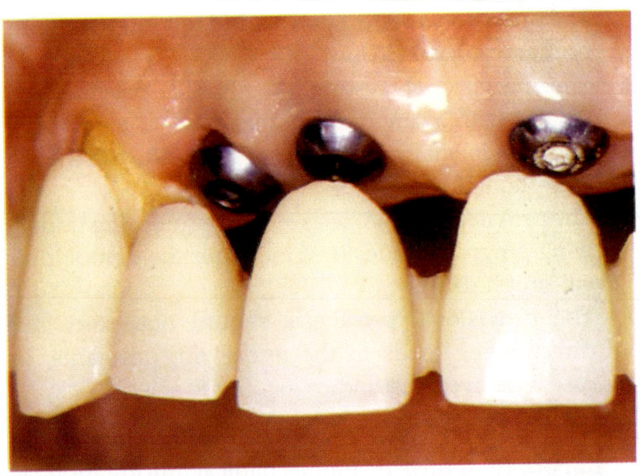

Figure 2.41. Using a duplicate of an old bridge as a provisional prosthesis.

Removable Partial Dentures

One of the easiest forms of provisionalization between stage one and stage two implant surgery is the use of a removable prosthesis that is typically fabricated as an interim restoration for partially (bounded and free-end saddles) or fully edentulous patients. It is simply fabricated by making an impression, casting it, and drawing the design of the saddle. The laboratory technician then constructs a removable partial denture accordingly. The removable prosthesis can be an advantage during multiple surgical interventions. The partial denture can be removed and then replaced after the procedure has been completed without clinical complexity. Removable dentures also might stimulate bone remodeling around dental implants in totally edentulous patients and can be used to confirm osseointegration before the final prosthesis is constructed (Lewis et al. 1995).

This type of provisional solution provides an inexpensive provisional modality that can be considered in any treatment plan, based on the patient's financial status. The patient may feel psychologically improved with the edentulous area temporarily restored and other related facial structures supported. However, the patient should be reminded that the prosthesis is only a temporary alternative for the missing space. Removable partial dentures can be limiting in their function, especially during speaking or chewing, due to their instability. Furthermore, some clinical precautions need to be observed when removable partial dentures are used as a provisional modality for totally or partially edentulous patients. The appliance should be relieved from its fitting surface on top of the implant heads to avoid any biting load being exerted on the implants during the healing period and to allow undisturbed soft tissue healing. The patient is advised to use the denture primarily for social reasons rather than for masticatory purposes.

In addition, when the partial denture is relined, the lining material tends to dry and become stiff over time, usually one to two months. This can be handled by changing the lining material at monthly intervals to keep the fitting surface of the denture elastic. A removable provisional prosthesis can influence the underlying gingival tissues at the pontic areas to create and simulate a natural gingival architecture of the implant-supported restorations. This can be achieved by adding acrylic resin to the fitting surface of the pontic at the specific areas to be stimulated to press and conform the alveolar mucosa to the required shape and contour, as shown in Figure 2.42, 2.43A–B.

Adhesive Bridges

An alternative conservative treatment option that has been suggested in restoring missing dentition in the esthetic zone is adhesive bridges, which eliminate the need for substantial destruction of natural abutments. Adhesive bridges were originally introduced by Rochette to be used as periodontal splints (Rochette 1986). When used as provisional prostheses, adhesive bridges help to restore esthetics, maintain occlusion, and free the implant from biting loads (Hussey et al. 1991). Adhesive bridges, unlike removable partial dentures, do

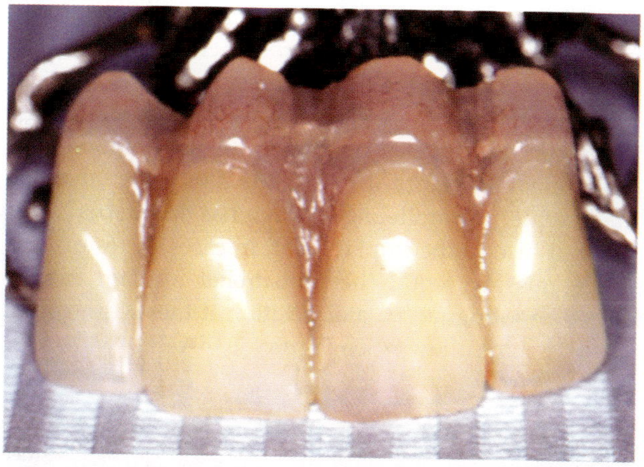

Figure 2.42. Removable partial denture is used to provisionally restore four missing anterior teeth during the grafting and implant integration period.

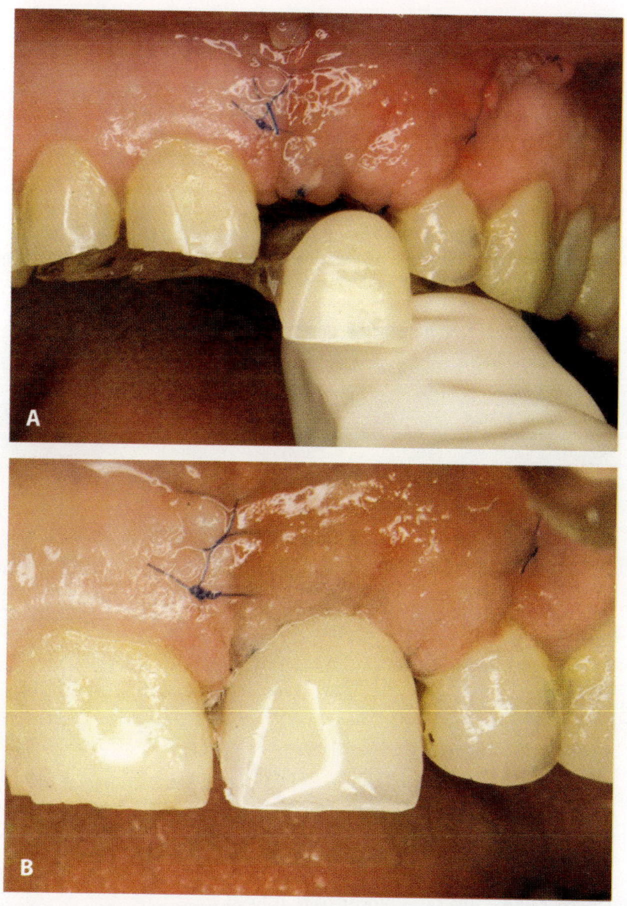

Figure 2.43A, B. A temporary partial denture used to restore esthetics.

not exert any pressure on the implant area. They are better tolerated by the patient and may be more reassuring than a removable partial denture because of the improved esthetic results, stability, and fixation. However, a resin-bonded bridge can be a deterrent when multiple reentries to the surgical site are required.

The prosthesis is totally tooth-supported and retained by acid etching the adjacent teeth and cementing using composite resin. However, adhesive bridges require greater clinical skills than do conventional bridges, and there is the possibility of recurrent dental caries occurring around the margins and line angles. Debonding tendency occurs with a frequency as high as 25% to 31% (Williams et al. 1989), which requires the recementation every time it occurs. This provisional method can be used when patients are extremely concerned with their social appearance or their work includes speaking in front of the media, so they cannot afford any movable devices in their mouth (See Figure 2.44).

Transitional Implants

Transitional implants were introduced as treatment alternatives in 1993 (MTI, Dentatus New York, NY, USA). This procedure, involving the placement of miniature titanium implants to restore fixed or removable temporary restorations (Petrungaro et al. 1999, Froum et al. 1997, Sendax 1996), really brought provisionalization in to a new era. Using temporary implants has solved many clinical problems, especially for totally edentulous patients. They offer a stable, nonmobile, esthetic provisional restoration. All types of temporary implants or transitional implants use self-tapping screws that have diameters ranging between 1.8 mm and 2.8 mm and come in an assortment of lengths. They are fabricated from either grade one commercially pure titanium or tritium alloy. They are inserted via a one-stage drilling procedure (only a pilot drill) with minimal surgical intervention. They should be placed at a distance 1 mm to 2 mm from

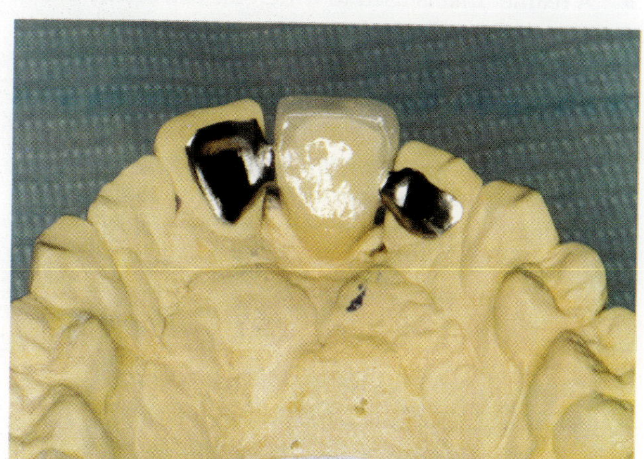

Figure 2.44. Two resin-bonded bridges on the cast.

the site of the permanent implants to avoid interrupting osseointegration around the implant-bone interface.

Transitional implants require a bone height of at least 7 mm to allow for initial stability, and an interocclusal space of at least 6 mm to 9 mm should be available. The implants can be easily removed after the completion of the healing period by reversed torque on a counter-clockwise rotation using the supplied retrieval tool or trephined by using a small diameter trephine drill.

Transitional implants satisfy the patient's expectations by providing a retentive, esthetic, and functional restoration on the day of the surgery (Petrungaro 1997), and they allow the patient to tolerate the overall implant treatment (El Attar et al. 1999). Transitional implants eliminate the accidental premature loading that removable prostheses can exert over the permanent implants or augmented bone, therefore allowing uninterrupted healing. They also can be used in "rescue and repair" situations (Bichacho et al. 1999) in which guided bone regeneration is required for potential future implant site development. Transitional implants can then be used to support a temporary prosthesis to avoid any undesirable loads on the regenerating tissues.

The clinician must be cautious when dealing with transitional implants, because they may interfere with the osseointegration of the permanent implants if they are too close. Also, if the implants are placed close to natural roots, they might disrupt the harmony of the periodontal environment. Transitional implants fail quickly upon neglected oral hygiene, as do permanent implants.

The implants must be sterilized prior to the surgery with autoclaving (See Figure 2.45). The basic transitional implant kit includes the following:

- Implants (MTI, Dentatus, New York, NY, USA) that are notched at their heads to accommodate the cross-bar of the singular coping placement
- A drill, 1.3 mm in diameter and laser marked to the corresponding implant lengths
- A reamer that is used to widen the osteotomy site in case of D1 or D2 bone
- The manual socket key that is used to drive the implant to the osteotomy full depth because the MTI has a self-threading feature
- The singular coping with the stabilizing cross bar
- A plastic gingival protective spacer that protects against any ingression of the polymerizing restorative material at the implant neck level

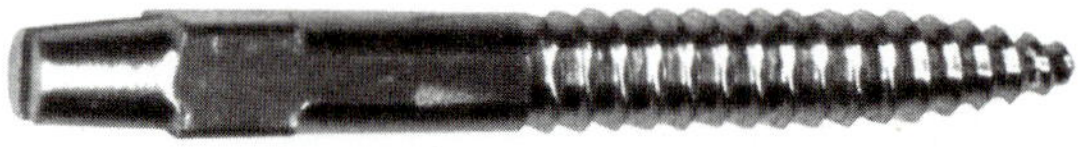

Figure 2.45. MTI temporary implant.

To install transitional implants, drilling is performed after flap reflection, site preparation, and permanent implant placement. The drilling is performed in a single step. The depth of the osteotomy should be limited to the half-length of the transitional implant, to allow a self-tapped placement to the final position with primary mechanical retention. It is placed manually with a finger wrench and ratchet to verify initial stability. After the osteotomies are prepared, the MTI implants are placed with the manual socket key with the cross bar for aligning the implant slots with the crest of the ridge. After transitional implants are seated in place, parallelism is then checked. If any correction in the angulation of the transitional implants is required, tilting can then be made with the paralleling rod that has an internal cross bar that bisects the implant slot. In cases of restoring a single missing tooth, the transitional implant can be placed in a lingual/palatal position if the width of the alveolar ridge allows (See Figures 2.46A–B).

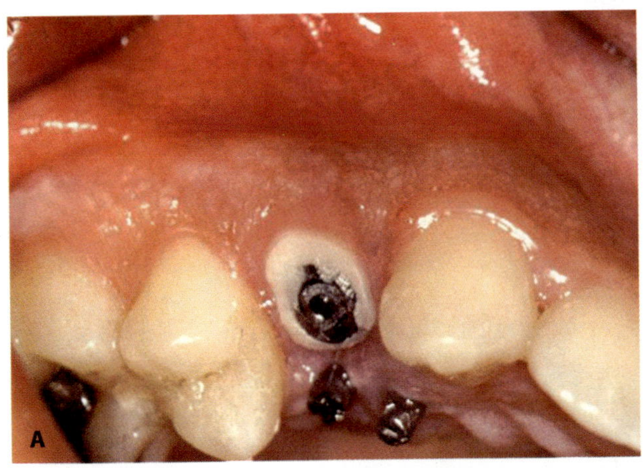

Figure 2.46A. Two transitional implants positioned palatally to restore missing single tooth.

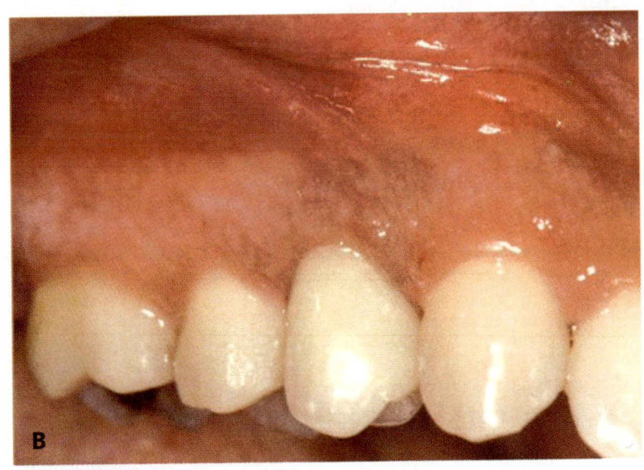

Figure 2.46B. The cases provisionally restored.

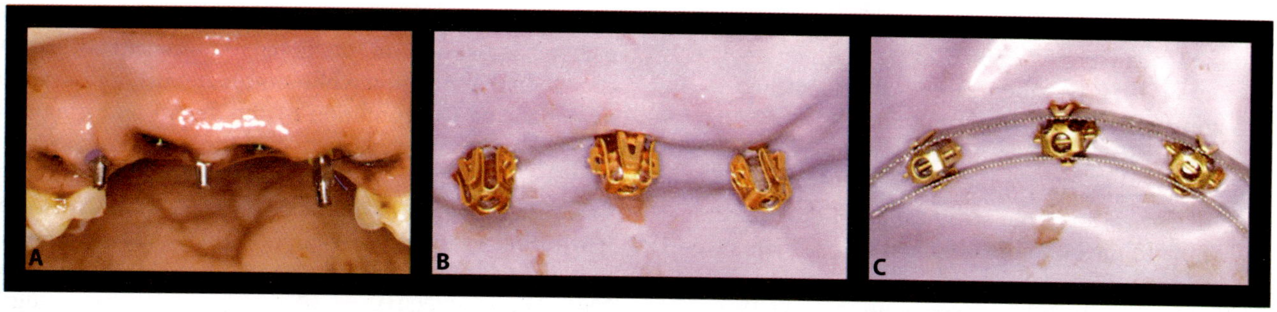

Figure 2.47. **A.** Transitional implants placed 2 mm away from the permanent implants with the plastic spacers positioned around the necks of the transitional implants. **B.** Singular copings in place with its crossbar adapted in the MTI transverse slots and the tabs are positioned buccolingually. **C.** Flexible titanium bars are placed in the buccolingual tabs of the copings.

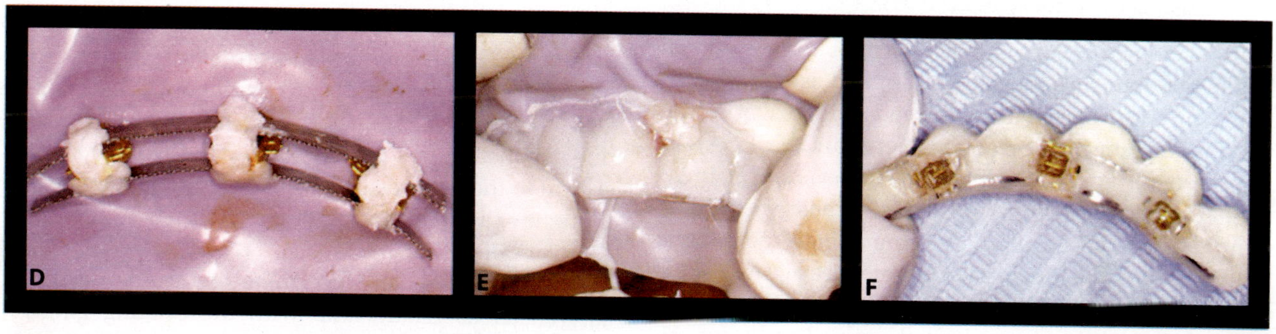

Figure 2.47. **D.** The coping-bar attachments covered with self-curing acrylic resin. **E.** Vacuum formed resilient acrylic shell filled with self-curing acrylic resin fitted on the prosthetic assembly. **F.** The acrylic bridge-splint restorative unit trimmed to the desirable contour.

The prosthetic procedure follows. After the wound closure, a rubber dam or a thin tape is placed over the MTI fixtures to help prevent the ingression of the acrylic resin in the wound edges or to adhere to the sutures. Plastic gingival sleeves are then placed over the MTI implant extension to isolate the neck of the implant from the wound area. The sleeves should be removed prior to cementation of the provisional restoration. Modular copings are then seated over the implants and the bar and pushed downward, locking the coping assembly in place. The titanium bar is then tailored to the proper length to join the transitional implants from labial and lingual sides on the sides of the modular copings. A clear vacuum template full of self-curing resin is placed over the titanium bar and modular assembly and then removed when totally cured. Then the assembly is taken out of the mouth, finished and polished, then returned to the mouth for cementation, as shown in Figures 2.47A–G.

The literature has confirmed that transitional implants that were placed and functional and fully loaded for a period of eight months have shown excellent bone adaptation and normal soft tissue conditions (Brown and Tarnow 2001). They also can be placed between the permanent implants and restored at the time of the surgery either by direct technique using an acrylic shell previously prepared in the laboratory on the study cast or by indirect technique (Keller 2001).

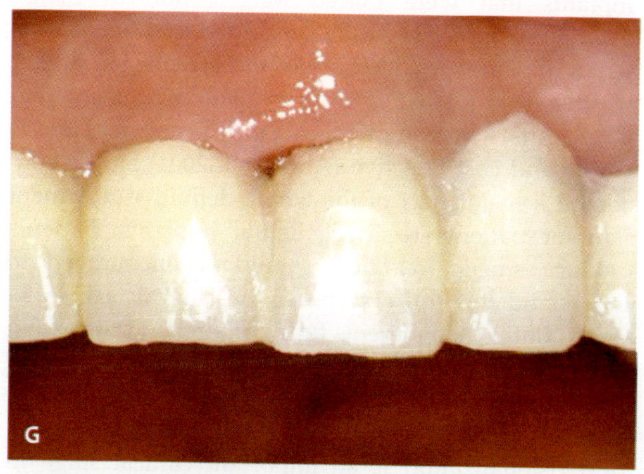

Figure 2.47G. The assembly is cemented in place.

Transitional implants require some clinical precautions:

1. Excessive loading or placement of the transitional implant fixtures in bone of inadequate volume may result in potential fracture or premature loss of the implant fixture.
2. Depending on the system used, transitional implants require at least 7 mm of bone for placement

and therefore are contraindicated where there is inadequate bone depth.
3. Because the prosthetic abutment is attached to the implant body, the amount of interarch space cannot be less than 6 mm (4 mm for the abutment component and 2 mm for the coping and restorative material).
4. To provide an initial stabilization of the transitional implant, the bone quality must be adequate (type 1 or type 2 bone).
5. In partial edentulous cases with straight line temporization, the implants are at high risk for torque with subsequent fibrous encapsulation (Froum et al. 1997, Petrungaro 1997, Rossein and Boris 2001, Minsk 2001, Zubery et al. 1999).

Transitional implants are now available from several manufacturers, and they can be applied as an overdentures protocol or fixed crown and bridge work. The ANEW Implants (MTI, Dentatus New York, NY, USA) are considered a new version of the MTI screws and claim to be permanent or semipermanent solutions. This procedure claims to be useful for restoring a single tooth (non-fully loaded) for a long period of time (See Figure 2.48).

A study evaluated the efficacy of 27 provisional transitional dental implants loaded immediately for 11 patients. The diameter of the implants was 1.8 mm (IMTEC Corp., OK, USA). The lengths of the minidental implants that were placed were 13 mm to 18 mm (average 15 mm). The study concluded that transitional dental implants provided stable and esthetic temporary prostheses immediately after implant placement and bone grafts. The use of transitional dental implants is simple and cost effective (Ahn et al. 2004) and is considered a major part of the whole definitive treatment plan for patients receiving dental implants. Patients seeking esthetic treatment should be encouraged to understand the entire scope of the clinical task to be carried out. When patients fully comprehend the extent of the work entailed, they will be able to appreciate it and accept the difficulties that might occur during treatment (Froum et al. 1997, Brown and Tarnow 2001).

Provisionalization is an important clinical stage in implant therapy that should be carefully designed in the presurgical stage. Various provisionalization techniques are available to achieve function and esthetics. It is the responsibility of the clinician to decide the proper technique that fulfills the patient's expectations and provides successful osseointegrated implant results. The members of the treatment team should be able to restore esthetic, phonetic, and functional requirements from the provisional restoration while simultaneously preserving or enhancing the condition of the dental and gingival tissues until the reconstruction of the final prosthesis is completed. Therefore, the primary goal of establishing a final restorative result should be no more successful than fabricating a functional esthetic provisional prosthesis that precedes it (Froum et al. 1997, Brown and Tarnow 2001, Ahn et al. 2004).

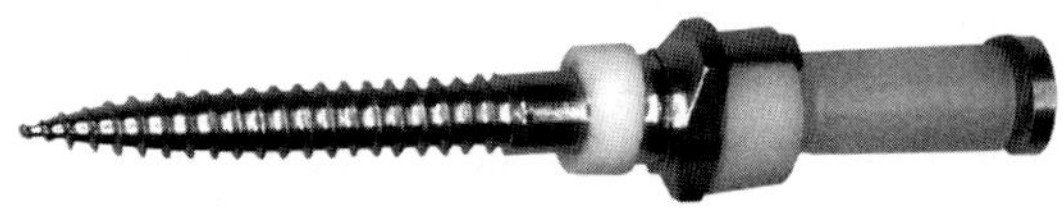

Figure 2.48. Anew Dentatus implant.

Establishing Esthetic Subgingival Profiles

Esthetic implant-supported restorations should duplicate the original contours and profile characters of the natural teeth from all aspects (Higginbottom and Wilson 2002, Sullivan 2001, Garber and Belser 1995). Consequently, the implant position within the alveolar ridge is critical to the final result, because the implant should be thought of as an extension of the clinical crown into the alveolar bone.

Several factors help determine the implant position as well as its relationship with the existing gingival contours. A number of factors also might influence the resultant emergence profile—the tissue biotype, the original tissue volume available prior to surgery, the accurate fabrication of the surgical template, the condition of the remaining natural teeth, and the ability of the dental technician to develop natural-looking prosthetic contours. Furthermore, achieving a flat emergence profile around implant-supported prostheses warrants obtaining sufficient information about the type of future prosthetic components that will be used. Because an implant fixture differs from a natural tooth in its morphological characteristics, the cylindrical or screw shape of the implant must be influenced within the subgingival compartment; for example, a central incisor, with a mesiodistal dimension of 6.4 mm at the CEJ level, and 5.5 mm at 2 mm apical to the CEJ, in contrast to the available known implant dimensions that are commonly used. Therefore, development of the proper emergence profile begins after stage-two surgery, with the placement of a properly contoured provisional restoration that allows expansion pressure on the surrounding peri-implant tissues. This facilitates ideal gingival scalloping and papillae reformation while creating a natural emergence profile that will be supported by the final restoration (See Figures 2.49A–B) (Belser et al. 1996).

The clinician must compensate for this dimensional discrepancy by developing the soft tissue margins and influencing them with the precise fabrication of a provisional restoration that transfers the cylindrical shape of the implant to the cross-sectional shape of the root of the natural tooth at the gingival margin, until it gradually

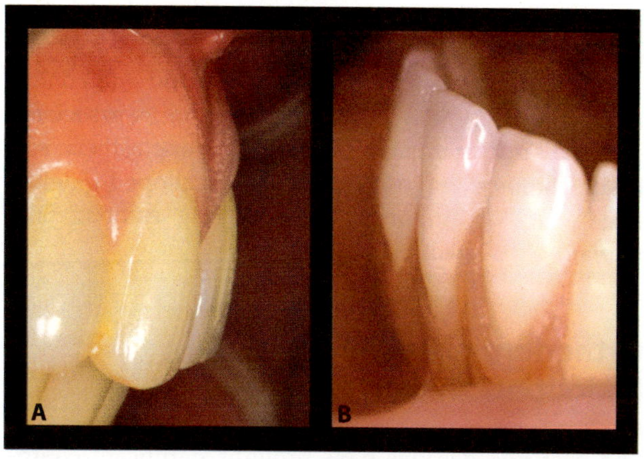

Figure 2.49. **A.** Flat emergence profile of the natural maxillary anterior teeth. **B.** Flat emergence profile of the natural mandibular anterior teeth.

shapes the peri-implant soft tissue to the desired configuration (Weisgold et al. 1997). Developing an optimal emergence profile is critical to achieving a final restoration that has soft tissue margins closely mimicking those of adjacent natural teeth.

The ability of the clinician to duplicate the emergence of the natural teeth to the implant-supported restorations becomes a vital factor in achieving natural esthetics. As the teeth emerge from the gingival area in a flat profile, this flat profile should be duplicated with the aid of the provisional restoration. Prior to implant installation, the clinician should evaluate the crestal bone-to-implant interface closely via the available versatile radiographic views to ensure the absence of any crestal bone deficiency. In the case of any suspected or confirmed facial bone loss, the dentist should directly evaluate the soft tissue. The treatment of the osseous deficiency is determined according to the type of bone defect, whether vertical or horizontal, or one wall, two walls, or multi-dimensional osseous deficiency. After the second-stage surgery, the final abutment and temporary restoration are inserted. The soft tissues are allowed to achieve full maturation along the contours of the provisional restoration before making the final restoration (Misch et al. 2004).

An anatomical cast may be fabricated by transferring the subgingival contours of the provisional restoration to the working cast. This may be accomplished with a custom impression coping or by retrofitting the provisional to the working cast. The optimal 3-D implant position of the implant head should be within 2 mm apical to the gingival zeniths of the adjacent natural teeth, with a buccal bone wall of at least 1 mm to 2 mm in thickness. Gingival augmentation procedures can be preformed at any time to resolve deficient gingival and mucosal contours, enhance existing thin facial tissues, and mask any metal that might show, ultimately creating a satisfactory treatment outcome.

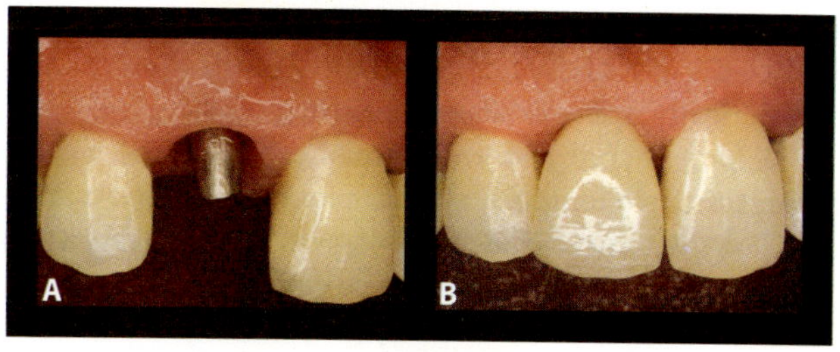

Figure 2.50. **A.** Gingival tissues opposite from the maxillary right central incisor. **B.** The flat emergence profile is being replicated via gingival stimulation and case restored.

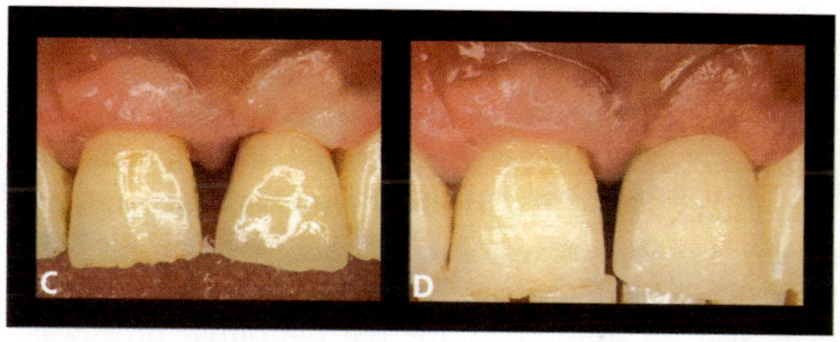

Figure 2.50. **C.** Implant-supported restoration restoring the maxillary left central incisor, showing deficient prosthetic dimensions that do not achieve an optimal emergence profile. **D.** The enhancements of the restoration lead to the correction of the emergence profile.

Developing a natural emergence profile starts when the position of the gingival margin following stage-two surgery is in a collapsed state and ends when it finds support by the prosthetic components against which it comes to rest (Potashnick and Rosenberg 1982). The gingival tissues around dental implant components should be enhanced, influenced, and developed to acquire the same dimensions and configurations of the original tissues around natural dentition. The original soft tissue configuration around dental implants attains a flat profile where they emerge from the free gingival margin (See Figures 2.50A–D) (Perel 1993, Croll 1989).

The subgingival area, and particularly the biological width, is the area that harbors the development of the emergence profile of the final prosthesis that should match the dimensions of the tooth to be replicated. The use of an accurately fabricated surgical template can help ensure accurate implant positioning in relation to the adjacent dentition, which directly influences the resultant emergence profile (Touati 1997b). Therefore, precise implant placement and careful soft-tissue manipulation will enable the clinician to enhance the peri-implant soft-tissue contours with the use of provisional restoration. Provisional restoration encourages gingival maturation via mild constant pressure to provide an ideal frame for the implant-supported prosthesis. The cervical third of the labial aspect of the provisional prosthesis is responsible for stimulating peri-implant tissues and developing the natural emergence. This process establishes a natural and esthetic soft tissue form that will set guidelines for laboratory fabrication of an anatomically appropriate soft tissue model.

The provisional restoration may be fabricated in the laboratory on a temporization coping. The clinician may also use the temporization coping chairside to fabricate a screw-retained provisional restoration or a cemented abutment may be used to support a cemented provisional restoration. There are many clinical methods available to duplicate the original emergence profile.

One method is used to create a provisional restoration that exactly represents the amount of profiling and reduces gingival trauma by eliminating the intraoral use of resin monomer and minimizes gingival surgical procedures by using properly contoured provisional restorations. This eliminates the possible heat from the polymerization process introduced (Macintosh and Sutherland 2004). The method entails the preparation of the provisional restoration emergence profile after the second-stage surgery, so that the developed shape may also be duplicated for the definitive prosthesis. The silicone soft-tissue substitute (Gingifast, Zhermack, Badia Polsine, Italy) or the gingival substitute is to be injected around the impression coping until the level of the substitute extends beyond the impression coping-abutment replica junction so the definitive cast can be placed and removed on the cast to allow access to view margins and the emergence profile. Then the internal emergence profile is shaped in the soft tissue substitute with a bur between the outer occlusal facing margin of the abutment replica and the free gingival margin. The soft tissue substitute can be removed and replaced on the cast to reduce the chance of damaging the abutment replica. Then a negative index of the diagnostic wax-up is made for making an indirect heat-polymerized provisional restoration. A provisional cylinder is to be placed on the abutment replica and trimmed so that the silicone index is seated completely; the resultant space between the soft tissue index and the provisional cylinder is the actual space for optimal emergence. An acrylic resin will then be poured (Duralay, Reliance Dental Manufacturing Co., Worth, IL, USA) into the index and onto the provisional cylinder, and the cast inverted into the index.

The entire assembly is then placed into a pressure vessel at 10 pounds psi, and the index is removed when polymerization is completed. The method provides a completed provisional restoration that only requires polishing and finishing with no discontinuities to fill. A natural flat emergence profile of any esthetic implant-supported restoration is important for hygiene, gingival health, and appearance. The vertical length of the subgingival portion of the restoration is particularly important because guided gingival growth is indirectly proportional to the submergence depth of the implant (Stein and Nevins 1996).

The ability of the clinician to understand and control the relationship between the implant and its associated gingival structures can lead to establishing esthetic soft tissue contours and a harmoniously scalloped gingival line, which is important in achieving esthetic final implant-supported restoration.

Orthodontic, Periodontic, and Endodontic Factors

The past two decades have brought significant contributions from orthodontics to today's implantology. Treatment is no longer restricted to juvenile and adolescent age groups. The advent of more esthetic and socially acceptable brackets and advancements in wire technology resulting in longer appointment intervals have significantly broadened the age spectrum as well as the scope of orthodontic treatment. On one end of this spectrum, orthodontic treatment is beginning at a much younger age than ever before; on the other end, adults and even the elderly are seeking orthodontic treatment as a solution to their overall oral rehabilitation. Implants have not only become a viable restorative option to replace missing teeth, but have also opened up many orthodontic possibilities. For example, implants can be used to provide anchorage in the edentulous spaces to make tooth movement possible and easier.

There has been a major paradigm shift in orthodontic diagnosis and treatment planning. The goal of the orthodontist is no longer just to fit the teeth within the dental arches to the best alignment. Contemporary orthodontists now strive to attain facial esthetics, dental esthetics, periodontal health, optimum functional occlusion, temporomandibular joint health, and long-term stability. This helps solve certain clinical dilemmas and reduce the tendency for performing invasive surgical procedures. Advances in digital imaging and radiography have significantly facilitated diagnosis and treatment planning. Many orthodontic software programs have been developed to aid orthodontists in simulating various treatment possibilities, allowing them to better educate their patients. These simulations, referred to as *visualized treatment objectives*, which were quite tedious to perform before computerization, test the feasibility of various treatment plans and the effect of the proposed treatments on appearance.

Proximal drifting of the remaining teeth occurs as a result of tooth loss, especially that due to premature extraction of deciduous dentition. The crowded dentition and the insufficient space do not allow for restoring teeth predictably (Salama and Salama 1993). Restoring lost space to its original optimal dimensions is becoming a valuable treatment factor that influences the final treatment outcome (Zaher 2000). Space developing is the optimal clinical solution to such cases. It requires a fairly long treatment time, but it is minimally invasive and provides more natural tissue contours.

Salama and others (1996) were the first to describe the applications of the conventional orthodontic techniques to facilitate implant placement. They made use of so-called restorative orthodontics to develop the supragingival restorative space (space development). They applied this technique in situations in which the residual space was not sufficient for placing a dental implant.

Periodontic-orthodontic management is yet another benefit of the modern orthodontics that is suggested for achieving greater osseous support (Ingber 1974, Brown 1973). This method entails forced eruption of unsalvageable residual roots that are scheduled to be replaced by dental implants. In other words, soft and hard tissues may be manipulated to favor the placement of an esthetic restoration (Bruskin et al. 2000).

Orthodontic extrusive remodeling or extrusion combined with tooth extraction is currently used in regular orthodontic treatments (Salama and Salama 1993). This procedure was originally performed to gain access to deep carious cavities or in the treatment of crown and root fractures below gingival margins. In this technique, slow eruption of teeth using a light eruptive force of 25 g to 30 g results in a coronal migration of the entire attachment apparatus (Beitan 1967). As a result, new bone is deposited in the apical area above the root apex, and is accompanied by an increase in the width of the attached mucosa and the proximal papillae at the cervical area (See Figure 2.51) (Perel 1993).

Orthodontic extrusion resembles forced tooth eruption or extrusion, because the tooth is moved coronally in both techniques. The main difference between these two techniques relies on the use or nonuse of supracrestal fiberotomy procedures. Supracrestal fiberotomy aims to detach the supracrestal periodontium from the tooth surface, minimizing coronal migration of these tissues. Because the present goal is not only to extract the tooth but also to develop both hard and soft tissues, no supracrestal fiberotomy procedures are performed. The tooth is coronally moved until extraction can be easily achieved and implant site development is achieved. Four months after orthodontic extrusion, both soft tissue and bone are moved coronally, as demonstrated clinically and radiographically. The alveolar bone attached to the root surface by periodontal fibers migrates along with the investing soft tissues in an incisal direction. Thus an increase in the available alveolar bone height is to be observed (Meyer and Bruce 2000). Subsequently, the coronal migration of the attachment complex promotes regeneration of the papilla and adjacent gingival contours, thus giving more freedom to surgical and esthetic implantology work. The tooth to be removed must be allowed to move only in an axial direction without tipping, which might cause penetration of the labial plate. Extrusion should be brought about at a speed that does not exceed the rate of bone deposition. It usually requires three to four months to occur; however, it requires only half the waiting time for a bone grafting procedure. Forced extrusion is less traumatic to the patient; however, patient selection and motivation are important factors to be considered before undertaking these procedures (See Figures 2.52A–C).

The local surrounding environment of the proposed implant sites can be an issue of concern during the

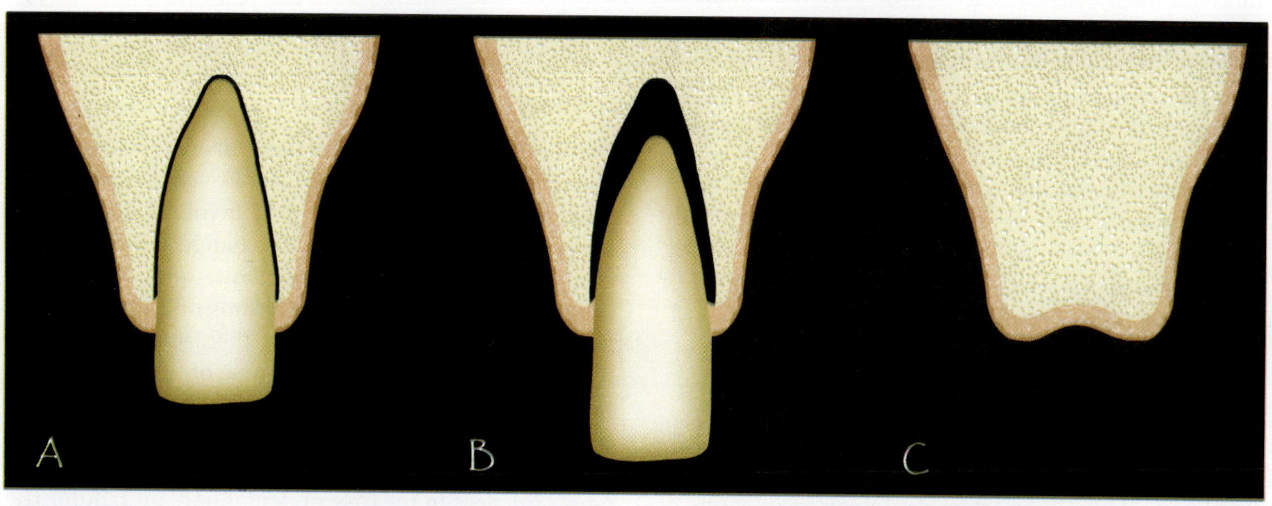

Figure 2.51. Illustration showing forced eruption sequence.

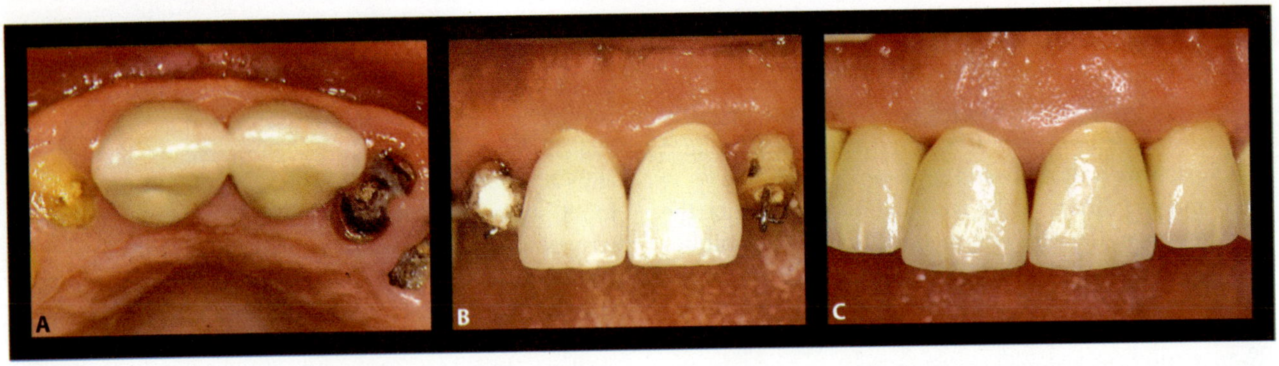

Figure 2.52. **A.** Intraoral view of unsalvageable severely compromised anterior teeth with loss of the natural height of the interdental papillae. **B.** The orthodontic appliance in action. Note the hook with the rings attached together. Note that forced eruption occurred to the roots with remarkable movement of the interdental papillae in an incisal direction. **C.** The case restored finally.

presurgical phase of implant therapy. Any endodontic lesion should be eliminated prior to implant surgery, because it can lead to implant failure (El Askary et al. 1999a). The implant can be particularly vulnerable if it is placed closer to an endodontic pathological lesion during the initial stage of osseointegration (Sussman and Moss 1993). This concern was raised in a case report by Sussman (1997) in which he suggested that an implant does not have the ability to withstand any bacterial challenge during the healing period.

However, Novaes and Novaes (1995) later argued that placement of an implant into a socket that has a chronic endodontic lesion does not necessarily result in failure, provided certain precautions are taken. The authors suggested complete removal of the causative factor (the unsalvageable tooth) with careful and thorough debridement of the socket, administration of antibiotics at least two days prior to surgery, and maintenance 10 days postoperatively. This was intended to reduce or eliminate the likelihood of bacterial contamination and allow the host cells to take control after the course of antibiotics was completed.

The decision whether to remove the lesion before or with the implant placement depends on the clinician's judgment. It is obvious that modern orthodontics has contributed immensely to implant dentistry. We currently benefit from this contribution; however, in some cases, implants must be disregarded. This is especially true when a space may not be created orthodontically, either because orthodontic treatment is not indicated or because the patient refuses to go through with it.

Decision Making in Esthetic Implantology Cases

Decision making in dental implantology cases is one of the clinician's delicate activities. The decisions include selecting a particular treatment method, specific surgical protocols, and particular materials, and they can influence the treatment's final outcome. Factors that affect the decisions in any treatment plan involving dental implant therapy are numerous, including time, cultural and ethnic background, physical appearance, age, profession, cost, lifestyle requirements, personality of the patient, intraoral condition, facial condition, skillfulness of the clinician, available modern diagnostic tools, and many others (Stein and Kuwata 1977, Frush and Fisher 1958).

Current data, statistical analysis methods, and technological advancements give the practitioner the ability to select a specific treatment path in a more thorough and predictable manner than ever before. When esthetics is a priority, the patient will preferably be actively involved in the details of the treatment plan, so the clinician can accurately ascertain their expectations. It is crucial to conceive and comprehend what is in the patient's best interest before any esthetic reconstructive methods are undertaken to avoid any future disappointments.

Financial Topics

Prior to the final selection of the course of treatment, the patient must be informed about the overall approximate financial cost as well as the time involved. One reason for patient dissatisfaction is the change of the financial plan, which leads to mistrust and questions. The budget should include detailed descriptions of all of the treatment elements. In addition, the patient should be told of the possibility of altering the course of treatment at any time and any related financial consequences and implications.

One of the most critical aspects of dental implantology is finances in the case of dental implant failure. The assignment of each party's responsibility and involvement becomes an important issue. Some clinicians prefer to completely cover the implant expense when implants fail during the first year postrestorative (if the clinicians complete the prostheses in their offices), whereas some prefer that the patient share in the responsibility for the failure. Yet others give lifetime warranties for their work. A common dilemma occurs when the surgical part of the dental implant service is conducted in one office and the prosthetic work is performed in another office. The ultimate responsibility for the cost of implant failure would be determined according to an agreement between the clinician and the patient that is made before treatment begins, or the responsibility lies with the restorative office, which may sometimes be unfair.

Fabricating an esthetic implant-supported prosthesis is unlike fabricating a merely functioning implant-supported prosthesis. The first scenario may involve higher treatment costs due to the possibility of using tooth-colored or laser-milled abutments or performing extra corrective surgeries. The fact that some clinicians charge more for esthetic rehabilitative cases than for regular cases requires an explanation to the client. An anterior implant-supported prosthesis invariably requires that the clinician spend more time, effort, and skill than they would on replacements in the posterior zone.

The clinician has probably participated in specific educational courses to learn more about restoring patients with esthetically predictable results; consequently, the overall cost of a single anterior implant-supported restoration can be up to one-third higher than the total cost of a posterior restoration. In fact, the time required for treatment may be doubled. Therefore, the most accurate estimate of the time and cost required for each treatment option should be a distinctive part of the doctor-patient preoperative conversation, and it should be confirmed with a singed consent by the patient.

It is also possible for the dentist to select a particular treatment plan, rather than follow an objective approach (Hebel et al. 2000). Just because the clinician is capable of performing some procedures better than others, it is the clinician who is, in the end, responsible for the treatment choice and its consecutive results. Therefore, the clinician is urged to select a reasonable treatment option that both suits the patient's best interests and matches the clinician's skills and training. This results in an individualized approach for each patient.

Treatment planning and acceptance of a proposed plan are influenced to a large degree by the cost of treatment and corresponding insurance coverage in some countries. The proposed treatment plan must be affordable to the patient and remunerative to the provider. In many situations, the treatment sequence is conducted in stages to maximize insurance coverage. While staged or quadrant dentistry has become the normal when treating patients who want to maximize insurance benefits, it does not always reflect the ideal approach or proper treatment sequence. For example, a patient with extensive dental needs and limited insurance benefits may desire to have the more visible anterior crowns completed first, although the posterior crowns may have a higher functional priority. Treating the anterior teeth first may be a mistake, especially if the patient does not follow through with the posterior crowns.

A rational treatment plan cannot be subverted to meet unrealistic patient demands or to maximize insurance benefits. The public perception is that dental insurance should pay for the treatment of dental diseases; however, the reality is that most insurance plans provide inadequate benefits for effective treatment of dental diseases, whether the treatment is innovative or even considered to be standard, such as implants. The increase in the number of insurance plans and third-party payers clearly influences (and will continue to influence) the treatment planning process in many countries.

A recent study (Bragger et al. 2005) assessed and compared economic parameters of two treatment options in patients requiring single-tooth replacements. Thirty-seven patients received 41 conventional three-unit fixed partial dentures (FPD). Fifty-two patients received 59 single crowns on implants. Economic parameters were noted for the preparatory phase, the actual reconstruction, and treatment of biological and/or technical complications thereafter for a period of one to four years. This included the number of visits, chair-side time, treatment costs, costs for implant components, and laboratory work.

The results showed that the total treatment time was similar. Laboratory costs were higher for FPD, and costs for treatment of technical and biological complications were similar. Even when considering opportunity costs for each visit, the implant solution was less expensive. Costs for treatment of complications were similar in both situations. The study concluded that over a short observation period, implant reconstruction demonstrated a more favorable cost-effectiveness ratio. Especially in clinical situations involving no restored teeth, minimally restored teeth, or sufficient bone, implant reconstruction should be recommended from an economical point of view.

Selecting Suitable Treatment Options

Various methods for restoring lost anterior teeth include conventional bridges, resin-bonded bridges, implant-supported restorations, removable partial dentures, or a combination of all of these options.

Conventional Fixed Bridges

Conventional fixed bridges have long been considered the most ideal treatment modality for restoring natural dentition. They have exhibited clinically proven high success rates with their excellent esthetics and long-term functional serviceability, even if the structure of the remaining natural teeth was compromised (Meyenberg 1995). However, in spite of their outstanding clinical performance, there is a significant variation in their success rates, documented in the literature as ranging from 97 to 80% (Palmquist and Swartz 1993, Schwartz et al. 1970).

These variations are probably due to differences in clinical performance, precision of the bridge fabrication, and the type of metal alloy used. Conventional single-tooth replacement with fixed partial dentures involves several biological and technical risks, such as endodontic complications, secondary caries, difficult access for plaque control resulting in periodontal complications, loss of retention, and fractures of abutment teeth. The main reason for failure of conventional bridges is attributed to endodontic failure of the abutment teeth after an unknown period of time (Meyenberg and Imoberdof 1997). The extensive destruction of the abutment teeth through tooth preparation for conventional bridges is now considered to be a clinical drawback, especially when the teeth are sound. The immense loss of tooth structure during tooth preparation can be the actual reason for unsatisfactory results that result from this treatment option.

With the evolution of dental implants, there is greater emphasis on the preservation of natural teeth that would normally be used to serve as abutments for a fixed bridge. In other words, dental implants have led to increased preservation of remaining natural teeth. Dental implants are used to replace missing teeth without resorting to including adjacent abutment teeth that are in relatively good condition. Using general standards in the literature, the average lifetime of a fixed bridge is 8.3 years to 10.3 years (Koth 1982, Silness 1970). This might raise the question of how many restorations a young patient might require over a lifetime. Alternatively, if the teeth adjacent to an edentulous space have either severe attrition or a gross restoration, dental implants may not be the preferred treatment option. In this case, it is better to consider protecting and splinting these compromised teeth within a bridge framework. Thus, the condition and number of the remaining dentition, parafunctional habits, type of occlusion, and leverage are all factors that help determine the appropriateness of this treatment modality.

Adhesive Bridges

Adhesive bridges, which eliminate the need for substantial destruction of natural abutments, are another option. Adhesive bridges were originally introduced by Rochette (1986) to be used as periodontal splints. However, adhesive bridges require greater clinical skills than do conventional bridges, and there is the possibility of recurrent dental caries occurring around the bridge margins and line angles. Debonding of adhesive bridges, which leads to loosening of the bridge, tends to occur at a frequency rate as high as 25% to 31% (Hussey et al. 1991, Williams 1989). The debonding tendency is considered to be the major complication of this type of bridge, which limits its regular daily use.

Resin-bonded restorations have shown a wide range of clinical results, as cited in the literature, from a failure rate of 54% in 11 months (when used in the absence of mechanical retentive methods) to a success rate of 92.9% in 127 cases (with a mean longevity of five years) (Hansson 1994, Barrack and Bretz 1993). Resin-bonded bridges are only suggested for patients seeking a temporary, inexpensive esthetic solution for a particular period of time. The specific nature of this treatment option should be explicitly explained.

Dental Implants

Unlike the previous treatment alternatives, dental implants have been exhaustively investigated under controlled parameters as treatment options, especially for completely edentulous patients (Priest 1996, Haas et al. 1995, Jemt et al. 1990). Since the late 1980s, continuous research and sophisticated statistical analyses have shown dental implants to be a predictable treatment option for dental restoration in totally and partially edentulous patients.

The scope of dental implants was later expanded to include the treatment of missing single teeth. This treatment has shown consistent success rates ranging from 91% to 97.4% over a three- to six-year period (Haas et al. 1995, Jemt et al. 1990). However, a few complications were encountered with this treatment modality; screw loosening has been reported most often in single-tooth implant-supported restorations (Schwarz 2000). This drawback has been overcome greatly by the introduction of new implant-abutment connections that provide greater surface areas, stability against lateral displacement, and a predictable retention.

Implant dentistry has dramatically changed the conventional routine of restorative dentistry. It has inspired many clinicians who, in turn, have contributed to improving the clinical esthetic outcome of this treatment modality. New soft and hard tissue augmentation procedures were developed to optimize the long-term esthetic outcome of dental implants (Grunder et al. 1996). In partially edentulous patients, dental implants offer the advantage of eliminating the natural abutment preparation. These procedures are considered to be the best tooth replacement alternatives for both young and old patients because they preserve the structural integrity of the natural dentition. The cumulative survival rate of oral implants supporting FPDs was 95.4% after five years of function and 92.8% after 10 years. This evidence is derived from 10 prospective and five retrospective cohort studies with a mean of five years of follow-up and six prospective cohort studies with a mean 10-year follow-up (Lang et al. 2004). The cumulative survival rate of FPDs supported by oral implants was 95% after five years of function and 86.7% after 10 years. This evidence is derived from 14 studies including 1,289 FPDs after five years and three studies including 219 FPDs after 10 years (Lang et al. 2004).

If the dental implant treatment fails at any time, other treatment options are still available, which makes this modality unique. Moreover, retrospective and prospective studies have reported that dental implants have a positive effect on the recipient's well-being and quality of life, which has added a new social dimension to this treatment modality (Bloomberg and Linquist 1983).

Removable Partial Dentures

Designing a removable partial denture (RPD) is much more than a mechanical exercise in selecting from a list of clasps, rests, major connectors, and other components that are assembled within the framework. It is sometimes a tedious procedure to fabricate a properly designed partial denture. Insight on the intraoral condition should include the evaluation of the following factors:

- Health of the periodontium
- Length of the tooth roots and the crown-root ratio
- Whether a tooth will stand alone or should be splinted to another tooth by a complex double clasp or fixed restoration
- Character of supporting soft tissue
- Health and condition of the adjacent tooth
- Whether the ridges are well healed
- Whether the soft tissue is firm or flabby
- Nature and strength of the teeth, including the type of materials used in restorations
- Health of the natural tooth structure
- Location and condition of the amalgam, that is, composite, gold, and/or ceramic restorations for any occlusal rest usage
- Whether the patient will accept the display of any metal components
- Understanding the psychological needs and desires of the patient

RPDs have been the treatment of choice when there are multiple missing teeth that may be dispersed throughout the dental arch and that are not necessarily next to each other. This option is also indicated when the remaining teeth are mobile and future extractions are expected. In addition, when patient resources are limited and the cost of treatment is a determining factor, the relative inexpensiveness of removable partial dentures becomes a good incentive for choosing this treatment. However, as with other treatment options, partial dentures have a fairly high number of drawbacks. The possibility of periodontal disease and natural tooth decay adjacent to the abutment teeth is one of the major disadvantages. Resorption of the alveolar ridge due to pressure from the fitting surface is another (Tuominen et al. 1989, Wright et al. 1992, Witter et al. 1989). In addition, certain parts of the denture framework or acrylic resin can sometimes become visible while talking or smiling, which may not be esthetically pleasing and thus may negatively contribute to the social dimension (Cowan et al. 1991). The esthetic and functional outcome of fixed partial dentures, that is, conventional bridges, is usually considered to be superior to that of a removable partial denture (Budtz-Jg̊ensen and Isidor 1987).

Selecting Suitable Treatment Techniques

The optimal implant placement technique will preserve the alveolar ridge, provide satisfactory esthetic results, and enhance esthetic soft tissue contours around dental implants, especially when the anterior maxilla is involved. The decision whether to insert the implant immediately after tooth extraction or delay its placement until total socket healing occurs is based on many factors (Tarnow and Fletcher 1993). These include soft tissue health and integrity, tissue biotype, the need to preserve interdental papillae, prevention of alveolar ridge resorption, the pathological and morphological condition of the alveolar socket immediately after extraction, patient demands, and the predictability of osseointegration. It must be duly noted that the decision on the timing of dental implant placement is critical and can significantly affect treatment results from the esthetic standpoint and/or that of serviceability.

The standard protocol for placing dental implants requires an alveolar ridge that is completely healed before inserting the implant fixture (Laney 1986). This is called the *delayed implant placement protocol* and requires a healing period varying between five and nine months post-tooth extraction before implant placement (Adell et al. 1981). The healing period not only allows the placement of the implant fixture in mature osseous architecture, but also permits the maturation of the associated soft tissue in the future implant site. This ultimately minimizes the need for excessive soft tissue manipulative procedures that are required to achieve primary soft tissue closure. The need for bone-grafting procedures is also minimized, especially in the posterior areas, because greater implant-bone contact is ensured. This in turn eliminates the possibility of epithelial down-growth into the osteotomy site.

However, delayed implant placement may not be the treatment of choice in all regions. In the maxillary anterior zone, in particular, delaying implant placement results in alveolar ridge resorption, both in the buccolingual and apicoincisal directions (Atwood and Coy 1971), which usually necessitates the use of guided tissue regenerative techniques to provide maximum esthetics. Furthermore, studies have shown that as much as 3mm to 4mm of alveolar ridge resorption can occur during the first six months after tooth extraction (if no bone-grafting procedures have been performed at the time of tooth extraction) (Johnson 1963). Other reports have indicated that 23% of the anterior alveolar ridge resorption takes place within the first six months following tooth extraction (Carlsson et al. 1967). This process significantly affects the topography of the hard and soft tissues, which in turn may hinder the esthetic 3-D positioning of the implant.

Some clinicians prefer the delayed implant placement technique; their reasons include reducing the risk of infection and reducing soft tissue manipulations (Misch et al. 1999). Postextraction bone resorption remains a controversial issue to be considered.

On the other hand, immediate implant placement has been extensively documented in the literature (Brazilay 1988, Becker and Becker 1990, Lazzara 1989). In this approach, the implant fixture is inserted immediately following the unsalvageable tooth extraction. This procedure may be performed with or without bone grafting of the space between the implant body and the alveolar socket walls. Immediate implant insertion can be an effective method to prevent the alveolus from undergoing postextraction resorption (Dennisen et al. 1993, Sclar 1999).

One solid reason for the increasing popularity of immediate implant placement is its proven success rate. Several studies have shown success rates using immediate implants that are comparable to those of implants inserted into healed sites (Mensdorff-Pouilly et al. 1994, Watzek et al. 1995, Rosenquist and Grenthe 1996). This technique's credibility has been further increased by the absence of infection, good mechanical anchorage and primary stability of the implant fixture, traumatic removal of the unsalvageable tooth with preservation of the labial plate of bone, use of the appropriate implant size and design that corresponds to the existing socket's configuration, and proper implant placement in terms of angulation and position. Unfortunately, most of the studies have measured success in terms of osseointegration, but have not considered soft tissue changes.

The soft tissue compromise that results from attempting the primary closure on top of the freshly extracted tooth socket, which directly influences the final esthetic soft tissue outcome, is the primary concern associated with this technique. A recent study recommended that wide-diameter implants be used with caution in esthetically demanding areas (Small et al. 2001). This was based on the conclusion that after the second stage of surgery the soft tissue receded an average of 1.58mm around wide-diameter implants, compared with a recession of 0.57mm around small-diameter implants (Small et al. 2001).

Extraction of a tooth leaves behind a socket that has its own characteristics. Many authors have classified extraction sites at the time of implant placement and have suggested clinical solutions for each class (Salama and Salama 1993, Gelb 1993, Ashman et al. 1995, Meltzer 1995, Tehemar 1999). The classifications of the socket condition can provide the clinician with an accurate diagnostic tool to deal with the different clinical situations. Salama and Salama (1993) have classified the socket state as follows:

- Class One describes a socket that has intact walls and is favorable for immediate implant placement with or without bone grafting.
- Class Two has a socket with a missing labial wall, necessitating the use of guided tissue regeneration (GTR) and a bone graft in conjunction with implant placement.
- Class Three refers to a socket that does not provide any implant anchorage and requires the application of a staged implant insertion as well as bone-grafting procedures.

Garber and Belser (1995) have categorized immediate implant sites after tooth extraction as follows:

- Type I is a socket having dehiscence of less than 5mm; this type is almost equivalent to the first class in Salama and Salama's classifications.
- Type II is a socket that has a dehiscence equal to 5mm; it requires autogenous bone grafting and GTR.
- Type III is a socket with a dehiscence of more than 5mm; it offers no primary stability for the implant fixture and warrants a staged approach for implant insertion and bone-grafting procedures.

Meltzer (1995) described four classes of socket conditions:

- A Class I socket possesses intact walls all over.
- A Class II socket has a fenestrated wall.
- A Class III socket has sufficient bone height, but not enough width, or has two missing osseous walls.
- A Class IV socket has insufficient or no vertical dimension.

The soft tissues surrounding the immediate dental implants also can be classified. This classification yields a more accurate description of the status of the socket at the time of immediate implant placement (Tehemar 1999). An immediate implant procedure offers many advantages, including optimal implant placement (i.e., the original tooth place), which thus minimizes the need for severely angulated abutments, and alveolar ridge preservation due to prevention of the postextraction resorption, which permits the use of longer and wider implants. Other advantages are (1) minimizing the possibility for injury of anatomical landmarks, (2) limiting postdrilling bone resorption by reducing heat generation during drilling, and (3) reducing treatment time to almost half. There is also a positive psychological impact on the patient in relation to dental implants because immediate replacement of the extracted root/tooth takes place without a delay while the patient waits for socket healing.

A nonsubmerged protocol for immediate implantation was proposed by Saadoun and La Gall (1998). In this protocol, the implant and healing abutment are connected at the time of implant placement without attempting any soft tissue modifications. This technique minimizes soft tissue trauma and plays a significant role in the maturation of the soft tissue around the site. Using an implant diameter that corresponds to the socket orifice will eventually reduce the need for bone grafting and prevent the in-growth of soft tissue along the socket walls (Wheeler et al. 2000).

However, soft tissue closure is still questionable in terms of predictable osseointegration. Lack of direct visibility of the labial plate of the alveolar bone raises some serious concerns over this procedure and its clinical success. The immediate delayed protocol of implant placement, on the other hand, permits soft tissue granulation on the socket orifice. Soft tissue requires six to 10 weeks after tooth extraction to mature. This approach aids in developing a soft tissue seal on top of the socket by secondary intention, after which the implant is placed, as is the case of the standard delayed method. The newly formed keratinized tissue helps minimize soft tissue complications that might arise from excessive surgical manipulations made to achieve primary closure in cases of immediate implant placement. Interestingly, a study by Osigo and others (1995) described another method for delayed implantation. This technique employs an implant osteotomy followed by wound closure without actually inserting the implant. Two weeks later, the patient undergoes another surgery to place the implant. The authors found that many new thin trabeculae and capillaries formed around the osteotomy walls during the waiting period, and the surrounding fibrous tissue encapsulation appeared to a lesser extent, thus enhancing osseointegration. This approach makes the technique clinically and practically inapplicable.

Another implant placement protocol is the one-stage implant placement technique. This refers to the insertion of a one-piece implant in a single surgical procedure, eliminating the second-stage surgery. The technique is similar to the nonsubmerged protocol of implant placement. The implant penetrates the soft tissue through the flared implant neck itself. The method can be used in both delayed and immediate cases. The use of nonsubmerged, one-piece implants has shown immense clinical success, especially at the functional level, with the ease of prosthetic management (Buser et al. 1997, Buser et al. 1999). The one-stage system eliminates the possibility of microgap formation between the abutment and the implant fixture at the level of the bone crest. These advantages certainly increase the popularity of this type of implant. It must be noted that the technique is restricted to areas where esthetics are not of chief concern (See Figures 2.53A–C) (Cornelini et al. 2000).

Diagnostic Checklist

A complex decision-making process will influence the choice of treatment path, such as the clinician's access to technology, level of skill, education, philosophy, evi-

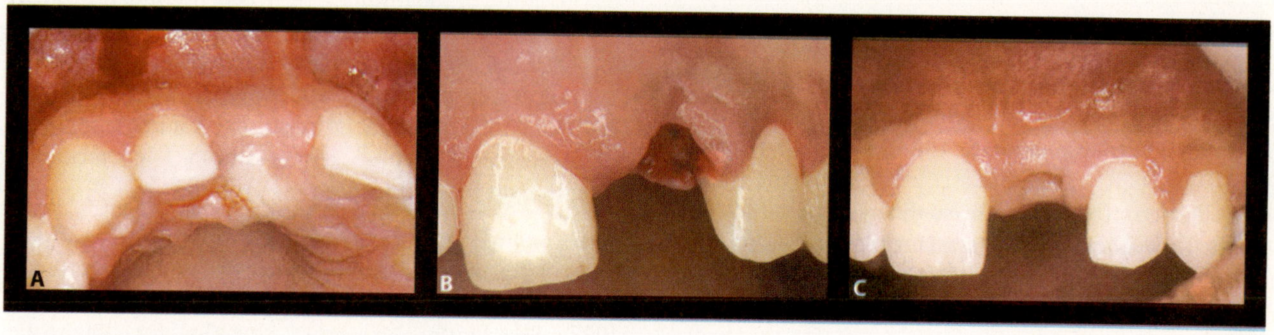

Figure 2.53. **A.** Healed osseous site that is scheduled for delayed implant placement protocol. **B.** Fresh extraction site that is scheduled for immediate implant placement. **C.** Partially healed site (i.e., the soft tissue is only healed but not the bone; the case is scheduled for delayed immediate implant therapy).

dence from the literature, and financial aspects (such as costs, investment, and amortization). In addition, patient preferences, treatment time, the number of visits, comfort, pre- and postoperative complications, and reluctance to undergo surgery are all factors to be considered. Patients seeking esthetic treatment should be encouraged to understand and evaluate the entire scope of the clinical task. When patients fully comprehend the extent of the work entailed, they are able to appreciate it and convey a positive impression to their personal contacts. In other words, the patient's positive attitude and greater willingness to cooperate during the treatment surely lead to a better working environment for the entire dental team.

Restoring function is and will continue to remain the primary goal of oral implantology. The functional aspect of the implant-supported prostheses should be emphasized and predicted first, because dental implants should be placed for long-term survival. Esthetics should be viewed as a complementary clinical benefit. Any planned implant-supported restorations in the esthetic zone should fulfill both functional and esthetic goals, but function should not be jeopardized due to overemphasizing esthetics. Any esthetic implant-supported restoration that fails to meet the functional goal cannot be considered a success, and vice versa. The delicate balance between function and esthetics must be maintained because they both complement the treatment outcome, which emphasizes the value of the presurgical stage as an integral part of the treatment. Misch (1999d) stated that too often the profession concentrates only on esthetics and soft tissue contours that might be accomplished at the expense of the sulcular health. Therefore, any excessive manipulations that focus only on the soft tissue appearance regardless of the osseous support will be disqualified. In other words, solid criteria for patient selection, aseptic surgical techniques, biomechanical concepts, and rigorous maintenance should be carefully regarded in any definitive treatment plan.

An interesting consensus has been published recently that evaluated the Clinical Procedures Regarding Esthetics in Implant Dentistry (Belser et al. 2004). In this consensus, the esthetic zone was defined objectively by Belser and others (2004) as any dentoalveolar segment that is visible upon full smile. Subjectively, the esthetic zone can be defined as any dentoalveolar area of esthetic importance to the patient. The consensus discussed three aspects: (1) outcome analysis of implant restorations located in the anterior maxilla, (2) anatomical and surgical considerations of implant therapy in the anterior maxilla, and (3) practical prosthodontic procedures related to anterior maxillary fixed implant restorations. However, the authors stated that most of these studies do not include well-defined esthetic parameters. The success rate of dental implants placed and restored in the esthetic zone have success rates similar to those reported for other segments of the jaws. Single anterior tooth replacement therapy revealed that predictable treatment outcomes, including esthetics, can be achieved because tissue support is provided by adjacent teeth. Multiple adjacent teeth replacement in the esthetic zone with fixed implant restorations was poorly documented, and esthetic restoration is not predictable, particularly regarding the contours of the interimplant soft tissue.

The consensus stated that implant therapy in the anterior maxilla is considered an advanced or complex procedure and requires comprehensive preoperative planning and precise surgical execution based on a restoration-driven approach. Patient selection should be approached with caution, because esthetic results are less consistent in smoking as well as systemically involved patients. Implant size and morphology selection should be conducted to favor soft tissue health and integrity, as well as the optimal 3-D implant positioning that is essential for any esthetic treatment outcome which results in an implant shoulder located in an ideal position, allowing for an esthetic implant restoration with stable, long-term peri-implant tissue support.

Another recommendation (Chiche and Aoshima 1997) for achieving optimal esthetic implantology results stated that sufficient horizontal and vertical bone volume is essential to obtain esthetic results. When deficiencies exist, appropriate hard and/or soft tissue augmentation procedures should be preformed. However, vertical bone deficiencies often lead to esthetic shortcomings. The esthetic peri-implant tissues, including health, height, volume, color, and contours, must be in harmony with the adjacent dentition. The restoration should imitate the natural appearance of the missing dental unit(s) in color, form, texture, size, and optical properties. Use of provisional restorations to optimize esthetic treatment outcomes is recommended to guide and shape the peri-implant tissue prior to definitive restoration. The esthetic-related soft tissue parameters that are clinically valid include:

1. Location of the midfacial mucosal implant margin in relation to the incisal edge or implant shoulder
2. Distance between the tip of the papilla and the most apical interproximal contact point
3. The width of the facial keratinized mucosa
4. Assessment of mucosal conditions (e.g., modified gingival index, bleeding on probing)

In conclusion, esthetics and function must be monitored and restored simultaneously when significant esthetic alterations are performed (Chiche and Aoshima 1997). See Figure 2.54 for a checklist for diagnostic elements to be considered in the treatment plan. The

Bone	Height	
	Width	
K.Tissue	Same Level With Contra Lateral	
	0.5 mm Less	
	1.0 mm Less	
Socket condition	Fresh Socket	
	Healed Socket	
	Partially healed Socket	
Natural teeth centric relation	Coinciding	
	Not coinciding	
Dynamic Condition of the teeth	Canine guidance	
	Incisal guidance	
	Group function	
Inter arch space (vertical)	Optimal	
	Defective	
	Excessive	
Available inter-dental spaces(horizontal)	Optimal	
	Defective	
	Excessive	
Arch form	Square	
	Ovoid	
	V Shaped	
Tissue bio type	Thin scalloped	
	Thick flat	
Opposing dentition	Natural teeth	
	Fixed bridge	
	Removable denture	
	Implants supp.	
Soft tissue pigmentation	Pigmented	
	Not Pigmented	
Tooth shape	Square	
	Cylinder	
	Triangular	
Related anatomical structures		
Missing teeth number	Single	
	Multiple	Adjacent
		Scattered
Soft tissue volume (labial)	Optimal level	
	Deficient	
Bone density	D1	
	D2	
	D3	
	D4	
Socket condition	Suppuritive	
	Healthy	
	Chronic infection	
Adjacent teeth	Periodontally involved	
	Apical Pathosis	
	Carious	
	Sound	
Scar tissue	Exists	
	Don't Exist	
Para function	Free	
	Clenching	
	Bruxing	
	Tapping	
	Tongue Thrusting	

Position of the inter-dental papilla	filling	
	Partially filling	
	Not filling	
Condition of the existing papilla(Nordland)	Class I	
	Class II	
	Class III	
(Predictability of the peri-implant papilla. Tarnow) Distance from the contact point of the natural tooth to the crest of the bone	5 mm	
	6 mm	
	7 mm or more	
(Predictability of the inter-implant papilla. Salama)	Class I IHB	
	Class II IHB	
	Class III IHB	
Lower lip position	Covered	
	Touching	
	Not Touching	
Upper lip position	High	
	Average	
	Low	
Upper lip curvature	Upward	
	Straight	
	Downward	
Smile arc	Parallel	
	Straight	
	Reversed	
Smile reveal	Max. teeth	
	Max.teeth+3 mm gingiva	
	Max. & Mand.	
	Mand. Only	
	Nor Mand. nor Max.	
Smile line	High	
	Medium	
	Low	
Midline Relationship of teeth (Central Incisor) to face(philtrum)	Symmetric	
	Right of center	
	Left of center	
Nasolabial angle	Prominent Maxilla < 90	
	Normal Apprx. 90	
	Retruded Maxilla > 90	
Rickets E-Plane	WNL	
	Convex	
	Concave	
Midline-Skewing to left or right	Right	
	Left	
	Straight	
Bilateral negative Space	Normal	
	Increased	
Teeth Symmetry	Symmetrical	
	Not Symmetrical	
Gingival Pigmentation	Physiologic	
	Non-physiologic	pathologic
		non-pathologic

Figure 2.54. A checklist for diagnostic elements to be considered in the treatment plan.

successful clinician working in the esthetic zone should have a good biologic understanding of tissue response to implant placement, a thorough surgical education enabling performance of precise and low-trauma surgical procedures, and a large patient pool providing sufficient surgical experience with esthetic implant placement (Buser et al. 2004).

References

Adell, R., U. Lekholm, B. Rockler, and P.I. Brånemark. 1981. A 15-year study of osseointegrated implants in the treatment of the edentulous jaw. *Int J Oral Surg*, (10), pp. 387–416.

Ahn, M., K. An, J. Choi, et al. 2004. Immediate Loading with Mini Dental Implants in the Fully Edentulous Mandible *Implant Dent*, 13, pp. 367–372.

Albrektsson, T. 1988. A multicenter report on osseointegrated oral implants. *J Prosthet Dent*, 60, pp. 75–84.

Ashman, A., I. LoPoint, and J. Rosenlicht. 1995. Ridge augmentation for immediate post-extraction implants: Eight year retrospective study. *Prct Periodont Aesthet Dent*, (7), pp. 85–95.

Atwood, D.A., and D.A. Coy. 1971. Clinical, cephalometric and ensitometric study of reduction of residual ridge. *J Prosthet Dent*, (26), pp. 280–293.

Bain, C.A. 1996. Smoking and implant failure–A smoking cessation protocol. *Int J Oral Maxillofac Implants*, 11, pp. 756–759.

Bain, C.A., and P.K. Moy. 1993. The association between the failure of dental implants and cigarette smoking. *Int J Oral Maxillofac Implants*, (8), pp. 609–615.

Balshi, T.J., and D.G. Garver. 1986. Osseointegration: The efficacy of the transitional denture. *Int J Oral Maxillofac Implants*, (1), pp. 113–118.

Barrack, G., and W.A. Bretz. 1993. A long-term prospective study of the acid etched-cast restoration. *Int J Prosthodont*, (6), pp. 428–434.

Becker, W., and B.E. Becker. 1990. Guided tissue regeneration for implants placed into extraction sockets and for implant dehiscences: Surgical techniques and case reports. *Int J Periodont Rest Dent*, (10), pp. 377–391.

Becker, C.M., and D.A. Kaiser. 2000. Surgical guide for dental implant placement. *J Prosthet Dent*, (83), pp. 248–251.

Becker, W., B.E. Becker, M.G. Newman, and S. Nyman. 1990. Clinical and microbiologic findings that may contribute to dental implant failure. *Int J Oral Maxillofac Surg*, 5, pp. 31–38.

Bedrossian, E. 2000. Veneer Grafting: A technique for augmentation of the resorbed alveolus prior to implant placement. A clinical report. *Int J Oral Maxillofac Implants*, 15, pp. 853–858.

Beitan, K. 1967. Clinical and histological observations on tooth movement during and after orthodontic treatment. *Am J Orthod*, (53), pp. 721–745.

Belser, U.C., J.P. Bernard, and D. Buser. 1996. Implant-supported restorations in the anterior region: prosthetic considerations. *Pract Periodontics Aesthet Dent*, 8, pp. 875–883, quiz 884.

Belser, U., D. Buser, and F. Higginbottom. 2004. Consensus Statements and Recommended Clinical Procedures Regarding Esthetics in Implant Dentistry. *Int J Oral Maxillofac Implants*, 19, pp. 873–874.

Bengazi, F., L. Wennstrom, and U. Lekholm. 1996. Recession of the soft tissue margin at oral implants: A 2-year longitudinal prospective study. *Clin Oral Implant Res*, (7), pp. 303–310.

Berglundh, T., and J. Lindhe. 1996. Dimension of the peri-implant mucosa: Biological width revisited. *J Clin Periodontol*, (23), pp. 971–973.

Bergström, J., and H. Preber. 1994. Tobacco as a risk factor. *J Periodontal*, 65 (May suppl.), pp. 545–550.

Bezzon, O.L. 1993. Allergic sensitivity to several base metals: A clinical report. *J Prosthet Dent*, (70), pp. 109–110.

Bichacho, N., C.J. Landsberg, M. Rohrer, et al. 1999. Immediate fixed transitional restoration in implant therapy. *Pract Periodontics Aesthet Dent*, 11, (1), pp. 45–51.

Biggs, W.F. 1996. Placement of a custom implant provisional restoration at the second-stage surgery for improved gingival management: A clinical report. *J Prosthet Dent*, (75), pp. 231–233.

Bloomberg, S., and L. Linquist. 1983. Psychological reactions to edentulousness and treatment with jaw bone-anchored bridges. *Acta Psychiatr Scand*, (68), pp. 251–262.

Bombonato, K., G. Brentegani, A. Thomazini, et al. 2004. Alcohol intake and Osseointegration around Implants: A Histometric and Scanning Electron Microscopy Study. *Implant Dent*, 13, pp. 238–244.

Bragger, U., P. Krenander, and N.P. Lang. 2005. Economic aspects of single-tooth replacement. *Clin. Oral Impl.* Res. 16, pp. 335–341.

Brazilay, I. 1988. Immediate implantation of pure titanium threaded implants into extraction sockets. *J Dent Res*, (67), p. 234.

Breeding, L.C., and D. Dixon. 1992. Compression resistance of four interocclusal recording materials. *J Prosthet Dent*, 68, p. 876.

Brown, M., and D. Tarnow. 2001. Fixed provisionalization with transitional implants for partially edentulous patients: A case report. *Pract Periodontics Aesthet Dent*, 13, (2), pp. 123–127.

Brown, I.S. 1973. The effect of orthodontic therapy on certain types of periodontal defects. *J Periodontol*, 44, (12), pp. 742–756.

Bruskin, R., P. Castellon, and J. Hochstedler. 2000. Orthodontic extrusion and orthodontic extraction in preprosthetic treatment using implant therapy. *Pract Periodont Aesthet Dent*, (12), pp. 213–221.

Budtz-Jǧensen, E., and F. Isidor. 1987. Cantilever bridges or removable partial dentures in geriatric patients: A two-year study. *J Oral Rehab*, (14), pp. 239–249.

Buhler, H. 1988. Evaluation of root resected teeth. Results after 10 years. *J Periodontol* 59, pp. 805–810.

Buser, D., R. Mericske-Stern, J.P. Bernard, A. Behneke, N. Behneke, H.P. Hirt, U.C. Belser, and N.P. Lang. 1997. Long-term evaluation of non-submerged ITI implants. Part 1: Eight-year life table analysis of a prospective multimember study with 2,359 implants. *Clin Oral Implant Res*, (8), pp. 161–172.

Buser, D., R. Mericske-Stern, K. Dula, and N.P. Lang. 1999. Clinical experience with one-stage, non-submerged dental implants. *Adv Dent Res*, (13), pp. 153–161.

Buser, D., W. Martin, and U. Belser. 2004. Optimizing Esthetics for Implant Restorations in the Anterior Maxilla: Anatomic and Surgical Considerations. *Int J Oral Maxillofac Implants*, 19, pp. 43–61.

Carlsson, G.E., B. Bergman, and B. Headegard. 1967. Changes in contour of the maxillary alveolar process under immediate dentures. A longitudinal clinical and x-ray cephalometric study covering 5 years. *Acta Odontol Scand*, (25), pp. 45–75.

Cehreli, M., C. Calis, and S. Sahin. 2002. A dual-purpose guide for optimum placement of dental implants. *J Prosthet Dent*, 88, pp. 640–643.

Cenrell, M.C., and S. Sahin. 2000. Fabrication of a dual-purpose surgical template for correct labiopalatal positioning of dental implants. *Int J Oral Maxillofac Implants*, (15), pp. 278–282.

Chai, Y., and H.C. Slavkin. 2003. Prospects for tooth regeneration in the 21st century: a perspective. *Microsc Res Tech*, April, 60, (5), pp. 469–479.

Chiche, G.J., and H. Aoshima. 1997. Functional versus aesthetic articulation of maxillary anterior restorations. *Pract Periodont Aesthet Dent*, 9, (3), pp. 335–342.

Cornelini, R., A. Scarano, U. Covani, G. Petrone, and A. Piattelli. 2000. Immediate one-stage post extraction implant: A human clinical and histologic case report. *Int J Oral Maxillofac Implants*, (15), pp. 432–437.

Cowan, P.W. 1990. Surgical templates for the placement of osseointegrated implants. *Quintessence Int*, (2), pp. 391–396.

Cowan, R.D., J.A. Gillbert, D.A. Elledge, and F.D. McGlynn. 1991. Patient use of removable partial dentures: Two- and four-year telephone interviews. *J Prosthet Dent*, (65), pp. 668–670.

Cox, J.F., and G.A. Zarb. 1987. The longitudinal clinical efficacy of osseointegrated dental implants: A 3-year report. *Int J Oral Maxillofac Implants*, (2), pp. 91–100.

Croll, B.M. 1989. Emergence profiles in natural tooth contour. Part 1: Photographic observations. *J Prosthet Dent*, (62), pp. 374–379.

Curtis, D., A. Lacy, R. Chu, et al. 2002. Treatment planning in the 21st Century: What's New? *J Cal Dent Assoc*. Jul; 30(7), pp. 503–510.

Dawson, P.E. 1974. *Evaluation, Diagnosis and Treatment of Occlusal Problems*. St Louis, Mosby.

De Bruyn, H., and B. Collaert. 1994. The effect of smoking on early implant failure. *Clin Oral Implant Res*, (5), pp. 260–264.

De Carvalho, P.S., L.W. Vasconcellos, and J. Pi. 2000. Influence of bed preparation on the incorporation of autogenous bone grafts: a study in dogs. *Int J Oral Maxillofac Implants*. Jul–Aug, 15, (4), pp. 565–570.

Dennisen, H.W., W. Kalk, H.A.H. Veldhusis, and M.A.J. Van Waas. 1993. Anatomic consideration for preventive implantation. *Int J Oral Maxillofac Implants*, (8), pp. 191–196.

Dorfman, H.S., J.E. Kennedy, and W.C. Bird. 1980. Longitudinal evaluation of free autogenous gingival autografts. *J Clin Periodontol*, (7), pp. 316–324.

DuBrul, E.L. 1982. *Sicher's Oral Anatomy*, St Louis, Mosby.

Dula, K., R. Mini, P.F. Van der Stelt, and D. Buser. 2001. The radiographic assessment of implant patients: Decision-making criteria. *Int J Oral Maxillofac Implants*, (16), pp. 80–89.

El Askary, A.S., R.M. Meffert, and T. Griffin. 1999a. Why Do Dental Implants Fail? Part I. *Implant Dent*, 8, pp. 173–185.

El Askary, A.S., R.M. Meffert, and T. Griffin. 1999b. Why Do Dental Implants Fail? Part II. *Implant Dent*, 8, pp. 265–277.

El Askary, A.S., and A. Shawkat. 2003. Provisionalization in Aesthetic Implant Dentistry. *International magazine of oral implantology*, 4, (2), pp. 8–13.

El Attar, M.S., D. el Shazly, S. Osman, et al. 1999. Study of the effect of using mini transitional implants as temporary abutments in implant over denture cases. *Implant Dent*, 8, (2), pp. 152–156.

Engelman, M.J., J.A. Sorensen, and P. Moy. 1988. Optimum placement of osseointegrated implants. *J Prosthet Dent*, (59), pp. 467–473.

Esposito, M., A. Ekestubbe, and K. Gröndahl. 1993. Radiological evaluation of marginal bone loss at tooth surfaces facing single Brånemark implants. Clin Oral Implant Res, (4), pp. 151–157.

Farman, A.G., and T.T. Farman. 1999. Radiovisiography-ui: A sensor to rival direct exposure intra- oral x-ray film. *Int J Computerized Dent*, 2, (3), pp. 183–196.

Fieding, A.F., and E.R. Hild. 1993. Maintaining the quality of life in the HIV patient through osseointegrated implants. Abstract. *Second International Workshop on the Oral Manifestations of HIV Infection*. San Francisco, Jan. 31–Feb. 3.

Flanagan, D. 2005. Arterial Supply of Maxillary Sinus and Potential for Bleeding Complication During Lateral Approach Sinus Elevation. *Implant Dent*, 14, pp. 336–339.

Froum, S., S. Emetiaz, and M.J. Bloom. 1997. The use of transitional implants for immediate fixed temporary prosthesis in cases of implant restorations. *Pract Periodontics Aesthet Dent*, 10, (6), p. 737.

Frush, J.P., and R.D. Fisher. 1958. The dynesthetic interpretation of the dentogenic concept. *J Prosthet Dent*, (8), pp. 558–581.

Ganz, C.H., S.A. Brisman, and V. Tauro. 1989. Computer video imaging: Computerization, communication, and creation. *QDT Yearbook*, 13, p. 64.

Garber, D.A. 1995. The esthetic dental implant: Letting the restoration be the guide. *J Am Dent Assoc.*, (126), pp. 319–325.

Garber, D.A., and U.C. Belser. 1995. Restoration-driven implant placement with restoration-driven site development. *Compend Contin Educ Dent*, 16, pp. 796–804.

Garg, A.K., and A. Vicari. 1995. Radiographic modalities for diagnosis and treatment planning in implant dentistry. *Implant Soc*, (5), 7–11.

Gargiulo, A.W., F.M. Wentz, and B. Orban. 1961. Dimensions and relations of the dentogingival junction in humans. *J Periodontol*, (32), pp. 261–267.

Gelb, D.A. 1993. Immediate implant surgery: Three-year retrospective evaluation of 50 consecutive cases. *Int J Oral Maxillofac Implants*, (8), pp. 388–399.

Genco, R.J. 1992. Host responses in periodontal diseases: Current concepts. *J Periodontol*, 63, pp. 333–338.

Glickman, I. 1972. *Clinical Periodontology*, 4th ed. W.B. Saunders, Philadelphia.

Goldstein, R.E., and C.E. Goldstein. 1988. Is your case really finished? *J Clin Orthod*, 702, p. 22.

Gorman, L.M., P.M. Lambert, H.F. Morris, S. Ochi, and S. Winkler. 1994. The effect of smoking on implant survival at second stage surgery: DICRG interim report. *Implant Dent*, (3), pp. 165–168.

Green, E.N. 1986. Hemisection and root amputation. *J Am Dent Assoc* 112, pp. 511–518.

Gher, M.E., and A.C. Richardson. 1995. The accuracy of dental radiographic techniques used for evaluation of implant fixture placement. *Int J Periodont Rest Dent*, (15), pp. 268–283.

Goaslind, G.D., P.B. Robertson, C.J. Mahan, et al. 1977. Thickness of facial gingiva. *J Periodontol*, 48, pp. 768–771.

Goldstein, R. 1997. *Change your Smile*. 3rd ed. Quintessence, Chicago, pp. 2–3.

Goodson, W.H., and T.K. Hunt. 1979. Wound Healing and the Diabetic Patient. *Surg Gyn Obstet*, 149, pp. 600–608.

Gouvoussis, J., D. Sindhusake, and S. Yeung. 1995. Cross infection from periodontitis sites to failing implant sites in the same mouth. *Int J Oral Maxillofac Implants*, 12, pp. 666–673.

Grossi, S.G., J. Zambon, E.E. Machtei, R. Schifferle, S. Adreana, R.J. Genco, D. Cummins, G. Harrap, et al. 1997. Effects of smoking and smoking cessation on healing after mechanical periodontal therapy. *J Am Dent Assoc*, (128), pp. 599–607.

Grunder, U., H.-P. Spielman, and T. Gaberthuel. 1996. Implant supported single tooth replacement in the aesthetic region: A complex challenge. *Pract Periodont Aesthet Dent*, 8, (9), pp. 835–842.

Haas, R., N. Mensdorff-Pouilly, G. Mailath, and G. Watzek. 1995. Brånemark single tooth implants: A preliminary report of 76 implants. *J Prosthet Dent*, (73), pp. 274–279.

Halstead, C., ed. 1982. *Physical Evaluation of the Dental Patient*. Mosby, St. Louis, pp. 74–81.

Hansen, P.A., and L.A. West. 1997. Allergic reaction following insertion of a Pd-Cu-Au fixed partial denture: A clinical report. *J Prosthod*, (6), pp. 144–148.

Hansson, O. 1994. Clinical results with resin-bonded prostheses and an adhesive cement. *Quintessence Int*, (25), pp. 125–132.

Hebel, K., R. Gajjar, and T. Hofstede. 2000. Single-tooth replacement: Bridge vs. implant supported restoration. *J Can Dent Assoc*, (66), pp. 435–438.

Henemyre, C., D. Scales, D. Hokett, et al. 2003. Nicotine Stimulates Osteoclast Resorption in a Porcine Marrow Cell Model. *J Periodontal*, 74, pp. 1440–1446.

Higginbottom, F.L., and T.G. Wilson. 2002. Successful implants in the esthetic zone. *Tex Dent J*, 119, pp. 1000–1005.

Holmes, D.C., and J.T. Loftus. 1997. Influence of bone quality on stress distribution for endosseous implants. *J Oral Implantol*, (23), p. 104.

Hussey, D.L., C. Pagni, and G.L. Linden. 1991. Performance of 400 adhesive bridges fitted in a restorative dentistry department. *J Dent*, (19), pp. 221–225.

Ingber, J.S. 1974. Forced eruption, Part I. A method of treating isolated one and two wall infrabony defects—Rationale and case report. *J Periodontol*, 45, (4), pp. 199–206.

James, R.A., J.L. Lozada, and H.P. Truitt. 1991. Computer tomography (CT) applications in implant dentistry. *J Oral Implantol*, (17), pp. 10–15.

Jansen, C.E., and A. Weisgold. 1995. Presurgical treatment planning for the anterior single-tooth implant restoration. *Compend Cont Educ Dent*, (16), pp. 746–762.

Jemt, T., U. Lekholm, and K. Grondahl. 1990. Three-year follow-up study of early single implant restorations ad modum Brånemark. *Int J Periodont Dent*, (10), pp. 340–349.

Jin, Q., O. Anusaksathien, S.A. Webb, et al. 2004. Engineering of tooth-supporting structures by delivery of PDGF gene therapy vectors. *Mol Ther*, 9, 5, pp. 19–26.

Jisaander, S., B. Grenthe, and P. Alberius. 1997. Dental implant survival in the irradiate jaw: A preliminary report. *Int J Oral Maxillofac Implants*, 12, pp. 643–648.

Johnson, K. 1963. A study of the dimensional changes occurring in the maxilla after tooth extraction. Part 1: Normal healing. *Aust Dent J*, (8), pp. 428–433.

Jovanovic, S.A. 1997. Bone rehabilitation to achieve optimal aesthetics. *Pract Periodont Aesthet Dent*, 9, (1), pp. 41–52.

Kao, R.T., D.A. Curtis, D.W. Richards, and J. Preble. 1995. Increased interlukin-1 beta in the crevicular fluid of diseased implants. *Int J Oral Maxillofac Implants*, 10, pp. 696–701.

Kazor, C.E., K. Al-Shammari, D.P. Sarment, et al. 2004. Implant plastic surgery: a review and rationale. *J Oral Implantol.*, 30, (4), pp. 240–254.

Keller, E.E. 1997. Placement of dental implants in the irradiated mandible: a protocol without adjunctive hyperbaric oxygen. *J Oral Maxillofac Surg*, 55, pp. 972–980.

Keller, W. 2001. Temporarily Replacing Congenitally Missing Maxillary Lateral Incisors in Teenagers Using Transitional Implants, *Implant News and Views*, 3, (1), Jan/Feb, pp. 1, 4, 5, 10.

Kennedy, J., W. Bird, K. Palcanis, and H. Dorfman. 1985. A longitudinal evaluation of varying widths of attached gingiva. *J Clin Periodontol*, 1985, 12, pp. 667–675.

Kennedy, B.D., T.A. Collins, and P.C. Kline. 1998. Simplified guide for precise implant placement: A technical note. *Int J Oral Maxillofac Implants*, (13), pp. 684–688.

King, M.A., G.W. Casarett, and D.A .Weber. 1979. A study of irradiated bone: Histologic and physiologic changes. *J Nucl Med*, 20, pp. 1142–1149.

Kinsel, R., and R. Lamb. 2002. Development of gingival esthetics in the edentulous patient prior to dental implant placement using a flangeless removable prosthesis: A case report. *Int J Oral Maxillofac Implants*. 17, pp. 866–872.

Klein, M., and M. Abrams. 2001. Computer-guided surgery utilizing a computer-milled surgical template, *Pract Proced Aesthet Dent*, (13), pp. 165–169.

Koth, D.L. 1982. Full crown restorations and gingival inflammation in a controlled population. *J Prosthet Dent*, (48), pp. 681–685.

Lam, R.V. 1967. Contour changes of the alveolar process following extraction. *J Prosthet Dent*, (17), pp. 21–27.

Laney, W.R. 1986. Selecting edentulous patients for tissue-integrated prosthesis. *Int J Oral Maxillofac Implants*, (1), pp. 129–138.

Lang, N.P., and H. Löe. 1972. The relationship between the width of keratinized gingival and gingival health. *J Periodontol*, (43), pp. 623–627.

Lang, N., T. Berglundh, H. Mayfield, et al. 2004. Consensus Statements and Recommended Clinical Procedures Regarding Implant Survival and Complications. *J Prosthet Dent*, 19, pp. 150–154.

Langer, B., S.D. Stein, and B. Wagnenberg. 1981. An evaluation of root resections. A ten-year study, *J Periodontol* 52, pp. 719–722.

Latta, G.H., Jr., S. McDougal, and W.F. Bowles. 1993. Response of known nickel-sensitive patient to a removable partial denture with a titanium alloy framework: A clinical report. *J Prosthet Dent*, (70), pp. 109–110.

Lazzara, R.J. 1989. Immediate implant placement into extraction sites: Surgical and restorative advantages. *Int J Periodont Rest Dent*, (9), pp. 333–343.

Lekholm, U., and G.A. Zarb. 1985. Patient selection and preparation. In: Brånemark, P.I., Zarb, G.A., Albrektsson, T. (eds): *Tissue Integrated Prosthesis—Osseointegration in Clinical Dentistry*, p. 199. Chicago, Quintessence Publishing Co.

Lewis, S., S. Parel, and R. Faulkner. 1995. Provisional implant supported fixed restorations. *Int J Oral Maxillofac Implants*, (10), pp. 319–325.

Lindholm, J., T. Steinlche, E. Rasmussen, et al. 1991. Bone disorder in men with chronic alcoholism: a reversible disease? *J Clin Endocrinol Met.*, 73, pp. 118–124.

Little, J.W., and D.A. Falace, eds. 1993. *Dental Management of the Medically Compromised Patient*, 4th ed. Mosby, St Louis.

Macintosh, D., and M. Sutherland. 2004. Method for developing an optimal emergence profile using heat-polymerized provisional restorations for single-tooth implant-supported restorations, *J Prosthet Dent*, 91, pp. 289–292.

Malamed, S.F. 1995. Physical and psychological evaluation. In: Malamed, S.F, ed. *Sedation: A Guide to Patient Management*, 3rd ed. Mosby St. Louis, pp. 32–62.

Marizola, R., K. Derbabian, T. Donovan, and A. Arcidiacono. 2000. The science of communicating the art of esthetic dentistry. Part I: Patient-dentist-patient communication. *J Fsthet Dent*, (12), pp. 131–138.

Marx, R.E., and R.P. Johnson. 1987. Studies in the radiobiology of osteoradionecrosis and their clinical significance. *Oral Surg Oral Med Oral Pathol*, 64, pp. 379–390.

Marx, R.E., Y. Sawatari, M. Fortin, et al. 2005. Bisphosphonate-induced exposed bone (osteonecrosis/osteopetrosis) of the jaws: risk factors, recognition, prevention, and treatment. *J Oral Maxillofac Surg.*, Nov, 63, (11), pp. 1567–1575.

Melamed, B.G. 1989. Psychological considerations for implant patients. *J Oral Implantol*, 15 (4), pp. 249–254.

Meltzer, A. 1995. Non-resorbable membrane-assisted bone regeneration: Stabilization and the avoidance of micromovement. *Dent Implantol Update*, (6), pp. 45–48.

Mensdorff-Pouilly, N., R. Haas, G. Mailath, and G. Watzek. 1994. The immediate implant: A retrospective study comparing the different types of immediate implantation. *Int J Oral Maxillofac Implants*, (9), pp. 571–578.

Meyenberg, K.H. 1995. Modified porcelain-fused-to-metal restorations and porcelain laminates for anterior aesthetics. *Pract Periodont Aesthet Dent*, 7, (8), pp. 33–44.

Meyenberg, K.H., and M.J. Imoberdof. 1997. The aesthetic challenges of single tooth replacement: A comparison of treatment alternatives. *Pract Periodont Aesthet Dent*, 9, (7), pp. 727–735.

Meyer, M.D., and D.M. Bruce. 2000. Implant site development using orthodontic extrusion: A case report. *N Z Dent J*, (96), pp. 18–20.

Minoretti, R., B.R. Merz, and A .Triaca. 2000. Predetermined implant positioning by means of a novel guide template technique. *Clin Oral Implant Res*, (11), pp. 266–272.

Minsk, L. 2001. Interim Implants for Immediate Loading of Temporary Restorations. *Compendium*, 22, (3), pp. 186–196.

Misch, C.E. 1982. Medical evaluation of the implant candidate. Part II. *Int J Oral Implant*, (2), pp. 11–18.

Misch, C.E. 1990. Divisions of available bone in implant dentistry. *Int J Oral Implant*, 7, pp. 9–17.

Misch, C.E. 1999a. Diagnostic casts, preimplant prosthodontics, treatment prostheses, and surgical templates. In: Misch C.E., ed. *Contemporary Implant Dentistry*, Mosby, St. Louis, pp. 135–149.

Misch, C.E. 1999b. Divisions of available bone. In: Misch, C.E., ed. *Contemporary Implant Dentistry*. Mosby, St. Louis, pp. 89–108.

Misch, C.E. 1999c. Bone density: A key determinant for clinical success. In: Misch, C.E., ed. *Contemporary Implant Dentistry*, Mosby, St. Louis, pp. 109–118.

Misch, C.E. 1999d. Single tooth implant. In: Misch C.E., ed. *Contemporary Implant Dentistry*. Mosby, St. Louis, pp. 397–428.

Misch, C.E., F.D. Misch, and C.M. Misch. 1999. A modified socket seal surgery with composite graft approach. *J Oral Implantol*, (4), pp. 244–250

Misch, C.E., K.E. Al-Shammari, and H.L. Wang. 2004. Creation of interimplant papillae through split finger technique, *Implant Dent*, 13, pp. 20–27.

Murray, C.G., J. Harson, T.E. Daly, and S. Zimmerman. 1980. Radiation necrosis of the mandible: a 10-year study. Part II. Dental factors: onset, duration and management of necrosis. *Int J Radiat Oncol Biol Phys*, 6, pp. 549–553.

Novaes, Jr., A.B., and A.B. Novaes. 1995. Immediate implants placed into infected sites: A clinical report. *Int J Oral Maxillofac Implants*, (10), pp. 609–613.

Oates, T., S. Mailer, J. West, et al. 2005. Human Gingival Fibroblast Integrin Subunit Expression on Titanium Implant Surfaces. *J Periodontol*, 76, pp. 1743–1750.

Ochsenbein, C., and S. Ross. 1973. A concept of osseous surgery and its clinical applications. In: Ward, H.L. and Chas, C., eds. A Periodontal Point of View. Charles C. Thomas, Springfield, IL.

Ogiso, M., T. Tabata, R. Ramonito, and D. Borgese. 1995. Delay method of implantation enhances implant-bone binding: *Maxillofac Implants*, (10), pp. 415–420.

O'Leary, T.J., R.B. Drake, P.P. Crump, and M.F. Allen. 1971. The incidence of recession in young males: A further study. *J Periodontol*, 42, pp. 264–267.

Olson, M., and J. Lindhe. 1991. Periodontal characteristics in individuals with varying forms of the upper central incisors. *J Clin Periodontol*, (18), pp. 78–82.

Palacci, P. 2001. Optimal implant positioning. In: Palacci, P., and Erecsson, I. *Esthetic Implant Dentistry. Soft and Hard Tissue Management*. Quintessence, Berlin, pp. 101–135.

Palmquist, S., and B. Swartz. 1993. Artificial crowns and fixed partial dentures 18 to 23 years after placement. *Int J Prosthodont*, (6), pp. 279–285.

Parkinson, C.F. 1978. Similarities in resorption patterns of maxillary and mandibular ridges. *J Prosthet Dent*, (39), pp. 598–602.

Perel, M. 1993. Achieving critical emergence profile for the anterior tooth implant. *Dent Implantol Update*,(4), pp. 88–92.

Perint, J. 1949. Surgical anatomy and physiology: detailed roentgenologic examination of the blood supply in the jaws and teeth by applying radiopaque solutions, *J Oral Surg*, 2, pp. 2–20.

Persson, L., J. Bergström, and A. Gustafsson. 2003. Effect of Tobacco Smoking on Neutrophil Activity Following Periodontal Surgery. *J Periodontal*, 74, pp. 1475–1482.

Petrungaro, P.S. 1997. Fixed temporization and bone augmented ridge stabilization with transitional implants. *Pract Periodontics Aesthet Dent*, 9, (9), pp. 1071–1078.

Petrungaro, P.S., M.D. Smilanich, and T.J. Adams. 1999. Altering concepts of implantology for the 21st century. *Contemp Aesthet Restorative Pract*, March 2–7.

Phillips, G.E., and V. John. 2005. Use of a Subepithelial Connective Tissue Graft to Treat an Area Pigmented With Graphite, *J Periodontal*, 76, pp. 1572–1575.

Pietrokovski, J., S. Sorin, and Z. Hirschfeld. 1967. The residual ridge in partially edentulous patients. *J Prosthet Dent*, (36), pp. 150–157.

Potashnick, S.R., and E.S. Rosenberg. 1982. Forced eruption: Principles in periodontics and restorative dentistry. *J Prosthet Dent*, (48), pp. 141–148.

Potter, B.J., M.K. Shrout, C.M. Russell, and M. Sharawy. 1997. Implant site assessment using panoramic cross-sectional tomographic imaging. *Oral Surg Oral Med Oral Pathol Oral Radiol Endod.*, (84), pp. 436–442.

Priest, G.F. 1996. Failure rates of restorations for single-tooth replacement. *Int J Prosthodont*, (9), pp. 38–45.

Proceedings of the 1996 World Workshop in Periodontics. 1996. Consensus Report. Implant Therapy II. Ann Periodont, 1, pp. 816–820.

Quinlan, P., C.R. Richardson, and E. Hall. 1998. A Multipurpose Template for Implant Placement. *Implant Dent*, 7, pp. 113–121.

Reddy, M.S., T. Donahoo, F.J. Vanderven, et al. 1994. A comparison of the diagnostic advantages of panoramic radiography and computed tomography scanning for placement of root from dental implants. *Clin Oral Implant Res*, (5), pp. 229–238.

Reddy, M.S., and I.C. Wang. 1999. Radiographic determinants of implant performance. *Adv Dent Res*, (13), pp. 136–145.

Rees, T.D., D.M. Liverett, and C.L. Guy. 1984. The effect of cigarette smoking on skin-flap survival in the face lift patient. *Plast Reconstr Surg*, (73), pp. 911–915.

Reynolds, M.A., and G.M. Bowers. 1996. Fate of demineralized freeze dried bone allografts in human intrabony defects. *J Periodontol*, 67, pp. 150–157.

Rifkin, L., and D. Materdomini. 1993. Facial/lip reproduction system for anterior restorations. *J Esthet Dent*, (5), pp. 126–131.

Robertson, P.B., M. Walsh, J. Greene, et al. 1990. Periodontal effects associated with the use of smokeless tobacco. *J Periodontol*, 61, pp. 438–443.

Rochette, A.L. 1986. Attachment of a splint to enamel of lower anterior teeth. *J Prosthet Dent*, (56), pp. 416–421.

Roge, M., and J.D. Preston. 1987. Color, light, and perception of form. *Quintessence Int.* (18), pp. 391–396.

Rosenberg, E.S., J.P. Torosian, and J. Slots. 1991. Microbial differences in two clinically distinct types of failures of osseointegrated implants. *Clin Oral Implants Res*, 2, pp. 134–144.

Rosenquist, B., and B. Grenthe. 1996. Immediate placement of implants into extraction sockets: Implant survival, *Int J Oral Maxillofac Implants*, (11), pp. 205–209.

Rossein, K., and F. Boris III. 2001. Stabilizing a Full Denture with a Transitional Implant-Supported Splint. *Contemporary Esthetics and Restorative Practice*, 5, (3), pp. 68–74.

Saadoun, A.P., and M. La Gall. 1998. Periodontal implications in implant treatment planning for aesthetic results. *Pract Periodont Aesthet Dent*, (11), pp. 655–664.

Sabes, W.R., S. Green, and C. Craine. 1970. Value of medical diagnostic screening tests for dental patients. *J Am Dent Assoc*, (80), pp. 133–136.

Salama, H., and M. Salama. 1993. The role of orthodontic extrusive remodeling in the enhancement of soft and hard tissue profiles prior to implant placement: A systematic approach to the management of extraction site defects. *Int J Periodont Rest Dent*, (13), pp. 313–333.

Salama, H., M. Salama, and J. Kelly. 1996. The orthodontic-periodontal connection in implant site development. *Pract Periodont Aesthet Dent*, (8), pp. 923–932.

Sampson, H.W., N. Perks, T.H. Champney, et al. 1996. Alcohol consumption inhibits bone growth and development in young actively growing rats. *Alcohol Clin Exp Res*, 20, pp. 1375–1384.

Sanz, M., J. Alandez, P. Lazaro, et al. 1991. Hiastopathologic characteristics of peri-implant soft tissues in Båanemark implants with 2 distinct clinical and radiological patterns. A histometric and ultrastructural study. *Clin Oral Implants Res*, pp. 128–134.

Scaf, G., A.G. Lurie, K.M. Mosier, et al. 1997. Dosimetry and cost of imaging osseointegrated implant with film-based and computed *Radiol Endod*, (83), pp. 41–48.

Schartz, M.S., S.L. Rothman, W. Chavetz, and M. Rhodes. 1989. Computed tomography in dental implant surgery. *Dent Clin North Am*, (33), pp. 565–597.

Schwartz, N.L., L.D. Whitsett, T.G. Berry, and J.L. Stewart. 1970. Unserviceable crowns and fixed partial dentures: Lifespan and causes of loss of serviceability. *J Am Dent Assoc*, (81), pp. 1395–1401.

Schwarz, M.S. 2000. Mechanical complications of dental implants. *Clin Oral Implant Res*, 11, (Suppl. 1), pp. 156–158.

Sclar, A.G. 1999. Ridge preservation for optimum esthetics and function: The "Bio-Col" technique. *Postgrad Dent*, (6), pp. 3–11.

Sendax, V.I. 1996. Mini-implants as adjuncts for transitional prosthesis. *Dent Implantol Update*, 7,(2), pp. 12–15.

Sharawy, M. 1990. *Companion of Spplied Snatomy*, 2nd ed, pp. 1–103, Augusta, GA, Medical College of Georgia Printing Service.

Shavell, H.M. 1979. Mastering the art of provisionalization. *CDA Journal*, pp. 44–51.

Shelby, D.S. 1977. Communication with the laboratory technician. In: Yamada, H.N., and Grenoble, P.B. (eds). *Dental Porcelain the State of the Art.* Univ of Southern California, School of Dentistry, Los Angeles, p. 269.

Shepherd, N.J. 1996. A general dentist's guide to proper implant placement from an oral surgeon's perspective. *Compend Cont Educ Dent,* (27), pp. 118–130.

Silness, J. 1970. Periodontal conditions in patients with dental bridges. The relationship between the location of the crown margin and the periodontal condition. *J Periodontol Res,* (5), pp. 225–229.

Small, P.N., D.P. Tarnow, and S.C. Cho. 2001. Gingival recession around standard-diameter implants: A 3- to 5-year longitudinal prospective study. *Pract Proced Aesthet Dent,* (13), pp. 143–146.

Smiler, D.G. 1987. Evaluation and treatment planning. *J Calif Dent Assoc,* (10), pp. 35–41.

Smith, R.A., S. Silverman, Jr., and O. Auclert. 1989. Recognition of malignancy and dysplasia in the dental implant patient. *J Oral Implantol,* 15, (4), pp. 255–258.

Smith, R.A., R. Berger, and T.B. Dodson. 1992. Risk Factors Associated with Dental Implants in Healthy and Medically Compromised Patients. *Int J Oral Maxillofac Implants,* 7, pp. 367–372.

Soballe, K., E.S. Hansen, H. Brockstedt-Rasmussen, C.M. Pedersen, and C. Bunger. 1990. Hydroxyapatite coating enhances fixation of porous coated implants. *Acta Orthop Scand,* 61, (4), pp. 299 306.

Spear, F.M. 1999. Maintenance of the interdental papilla following anterior tooth removal. *Pract Periodont Aesthet Dent,* 11, (1), pp. 21–28.

Spencer, H., E. Rubio, M. Indreika, and A. Seitam. 1986. Chronic alcoholism. Frequently overlooked cause of osteopenia. *Am J Med.,* 80, pp. 393–397.

Stein, R.S., and M.A. Kuwata. 1977. Dentist and a dental technologist analyze current ceramometal procedures. *Dent Clin North Am,* (21), pp. 729–749.

Stein, J.M., and M. Nevins. 1996. The relationship of the guided gingival frame to the provisional crown for a single-implant restoration. *Compend Contin Educ Dent,* 17, pp. 1175–1182.

Stetler, K.J., and N.F. Bissada. 1987. Significance of the width of keratinized gingival on the periodontal status of teeth with submarginal restorations. *J Periodontol,* (58), pp. 696–700.

Sullivan, R.M. 2001. Perspectives on esthetics in implant dentistry. *Compend Contin Educ Dent,* 22, pp. 685–695, quiz 694.

Sussman, H.I. 1997. Endodontic pathology leading to implant failure: A case report. *J Oral Implantol,* (23), pp. 112–115.

Sussman, H.I., and S.S. Moss. 1993. Localized osteomyelitis secondary to endodontic-implant pathosis: A case report. *J Periodontol,* (64), pp. 306–310.

Tallgren, A. 1972. The continuing reduction of the residual alveolar ridges in complete denture wearers. A mixed longitudinal study covering 25 years. *J Prosthet Dent,* (27), pp. 120–123.

Tarnow, D.P., and R.N. Eskow. 1995a. Preservation of implant esthetics: Soft and restorative considerations. *J Esthet Dent,* (8), pp. 12–19.

Tarnow, D.P., and R.N. Eskow. 1995b. Considerations for single unit esthetic implant restorations. *Compend Cont Educ Dent,* (16), pp. 778–788.

Tarnow, D., and P. Fletcher. 1993. The two to three months post extraction placement of root form implants: A useful compromise. *Implants. Clin Rev Dent,* (2), pp. 1–8.

Tarnow, D., A. Magner, and P. Fletcher. 1992. The effect of the distance from contact point to the crest of bone on the presence or absence of the interproximal papilla. *J Periodontol,* (63), pp. 995–996.

Tehemar, S.H. 1999. Classification and treatment modalities for immediate implantation. Part I: Hard and soft tissue status. *Implant Dent,* (8), pp. 54–60.

Touati, B. 1997a. The double guidance concept. *Pract Periodont Aesthet Dent,* (9), pp. 1089–1094.

Touati, B. 1997b. The double guidance concept. *Int J Dent Symp,* (4), pp. 4–9.

Tuominen, R., K. Ranta, and I. Paunio. 1989. Wearing of removable partial dentures in relation to periodontal pockets. *J Oral Rehab,* (16), pp. 119–126.

Ueda, M., Y. Yamada, R. Ozawa, and Y. Okazaki. 2005. Clinical case reports of injectable tissue-engineered bone for alveolar augmentation with simultaneous implant placement. *Int J Periodontics Restorative Dent.,* Apr, 25, (2), pp. 129–137.

Verdi, M.A., and S.M. Morgano. 1993. A dual-purpose stent for the implant-supported prosthesis. *J Prosthet Dent,* (69), pp. 276–280.

Wakley, G.K., and D.J. Baylink. 1988. Systemic influences on the bone response to dental and orthopedic implant, *J Oral Implant,* 14, pp. 285–311.

Watzek, G., R. Haider, N. Mensdorff-Pouilly, and R. Haas. 1995. Immediate and delayed implantation for complete restoration of the jaw following extraction of all residual teeth: A retrospective study comparing different types of serial immediate implantation. *Int J Oral Maxillofac Implants,* (10), pp. 561–567.

Weinberg, L., and B. Kruger. 1998. Three-Dimensional Guidance System for Implant Insertion: Part I. *Implant Dent,* 7, pp. 81–93.

Weisgold, A. 1977. Contours of the full crown restoration. *Alpha Omegan,* (10), pp. 77–89.

Weisgold, A.S., J.P. Arnoux, and J. Lu. 1997. Single-tooth anterior implant: A word of caution. *J Esthet Dent,* (9), pp. 225–233.

Wheeler, S.L., R.E. Vogel, and R. Casellini. 2000. Tissue preservation and maintenance of optimum esthetics: A clinical report. *Int Oral Maxillofac Implants,* (15), pp. 265–271.

Wilderman, M., B. Pennel, et al. 1970. Histogenesis of repair following osseous surgery. *J Periodontol,* 41, pp. 551–565.

Williams, V.D., K.E. Thayer, G.E. Denehy, and D.B. Boyer. 1989. Cast metal, resin bonded prosthesis: A 10-year retrospective study. *J Prosthet Dent,* (61), pp. 436–441.

Williams, P.L., and R. Warwick. 1980. *Gray's Anatomy,* 36th ed, WB Saunders, Philadelphia.

Wilson, D.J. 1989. Ridge mapping for determination of alveolar ridge width. *Int Oral Maxillofac Implants,*(4), pp. 41–46.

Winter, R. 1990. Achieving esthetic ceramic restorations. *J Calif Dent Assoc,* Sept. 21.

Witter, D.J., P. van Elteren, A.F. Kåyser, and M.J. van Rossum. 1989. The effect of removable partial dentures on the oral function in shortened dental arches. *J Oral Rehab*, (16), pp. 27–33.

Wood, R.E., and L. Lee. 1994. Systematic interpretation of pathologic conditions on oral radiographs. *Ontario Dentist*, (Jan/Feb), pp. 17–22.

Wright, P.S., P.H. Hellyer, D. Beighton, et al. 1992. Relationship of removable partial denture use to root caries in an older population. *Int J Prosthodont*, (5), pp. 39–46.

Zabalegui, J., J.A. Gil, and B. Zabalegui. 1990. Magnetic resonance imaging as an adjunctive diagnostic aid in patient selection for endosseous implants, preliminary study. *Int J Oral Maxillofac Implants*, (5), pp. 283–287.

Zaher, A. 2000. Personal communication, Alexandria, Egypt.

Zarb, G.A., and A. Schmitt. 1990. The longitudinal clinical effectiveness of osseointegrated dental implants: The Toronto study. Part III: Problems and complications encountered. *J Prosthet Dent*, (64), pp. 185–194.

Zitzmann, N., C. Marinello, and T. Berglundh. 2002. The ovate pontic design: A histologic observation in humans. *J Prosthet Dent*, 88, pp. 375–380.

Zubery, Y., N. Bichacho, O. Moses, et al. 1999. Immediate loading of modular transitional implants: a histologic and histomorphometric study in dogs. *Int J Periodontics Restorative Dent*, 19, (4), pp. 343–353.

Chapter 3
Contemporary Facial Evaluation

Abd El Salam El Askary

Human Face

The human face is a unique part of the human body. It is created with a very delicate, unique perfection; the result is a gathering of balanced, proportionate elements of various sizes. The proportional relationships between the dental anatomy and the morphological features of the face deserve attention from clinicians who seek perfect esthetic restorative therapy. The infinite variations of the human face, however, often pose a challenge. Emotional derivations combine to make the task even more complex.

The facial organs that constitute a human smile are likewise plentiful; the cheeks, nose, nasal bridge, chin, eyes, eyebrows, forehead, zygomatic arch, lips, and displayed teeth are considered the variable elements governing facial appearance. Race, skin tone, and character complete the overall picture. As a result of the many variations and elements, the overall clinical assessment for any smile is a mere personal perception rather than a step-by-step methodology.

Many attempts have been made to create a proportional relationship between dental anatomy and facial anatomy, concluding with a proportional relationship (Rufenacht 1990). Although these ratios have been practically applied in many cases, in reality they deviate in many other clinical instances, probably due to the unlimited variations of facial patterns. The orofacial complex still constitutes a prime challenge for both dentists and cosmetic surgeons. Many clinicians consider the facial complex as a separate entity from the dental complex, although they are closely linked. Whereas many dentists focus only on major esthetic reconstruction jobs related to the intraoral parameters, conversely, plastic surgeons focus only on the extraoral clinical parameters and the mere facial structure; as a result, the overall cosmetic job incomplete for both parties. Therefore, combining the two entities in one treatment plan becomes a logical request. In addition, any treatment plan should achieve the delicate balance and harmony of the relationship between the extraoral and the intraoral conditions.

Usually, patients who seek major reconstructive esthetic rehabilitation have certain personal expectations that revolve around the improvement in their appearance, specifically their smiles and how they can appear prettier, younger, and healthier. These patients do not particularly pay attention to the quality or the precision of the dental restoration itself, but rather to what it has done for their overall appearance (Ameed 2001). It is important to keep this attitude in mind when developing a successful comprehensive treatment plan. Achieving patients' desires requires meticulous assessment of the face and smile and must be part of the original treatment plan to maintain the oro-facial balance.

The evaluation and identification of the smile pattern becomes a prime concern in the treatment of major oral rehabilitation procedures. An in-depth analysis of facial morphology as it relates to the future dental assembly should be performed. This includes the lip anatomy (Hulsey 1970), thickness, line, and curvature; as well as the nasolabial angle, intercommissure line, smile arc, Burstone line (Burstone 1967); Steiner S line (Weickersheimer 1995); and Ricketts' E-plane (Viazis 1991), as shown in Figure 3.1.

Other elements that complement the facial beauty and constitute its character include the cheek size; nasal bridge continuity; overall nose size; chin shape and size; eye width, color, and volume; extent of the elevation the eyebrows; forehead size; and zygomatic arch prominence. Therefore, learning about the facial landmarks, identifying smile patterns, detecting the amount of teeth display, and observing most of this information in the detailed patient's facial composition analysis becomes valuable for esthetic restorative therapy. Most of this information should be gathered during verbal communication with the patient, preferably when the patient is not fully aware of the assessment procedure, because they sometimes exaggerate their facial reactions when they are asked to reveal them. Factors such as the patient's character, profession, social standing, and treatment expectations should be noted. This information

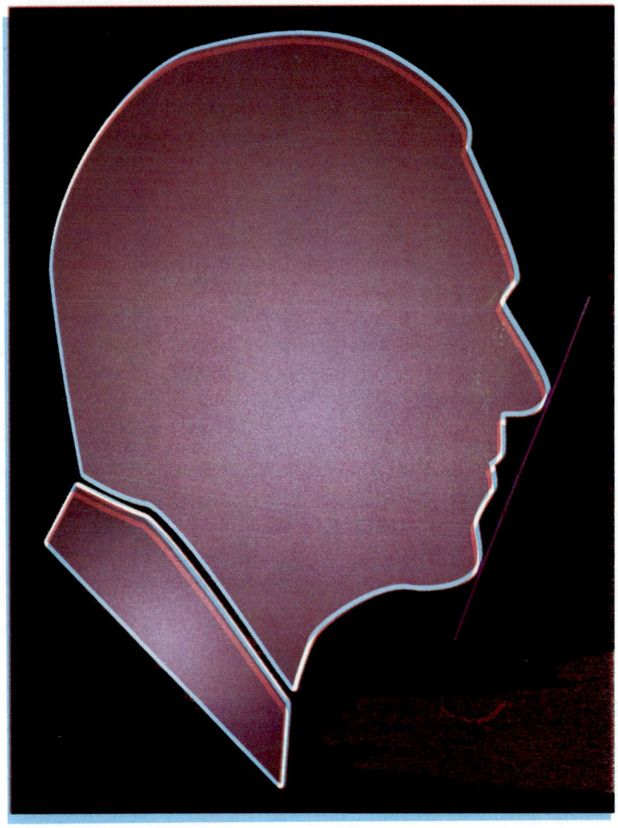

Figure 3.1. The Ricketts' E-plane.

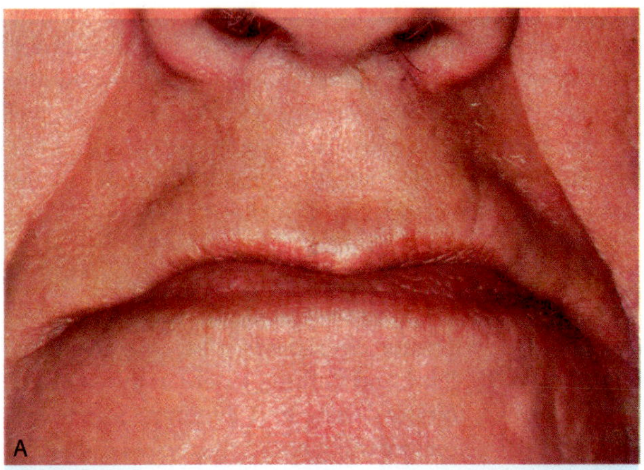

Figure 3.2A. The facial effect of teeth loss. Note the deep nasolabial fold.

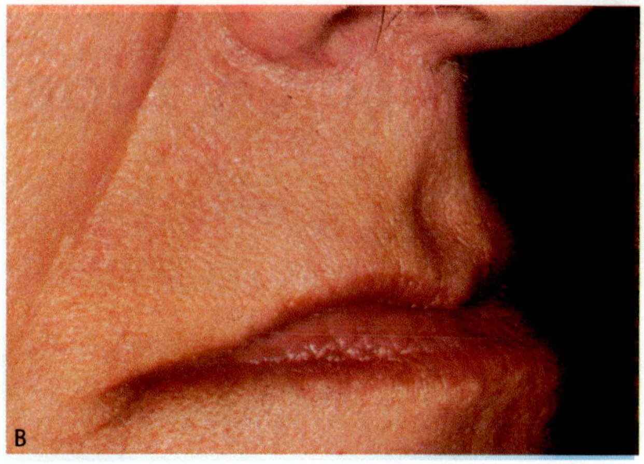

Figure 3.2B. The facial effect of teeth loss Note the loss of lip support.

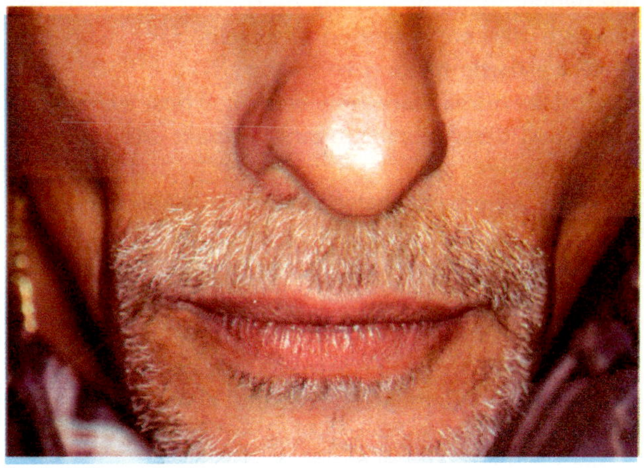

Figure 3.3. The facial effect of teeth loss. Note the cheek drop due to the lack of support of the buccinator muscle.

should assist in the overall assessment of the treatment protocol.

The effect of teeth loss on the facial features is the factor that relates the intraoral condition to the extraoral condition. The consequences of teeth loss on the face have been described by Misch (2005a) as a decrease in facial height, loss of labiomental angle, deepening of vertical lines of the face, forward rotation of the chin and creation of a prognathic facial appearance, a decrease in the horizontal labial angle at the corner of the lips, thinning of the vermillion border of the lips, the loss of overall tonicity of the muscles involved in facial expression, deepening of the nasolabial groove, and an increase in the depth in the Columella-Philtrum angle. This can make the nose appear larger, and the loss of muscle attachments lead to ptosis of the chin (witch's chin), reversed lip line, and increased lip angle under the nose. The effect of the teeth loss is cumulative as well; it is followed by bone loss, then muscle attachment alteration, and then soft tissue loss. See Figures 3.2A–B, 3.3, 3.4A–B, and 3.5A–B.

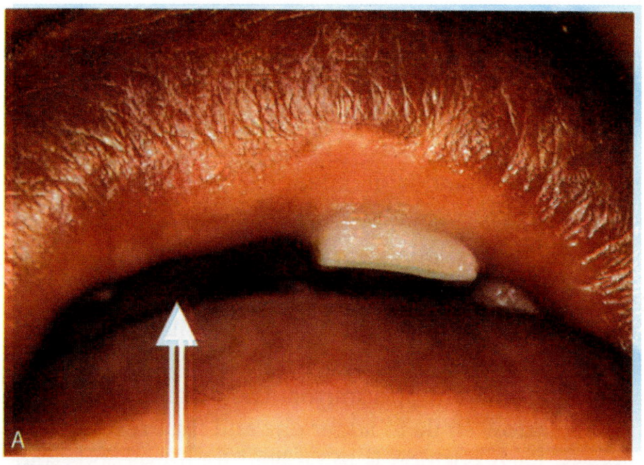

Figure 3.4A. Extraoral view showing missing right maxillary central incisor.

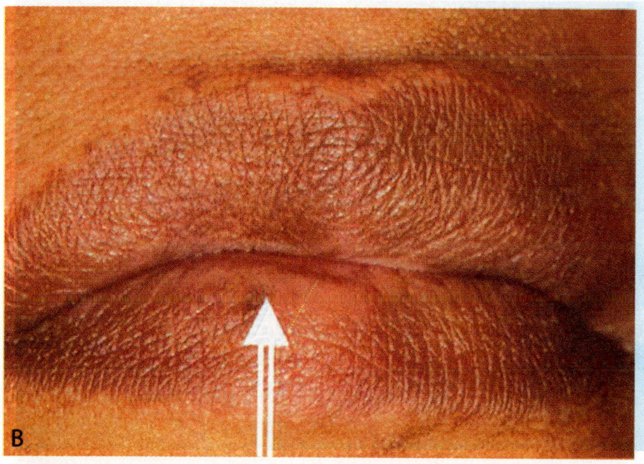

Figure 3.4B. Note the drop of the lip even in the case of only losing one tooth.

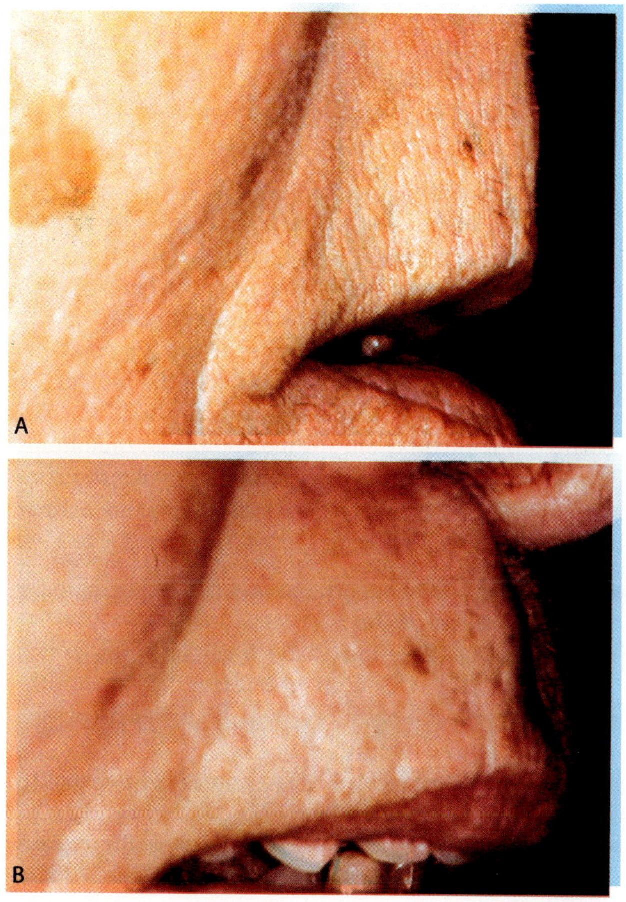

Figure 3.5A, B. Note the difference in the upper lip condition, in terms of support after implant-supported restorative treatment.

Human Smile

The human smile, one of the mercies that we acquire in the fetal stage, does not provide any financial consequence to anyone, although it offers many other benefits. A smile enriches the soul. Its effect consumes only a moment, but it can last for many years engraved in someone's memory. Its value can be felt when it fades away. A true smile creates happiness that does not differentiate between the intelligence and financial categories of the recipients. A smile melts barriers among humankind. The smile's profound psychological effect on human beings explains its value (Kent 1992). The smile is the most vivid of all our facial features because it is an extension and expression of the person as a whole. It is one of many facial expressions that are a part of our daily basic nonverbal communication (Renner 1985). The smile magnifies the beauty of the human face.

The smile also gives the face its glamour. How many times have you seen faces that lack vitality but when the person smiles, the vitality becomes apparent? A smile makes the person appear full of life, and it reflects the virtues of the person's character. The smile can convey countless emotions, from the small grin of embarrassment to the wider smile of happiness and enchantment to the full-teeth dazzling smile of exhilaration. It may last for a fleeting moment or remain intense for quite a while, but it reveals the emotions of happiness and joy (Matthews 1978). The human smile is defined in the literature as the changes in the facial musculature that occur as a result of the incumbent emotional state to the smile effect and the manner in which the lips, teeth, and silhouettes blend to create harmony that gives a smile its own unique magical character (Philips 1996).

The clinical assessment of the patient's smile that is to be reconstructed should include four major components that complement each other, as stated by Morley (1999):

1. Facial esthetics evaluates lips and facial muscles during speech, smiling, and laughter.
2. Gingival esthetics evaluates gingival health in terms of asymmetry or inflammation or blunted papillae.

3. Microesthetics evaluates tooth anatomy and location within the arch as well as shade and characterization.
4. Macroesthetics evaluates the relationship between the teeth and the orofacial structures.

When someone expresses joy, the joyful feeling is expressed by the muscles of the face accordingly. Specifically, the smile is expressed by muscular action around the lips in the inferior third of the face. Duchenne (1990) noted that the emotion of frank joy is expressed on the face by the combined contraction of the zygomaticus major muscle and the inferior portion of the orbicularis oculi muscle. The first muscle obeys the will, but the second is put into play only by the appropriate emotions. Fake joy or a deceitful laugh cannot provoke the contraction of the latter muscle. The muscles that are mainly responsible for the smile, as shown in Figure 3.6, follow:

- The levator labii superioris, which is responsible for raising the upper lip
- The zygomaticus major and levator anguli, which are responsible for lifting the corners of the mouth
- The depressor anguli oris, which pushes down the corners of the mouth
- The risorius, which pulls the corners of the mouth sideways while laughing
- The buccinator muscle, which pushes the cheeks against the teeth medially

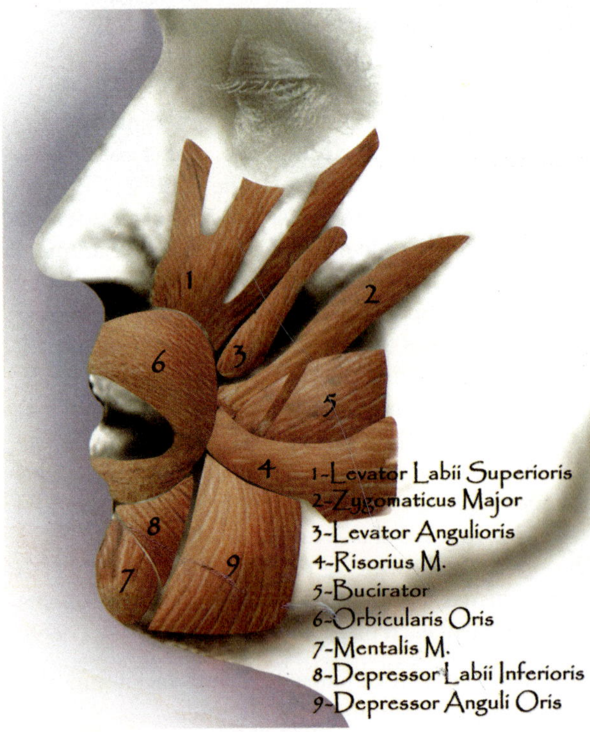

Figure 3.6. A sketch showing the facial muscles controlling the smile.

- The orbicularis oris, which provides the basis for the structure of the lips and the function for the opening-and-closing mechanism of the mouth
- The mentalis muscle, which is responsible for elevating the chin skin upward while laughing
- The depressor labii inferioris, which pushes the lower lip down

It is worth mentioning that Gibson (1989) has developed a smile exercise program to develop and control facial muscles to improve a person's smile. In Gibson's first smile exercise, the patient goes through the process of smiling in front of a mirror. The patient progresses from a narrow smile to larger one and then reverses the process. Each position is to be held for 10 seconds and repeated several times. In this isotonic exercise, the muscles are taken repeatedly through their entire range of movement. An isometric exercise involves closing the smile against the resistance of the fingers, which increases the tone and strength of the muscles around the mouth. The patient makes a full smile and holds the corners of the mouth firmly with the fingers, then slowly closes the lips back to no smile, against the resistance of the fingers.

Smile Patterns

The amount of teeth displayed during smiling determines the type of smile. This statement fits all classification systems for the smile pattern and should be kept in mind while evaluating someone's smile. The clinician should be able to learn how to detect the teeth revealed by any smile, thus distinguishing the type of smile. A group of people can share a smile upon any external stimulus, but they might differ in the amount of teeth displayed. This characterizes each individual smile as a separate entity. Factors that control teeth display during the smile are plenty, including age, the tonicity of the facial muscles, depth of the stimulant, length of the maxillary incisors, length of the lip, thickness of the lip, and class of skeletal and dental occlusion.

Ackerman and others (1998) have classified the smile according to its very nature, as shown in Figures 3.7A–B:

- Enjoyment smile that is used when experiencing real pleasure, is involuntary, attains maximum muscle contraction of the lips, and attains maximum gingival and tooth display
- Social smile that is used in greetings, is voluntary and unstrained, portrays a static facial expression, uses moderate lip muscle contraction, and attains a slight amount of teeth and gingival display

Another classification by Rubin (1974) identifies the smile according to the amount of teeth displayed, as shown in Figures 3.8A–E:

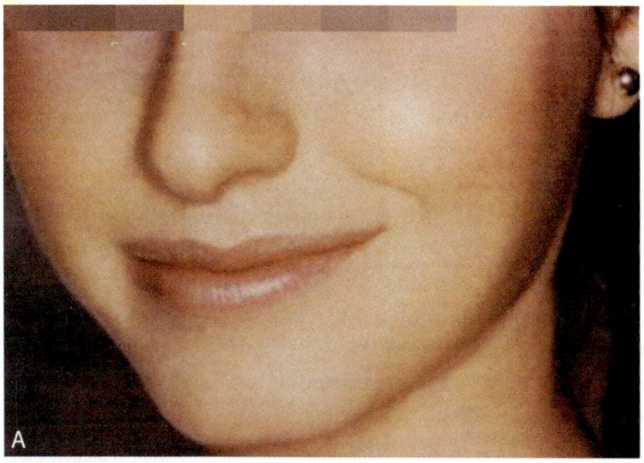

Figure 3.7A. A social smile.

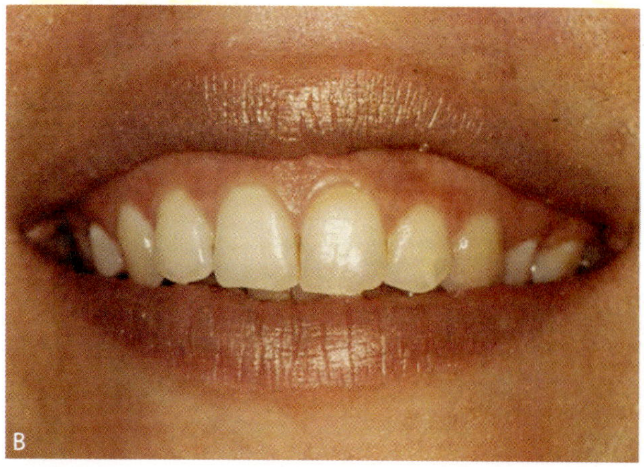

Figure 3.8B. Maxillary smile with 3 mm of the gingiva.

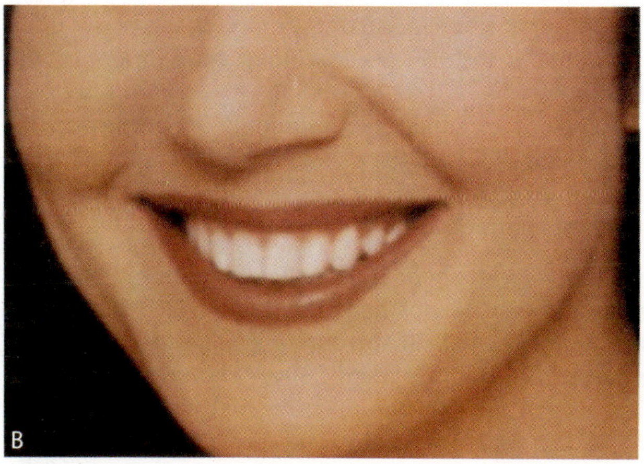

Figure 3.7B. An enjoyment smile.

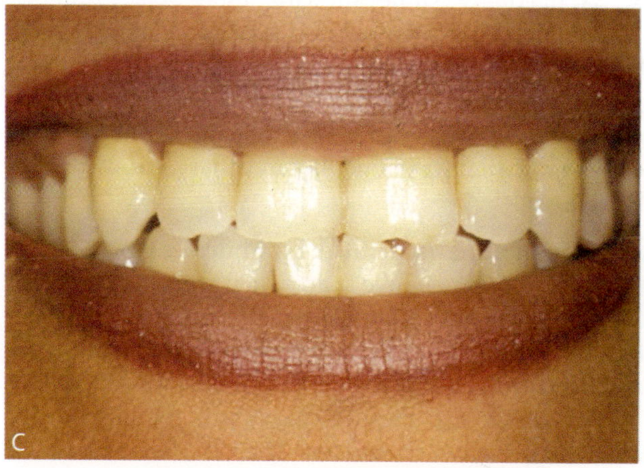

Figure 3.8C. Both maxillary and mandibular smile.

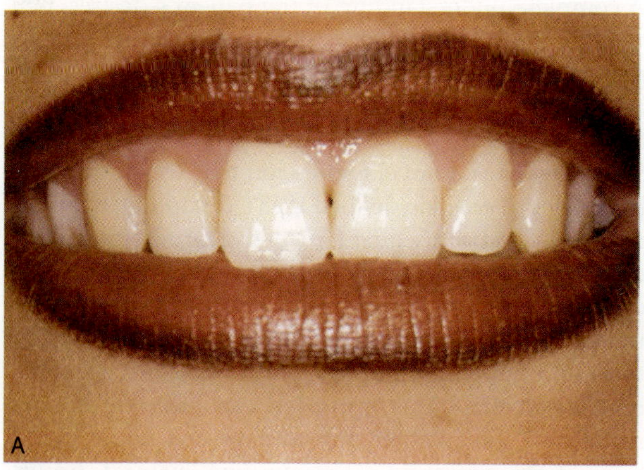

Figure 3.8A. Solely maxillary smile.

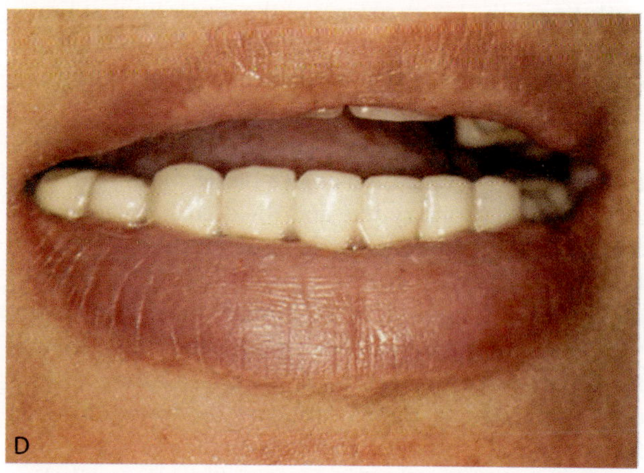

Figure 3.8D. Solely mandibular smile.

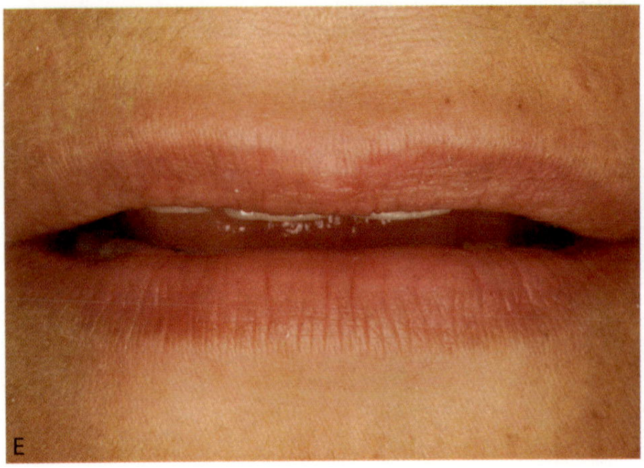

Figure 3.8E. Neither maxillary nor mandibular smile.

- A maxillary smile showing only the maxillary teeth
- A maxillary smile showing more than 3 mm of gingiva; also often referred to as a gummy smile
- A solely mandibular smile
- A smile with both maxillary and mandibular teeth appearing
- A smile that shows neither maxillary nor mandibular teeth

The smile line is defined by Philips as that which shows a dark or negative space when both jaws separate (Philips 1990). In other words, the silhouettes of the incisal edges of the maxillary teeth in comparison to the mandibular incisal edges can also define the smile line. The smile line can vary in shape; it is thought to frequently be convex in females. The development of the smile, from the quarter smile, to the half smile, to the full smile, in relation to the amount of tooth displayed will suggest to the clinician whether to display or hide the morphological deviation in tooth-gingival relationships (Hulsey 1970, Tjan and Miller 1984). Practically, the smile line is the lower margin of the upper lip that limits the visibility of the teeth. The smile line follows the edges of the maxillary anterior teeth and the curvature of the inner border of the lower lip.

Rufenacht (1990) described the ideal smile line as one that is achieved when the angles of the mouth are parallel to the bipupillary line and the occlusal plane, with the tips of the canines barely touching the lower lip. When the lower lip curves upward and posteriorly to the corner of the mouth where it meets the upper lip, the viewer's attention is drawn to the dentition that is framed in the upward curve of the lips. As the viewer's eye is attracted to the elevation of the lower lip, it is focusing on the occlusal and incisal planes.

Frush and Fisher (1985) have described the smile line as the harmony between the curvature of the incisal edges of the maxillary anterior teeth and the upper border of the lower lip. Hulsey (1970) found that the smile line ratio—the congruency of the arc of curvature of the upper border of the lower lip and the arc of curvature of the incisal edges of the maxillary anterior teeth—appeared to be important in an attractive smile, and that the most attractive smile displayed a smile line ratio of 1:1.25. Tjan and Miller (1984) reported that an average smile exhibits the full length of the maxillary anterior teeth, displays an incisal curve of the maxillary teeth that is parallel to the inner curvature of the lower lip, and displays the six maxillary anterior teeth and the premolars.

Rubin (1974) stated that there are three basic styles of smiles:

- A commissure smile is the most common type (67%); the corners of the mouth are initially pulled upward and outward, followed by rising of the upper lip to exhibit only the maxillary teeth.
- A cupid smile, occurring in 31% of the population, exposes the canines and then the corners of the mouth.
- A complex smile appears in only 2% of the population; it shows all the maxillary and mandibular teeth simultaneously during elevation of the upper lip and contraction of the lower lip.

Prior to any esthetic comprehensive therapy, the information about the position, shape, and size of the original dentition and its surrounding facial tissues that is vital in restoring a patient's smile should be collected. The role of the clinician in smile analysis is to comprehend the patient's desire and expectations from the treatment, then to gather information about the cause of the esthetic or the functional problem, such as trauma, faulty dentistry, pathological reasons, or others. Photography can be of great assistance in examining the facial features during speech and laughter in paused positions. A complete understanding of the patient's desires, personality, and psychological state will result in greater patient satisfaction (Levin 1988).

Smile Design

Smile design is a novel expression that was introduced by Morley (1997). He defined it as a discipline involving diagnosis and subsequent planning primarily for the esthetic component of the overall dental treatment. In other words, it is the enhancement of the amount of tooth displayed during smiling, using the available tools and applying the principles of design to anterior dental esthetics. This approach can turn an average restorative job into an outstanding one while at the same time preserving the existing natural beauty (Golub-Evans 1994).

Esthetic factors that contribute to smile design and can be influenced in the treatment include the incisal plane, size and inclination of the central incisors, midline position, axial alignment of the remaining teeth, size and form of the arch, lip line to the incisal edge position, form and morphology of the dentition, position of the contact points, gingival height, zenith color, and contour (Rufenacht 1990, Dickerson 1996, Moskowitz and Nayyar 1995). The patient's character and lifestyle also can influence the treatment to some extent.

The clinician's personal artistic abilities and subjective tools for making each treatment plan unique distinguish an excellent clinician from an average one. Therefore, smile design should focus on an individualized approach that allows each restoration to be designed according to a particular individual's needs, and that provides balance and harmony along with the functional demands. Smile harmony can be achieved when the various lines, proportions, and structures are in visual balance with each other (Gwinnett 1992). A smile can be changed slightly by altering these proportions, creating illusions, and minimizing the negative visual tension produced by improperly aligned teeth, gingiva, and the lips (Moskowitz and Nayyar 1995). When attempting to perform smile design, one must consider teeth not as a separate component but rather a part of the entire facial structure.

Smile Landmarks

Several clinical orofacial landmarks should be diagnosed and assessed when constructing a new smile or performing smile design operation. These landmarks are very influential to the treatment outcome, and they may assist to a great extent in achieving a natural smile and avoiding a misbalance between the intraoral and extraoral relationships. In any major reconstructive case, these landmarks should be carefully regarded if someone is willing to make a harmonious esthetic prosthesis.

Intercommissure Line

The intercommissure line (ICL) is an imaginary line that is drawn through the corners of the mouth. It connects the two corners of the mouth in paused smile. The amount of maxillary teeth that are revealed below the ICL can provide information on the patient's age. In youthful smiles 75% to 100% of teeth structure shows below this line. In youthful smiles, the amount of display can reach up to 10 mm to 13 mm from the incisal edge to that line. In aged patients, fewer maxillary teeth show below this line. Fewer teeth showing with age is attributed to: (1) loss of muscle tone of the face, and (2) attrition of the teeth.

The value of this line indicates the age of the patient and youthfulness. The more teeth-gingiva displayed, the younger the patient looks. Therefore, this line might become an important aspect of the treatment, especially in totally edentulous reconstructive procedures. (See Figures 3.9A–B.)

An interesting study (Choi and Demf 1991) has evaluated changes in the smile caused by aging. It measured the exposure of the maxillary and mandibular central incisors in both resting and smiling positions in 230 subjects (103 male, 127 female) 20 to 69 years of age. It reported that the amount of maxillary incisal exposure gradually decreased with age. This was accompanied by a gradual increase in mandibular incisal exposure in the smiling position. The mean amount of incisal exposure was 5.92 mm in the maxilla and 2.78 mm in the mandible.

Another study (Robinson 1969) regarding the amount of teeth revealed in relation to age stated that

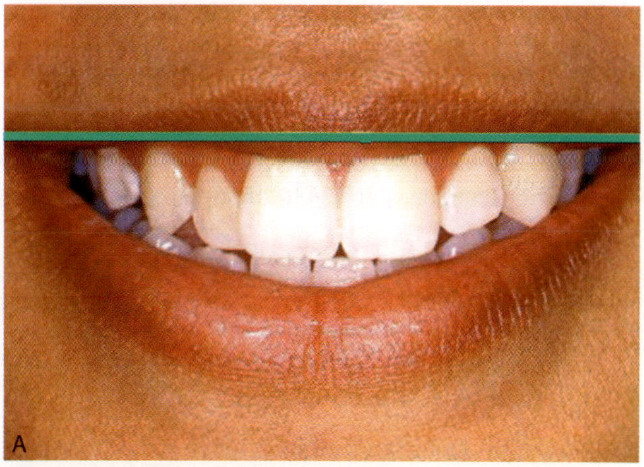

Figure 3.9A. Intercommissure line for a young patient revealing more vital structure beneath it.

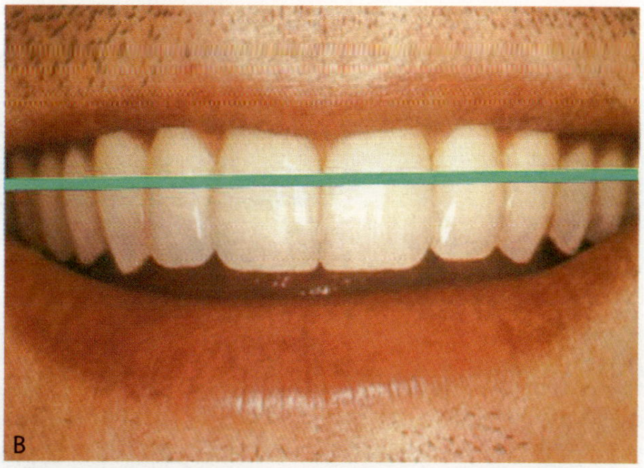

Figure 3.9B. Intercommissure line of an old patient showing less vital structure beneath it.

a 30-year-old patient exposes more than 3mm of the maxillary central incisors when the maxillary lip is at rest or repose. A 40-year-old shows 1.5mm of maxillary central incisors, a 50-year-old exposes less or equal to 1mm, and a 60-year-old exposes 0.5mm, while at the age of 80 years the lip margin is level with the incisal edges of the maxillary teeth. These rates are reversed with the relationship of the lower lip with the maxillary incisal edges.

Smile Arc

The relationship of the incisal edges of the maxillary incisors and canine tips to the curvature of the lower lip in the posed smile is called the *smile arc*. An ideal smile arc occurs when a line is drawn touching the incisal edges and the tips of the canines, another line touches the lower lip curvature, and these two lines are parallel to the infraorbital line and perpendicular to the facial midline. In other words, the ideal smile arc has the maxillary incisal edge curvature parallel to the curvature of the lower lip (Golub-Evans 1994, Moskowitz and Nayyar 1995, Sarver 2001). (See Figures 3.10A–C.) The parallelism of the maxillary anterior incisal curve with the lower lip was divided into three categories:

1. Parallel—when the incisal edges of the maxillary anterior teeth are parallel to the upper border of the lower lip
2. Straight—when the incisal edges of the maxillary anterior teeth are in a straight line
3. Reverse—when the incisal edges of the maxillary anterior teeth are curved in reverse to the upper border of the lower lip

A study by Dong and others (1999) concluded that there are many subjects with a parallel smile (60%), some with a straight smile (34%), and only a few subjects with a reverse smile (5%). Parallel and straight smiles received higher esthetic rankings than reverse smiles ($P < 0.05$), as shown in Figure 3.11.

The ideal smile has been described by another study (Yoon and Dong 1992) as one in which the upper lip curved upward or was straight when the full shape of the maxillary anterior teeth was displayed between the upper and lower lip, the maxillary anterior incisal curve was parallel to the lower lip, and the teeth were displayed to the first molar. (See Figures 3.12A–B.)

Vestibular Reveal

The vestibular reveal is the amount of teeth and/or gingival structure that shows in various lip positions throughout the buccal corridor when the teeth are viewed from the front. The amount of posterior teeth that shows during smiling can be called the vestibular reveal. In natural teeth, the maxillary teeth after the canine start to look smaller and darker, and become blurred. When fabricating any prostheses in the maxillary arch, this

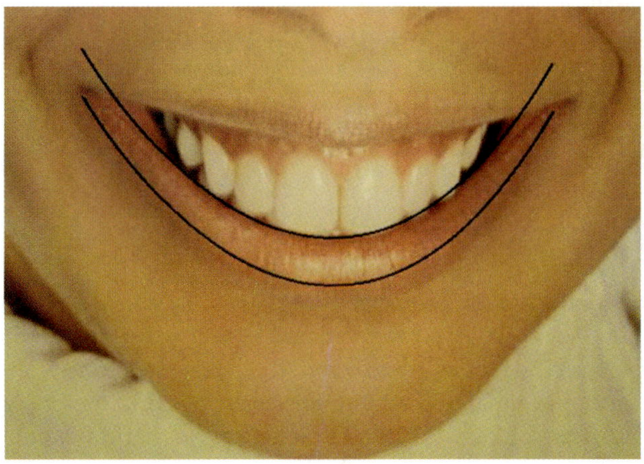

Figure 3.11. Ideal smile arc.

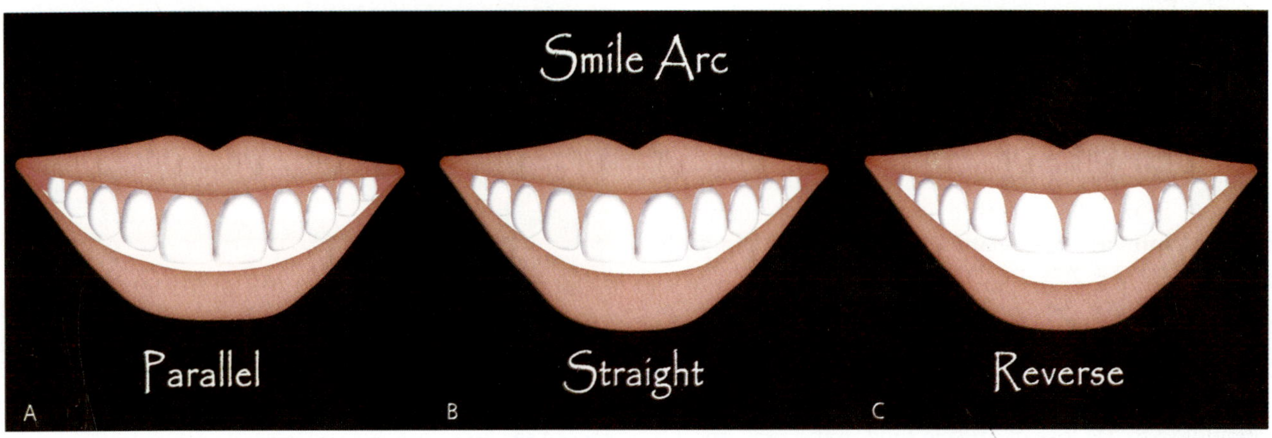

Figure 3.10. A sketch showing the different situations of the smile arc.

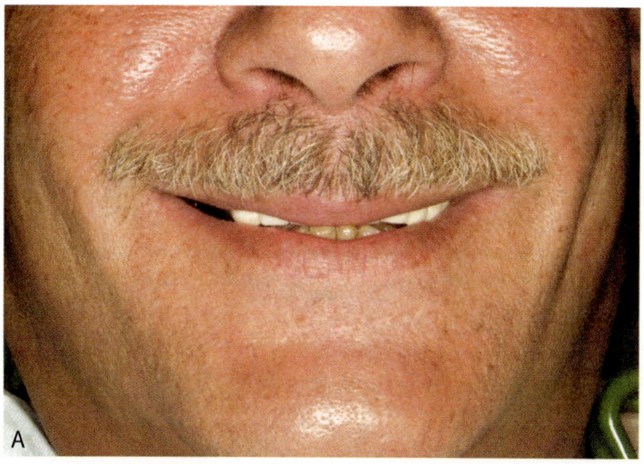

Figure 3.12A. A smile with reversed smile arc due to faulty dentistry.

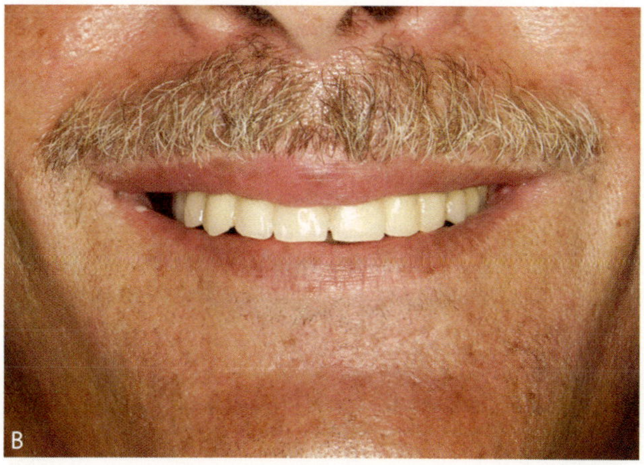

Figure 3.12B. Smile arc after being corrected.

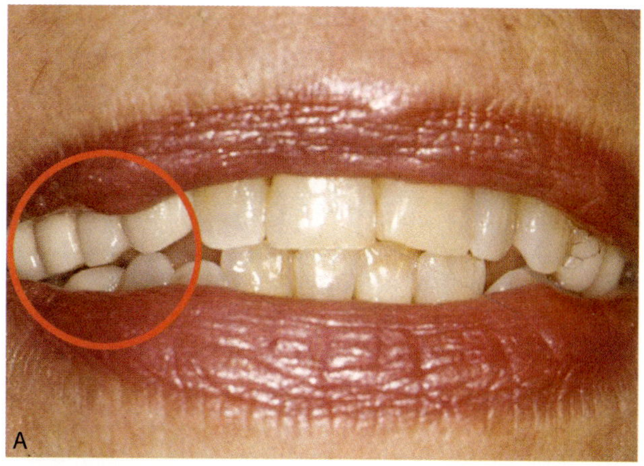

Figure 3.13A. Excessive vestibular reveal (EVR) in the maxillary right side of the patient.

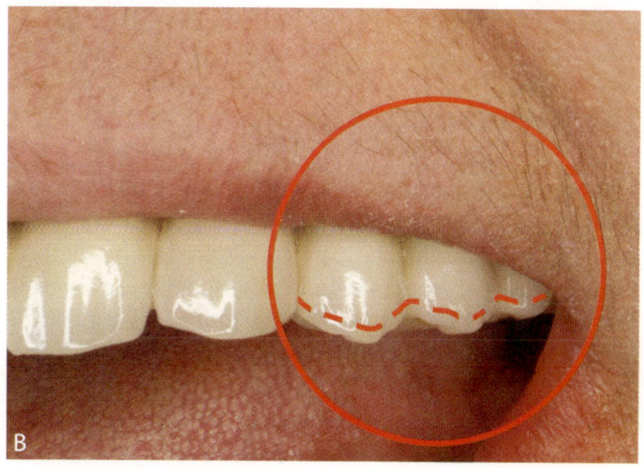

Figure 3.13B. EVR condition, the red interrupted line represents the optimal place of the prosthetic margins.

reveal should be duplicated and not violated. This condition is called deficient vestibular reveal (DVR) or excessive vestibular reveal (EVR) (Morley 1999).

To clinically detect the amount of teeth that are revealed, ask the patient, while seated in an upright position, to pronounce the letter "M" several times. After pronunciation ceases, the lips return to the relaxed resting position for evaluation, and a picture can be taken to detect the minimum tooth reveal. The patient is then asked to pronounce the letter "E" and to then pause to detect the maximum teeth reveal. By detecting these parameters, the clinician will gain an idea of the patient's amount of teeth that are revealed and duplicate it in the final prostheses. (See Figures 3.13A–B.)

The relationship between the opposing dental arches determines the length of the maxillary incisors and the length of the maxillary incisors plays an important role in the anterior guidance and phonetics of the patient. Some factors should be considered when detecting the extent of the maxillary incisors in fully edentulous cases: the length of the upper lip, age of the patient, and maximum or minimum teeth reveal. The maxillary teeth should be displayed halfway between the upper and lower lip lines in the maximum teeth reveal position (Vig and Brundo 1978). Also, the lingual tilt of the maxillary central incisor (the incisal third) determines the correct pronunciation of the letters "F" and "V." The maxillary central incisor should slightly press against the lower lip inner edge of the vermilion border, blocking the remaining air coming out of the mouth (Dawson 1983).

In fully edentulous cases, the determination of the optimal incisal edge position becomes randomized by many clinicians. Misch (2005b) has set his original methodological maxillary incisal edge position guidelines, noting that the canine position is more consistent and less affected by age than the other natural teeth within the arch in the frontal area. In general, the canine tip is in a lateral position to the lip bow and is usually

1 mm longer than the maxillary lip in repose (letter "M") from 20 to 40 years of age. The canine is in an even position with the lip line from 40 to 60 years, and the lip is 1 mm longer than the canine position at 60 to 80 years. Once the position of the canine tip is set, the other teeth can follow. Speech then can be checked with the pronunciation of the letter "F" to set the length of the labiolingual position and pronunciation of the letter "N" to set the incisal edge touching point with the lower border of the lip; it should lightly touch the wet-dry border of the lower lip, similar to the lower lip position during a broad smile (Heinlein 1980). He also stated that when the patient says "E," 50% to 70% of the space between the maxillary and mandibular lip should be occupied by the maxillary central incisors. If less than 50% of the space is occupied, the teeth usually can be lengthened, but if more than 70% of the space is occupied by maxillary centrals, lengthening the teeth usually is not indicated.

The Lip Influence

The lips' value complements both the face and the oral cavity because both upper and lower lips compose the frame of the mouth. They are considered to be the curtains that reveal what is behind when they are moved in any direction. Generally speaking, both lips contribute to both the shape of the face and the pronunciation of words. The lip frame, which surrounds natural dentition, contributes dramatically to dental esthetics. Consequently, the lips demand careful inspection and assessment (Hulsey 1970). The anatomy of the lips enclosing the orbicularis oris muscle that joins the lips superiorly to the base of the nose, laterally by the nasolabial sulci, and inferiorly by the mentolabial sulcus, vertical depression, called the "philtrum," is located on the upper lip. It proceeds superiorly on the facial skin from the tubercle of the upper lip and runs to the base of the nose. The philtrum is one of the most important landmarks when the placement of the dental midline is of concern (Vig and Brundo 1978). Different positions of head posture can easily change the vertical or horizontal display of lips as a result of the weaker muscle tone. The difference between a normal lip and a cleft lip can give an indication of the importance of the upper lip to the facial composition.

The lower lip has a tendency to be wider, fuller, longer, and more elastic (Renner 1985). The relationship between the upper and lower lips varies according to the skeletal class of the occlusion. The relationship plays an important role in determining tooth spatial alignment, and the degree of lip protrusion or retrusion affects the facial profile to a great extent (Tweed 1991).

Several authors have described the anatomical landmarks of the lip to diagnose facial deformities within the treatment plan; the Burstone line is a reference line that connects the subnasale point to the pogonion point. The upper and lower lips are compressed by this reference line (ideally +3.5 mm and +2.2 mm, respectively, above this line) (Burstone 1967). The Steiner S line is a line joining the midpoint of the nose to the chin, where the patient's lips touch this line (Weickersheimer 1995). The Ricketts' E-plane describes a line that extends from the tip of the nose to the chin, in which the maxillary and mandibular lip positions measure 4 mm and 2 mm, respectively (Viazis 1991). For the most favorable facial esthetics, the distance between the subnasale point (base of the nose) and the upper lip should be approximately half the distance from the lower lip to the menton (lowest chin) point (Rifkin 2000).

The upper lip position can be divided into three categories, taking into consideration that all of these positions were recorded in a full smiling position (Dong et al. 1999):

1. A higher lip position that reveals the total length of the maxillary anterior teeth and a contiguous band of gingiva
2. An average lip position that reveals 75% to 100% of the maxillary anterior teeth length and the interproximal gingiva only (which is equal to the maxillary smile)
3. A low lip position that reveals less than 75% of the anterior teeth height with no gingival tissues revealed

Another classification for the lip lines comprises the following three categories (Touati et al. 1999):

1. A low lip line hides the gingiva and a considerable portion of the anterior teeth where it is difficult to show the incisor tips when the lips are at a resting position. The anterior teeth may be displayed when the patient is in full smile. In this class, it may be necessary to perform crown lengthening to establish a balance between the length of the lip line when at rest and when smiling.
2. A medium lip line applies when 1 mm to 3 mm of the maxillary incisal edges are shown at a resting position.
3. A high lip line can be seen when more than 4 mm to 5 mm of the gingiva is displayed during a posed smile.

A medium lip line is considered to be the most preferable type in several oral rehabilitation procedures. (See Figures 3.14A–C.)

The upper lip curvature influences the smile directly. It can be divided into the following three categories, as shown in Figures 3.15A–C:

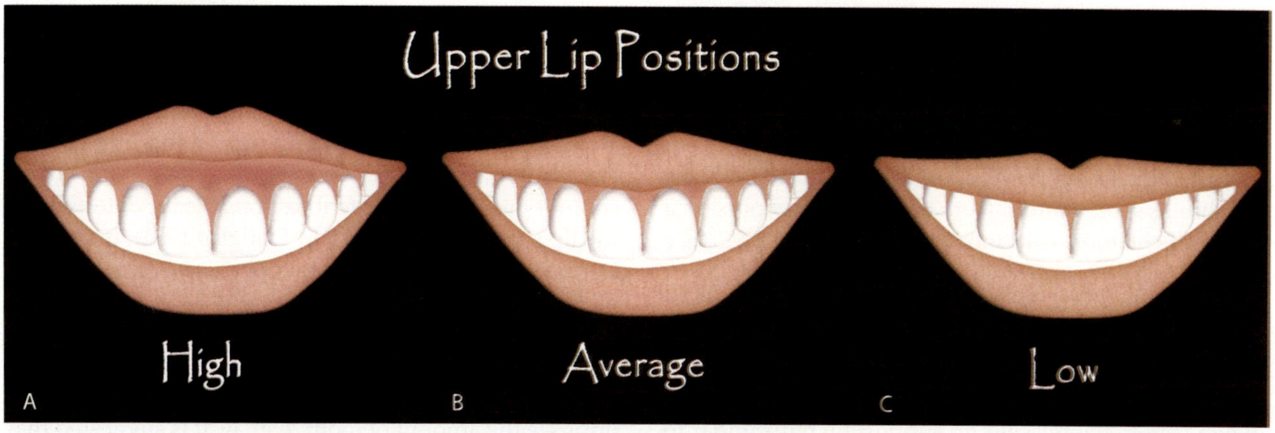

Figure 3.14. **A.** An illustration showing high upper lip position. **B.** An illustration showing average upper lip position. **C.** An illustration showing low upper lip position.

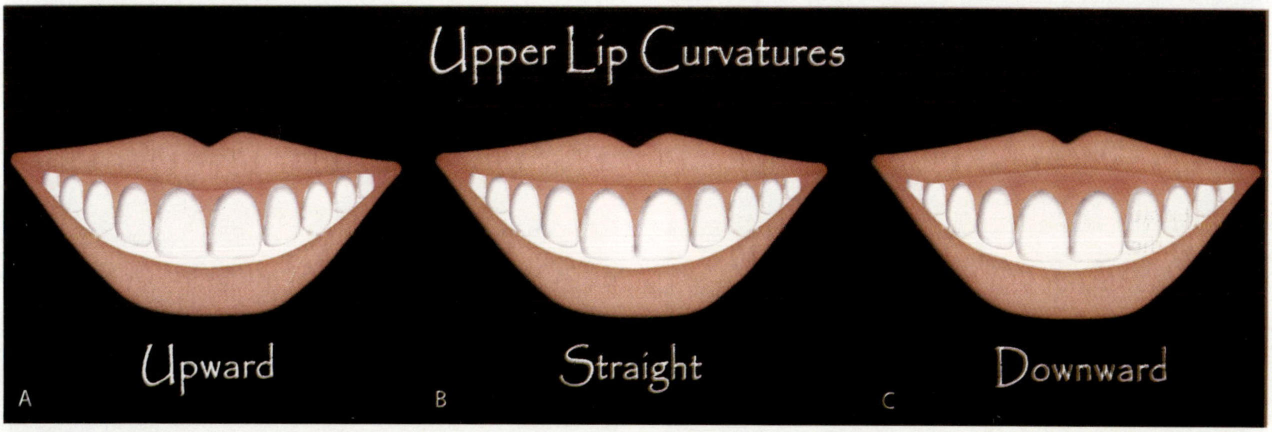

Figure 3.15. **A.** An illustration showing an upward lip curvature. **B.** An illustration showing a straight lip curvature. **C.** An illustration showing a downward lip curvature.

1. Upward curvature (12%), which occurs when the corner of the mouth is higher than the center of the lower border of the upper lip
2. Straight orientation (45%), which occurs when the corner of the mouth and the center of the lower border of the upper lip are in a straight line
3. Downward curvature (43%), which occurs when the corner of the mouth is lower than the center of the lower border of the upper lip (Dong et al. 1999)

The size of the lips can influence the treatment plan in terms of defining the amount of teeth display as well as the artificial teeth selection in most of the major oral rehabilitation procedures. Thick lips often do not reveal a greater amount of tooth-gingiva structure because of the amount of the lip tissues that hide the teeth behind it, as shown in Figure 3.16. It is worth mentioning that

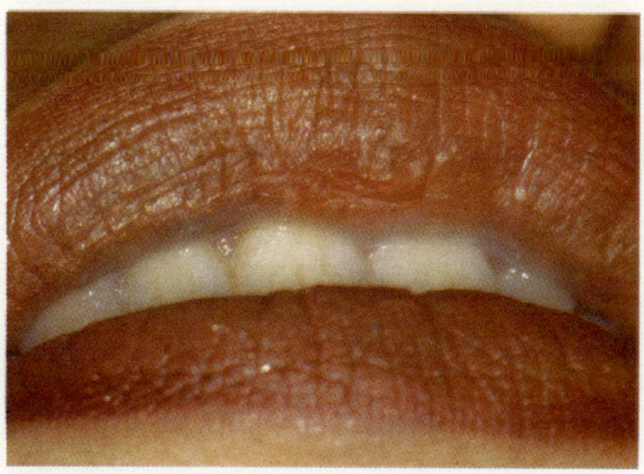

Figure 3.16. Thick lips reveal a lesser amount of teeth display in a posed smile.

thick lips can be more favorable than thin lips in cosmetic dental reconstruction because thick lips might hide any marginal prosthetic artifact (if it exists). On the other hand, when a thin lip contracts, it reveals most of the dentogingival complex. A thin lip requires meticulous attention to the prosthetic marginal details; in short and thin lips, the natural teeth behind usually possess a lingual inclination (Martone and Edwards 1978). (See Figure 3.17.)

In case of early teeth loss, the lips lose their support and drop medially toward the oral cavity. This can be a starting point for facial deformity and, subsequently, skin wrinkles. In such conditions, the dentist should be able to restore the missing lip support by returning it to its original place prior to teeth loss. Restoring missing teeth has proven to improve the facial appearance to a great extent. Teeth loss does not only affect lip support but also the cheek support, by removing its posterior support (the buccinator muscle). (See Figures 3.18A–C.)

In the case of severe alveolar ridge resorption, a carefully fabricated wax-up on the study cast will indicate the amount of osseous structure required facially to support the lip and return it to its original position, along with the prosthetic contours, taking into consideration that the cervical and middle thirds of the crown contour are to a great extent responsible for determining the lip support (Maritato and Douglas 1964). In cases of lip defects that might affect teeth display, the wise use of lip augmentation therapy might help improve the teeth display, as shown in Figure 3.19A–B. Because teeth are not well displayed in patients with thick upper lips, a lighter teeth shade selection is required to enhance and improve the amount of tooth display. It is suggested that the upper lip takes more responsibility in the control of the teeth display, while the lower lip plays a major role in pronunciation. Treatment of patients with a high upper lip line often becomes more complex and unpredictable; therefore, a careful evaluation of lip size, thick-

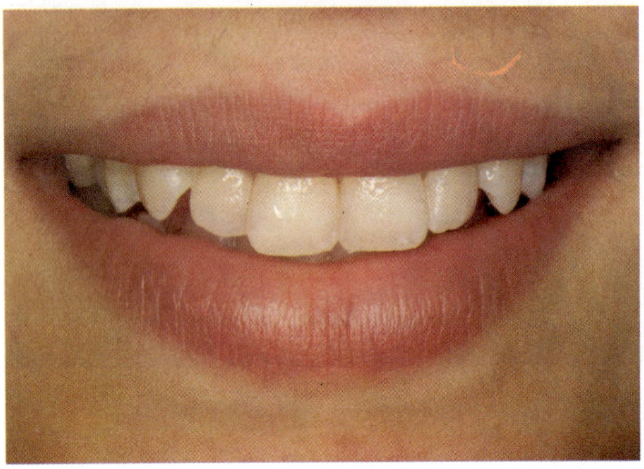

Figure 3.17. Thin lips exhibit shorter anterior teeth with lingually inclined incisal edges.

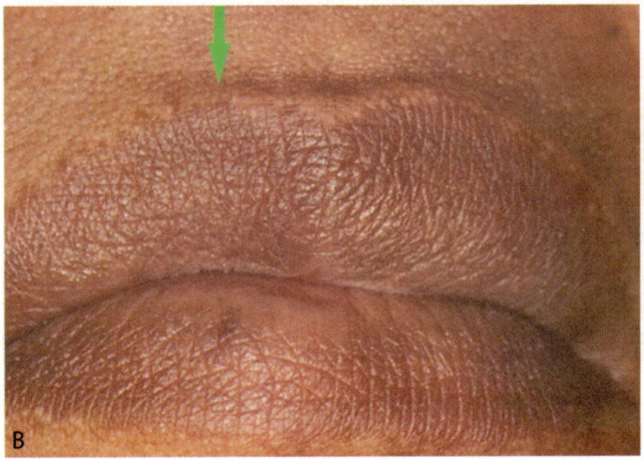

Figure 3.18B. Patient with missing central incisor, which leads to lip drop.

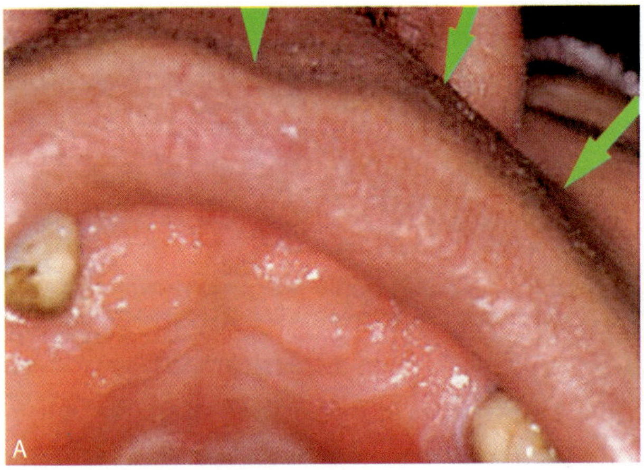

Figure 3.18A. Facial deformation due to loss of dental support due to teeth loss.

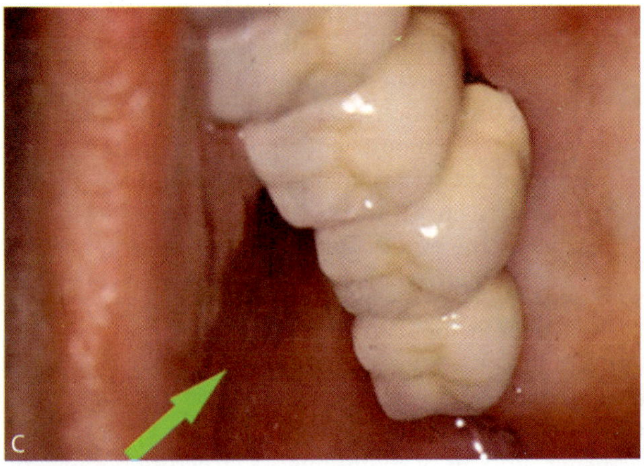

Figure 3.18C. Improper posterior buccal contour of the implant-supported prosthesis, which leads to the deficient support of the buccinator muscle.

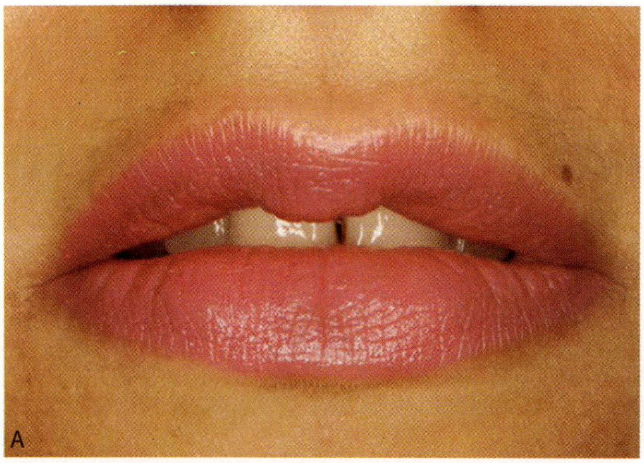

Figure 3.19A. Insufficient teeth display due to upper lip deformity that warrants correction.

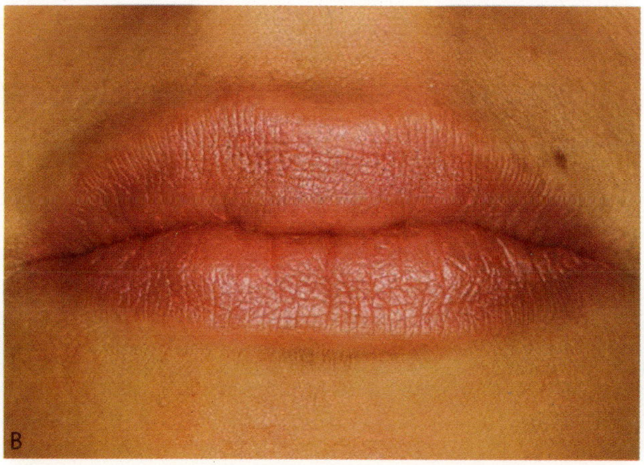

Figure 3.19B. Corrected teeth display via lip augmentation therapy.

ness, and character will determine how much of the restoration should be displayed while smiling or with the lip in any other position.

Teeth Morphology

Attempts to solve esthetic problems in this age of scientific revolution led dentists to seek an evidence-based concept. This search for esthetic success with dental restorations was led by Williams (1914) but involved many other ideas and authors as well (Wavrin 1920, Young 1954). While credit is often given to Williams, Hall (1886) was the first to describe what he believed was a correlation between face form and tooth form. He stated that three basic forms of teeth existed: square, tapering, and ovoid (Stein 1936). The correlation succeeded due to its practicality and manufacturer support, and not because of any actual relationship (Young 1954). However, most of the research has shown that no significant correlation exists between facial form and tooth form (Sellen et al. 1998) because it is clinically complicated by different facial form appearances due to age, hairstyle, eyewear, and body mass changes. Furthermore, no significant correlation exists because of the vast variety of facial forms and the fact that the amazing face creation cannot be confined within limited forms and formulas. In all cases, the guidelines that will be reviewed within this topic are considered to be only relative guides to the overall appearance, rather than rules to be followed.

The correct understanding of the dental morphology of humankind allows us to create natural looking implant-supported prostheses. Lombardi (1973) detailed the artificial teeth characters and their impact on the smile design and final treatment results. Studying the standard anatomical object characters of natural teeth with which people are born has led the way to a wealth of knowledge and information that can be valuable in any esthetic reconstructive procedure. Age, gender, personality, habits, tooth position, shade, illumination, and illusion all influence the selection of the shape of the anterior maxillary teeth either in fully or partially edentulous cases. In cases of restoring missing maxillary teeth in the esthetic zone with or without dental implants, the clinician should strive to fabricate identical restorations that almost replicate natural missing dentition. If the missing teeth cannot be used as a reference due to their absence, then other references may be used as a guide. Therefore, the relationship between teeth form and the human face becomes poorly evidenced while the relationship between teeth, characters, and extraoral or intraoral factors become more logical.

Age

The morphological characters of anterior maxillary teeth are strongly influenced by the patient's age. In young individuals, the central and lateral incisors are long and rectangular, which emphasizes youthfulness. (See Figures 3.20A–B.) In older individuals, the front teeth often get worn and lose their rectangular shape, become square in shape due to incisal micro- or macrocracks, and sometimes attain up-fractions. The central incisors grow shorter due to parafunction, gingival recession, enamel cracks, and faulty dentistry. Less tooth structure will be visible when smiling. Small-sized incisal embrasures occur, whereas the gingival embrasures widen as a result of the recession of the gingiva (Goldstein 1998). Flat broad incisal edges and functional or parafunctional generalized attrition results in posterior wear of the dentition. This excessive wear can eventually lead to

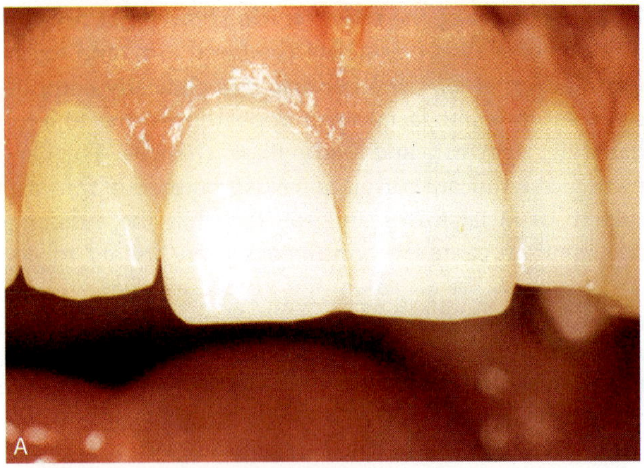

Figure 3.20A. Two central incisors characterize younger look, by its long and rectangular shape.

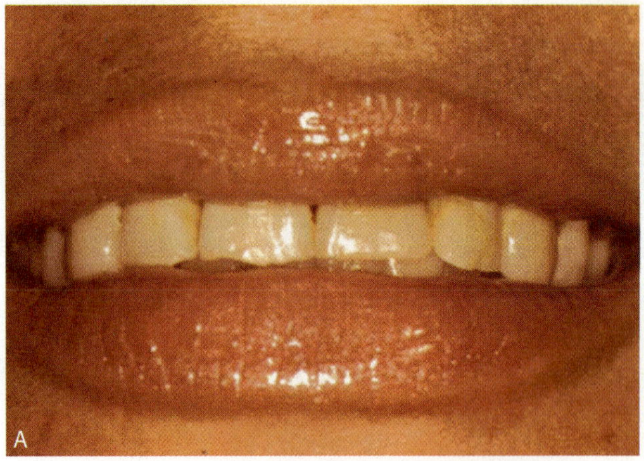

Figure 3.21A. An older smile that possesses worn central incisors.

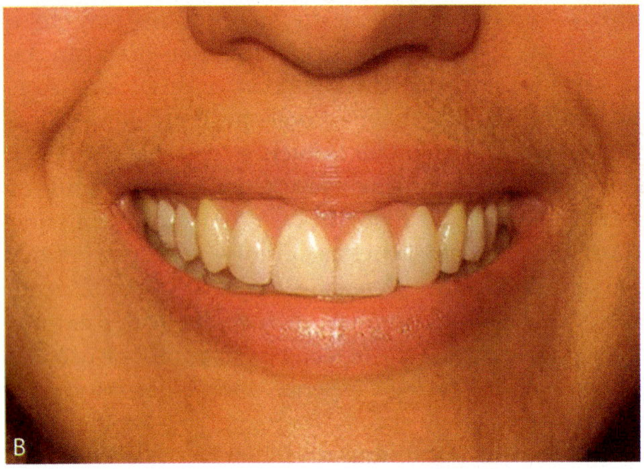

Figure 3.20B. A young female with a typical shape of youthful central incisors.

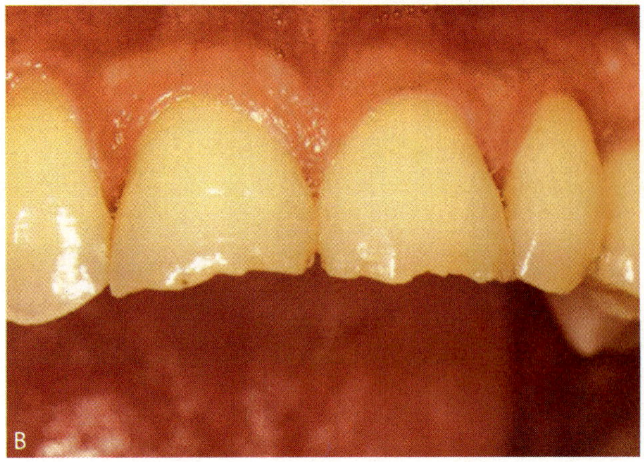

Figure 3.21B. Two central incisors exhibit wear and attrition due to parafunction.

shortening of the teeth. The incisal edges of the maxillary central incisors tend to wear more cervically, affecting the lingual, rather than the labial enamel. Eventually, the maxillary central and lateral incisors will exhibit the same incisogingival length (Yamamoto et al. 1990/1991). (See Figures 3.21A–B.) When the mouth is slightly open, approximately 3.5 mm of the incisal portion of the maxillary teeth is visible in a 20-year-old person, while the mandibular teeth are barely visible. Between the ages of 30 and 40 years, mandibular incisor exposure increases while the maxillary tooth length exposure decreases (Vig and Brundo 1978).

The maxillary central incisor is the key tooth in the oral cavity; it dominates the composition of the oral cavity by its size and location, and it brings order and coherence to the oral cavity (Frush and Fisher 1956). Sometimes the central incisors are not visible when the lips are at rest, but can be seen when smiling. This tends to render an older appearance to the dentition. If any morphological deviation exists in the original dimensions and counters, an interdisciplinary approach might be taken. (See Figure 3.22A–E.)

Hence, the importance of selecting the proper shape of the central incisor in major or minor implant-supported prosthetic cases is important. Many factors influence the selection of the shape of the central incisors, including (1) the amount of gingival display required, (2) lip line situation, (3) type of smile, (4) age of the patient, (5) amount of available interarch space, (6) the golden proportion, (7) the existing occlusion, and (8) the length and curvature of the upper lip (Chiche and Pinault 1994). Other factors that contribute to the selection of the shape of the maxillary central incisors include the lip muscle tone and skeletal build-up, and the incisal edge to the anterior guidance relationship (Qaltrough and Burke 1994).

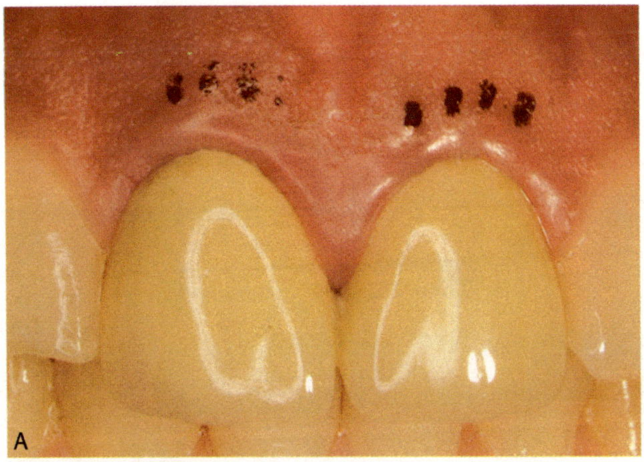

Figure 3.22A. Improper incisal-gingival position of the two central incisors. The black dots indicate the optimal position.

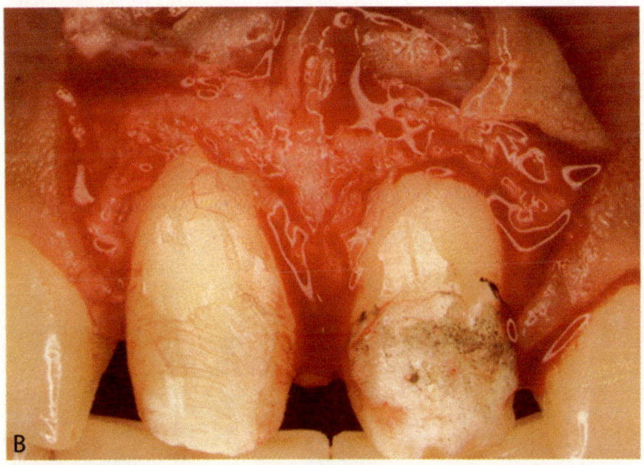

Figure 3.22B. Apical repositioning of the periodontium.

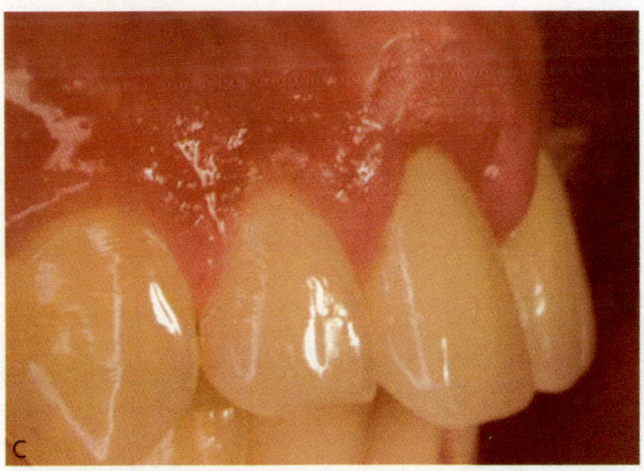

Figure 3.22C. The smile is enhanced after the correction of the incisal-gingival relationship.

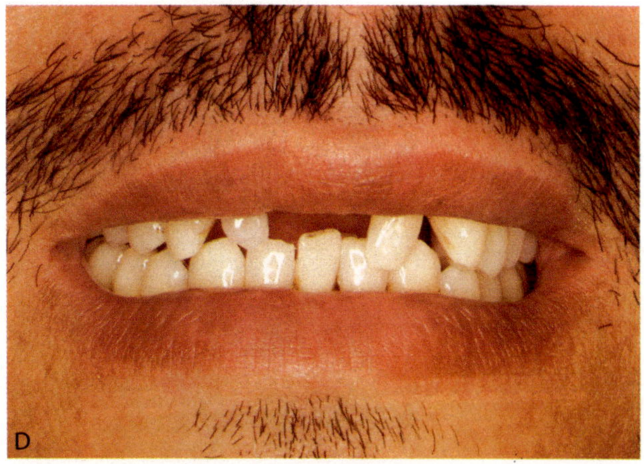

Figure 3.22D. Disfigured smile due to front teeth loss. Note the lost landmark for the extent of the central incisor height.

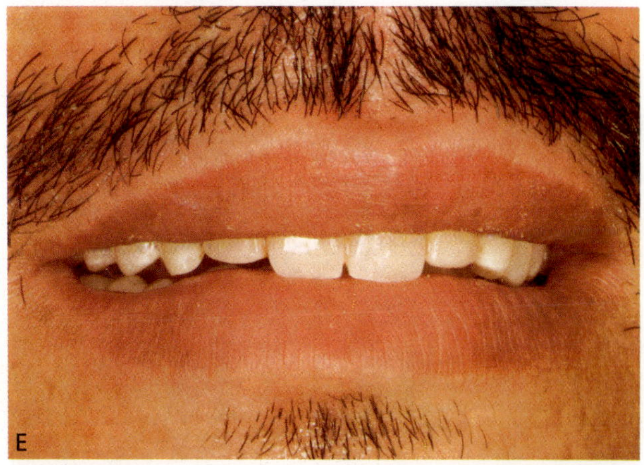

Figure 3.22E. The implant-supported provisional prosthesis in place to offering a proposed central incisor height that reflects harmony with the lower lip as well as optimal youthful display.

When performing major esthetic implant-supported restorations in totally edentulous patients, the selection of the shape of the anterior maxillary teeth and the amount of teeth display during smiling becomes extremely important to the overall prognosis of the treatment plan. The incisal edge of the maxillary central incisor is the most important factor in the fabrication of the artificial teeth set up. Once that is set, it determines the proper teeth proportion to follow and related gingival levels; therefore, the improper placement of the central incisor can lead to inadequate tooth display, or a displeasing tooth or crown proportion. (See Figures 3.23A–F.)

In a few clinical instances, shortening the incisal edge may be required to compensate for excessive display resulting from generalized gingival recession, especially in high smile line patients. The self-image of the patient and their desire for a dynamic and youthful appearance can help determine how prominent the dental arch can be. The average anatomic crown length for the maxillary

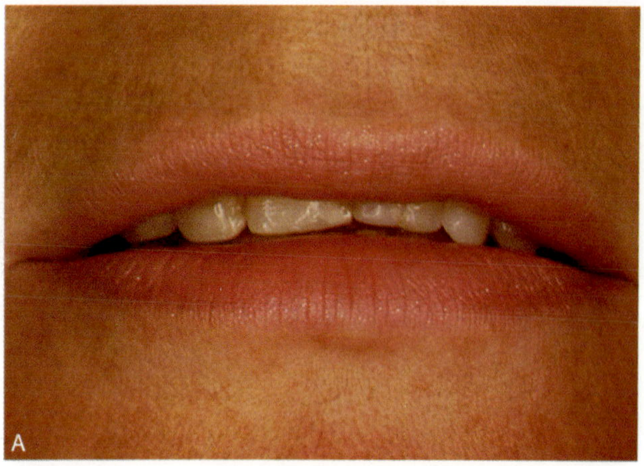

Figure 3.23A. A patient with an deficient smile due to decency of the central incisors.

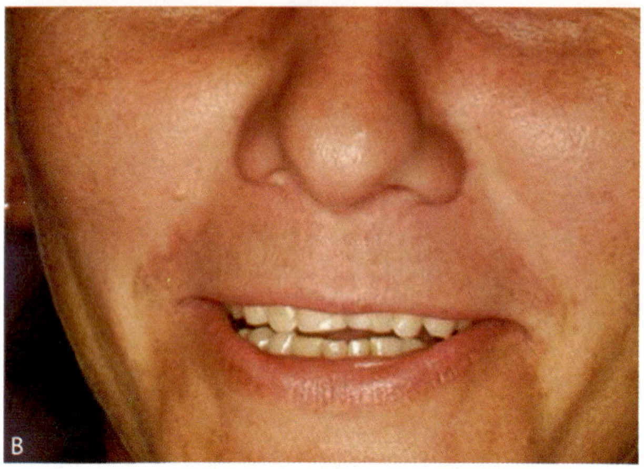

Figure 3.23B. The patient's face that reveals deficient smile.

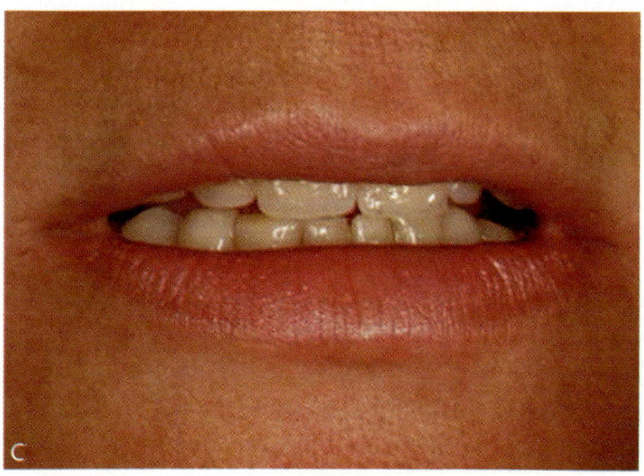

Figure 3.23C. The two central incisors being restored and the incisalgingival relationship corrected.

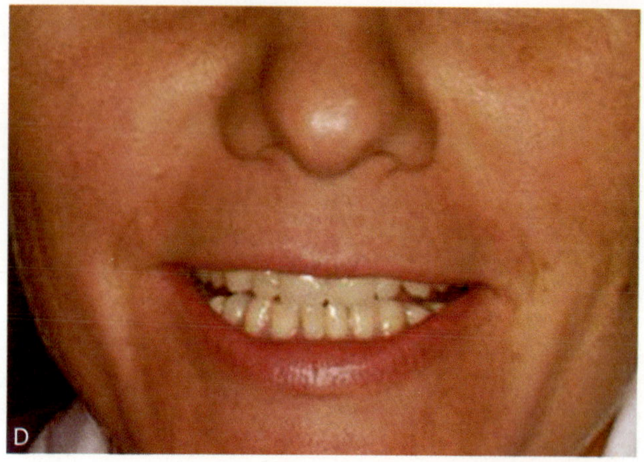

Figure 3.23D. The total smile improvement upon the teeth morphological correction.

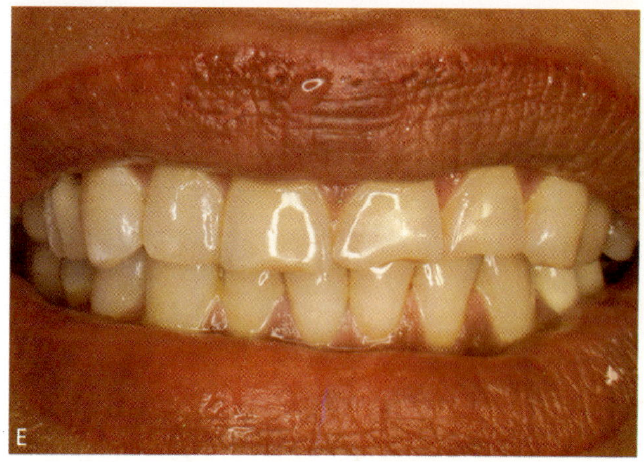

Figure 3.23E. Preoperative picture of an improper teeth reveal.

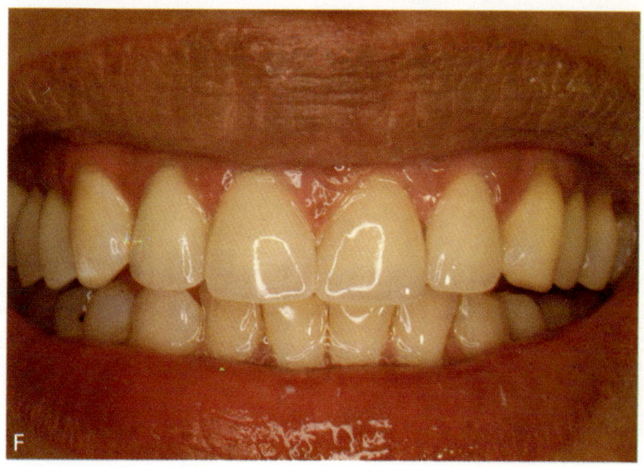

Figure 3.23F. Postoperative result postrestorative.

central incisor ranges from 10.4 mm to 11.2 mm. Treatment records might help to determine the original shape and height of the future prosthesis. Without this reference, determining the original shape and morphology of the missing teeth becomes a difficult task. When the treatment records do not exist, the clinician can use the upper lip position, the smile arc, and the remaining teeth as reference points. Therefore, the determination of the relationship between the lost central incisors and both lips mainly falls on the clinician's skills and prosthodontic experience, in addition to the previously mentioned factors.

The optimal position of the incisal edge of the maxillary teeth not only influences esthetics but also phonetics, because the lips and teeth attain a different position and relation for each sound that is made. The clinician asks the patient to say the letter "V" to determine the length and the lingual tilt of the incisal third of the maxillary central incisors and the letter "F" to determine the relationship of the maxillary teeth to the lower lip position. (See Figures 3.24A–B.) To emphasize the younger look of the artificial teeth, the cervical line might be set below the gingival margin, and the use of cylinder-shaped incisors might help. The enamel surface of a youthful dentition is semi-translucent, hard, and shiny, with a slightly irregular surface. Younger teeth often have white hypoplastic lines and have lower saturation and less characterization—a result of lower chroma—with a more textured, lighter, brighter, and higher value (Heymann 1987).

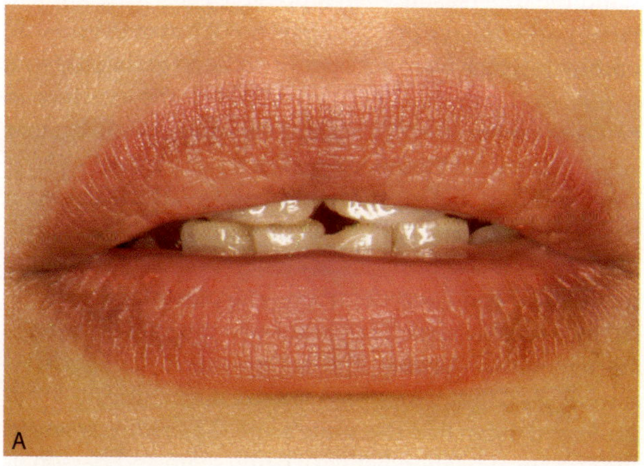

Figure 3.24A. A posed smile showing the minimum teeth reveal being detected by asking the patient to pronounce the letter "M."

Gender

The general teeth line angles in female dentition are more rounded than square. Femininity can be expressed in terms of delicacy and softness, whereas masculinity can be expressed in terms of vigor and angularity. The character in the female form appears as the roundness, smoothness, and softness that is typical in a woman. Masculinity, on the other hand, according to Frush and Fisher (1956) is the "cuboidal, hard, muscular, vigorous appearance, which is typical of men." For example, the shape of maxillary lateral incisors characterizes femininity to a certain extent. The feminine lateral incisor has rounded edges and possesses a constricted neck. On the other hand, the shape of the masculine lateral incisor is more rectangular and wider, and possesses sharp line angles (Lombardi 1973). The rotation of the lateral incisor's mesial surface, outward and beyond the distal surface of the central incisor, can create a more delicate or softer appearance of the lateral incisor when observed. On the contrary, the masculine lateral incisor appears square, with a flatter surface and sharper line angles. (See Figures 3.25 and 3.26.)

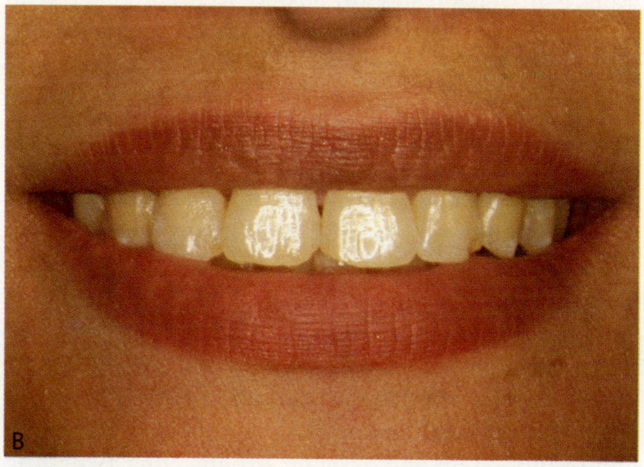

Figure 3.24B. The maximum teeth reveal is being detected by asking the patient to pronounce the letter "E."

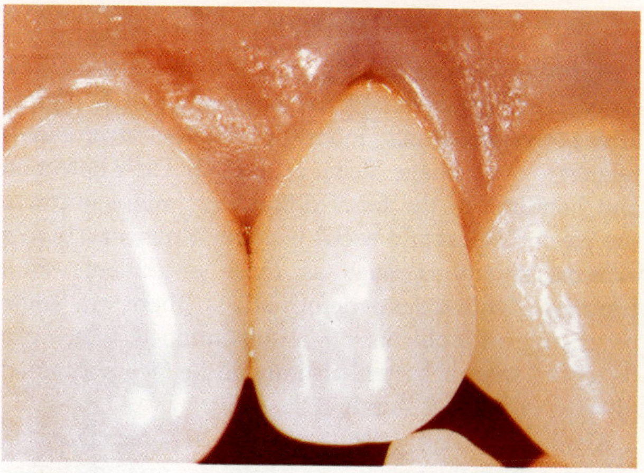

Figure 3.25. Feminine lateral incisor that is rounded in shape and possesses a constricted neck.

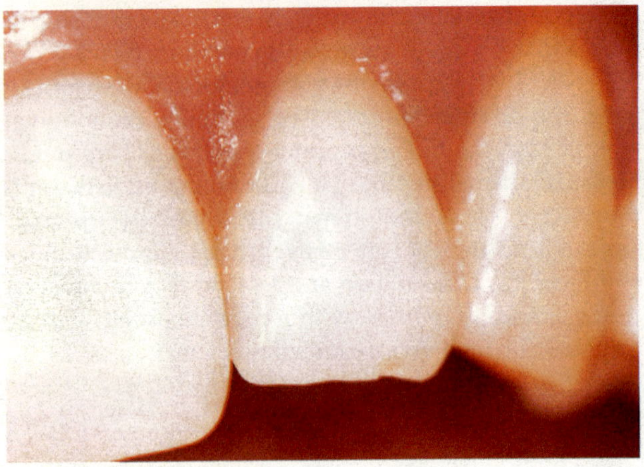

Figure 3.26. Masculine lateral incisor that is flat and has sharp line angles.

Personality

Major worries about physical attraction are concentrated on the face. Adults who are highly satisfied with their own faces normally feel more confident than others. Despite a lack of research supporting the connection between personality and facial features, it is a common perception that beautiful adults and children have more advantages in terms of social qualifications and intelligence than those considered to be ugly (Adams 1977, Adams 1978, Dion et al. 1972, Goldman and Lewis 1977). According to Proffit and White (1990), the psychological response of the patient to a malformation may be classified as follows:

1. A response of compensation (the patient takes on an attitude that allows him to overcome his disfigurement)
2. An inadequate response (the patient blames his malformation for certain difficulties in his life and relationships)
3. A pathological response (the patient appears to have some definite traits of neurosis and prepsychosis)

A negative body image may cause some serious defensive personal complexes that might slowly regress after correction; it may modify psychological problems related to body image (Belfer et al. 1982). Early detection and handling of the facial deformities might improve the psychological and social welfare of patients. In less extreme situations, such as those of patients with common dentoskeletal deformations, there are some psychological problems, often unmentioned, which can be solved when a better harmony of the face is attained (Strauss et al. 1988, Arndt et al. 1987).

Kiyak and Bell (1990) studied 977 teenagers to appraise the influence of dental esthetics on body image and social factors. There was a remarkable difference between those who had an intermaxillary discrepancy and those who did not. The more serious cases of intermaxillary discrepancy considerably affected self-esteem and body image. However, Kenealy and others (1989) examined 1,918 children aged 1 to 12 and did not find any psychological problems among children with intermaxillary discrepancy.

In general, patients are more satisfied with the improvement in their personality and appearance than they were with the improvement in their oral functions. In a longitudinal study, Wictorin, Hillerstrom, and Sorensen (1969) examined 95 patients before the operation and 49 patients one year after surgery: 96% were satisfied, 74% reported improvement in their social relationships, and 60% were found to be more confident. Laufer and others (1976) studied 25 patients two to six years after surgical correction of facial deformities. They found 84% to be satisfied and noted an improvement in personality. Despite the favorable outcomes, some patients were not satisfied. It is often difficult to understand the true reason, even if possible causes are known. Some patients have previous psychological or psychiatric problems which were not openly declared to the surgeon.

Kim and others (1995) investigated the correlation between personality factors and the smile, assuming that smile esthetics is closely related to an individual's physical condition and psychological state. They selected a panel of 30 male and 30 female students who had no missing teeth, no previous orthodontic or prosthodontic treatments, and good dentition. The personalities of the subjects were assessed by means of a questionnaire with 16 personality factors. The authors took standardized frontal photographs of each subject's face during a full smile and estimated the smile score. Then they assessed the statistical relation between smile score and personality. Warm, calm, enthusiastic, venturesome, self-assured, group-oriented, and relaxed personality traits were correlated with an attractive smile. Of the second-order personality factors derived from the primary personality traits, extroversion and low anxiety were correlated with an attractive smile. Interestingly, women's personalities were correlated to attractive smiles but men's personalities were not. The esthetic levels of women's smiles were correlated at statistically significant levels to four primary and two secondary personality traits. Among men, however, there were no statistically significant relationships between personality trails and smile esthetics.

The maxillary canines are the key teeth that provide the vigor of the personality effect because they may emphasize vigor of the personality (Lombardi 1973). A sharp, pointed incisal tip canine appears to add more vigor, while a flat tip cuspid may show no aggression at all in the personality. The passive cuspid may have a blunt rounded tip and a convex profile, often exhibiting large incisal embrasures between the laterals and canines that create a passive appearance (Morley 1997), as shown in Figures 3.27A–B. The shade of the teeth also

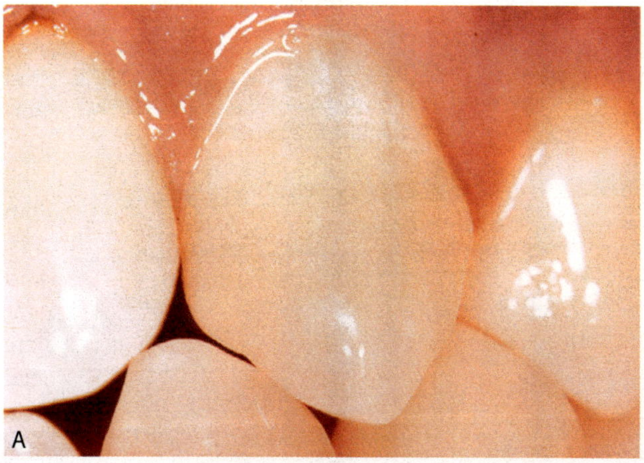

Figure 3.27A. Sharp canine tip that impacts the vigor of the personality.

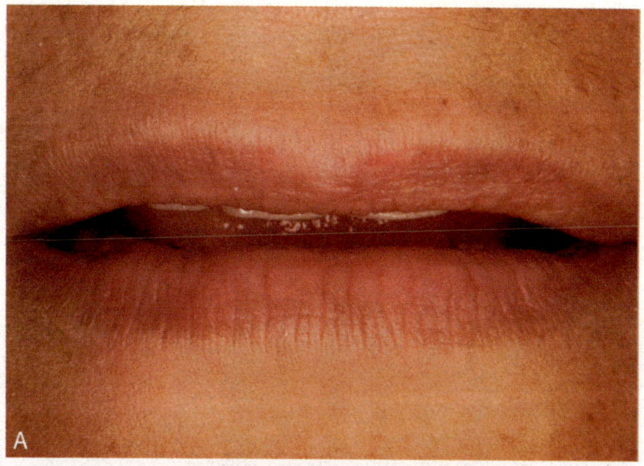

Figure 3.28A. A patient with defective teeth reveal.

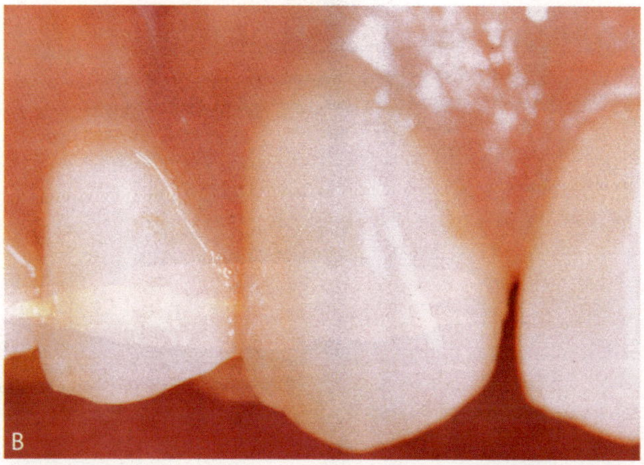

Figure 3.27B. A low profile tipped canine that indicates an average personality.

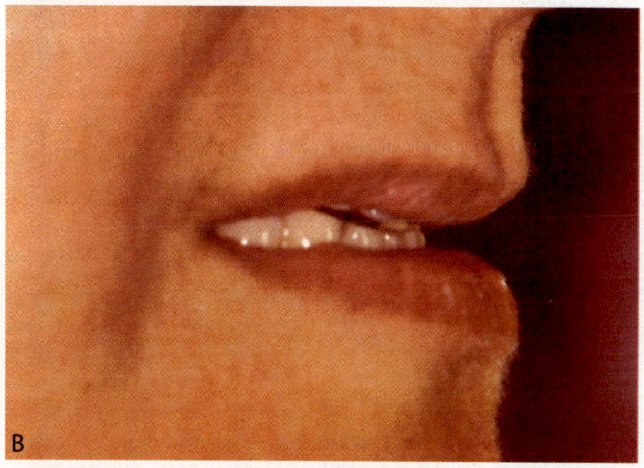

Figure 3.28B. The impact of the deficient teeth reveal on the profile.

can give an impression of the personality. In general, light teeth characterize a young, strong, and/or sharp personality, while darker teeth may sometimes reflect a workaholic, stressed, or loaded personality. Placing the maxillary anterior teeth slightly in a labial position can give an effect of youthfulness and an optimistic look. In addition, the slight increase in the incisal edge of the front teeth (in very limited microns) can improve the personal impact, as shown in Figures 3.28A–L.

Using sharp teeth line angles sharpens the look of the face. A consistent arch form and correct proportion to the facial morphology are essential factors in achieving pleasing dentition with a strong personal impact. The proportion must be in harmony with the strong or weak features of the face; this might be applied successfully to the central incisor length (Rufenacht 1990).

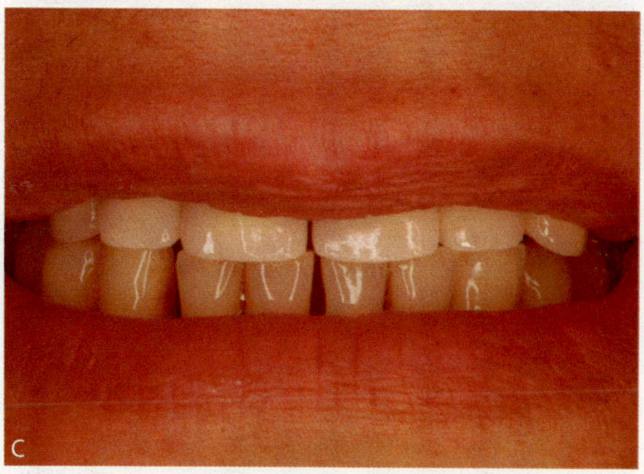

Figure 3.28C. Teeth reveal enhanced.

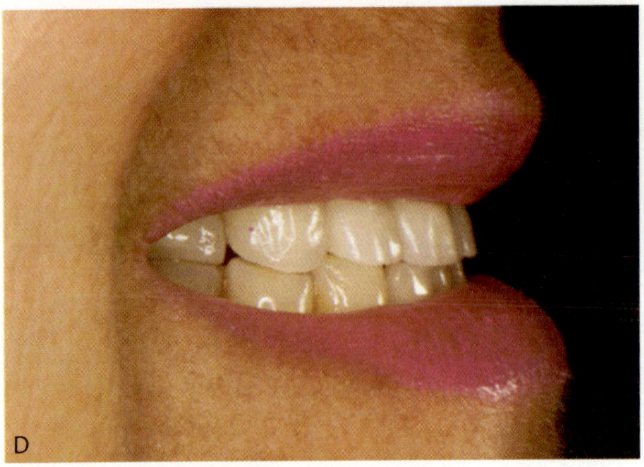

Figure 3.28D. The improvement of the patient profile.

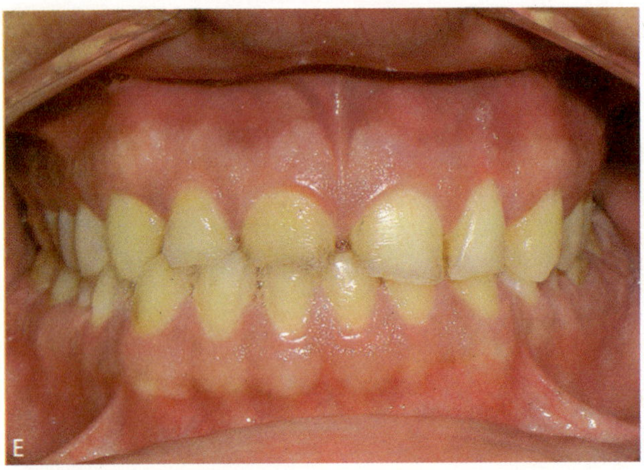

Figure 3.28E. Patient presented with bite collapse and improper incisogingival relationship at the incisors area. Note the level of the gingival margin of the central incisors in relation to the lateral incisors, which negatively influence the amount of teeth reveal within the smile.

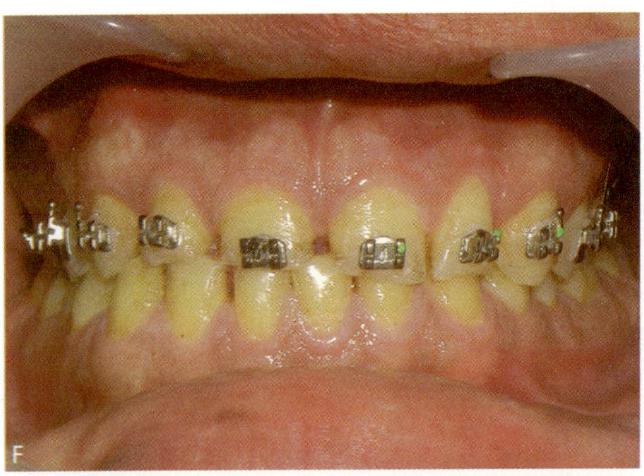

Figure 3.28F. The orthodontic brackets are positioned in a way that would regain the optimal incisogingival relationship (Abbas Zaher, personal communications, Alexandria, Egypt 2006).

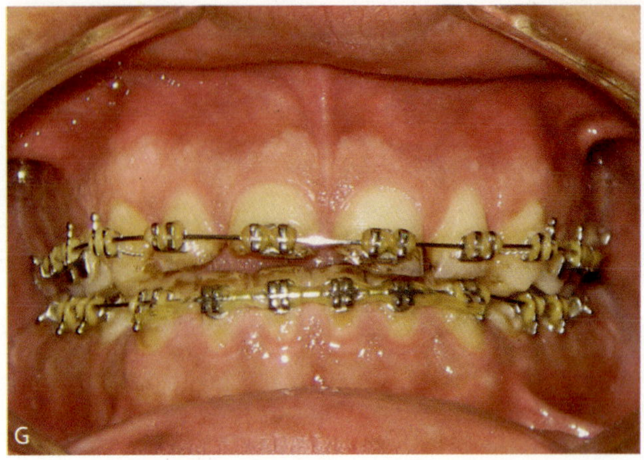

Figure 3.28G. Note the improvement in the bite level as well as the incisogingival relationship.

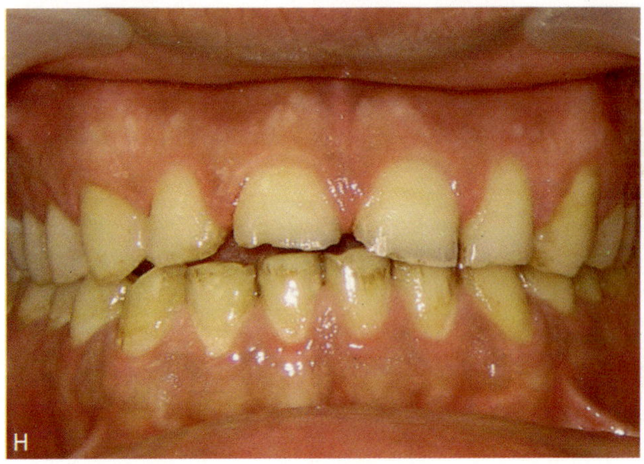

Figure 3.28H. The clinical condition post-orthodontic wires removal.

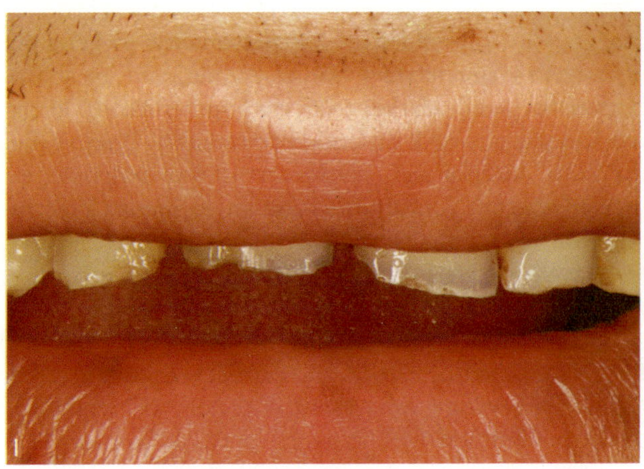

Figure 3.28I. The deficient teeth reveal that negatively influences the smile.

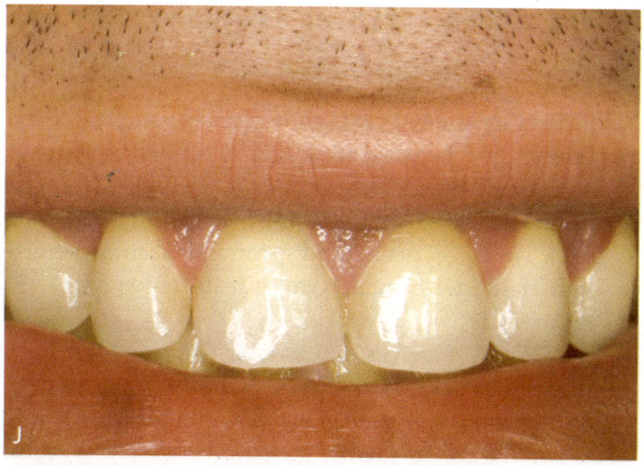

Figure 3.28J. The reveal is corrected to its critical limit.

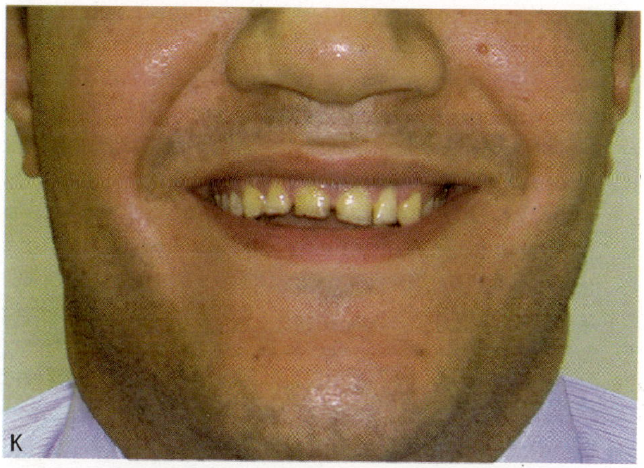

Figure 3.28K. Preoperative view of the patient smile.

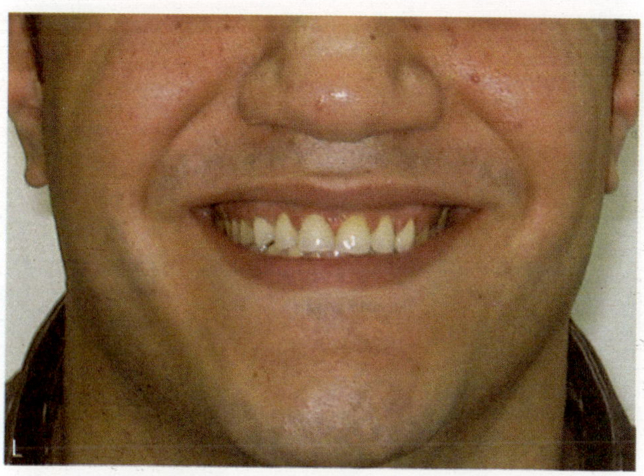

Figure 3.28L. Postoperative view of the smile improvement.

Prosthetic Shade

Shade is yet another vital factor in the symphony. Two methods are commonly used to analyze the color of natural teeth and shade guides: the first and most common method involves visual comparison, and the second method involves the use of an instrument such as a colorimeter. Unfortunately, both techniques have inherent inaccuracies. Visual examination requires trained and experienced individuals (Goodkind and others 1985), and shade selection can be affected by illumination and surrounding tissues. Instrumental measurements may be complicated by setup difficulty and heat produced by the instrument in repeated measurements, which could cause discomfort to the subject or failure of the instrument to maintain its calibration (Goodkind and Schwabacher 1987, Hasegawa et al. 2000). The teeth shade can be identified with the Munsell system of color identification:

- Hue refers to the dimension of color that distinguishes one family of color from another (red, blue, yellow, and so on).
- Value describes the dimension of color that denotes relative blackness or whiteness/brightness.
- Chroma is the dimension that describes the saturation, intensity, or strength of a hue (Ahangiri et al. 2002).

The shade of the artificial teeth is one of the most controversial aspects in dentistry; it is influenced by the patient's desires and the clinician's views. Nowadays the general population wants to have white teeth; however, white teeth often are not suitable for many patients. The shade of the prosthesis is strongly linked to many related clinical issues. For example, a female patient who wears red lipstick might attain some reddish pigments in her prosthesis to allow for color matching and white, cleaner, and fresher teeth might be desirable (Touati et al. 1999). Hence the proper shade and color matching of the prosthesis have a direct impact on the patient's overall well-being.

Reproduction of the original natural shade progression becomes a valuable tool in restoring a natural smile. (See Figure 3.29.) The shade of teeth uniquely progresses in individuals. A gradual dimming naturally occurs in the degree of shading (i.e., the central incisor is the lightest tooth in the maxillary arch followed by the lateral incisor that is similar in hue, but lower in color value). Then the canine becomes the darkest tooth in the oral cavity, thus forming the corners the mouth as it becomes darker with the highest chroma saturation and the lowest value. Then the premolars become lighter again (Goodkind and Schwabacher 1973). This unique natural shade progression allows for a natural look that does not obscure the vision.

Shade relates to lip size and gender, as well. When restoring a young patient with a thick lip, lighter shades might be considered. On the contrary, when restoring an older patient, darker shades that are lower in value and higher in chroma than those seen in younger adults could be used. The dentine begins to dominate the shade to simulate the natural effect of worn enamel. Some stains can be added to emphasize oral habits such as smoking or tooth up-fractions, because it is illogical to give an 80-year-old patient lighter teeth that do not match his facial characteristics or complexion at this particular age. This could make a natural-looking person look artificial. The perception of the teeth shade is influenced by the tooth's shape and its morphologic position within the arch, as well as the clinician's decision (Golub-Evans 1994). (See Figure 3.30.)

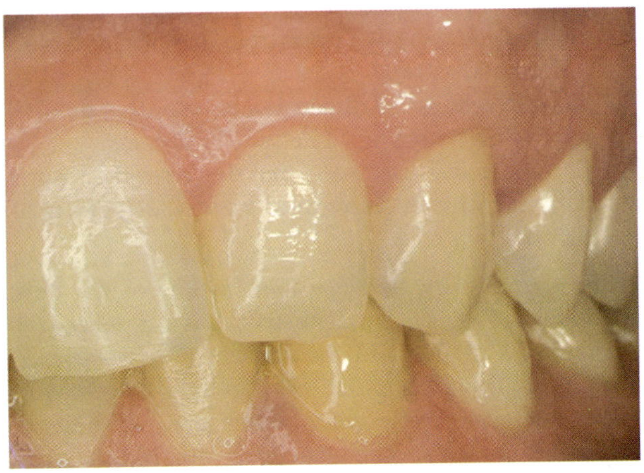

Figure 3.29. Natural shade progression.

Factors Influencing Shade Selection

Many factors influence artificial teeth shade selection:

1. Patient's personality: Lighter shades usually are recommended because they add a positive impact to someone's personality.
2. Facial features: Strong facial features such as wide eyes, a large nose, and prominent chin require lighter shades to match those features, as shown in Figure 3.31.
3. Skin color: A perception among clinicians has been that individuals with darker skin colors should have lighter shades of teeth. This perception is commonly explained by the greater contrast between skin color and tooth shade. Studies related to staining and altering tooth shades are abundant in the dental literature.

Ahangiri and others (2002) explored the possibility of a relationship between tooth shade and skin color in a study of 119 individuals aged 18 to 80 years. Two investigators trained to examine tooth shade performed all of the examinations. A Vita-Lumin shade guide was used to examine either the maxillary right or left central incisor, one of which had to be restoration- and caries-free for study inclusion. Tooth shades were divided into four categories according to value. Skin tones were also divided into four categories (fair, fair/medium, medium, and dark) with the use of L'Oreal True Illusion compact makeup shades as a guide. Categorical modeling with chi-square analysis and Fisher's exact tests was used to analyze the data. The study did not find any interaction among age, skin color, and tooth shade or gender, skin color, and tooth shade; however, age was associated with tooth shade. Older people were more likely to have teeth with lower values (darker). Among those aged 60 and older, 85% had teeth in the medium and low range values compared with 17%

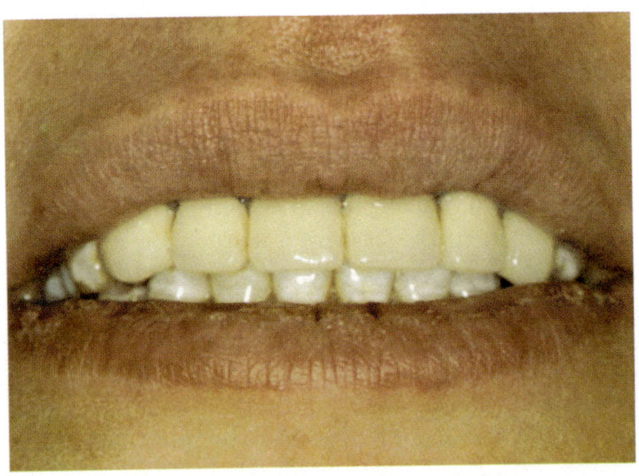

Figure 3.30. An implant-supported prosthesis that lacks teeth characterization and lacks shade progression.

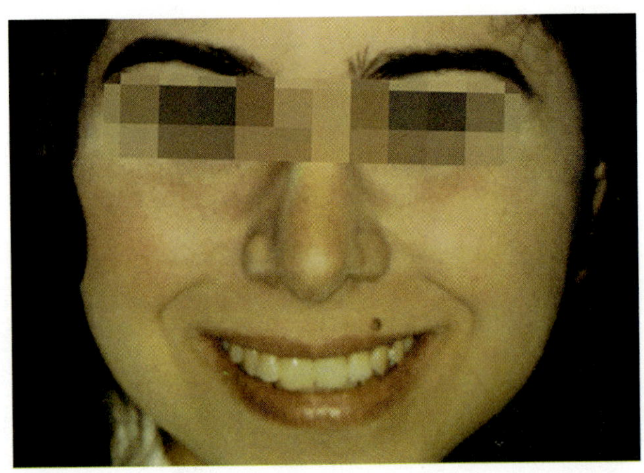

Figure 3.31. Strong facial features like prominent chin, wide black eyes.

of those younger than 31. Significant tooth shade differences were discovered among patients with different skin colors. Among those with low values (darker teeth), 50% were of fair complexion and 17% were of dark complexion.

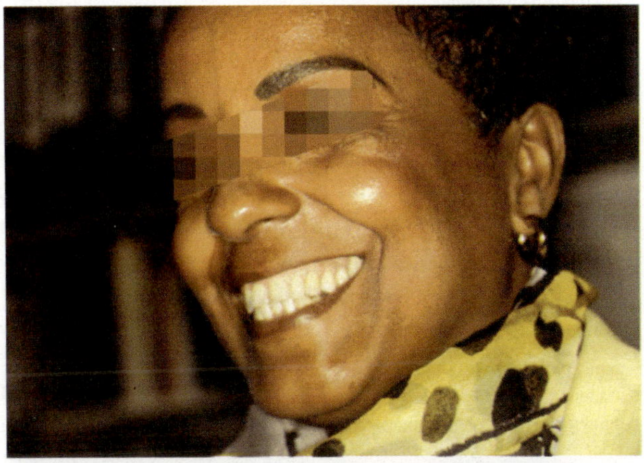

Figure 3.32. Dark skinned person that does not necessarily require a lighter shade.

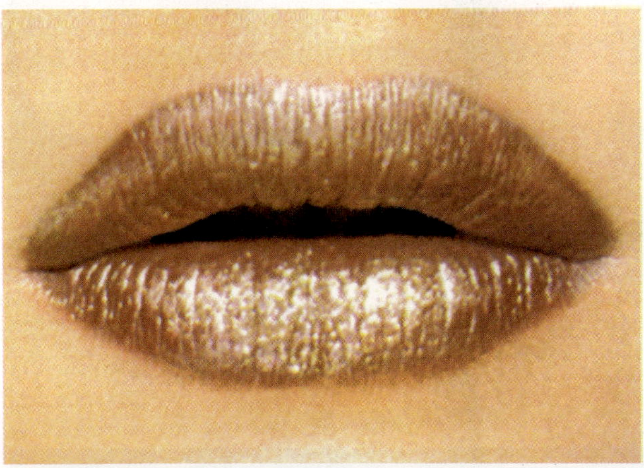

Figure 3.33. The mouth appears dark due to the overall smaller teeth surface area.

The study concluded that tooth shade value and skin color were inversely related. Older adults were more likely to have darker teeth (lower value). The study proposed that there is a significant relationship between tooth shade and skin color. People with medium-to-dark skin tones were more likely to have teeth with higher values (lighter), whereas individuals with lighter skin tones tended to have teeth with lower values (darker), regardless of gender or age. However, a dark-skinned person does not necessarily require lighter teeth, because the dark skin background reflects the shade more to appear lighter because the greater the contrast, the greater the visibility, as shown in Figure 3.32. It is also worth mentioning that wrinkled skin reflects less light than nonwrinkled skin.

4. Total exposed tooth area: Patients with reduced teeth size usually require maximum lighter shades to give an impact for the mouth. (See Figure 3.33.)
5. Size of teeth: Large teeth display requires slightly darker shades in cases in which the teeth need to appear smaller.
6. Tooth morphological effects: Rough surface texture allows the deflection and reflection of light from the dental surfaces, thus reducing light, as shown in Figures 3.34A–C.)

Illusion in Dentistry

Illusion is routinely used in dentistry to help hide some prosthetic artifacts (i.e., deficient papillae) or to pronounce clinical reality (i.e., buccal corridor). The rules of illusion that are commonly applied in dentistry are:

1. If two structures of the same size are placed at different distances, the closest one appears larger, as shown in Figure 3.35. This rule is applied in the oral cavity. As the teeth pass posteriorly, the light is reduced within the buccal corridor, giving a gradually darker shade, blurring the details and making

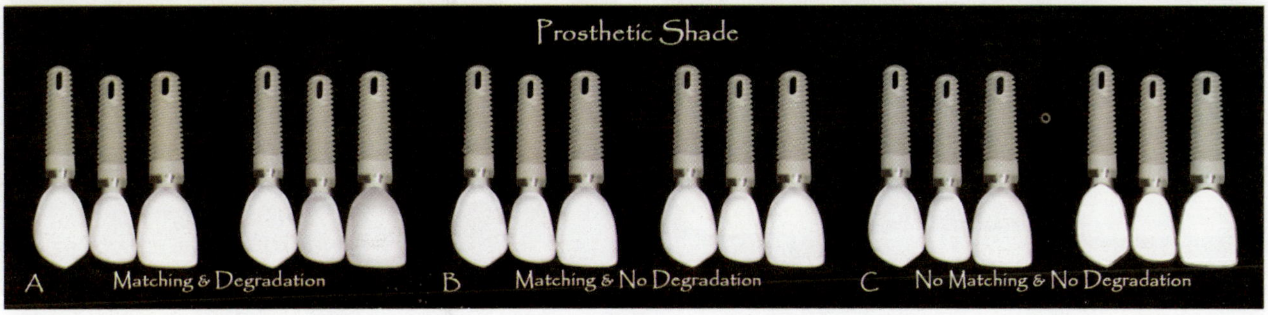

Figure 3.34A, B, C. Shade assessment parameters.

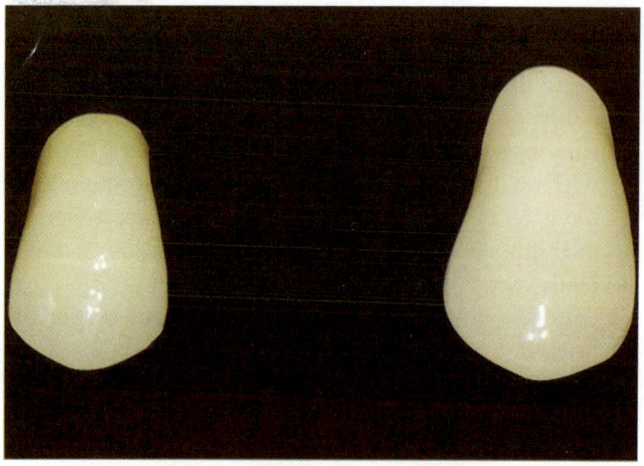

Figure 3.35. If two structures of the same size are placed at different distances, the closest one appears larger.

the teeth appear smaller as seen posteriorly, as shown in Figure 3.36.

2. Of two objects that are the same size and the same level, the lighter colored object will appear larger, as shown in Figure 3.37.
3. Teeth of equal widths but with different lengths appear to have different widths, as shown in Figure 3.38, because the smaller the tooth contour, the smaller the tooth appears.
4. As the amount of contrast increases, visibility increases accordingly, as shown in Figure 3.39. These rules are applied daily in our practice; for example, a tooth could be made to look wider than its original size by doing some alterations in its surface texture (horizontal lines). A tooth may be made to look narrower than it is by simply moving the proximal line angles medially, or the tooth can be made

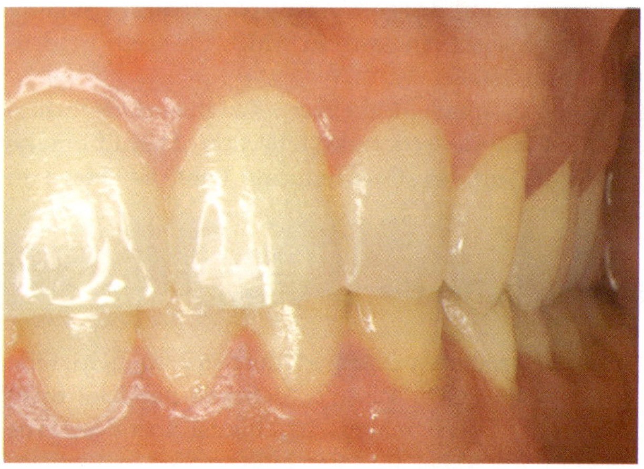

Figure 3.36. The natural teeth blur and get smaller as far as it goes posteriorly in the buccal corridor.

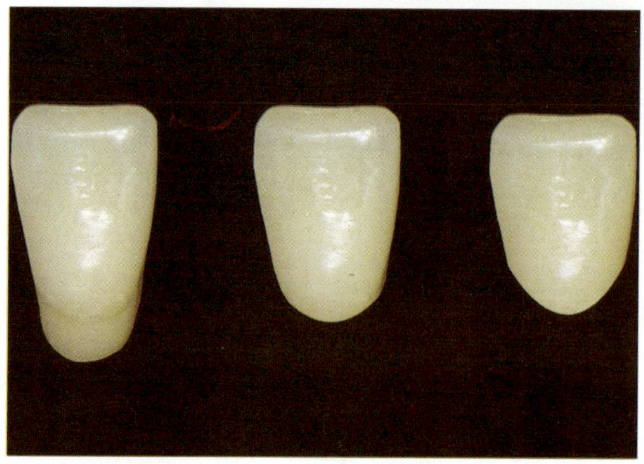

Figure 3.38. Teeth of equal widths but with different lengths appear to have different widths.

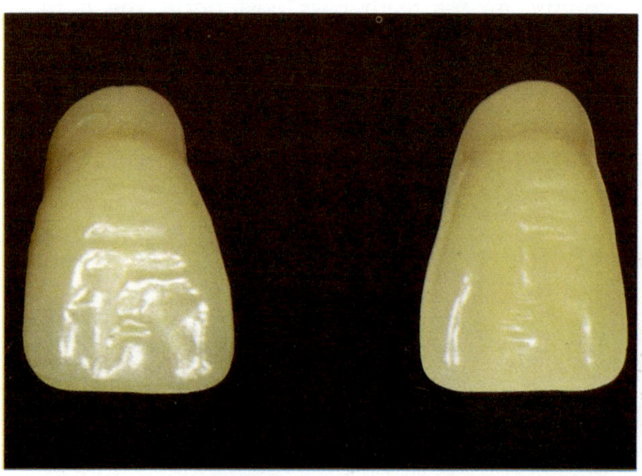

Figure 3.37. In two objects of the same size, the lighter will appear larger.

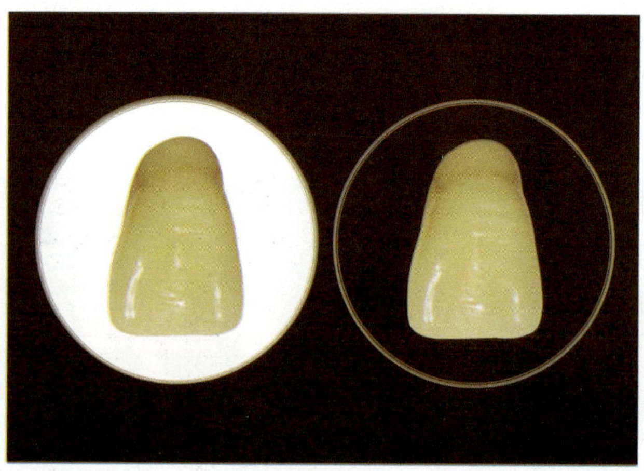

Figure 3.39. As the amount of contrast increases, visibility increases accordingly.

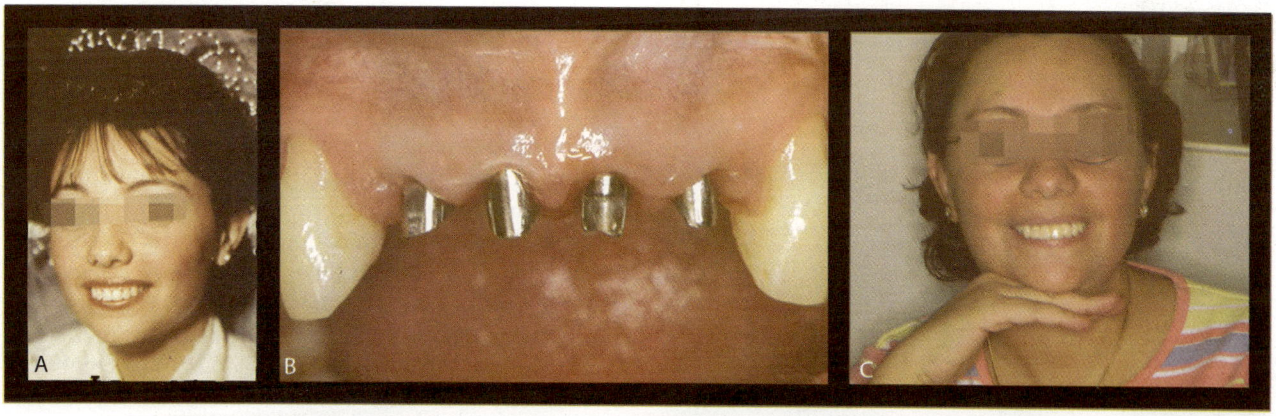

Figure 3.40. A. A female patient's preextraction picture (15 years prior to teeth loss). B. The implants in place and the abutments connected. C. The patient restored. Note the similarity between the teeth shape and reveal pre- and postteeth loss.

to look longer by adding vertical lines to it (Matthews 1978). The dark anterior "negative" space creates a clear contrast between the incisors and the lower lip in the anterior region, and this color contrast, in turn, adds a dynamic external appearance. Furthermore, if the artificial teeth lack characterization, they may appear more artificial, causing a high reflection of light (Matthews 1978). The light reflected by the dental surfaces alters the perception of the size and color and the perception of the depth of a tooth. A tooth will seem closer if an increased surface texture is added to it, and it will appear more distant, if the surface texture is kept as smooth as possible (Vanini 1996).

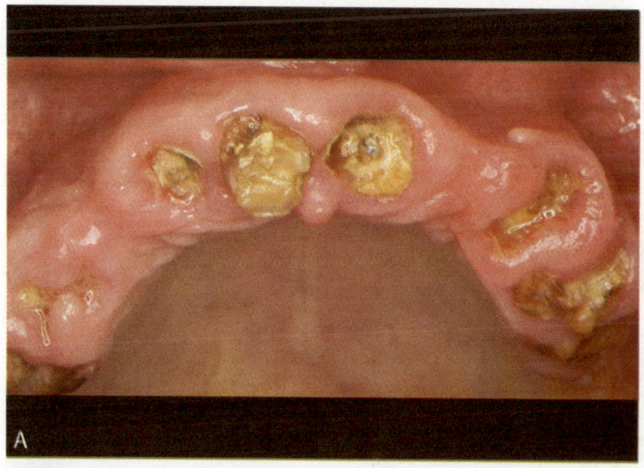

Figure 3.41A. An intraoral picture that indicates the loss of teeth shape and reveal.

Treatment Records

Data that is collected from an edentulous patient can be of great value to the treatment plan. Upon teeth loss, the reference to the original teeth shape is lost as well. The search for a reference is then important to give an idea on the shape of the teeth and their inherited surface characters (Baratieri 1998). The data can be collected from old photographs, slides, videotapes, etc. The problem for the clinician who is restoring lost teeth arises when there is no reference to imitate nor any original shape to duplicate. In that case, the patient might receive teeth that do not resemble their original shape or do not satisfy them psychologically. The data gathered from pictures can include the teeth reveal, teeth shape, teeth characters, the existence of diastema, smile arc pattern, and the relationship of the incisal edge to the lower lip. Photographs also may serve as proof of records for future referrals or for future comparison before and after the treatment. (See Figures 3.40A–C, 3.41A–D, and 3.42A–C.)

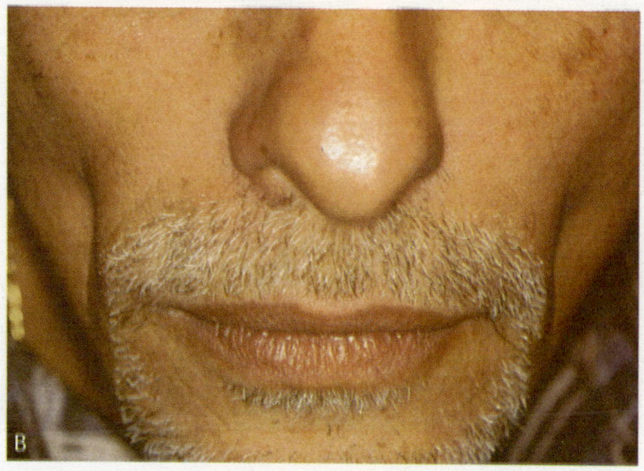

Figure 3.41B. The effect of teeth loss on the patient's face.

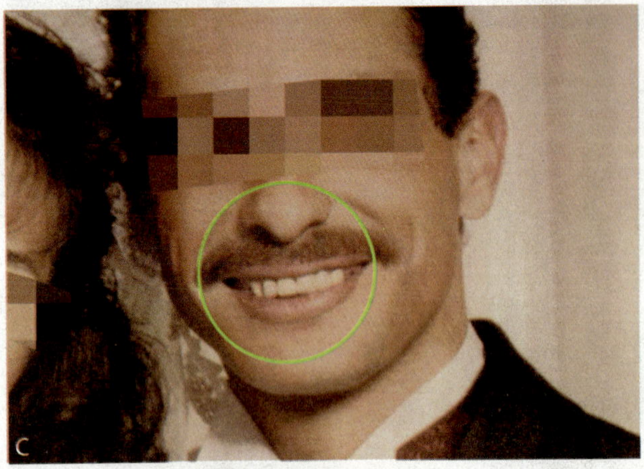

Figure 3.41C. An old picture of the patient that shows his original teeth shape and the amount of tooth display.

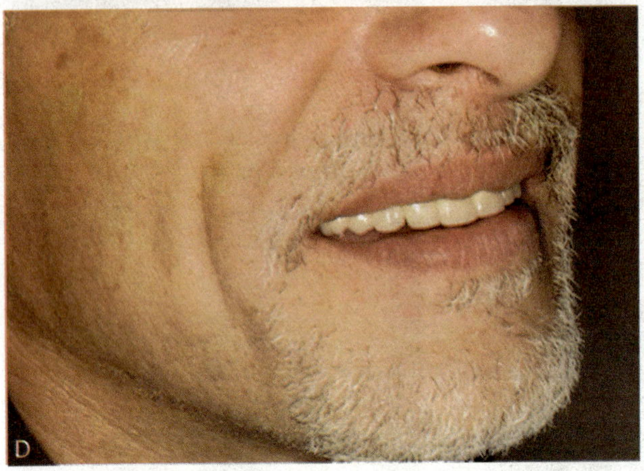

Figure 3.41D. The patient after being restored. Note the duplication of almost the same amount of tooth display and shape.

Symmetry

Symmetry and balance are interconnected requirements for any esthetic intraoral restoration that provides a pleasing look and does not annoy or obscure the natural feeling of an object. Among the factors that influence balance and symmetry in oral rehabilitation with dental implants are the determination of the correct occlusal or incisal plane and the midline. This helps to achieve the balance and symmetry of the oral mechanism and appearance (Strub and Turp 1999). Symmetry in the oral cavity indicates that the different elements are combined in harmony and with respect for each other. Any deviation from the natural known and created symmetry may lead to both esthetic and functional problems.

Balance is the stabilizing result of the exact adjustment of opposing forces (Goldstein 1984). Balance is observed while the eyes move distally starting from the center of an object, in contrast to symmetry, which is centrally located (Goldstein 1984). Good examples of poor symmetry are the disproportionate size of two adjacent central incisors or a case in which one of them is rotated facially or lingually. Poor balance is reflected in a deviated midline or an uneven implant-supported overdenture height. Lombardi (1973) noted that proper location of the dental midline is necessary for stability of the dental composition, because improper placement of the midline makes it impossible to balance the elements on either side of it. Tension is produced by induced forces that make the viewer feel that the line must move to its proper place to produce stability and permanence. (See Figures 3.43, 3.44A–B, and 3.45A–B.)

The rule of thirds can be a helpful way to determine the correct occlusal plane; it divides the lower third of the face into thirds. The ideal position of the occlusal

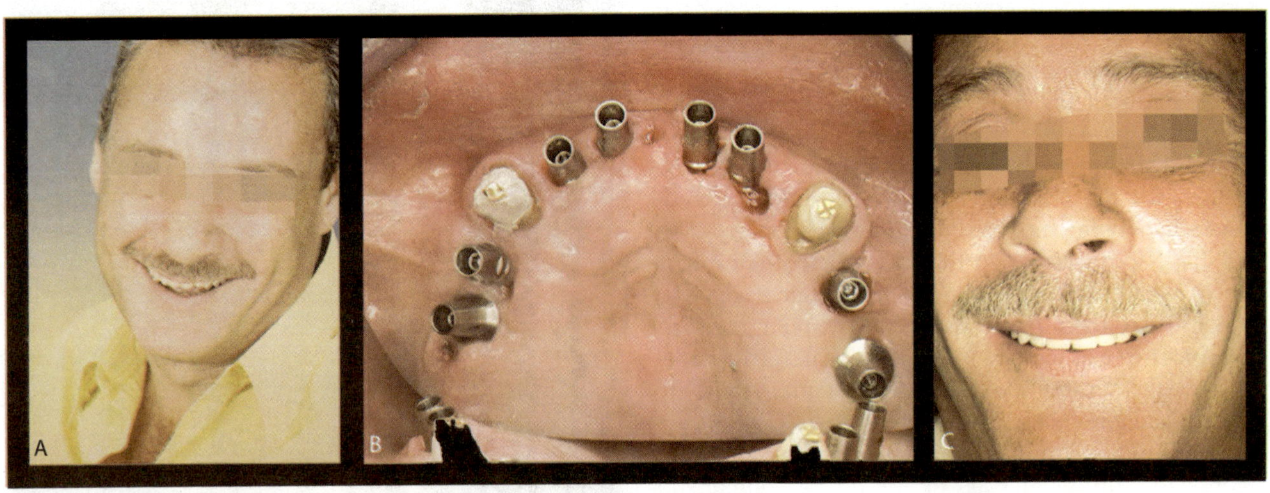

Figure 3.42. **A.** A male patient with his original teeth in place prior to teeth loss. **B.** The patient at the time of impression taking. **C.** The patient after being finally restored. Note the duplication of the smile arc of the patient prior to teeth loss.

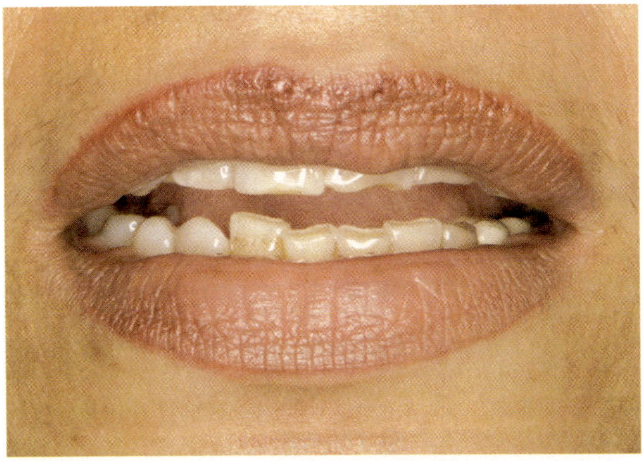

Figure 3.43. Poor asymmetry of teeth shape due to teeth wear.

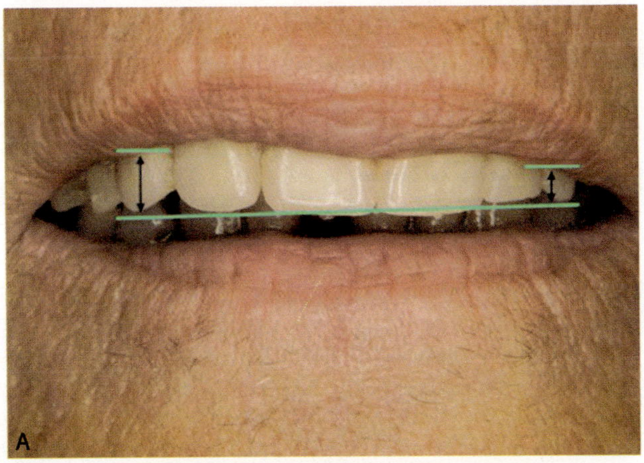

Figure 3.44A. An asymmetrical implant supported overdenture.

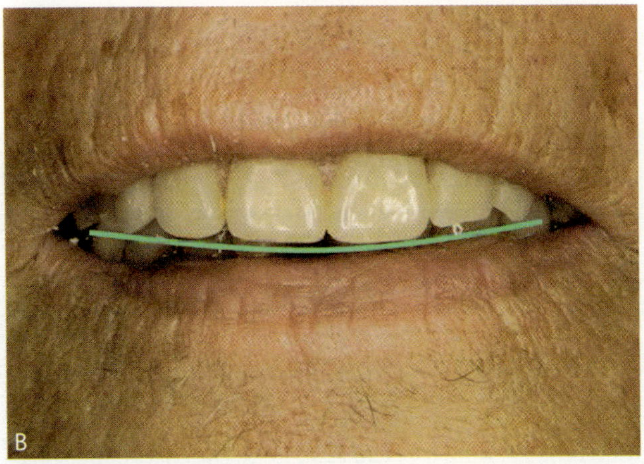

Figure 3.44B. The asymmetry is being corrected.

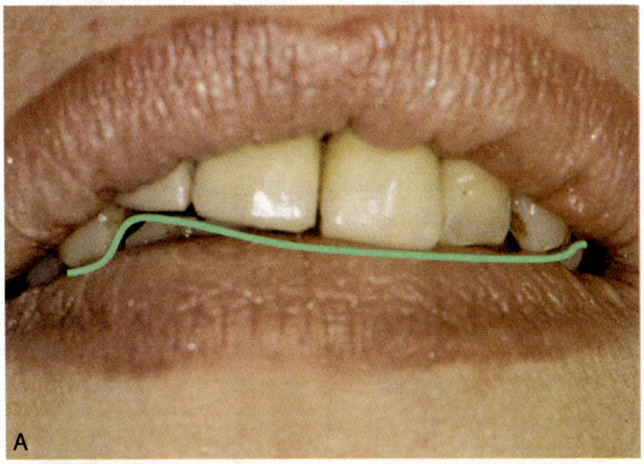

Figure 3.45A. Poorly made incisal plane.

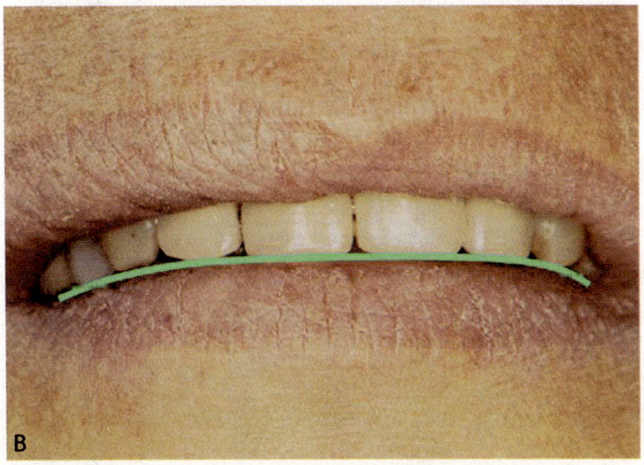

Figure 3.45B. The incisal plane is being corrected.

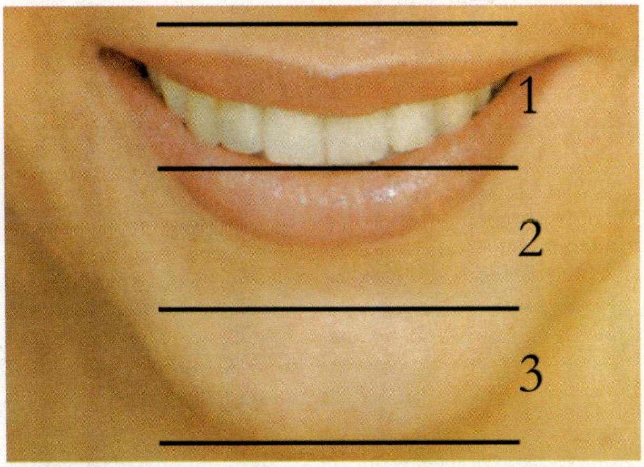

Figure 3.46. The rule of thirds.

plane is at the junction of the upper and middle thirds, as shown in Figure 3.46. The dental midline is an imaginary vertical line that does not necessarily coincide with the facial midline. Ideally, the papilla between the maxillary central incisors coincides with the midline of the face. This is not necessary, however, because not all patients have symmetrical faces; their chins or noses are not always centered, although they do not look disfigured (Johnston et al. 1999). Another example is when the right and left sides of the cheeks do not coincide; hence it is impossible to use them as landmarks for the facial midline (Rufenacht 1990).

The natural appearance of the face as a whole does not influence the visual perception of the dental midline. The dental midline should be right in line with the precise midline of where the smile appears, which is located in the center and coincides with the symmetry of the dental composition. In those cases where the dental and facial midlines do not coincide, the dental midline should be made perpendicular to the pupillary or horizontal lines to prevent the illusion of asymmetry. The composition, once it is vertical, will appear symmetrical or at least pleasing (Latta 1988).

References

Ackerman, J., M. Ackerman, C. Brensinger, and J. Landis. 1998. A morphometric analysis of the posed smile. *Clin Orth Res.* 1, pp. 2–11.

Adams, G.R. 1977. Physical attractiveness research: toward a developmental social psychology of beauty. *Hum Dev*, 20, pp. 217–230.

Adams, G.R. 1978. Racial membership and physical attractiveness effects on preschool teacher's expectations. *Child Study J*, 8, p. 29.

Ahangiri, A., S. Reinhardt, and R. Mehra. 2002. Relationship between tooth shade value and skin color: An observational study. *J Prosthet Dent*, 87, pp. 149–52.

Ameed, A. 2001. Personal communications, London, United Kingdom.

Arndt, E.M., E. Travis, A. Lefebvre, and I.R. Munro. 1987. Psychosocial adjustment of 20 patients with Treacher Collins syndrome before and after reconstructive surgery. *Br J Plast Surg*, 40, pp. 605–609.

Baratieri, L.N. 1998. Esthetics: *Direct Adhesive Restoration Fractured Anterior Teeth*, Sao Paulo: Quintessence, pp. 270–312.

Belfer, M.L., A.M. Harrison, F.C. Pillemer, and J.E. Murray. 1982. Appearance and the influence of reconstructive surgery on body image. *Clin Plast Surg*, 9, pp. 307–315.

Burstone, C.J. 1967. Lip posture and its significance in treatment planning. *Am J Orthod*, (53), pp. 262–284.

Chiche, G.J., and A. Pinault. 1994. *Esthetics of Anterior Fixed Prosthodontics*. Chicago: Quintessence, pp. 13–32, 53–74.

Choi, T.R., and I.K. Demf. 1991. A study on the exposure of maxillary and mandibular central incisor in smiling and physiologic rest position. *J Wonkwang Dent Res Instil*, 5, 371, p. 79.

Dawson, P.E. 1983. Determining the determinants of occlusion. *Int J Periodont Rest Dent*, 3, p. 9.

Dickerson, W. 1996. Trilogy of creating on esthetic smile, *Tech Update*, (1), pp. 1–7.

Dion, K., E. Berscheid, and E. Walster. 1972. What is beautiful is good. *J Pers Soc. Psychol*, 24, pp. 285–290.

Dong, K., T. Ho, H. Cho, et al. 1999. The Esthetics of the Smile: A Review of Some Recent Studies. *Int J Prosthodont*, 72, pp. 9–19.

Duchenne, G.B. 1990. *The Mechanism of Human Facial Expression*. New York: Cambridge Univ Press.

Frush, J.P., and R.D. Fisher. 1956. How dentogenic restorations interpret the sex factor. *J Prosthet Dent*, (6), pp. 160–17.

Frush, J.P., and R.D. Fisher. 1985. The clynasthetic interpretation of the clentogenic concept. *J Prosthet Dent*, 8, pp. 518–531.

Gibson, R. 1989. Smiling and facial exercise. *Dent Clin North Am*, 33, pp. 139–144.

Goldman, W., and P. Lewis. 1977. Beautiful is good: evidence that the physically attractive are more socially skillful. *J Exp Psychol General*, 13, p. 125.

Goldstein, R.E. 1984. *Change your Smile*. 1st ed. Chicago: Quintessence.

Goldstein, R.E. 1998. *Esthetics in Dentistry*. 2nd ed. Hamilton, ON: BC Decker Inc, pp. 133–186.

Golub-Evans, J. 1994. Unity and variety: Essential ingredients of a smile design. *Curr Opin Cosmet Dent*, pp. 1–5.

Goodkind, R.J., and W.B. Schwabacher. 1973. Use of a fiber-optic colorimeter for in vivo measurements of 2830 anterior teeth. *J Prosthet Dent*, 29, pp. 358–382.

Goodkind, R., and W.B. Schwabacher. 1987. Use of a fiber-optic colorimeter for in vivo color measurements of 2830 anterior teeth. *J Prosthet Dent*, 58, pp. 535–42.

Goodkind, R.J., K.M. Keenan, and W.B. Schwabacher. 1985. A comparison of Chromascan and spectrophotometric color measurements of 100 natural teeth. *J Prosthet Dent*, 53, (1), 105–9.

Gwinnett, A.J. 1992. Moist vs. dry dentin: Its effect on shear bond strength. *Am J Dent*, 5, pp. 127–129.

Hall, W.R. 1886. Temperament in mechanical dentistry. *Dental Practitioner*, 4, pp. 49–54.

Hasegawa, A., I. Ikeda, and S. Kawaguchi. 2000. Color and translucency of in vivo natural central incisors. *J Prosthet Dent*, 83, pp. 418–23.

Heinlein, W.D. 1980. Anterior teeth: Esthetics and function. *J Prosthet Dent*, 44, pp. 389–393.

Heymann, H.O. 1987. The artistry of conservative esthetic dentistry. *J Am Dent Assoc*, (special issue), pp. 14E–23E.

Hulsey, C.M. 1970. An esthetic evaluation of lip-teeth relationships present in the smile. *Am J Orthod*, (57), pp. 132–144.

Johnston, C.D., D.J. Burden, and M.R. Stevenson. 1999. The influence of dental midline discrepancies on dental attractiveness ratings. *Eur J Orthod*, 21, pp. 517–522.

Kenealy, P., N. Frude, and W. Shaw. 1989. An evaluation of the psychological and social effects of malocclusion: some implications for dental policy-making. *Soc Sci Med*, 6, pp. 583–591.

Kent, G. 1992. Effect of osseointegrated implants on psychological and social well-being: A literature review. *J Prosthet Dent*, (68), pp. 515–518.

Kim, H.S., I.P. Kim, S.C. Oh, et al. 1995. The effect of personality on the smile. *Wonkwang Dent Res*, 29, pp. 311–314.

Kiyak, H.A., and R. Bell. 1990. Psychosocial considerations in surgery and orthodontics. In: Proffit, W.R., White, R.P., eds. St Louis: CV Mosby Co. *Surgical-orthodontic Treatment*. pp. 71–93.

Latta, G.H. 1988. The midline and its relation to anatomic landmarks in the edentulous patient. *J Prosthet Dent*, 59, pp. 681–683.

Laufer, D., D. Glick, D. Gutman, and A. Sharon. 1976. Patient motivation and response to surgical correction of prognathism. *Oral Surg Oral Med Oral Path Oral Radiol*, 41, pp. 309–313.

Levin, R.P. 1988. Patient personality assessment improves ca presentation. *Dent Ecom*, 78, pp. 49–50, 52, 54–55.

Lombardi, R.E. 1973. The principles of visual perception and their clinical application to denture esthetics. *J Prosthet Dent*, 29, pp. 358–382.

Maritato, F.R., and J.R. Douglas. 1964. A positive guide to anterior tooth placement. *J Proshet Dent*, (14), p. 848.

Martone, A.L., and L.F. Edwards. 1978. Anatomy of the mouth and related structures. Part 1. The face. *J Prosthet Dent*, (39), pp. 128–134.

Matthews, T.G. 1978. The anatomy of a smile. *J Prosthet Dent*, 39, (2), pp. 128–34.

Misch, E.C. 2005a. Rationale for dental implants. In: Misch, C.E., ed. St. Louis: Elsevier-Mosby, *Dental Implants Prosthetics*. pp. 10–12.

Misch, E.C. 2005b. Maxillary Denture Opposing Implant Prosthesis and Modified Occlusal Concepts. In: Misch C.E., ed. St. Louis: Elsevier Mosby. *Dental Implant Prosthodontics*. pp. 568–586.

Morley, J. 1997. Smile design—specific consideration. *J Calif Dent Assn*. 25:633–7.

Morley, J. 1999. The role of cosmetic dentistry in restoring a youthful appearance. *JADA*, 130.

Moskowitz, M., and A. Nayyar. 1995. Determinants of dental esthetics: A rational for smile analysis and treatment. *Compend Cont Educ Dent*, (16), pp. 1164–1186.

Philips, E.D. 1990. The classifications of smile patterns. *J Can Dent Assoc*, 65, pp. 252–254.

Philips, E.D. 1996. The anatomy of a smile, *Oral Health*, (86), pp. 7–9, pp. 11–13.

Qaltrough, A.J.E., and F.J.T. Burke. 1994. *A Look at Dental Esthetics*. Quintessence Int, 25, pp. 7–14.

Renner, R.P. 1985. *An Introduction to Dental Anatomy and Esthetics*. Chicago: Quintessence, pp. 125–166, 187–233, 241–272.

Rifkin, R. 2000. Facial analysis: A comprehensive approach to treatment planning in aesthetic dentistry. *Pract Periodont Asthet Dent*, (12), pp. 865–871.

Robinson, S.C. 1969. Physiological placement of artificial anterior teeth, *Can Dent J*, 35, pp. 260–266.

Rubin, L.R. 1974. The anatomy of a smile: Its importance in the treatment of facial paralysis. *Plast Reconstr Surg*, (53), pp. 384–387.

Rufenacht, C.R. 1990. *Fundamentals of Esthetics*. Chicago: Quintessence, pp. 9–48, 67–134.

Sarver, D. 2001. The importance of the incisor positioning in the esthetic smile: The smile arc. *Am Orthod Dentofacial Orthop*, 120, pp. 98–111.

Sellen, P.N., D.C. Jagger, and A. Harrison. 1998. Computer-generated study of the correlation between tooth, face, arch forms, and palatal contour. *J Prosthet Dent*, 80, pp. 163–8.

Stein, M.R. 1936. Williams' classification of anterior tooth forms. *J Am Dent Assoc*, 23, pp. 1512–8.

Strauss, R.P., Y. Mintzker, R. Fenerstein, M.R. Wexler, and Y. Rand. 1988. Social perceptions of the effects of Down syndrome: school-based study of ratings by normal adolescents. *Plast Surg Reconstr*, 81, pp. 841–851.

Strub, J.R., and J.C. Turp. 1999. Esthetics in dental prosthetics. In: Fischer, J., *Esthetics and Prosthetics*. Chicago: Quintessence, p. 11.

Tjan, A.H.L., and G.D. Miller. 1984. Some esthetic factors in smile. *J Prosthet Dent*, 51, pp. 24–28.

Touati, B., P. Miara, and D. Nathanson. 1999. *Esthetic Dentistry and Ceramic Restorations*. New York: Martin Dunitz, pp. 139–161.

Tweed, C.H. 1991. The diagnostic facial triangle in the control of treatment objectives. *Am J Orthod*, 55, p. 651.

Vanini, L. 1996. Light and color in anterior composite restorations. *Pract Periodont Aesthet Dent*, 8, pp. 673–682.

Viazis, A.D. 1991. A new measurement of profile esthetics. *J Clin Orthod*, (25), pp. 15–20.

Vig, R.G., and G.C. Brundo. 1978. The kinetics of anterior tooth display. *J Prosthet Dent*, 39, pp. 502–504.

Wavrin, J.A. 1920. A simple method of classifying face forms. *Dent Dig*, 26, pp. 331–5.

Weickersheimer, P.B. 1995. Steiner analysis. In: Jacobson, A., *Ed Radiographic Cephalometry*. Carol Stream, IL: Quintessence Publishing, pp. 83–85.

Wictorin, L., K. Hillerstrom, and S. Sorensen. 1969. Biological and psychosocial factors in patients with malformation of the jaws. *Scand J Plast Reconstr Surg*, 3, pp. 138–143.

Williams, J.L. 1914. The temperamental selection of artificial teeth fallacy. *Dent Dig*, 20, pp. 63–75.

Yamamoto, M., M. Miyoshi, and S. Kataoka. 1990/1991. Special Discussion. Fundamentals of esthetics: contouring techniques for metal ceramic restorations. *QDT*, 14, pp. 10–81.

Yoon, M.E., and J.K. Dong. 1992. A study on the smile in Korean youth. *J Korean Aciad l'rosthoc Jont*, 30, pp. 259–270.

Young, H.A. 1954. Selecting the anterior tooth mold. *J Prosthet Dent*, 4, pp. 748–60.

Chapter 4
Multidimensional Esthetic Implant Positioning

Abd El Salam El Askary

Balancing the dental implant dimension and the remaining osseous dimension is critical to achieving satisfactory esthetic results. The orientation of the dental implant within the remaining alveolar ridge is vital to any implant-supported restoration that has an esthetic potential. To be called successful, accurate implant positioning within the alveolar ridge should provide a delicate balance between esthetics and function.

The nature of the alveolar housing in the esthetic zone differs from the posterior functional areas of the oral cavity in terms of load concern (English 1993). Thus, implant positioning in the posterior alveolar ridge is governed by factors such as occlusion, biting loads, opposing dentition, parafunctional habits, quality and quantity of the available bone, and the existing location of the anatomical landmarks. Although the esthetic zone is governed by other factors such as smile line, lip support, lip thickness, facial symmetry, quantity and quality of the soft tissues, periodontal biotype, emergence profile, type of prosthetic components to be used, and the future contour of the final restoration, these factors in fact do not only ensure success, but also long-term stability of both esthetic and functional results. In other words, dental implant positioning maximizes esthetics without sacrificing function.

Ideally speaking, the dental implant should be installed in the exact location of the missing tooth to attain its original appearance. Unfortunately, inserting the implant in its natural predecessor's location frequently is not a clinical option due to postextraction alveolar ridge resorption (Atwood and Coy 1971, Johnson 1963, Carlsson et al. 1967). Alveolar bone resorption usually takes on a horizontal pattern in the anterior maxilla, which in turn deviates the placement of the implant palatal to the buccal contour of the extracted root (Potashnick 1998). In most cases, such a placement negatively affects surrounding gingival contours and the morphological characteristics of the final prosthesis. As a result, it is necessary to first reconstitute the lost supporting structures to their original size so that the original tooth position may be replicated at the time of implant placement (Jansen and Weisgold 1995). (See Figures 4.1A–I.)

Preliminary case design is mandatory to precisely positioning an implant in its osseous housing. This is performed by determining the exact location of the implant fixture. An accurate wax-up of the edentulous area on the study cast should first be fabricated to establish the original location of the missing dentition (Chiche and Aoshima 1997). An accurate surgical template is then fabricated from the wax-up, thereby identifying the optimal position of the implant relative to the proposed final prosthesis (Spiekerman 1995, Garber 1995, Palacci 2001). The main purposes of the surgical template are to allow two-dimensional (2-D) positioning of the implant and, in perfect conditions, three-dimensional (3-D) positioning, thus leading to a precise transfer of the preplanned position of the implant on the study cast to the surgical site.

Optimizing clinical results through esthetic implant positioning is predicated on several factors that cannot be ignored. These factors embrace two very important themes. First, clinicians should strictly adhere to clinical guidelines to achieving predictable osseointegration. These guidelines include using a relatively gentle surgical technique, preparing a precise osteotomy, exerting as little pressure as possible to the alveolar bone, minimizing heat generation to the bone, achieving primary implant stability (Buser et al. 1999, Burger and Klein-Nulend 1999, Herrmann 2000), and avoiding direct biting loads at the bone-implant interface during a sufficient healing period (Szmukler-Moncler et al. 1998, Block et al. 1997, Brunski et al. 2000).

Second, clinicians should exercise extreme care so they do not compromise sulcular depth or gingival biological health in an attempt to achieve optimal implant placement (Misch 1995). Consequently, implant placement in the esthetic zone should be approached with extra caution to provide a harmonious implant-supported restoration and to reduce the risks of morbidity and implant failure (El Askary et al. 1999a, El Askary et al. 1999b). Implant failure is not limited to

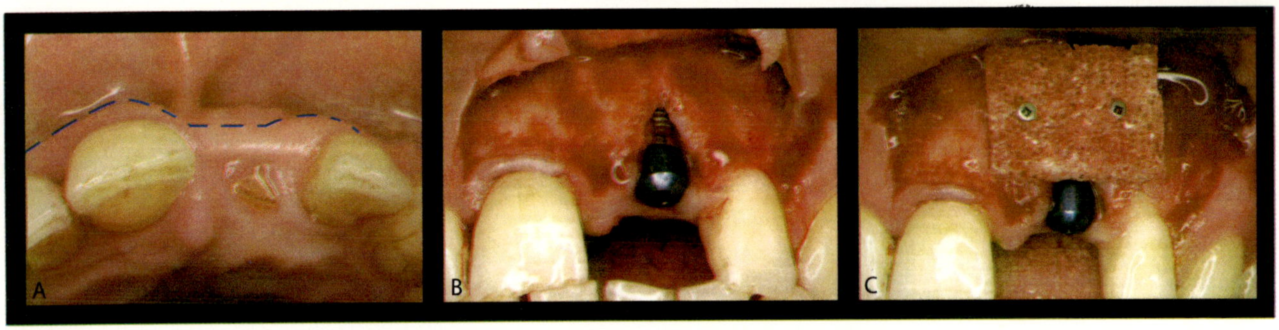

Figure 4.1. **A.** An intraoral view showing insufficient buccal restorative dimension. **B.** The implant is placed within the alveolar ridge. **C.** Xinograft bone-grafting block (Tutogen Medical GmbH, Neunkirchen, Germany) stabilized in place to restore the missing buccal contour.

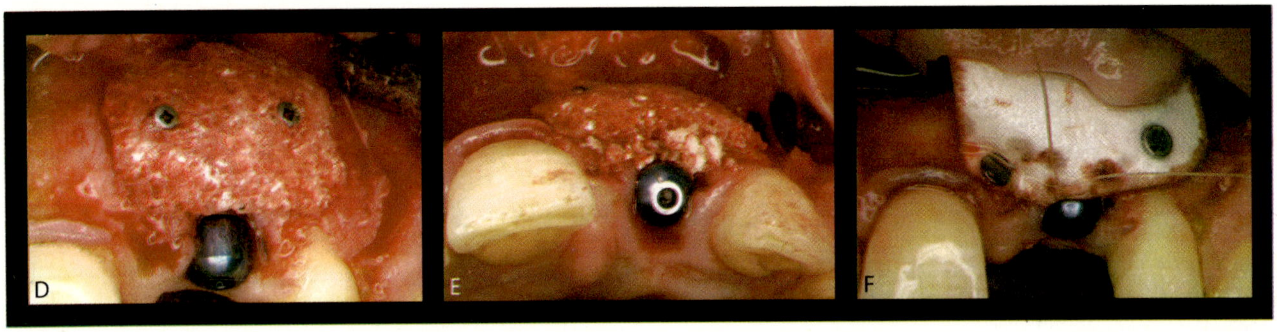

Figure 4.1. **D.** The bone block is being contoured and trimmed. **E.** The space voids are filled with particulated bone graft. **F.** The area was covered with BioMend collagen membrane (Zimmer Dental, Carlsbad, CA, USA). The membrane is stabilized with tacks and sutures to eliminate the dead space.

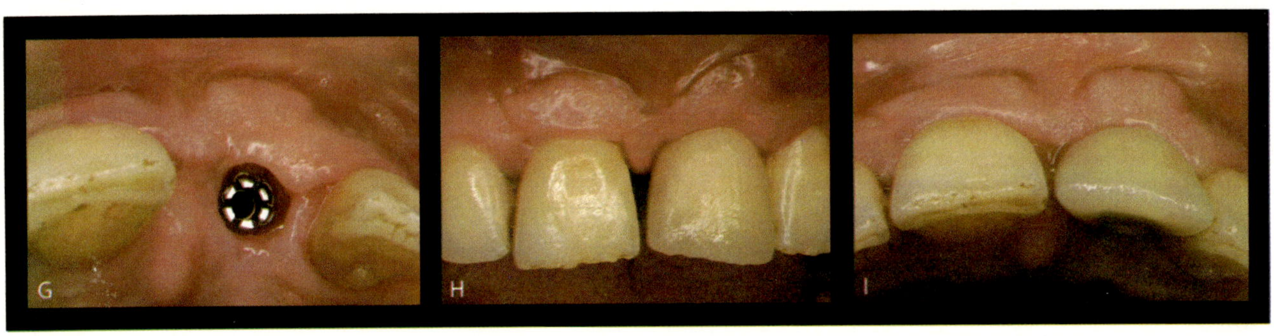

Figure 4.1. **G.** Note the improvement of the buccal contour. **H.** Postrestorative labial view of the case. **I.** Incisal view of the case.

the breakdown of the integration between the implant and investing bone, but also encompasses failure to achieve esthetic, functional, and phonetic goals. In other words, successful implant integration does not necessarily result in a satisfied patient (Meffert 1992).

Restorative Space Management

The available space after teeth extraction is called the *restorative space*; its boundaries are mesiodistal, buccolingual, and vertical dimensions. Factors that dictate the amount of the restorative space are teeth drifting, teeth over eruption, bone resorption, and malocclusion. The optimal management of the sufficient available restorative space or the insufficient restorative space becomes vital to the esthetic outcome. Insufficient restorative space often leads to many unsatisfactory clinical situations which begin when a clinician ignores the reasons for the deficit of the alveolar ridge and thus ignores the proper correction. Fortunately, modern implantology offers a vast array of techniques that enable the optimal correction of the deficient restorative space. An array of alternatives is now available with highly predictable clinical results. (See Figures 4.2A–B.) The available restorative space should be carefully optimized to host the implant fixtures and their related restorative components. (See Figure 4.3.)

Factors Influencing Implant Positioning

Several factors contribute to accurate implant positioning. These factors are not so much technical as they are treatment-related, and they help ensure predictable esthetic results. These factors follow:

1. **The grip**: During the drilling procedure, the grip of the hand-piece influences the implant's optimal position to a great extent. The control of the clinician's hand while drilling, using either a palm grip or pen-grasping grip, optimizes the positioning procedure. The palm grip sometimes provides better control over the other grips, especially in the maxillary premolars locations. It is the author's personal opinion that the palm grip offers greater control of the drilling procedure in the maxillary posterior areas. This preference is due to the nature of the drilling procedure, which differs from the regular turbine hand-piece grip that is used for cavity preparation. The nature of the slow speed and high torque during dental implantology procedures, as well as the bone resistance, allows the palm grip to assist in achieving better positioning control. (See Figures 4.4A–B.)
2. **Accuracy of the surgical template**: The more accurate the surgical template, the more accurate the implant positioning. New types of templates are being fabricated with computer-aided design/computer-aided manufacturing (CAD/CAM) technology that offers precise positioning in terms of locating the axial location of the implant head within the alveolar ridge. These precise surgical templates are being used with a computed tomography (CT) scan-based planning system (Tardieu et al. 2003) which allows the surgeon to select the optimal location for implant placement, taking into account specific anatomic characteristics of the patient and thus using the optimal bone densities. The precision of

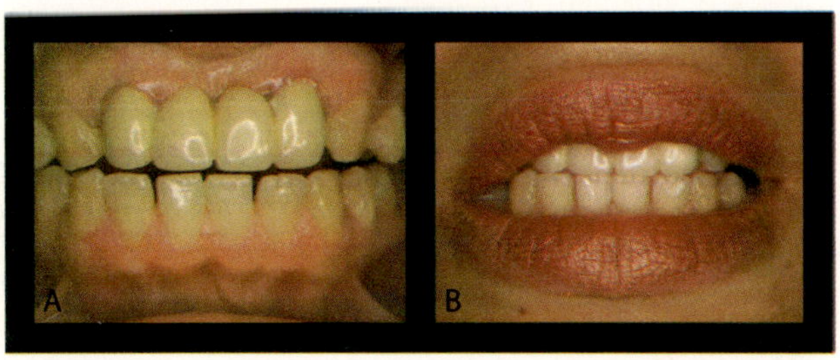

Figure 4.2. **A.** Intraoral picture of a poorly fabricated implant-supported prosthesis due to poor space management. **B.** Extraoral picture of the patient showing unpleasant smile.

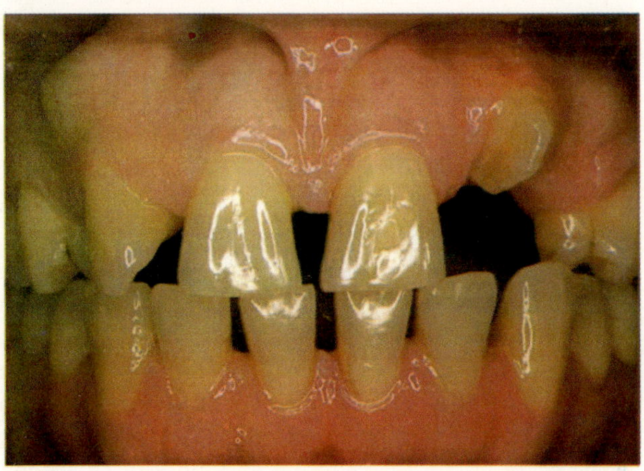

Figure 4.3. Insufficient restorative space that mandates space management protocol.

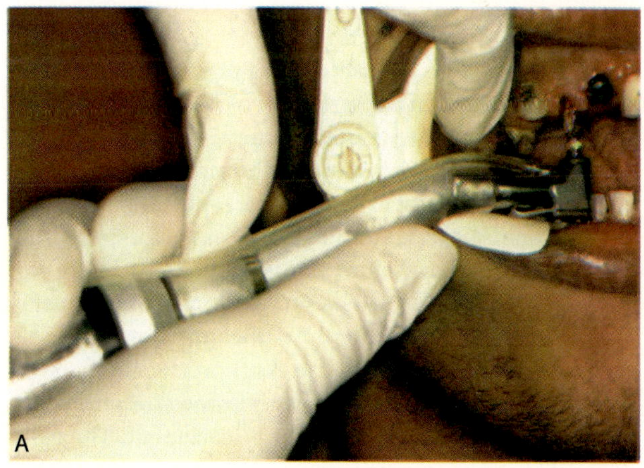

Figure 4.4A. A palm grip that controls the accuracy of implant position.

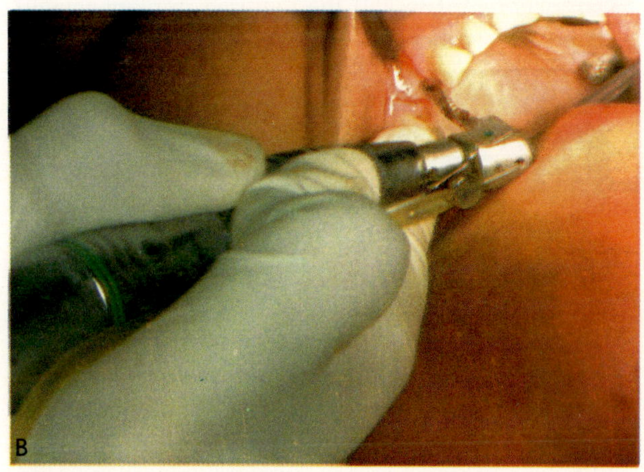

Figure 4.4B. A pen grasp grip.

the perpendicular reconstruction images along the axis of the arch (orthogonal frontal oblique sections) is almost 95%. Thus, the precision of these reconstruction sections is amply sufficient for clinical application in implant therapy.

The goal of this technology is to allow the clinician to use an individualized drill guide that fits exactly on the bone crest of the patient. A CAD/CAM program uses the shape of the scanning template and the 3-D information of the plan. A stereolithographic drill guide allows a physical transfer of the implant planning to the patient's mouth. The scannographic template is designed so that it can be transformed into a temporary fixed or final prosthesis for immediate loading.

Recently the NobelGuide® (Nobel Biocare AB, Göteborg, Sweden) system was introduced to maximize the implant positioning from the three dimensions. It also makes it possible to measure soft tissue height, which is considered an outstanding advantage, and the axial position of the dental implant. This subsequently transfers most of the surgical and prosthetic planning and fabrication outside the patient's mouth and allows the planning to be done prior to implant installation. This revolutionary treatment planning and surgical implementation system transfers extraoral planning into the mouth with accuracy and ease. Therefore, placing implants, abutments, and restorative components is simultaneous by using either conventional modeling or computer aided 3-D design. This system gives the exact position and depth of the implants prior to surgery. The laboratory can then produce a surgical template that guides the surgical procedure from the start to a completely successful placement. The case is planned in a computer based on CT scan data, which offers a more precise picture of anatomy, compared to model-based planning. A customized surgical template and the required implant-related components then can be ordered and used according to the preplanned case.

3. **Sharpness of the cutting drills**: Because drills become blunt with use, each implant manufacturer states the number of times a set of drills should be used, after which they should be discarded. The sharpness of the drill prevents it from wobbling in the surgical site and the subsequent deviation from the intended angulation or position. In fact, the sharpness of the rosette or the pilot drill that is used for the pilot oseotomy is the most valuable because it guides the primary path for the other drill to follow.
4. **The use of positioning devices**: Some positioning devices are now available to help keep an optimized distance between the implant and the natural teeth. A novel implant positioning system called IPS set (Storz am Markt GMBH, Emmingen-Liptingen, Germany) was introduced to assist in maintaining the proper implant position and angulation during the preparation of the surgical site. It consists of a series of sleeves and spreaders that maintain the proper interproximal dimensions and help determine the proper apical level of the implant head during surgery. The system facilitates selection of the implant diameter and axis, maintains exact spacing between the adjacent tooth and the implant or between adjacent implants, is compatible with any implant system, is useful for orthodontists in determining prospective implant positions in cases in which teeth are missing as a result of a congenital defect, and is suitable for use as seating tips in spacing templates (Iglhaut 2003). (See Figure 4.5.)
5. **The use of computerized navigation surgery**: Computerized navigation surgery is a developing technology for intraoperative tracking and guidance of surgical instruments to enhance minimally invasive procedures. It is considered to be a new era in perfecting implant positioning within the alveolar ridge, and it has evolved to facilitate minimally invasive procedures (Casap et al. 2005). This surgery, also called *image guided implantology*, can be used with flapless or flapped implant placement protocols in cases of flapless implant placement where the surgery may be perceived as a blind procedure that includes a risk of cortical plate perforation. The computerized navigation system provides real-time imaging of the drill and transforms flapless implant surgery into a fully monitored procedure. The surgeon can rely on the computerized navigation to

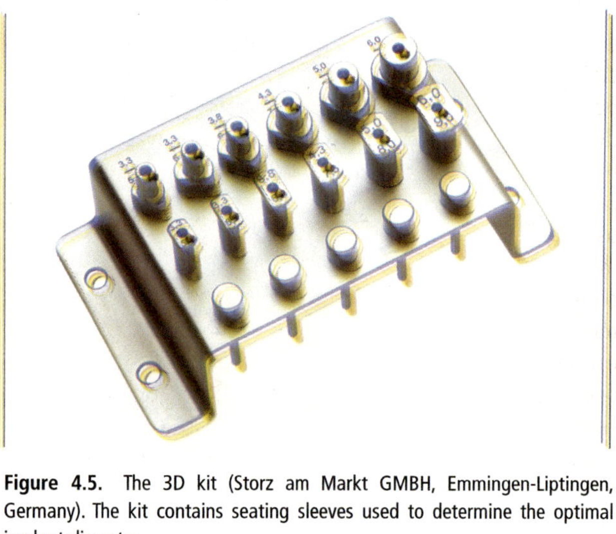

Figure 4.5. The 3D kit (Storz am Markt GMBH, Emmingen-Liptingen, Germany). The kit contains seating sleeves used to determine the optimal implant diameter.

adjust the position and angulation of the drill in absolute coordination with the presurgical digital implant plan. The highly accurate intraoperative navigation enables precise transfer of the detailed presurgical implant plan to the patient. Intraoperative computerized navigation in implant dentistry mandates that an interfacing template be firmly attached to the operated jaw throughout the surgery. In the partially edentulous patient, this template may be an acrylic resin splint that is mounted over the existing natural teeth, and in fully edentulous jaws, stabilizing bone screws might be used (Casap et al. 2005).

Implant Morphological and Design Considerations

Modern implant dentistry has versatile research dimensions, such as the implant design. The modern implant design has several additional morphological modifications than the original standard classic designs and was originally made to simulate the original tooth morphology in most of the designs. Unfortunately, all missing teeth in the same dental arch cannot be restored with the same implant design due to the unique and versatile nature of human tooth roots. Some roots possess antirotational characters, some have stronger anchorage characters, and still others have a greater load-bearing capacity. Therefore, the comparison between natural teeth and dental implants is unfair, and dental implants should not be called third dentition.

When restoring natural dentition with conventional prostheses, the anatomy of the existing natural teeth and periodontium serve as guides for replicating the original natural form and contours. Unfortunately, dental implants do not provide the same valuable guides that are available when restoring natural dentition, especially when multiple teeth are missing. Consequently, before inserting dental implants, the clinician should develop an imaginary picture that will act as a guide or reference during the treatment plan. This is accomplished by properly assessing the original shape of the osseous bed and the biological dimensions of the missing dentition and relating them to the restorative components that will be used. Understanding the basic morphology of the missing tooth in relation to the implant fixture design along with its related components becomes an absolute necessity for achieving successful esthetic results. (See Figure 4.6.)

Many scholars study the technical advancements in implant designs. As a result, a better understanding of bone behavior and cellular activities has led to the invention of new designs. The changes involved include implant surface treatments, predictable interface connections, versatile unique implant sizes, and new implant-related prosthetic components. The newly introduced dental implant designs have led many clinicians to dramatically improve the clinical outcome of dental implants from both the esthetic and functional standpoints and to take implant-supported restorations to new levels. Thus, selection of the optimum implant design and size is now an integral part of every treatment plan that seeks a superior esthetic outcome.

The elements of implant design are:

1. The implant surface topography (micro characters)
2. The overall physical geometry (macro characters), such as length, diameter, and macroscopic threads, vents, and grooves
3. The implant material composition

These factors contribute to the implant's overall design. The question inevitably arises regarding which design features best stabilize the implant in the receptor site, assist the implant mechanical anchorage in the bone, best distribute occlusal loads, and provide the maximum esthetic outcome (El Askary 2000).

Root form implant design should focus on several aspects when it is being used for the new modern loading modalities. For example, the cylinder implants and the finned implants press against the walls of the receptor site when the implant is tapped into place via a friction fit. These two particular designs cannot be used predictably for modern loading concepts due to the diminished initial bone-implant contact. In addition, they do not offer initial cortical bone engagement because they are not simply screwed in place; they are tapped in place. Therefore, the initial amount of bone that comes into direct contact with screw-type implants

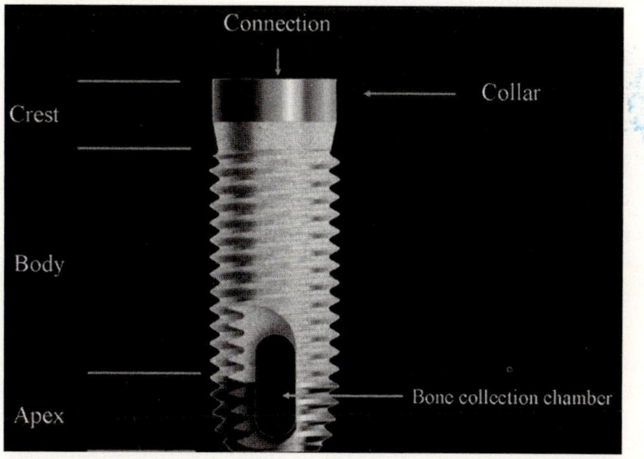

Figure 4.6. Implant morphology.

becomes important for the long-term survival of the implant (Johansson and Albrektsson 1987).

However, Sennerby and others (1992) observed that the removal torque of screw-type implants depends on the amount of available compact bone, rather than on the total amount of surrounding bone. Therefore, an ideal implant design should focus on achieving a maximum number of threads that should engage dense cortical bone for maximum stability. Also, the number of the threads increases the amount of area available to bear loading; hence, the greater the number of threads, the greater the functional surface area. Some threaded implants have a 1.5 mm distance between the threads, whereas others have a 0.4 mm distance. The smaller the distance between the threads, the greater the thread number and corresponding surface area (Misch et al. 2004).

The thread depth also influences the implant design; the greater the thread depth, the greater the functional surface area and mechanical anchorage. The thread depth can range from 0.2 mm to 0.42 mm (Misch et al. 2004). Thread geometry may affect the strength of early osseointegration and the bone implant interface. Osseointegrated implants either have a V-thread or a reverse buttress thread, or a square thread design. The V-shaped thread design offers 10 times greater shear force applied to bone when compared with other thread shapes. The V and reverse buttress thread geometry are similar in terms of bone maintenance around them, while the square thread demonstrates statistically significantly higher values of bone support (Misch et al. 2004). A tapered form for root-shaped implant design presents unique physical characteristics:

- It reduces the tendency for apical perforation when an immediate placement method is selected, as compared with those that are parallel-walled.
- It might avoid damaging the adjacent roots.
- It offers greater initial stability.
- It compresses bone against its walls.

In addition to threads, many root-form implants contain vents for bone anchorage to enhance posthealing mechanical fixation. Most of the screw-type implants have one or more vents in their apical regions (Gores et al. 1989). In addition, connecting screws are an integral part of any designed implant-retained prosthetic systems. Fatigue, loosening, and breaking of the screws are expected throughout the loading cycles intraorally.

A study by Yousef and others (2005) was designed to understand the parameters of screw loosening, using an *in vitro* model, which included torque, screw head rotation, changes in screw dimension, and distortion of the implant-abutment joint. Implants (4 mm × 10 mm) were potted in autopolymerizing blocks. Abutments were placed with screws tightened with a 35 Newton centimeter (Ncm) torque and standardized crowns were fabricated. Three implant systems were used: Nobel Biocare USA, Inc. (Yorba Linda, CA, USA), 3i Implant Innovations, Inc. (Palm Beach Gardens, FL, USA), and Bio-Lok International, Inc. (Deerfield Beach, FL, USA). Seven samples were tested for each system. The samples were loaded with 300 N loads for 50,000 cycles at 1 Hz. Torque turn audits were performed at 10,000, 25,000, and 50,000 cycles. At the conclusion of the loading, counterclockwise rotation of the abutment screw was measured. The screws were retrieved and measurements were made and compared with the controls. Finally, one sample from each group was embedded in resin, sectioned longitudinally, and examined under the standard error of the mean.

The Nobel Biocare system showed a 9.4 Ncm loss of torque from the loading protocol. This result was accompanied by a counterclockwise rotation of 7 degrees and a 200 μ elongation of the screw. Compression and distortion of the longitudinally sectioned joint architecture was observed with the standard error of the mean. No loss of torque, counterclockwise rotation, or lengthening of the screws were observed in the 3i and BioLok International systems. Intimate adaptation of the joint without distortion was seen in the longitudinal sections. Screw loosening appears to follow specific parameters that include counterclockwise rotation, lengthening of the screw, and distortion of the screw joint. This process is likely associated with both the physical properties of the screw as well as its configuration. This observation suggested that each implant screw joint "adapts" to its environment based upon its design and material characteristics.

The surface topography of the implant can range from relatively smooth, machined, rough, plasma sprayed, sand blasted, and acid etched to a porous form of hydroxyapatite (HA). There is a positive correlation between the degree of primary mechanical fixation of the implant and increasing roughness of the implant surface (Carlsson et al. 1988). This work was supported by Carlsson et al., which found that rough-surfaced titanium screws demonstrated a higher removal torque in comparison to smooth-surfaced duplicates after six weeks in rabbits (Carlsson et al. 1988).

The implant-abutment connection becomes an important element in implant design. It predicts the stability and fixation of the restorative components and helps minimize the marginal bone loss upon loading. It also resists rotation and future connecting screw loosening. Most implant connections consist of internal threads to both retain and facilitate the removal of the abutments. The main geometrical form of the common interlocking elements can be a hexagon or octagon, which mates with a complementary abutment to prevent rotation. The ideal abutment connection is internal with interlocking geometry to prevent rotation and for better load bearing.

A better understanding of the biological charters of the peri-implant tissues can also help attain better designs. Identifying the particular type of periodontium of the patient is relevant to the selection of the dental implant design, as are the future condition of its surrounding structures and the prognosis of the implant treatment. The unique human periodontium is divided into two basic biotypes: the thin scalloped biotype and the thick flat biotype (Seibert 1973, Oschsenbein and Ross 1973, Olsson and Lindhe 1991). Each biotype has its own particular tooth anatomy and osseous topography (Morris 1958).

Thin scalloped tissue biotype tooth anatomy is characterized by narrow, tapered roots and a triangular or cylindrical crown shape. The contact points are located more incisally; subsequently the interproximal papillae are located in an incisal position and they do not totally fill the whole embrasure space because of the further incisal location of the contact points. Due to the relatively small diameter and tapered form of the roots of the thin scalloped teeth biotype, the interradicular bone becomes wider than it does in the thick flat biotype (Wheeler 1961, Wheeler 1950, Glickman 1972, Seibert and Lindhe 1988). The thick flat tooth biotype is characterized by a bulbous root form and a square crown shape. In some areas, the wide root diameter of this biotype can have the same width as the widest part of the crown. Wide contact areas are located more apically, and eventually the interproximal papillae fill all of the embrasure space.

For these reasons, the final esthetic result of replacing a missing single tooth with thin scalloped tissue biotype characters with a dental implant might not be entirely predictable because recession of the interproximal papilla and its surrounding gingival structures is possible. This is due to the reduced amount of keratinized tissues and the fragile nature of the soft tissue that characterizes this biotype. Furthermore, the greater vertical distance of undulation between the edge of the implant's cervix and the interproximal bone margin stimulates mild bone resorption postoperatively, which leads to unsymmetrical peri-implant tissue margins when compared with the contralateral side (Wohrle 2003). Any additional osseous remodeling will result in further shortening of the already short papillae, thus complicating esthetics (Esposito et al. 1993).

Therefore, in immediate implant therapy, implant designs that have a narrow collar diameter due to the increased distance between the roots are preferable in thin scalloped tissue biotypes. In other words, a tapered implant morphology should be selected because of the increased bone thickness mesiodistally, to minimize the tendency for bone resorption with a narrower platform, and because the flapless implant placement is preferred in this type.

When it comes to prosthetic-related implant components, a limited flare is required. On the other hand, in the thick tissue biotype, the vertical undulation space located between the edge of the implant's cervix and the margin of the interproximal bone is minimized due to the larger space left after tooth extraction. This is not a serious clinical concern (Wohrle 2003). A wide implant diameter is valid in this treatment.

The thick flat tissue biotype certainly offers a more predictable esthetic treatment outcome than the thin scalloped biotype. Therefore, recognition and assessment of the tissue biotype before commencing implant therapy is important. The proper preoperative assessment of the tissue biotype will mandate a specific surgical approach that suits each type.

Root form implant design is used to restore missing teeth. The standard root form screw-type implant body is 3.75 mm in diameter, and the diameter of its platform might flare up to 4.1 mm. The cylinder design of endosseous implants usually has a 4 mm body diameter and the same platform dimensions as the screw type (Jansen and Weisgold 1995). The abutments for the cylindrical and screw-type implants start with the same diameter as the implant's platform and then flare out to 4.5 mm or 5 mm. While these dimensions might vary somewhat among implant manufacturers or due to laboratory modifications of the abutment, most of the standard implant diameters require a crown with a minimum diameter of 5.5 mm at the cementoenamel junction (CEJ) level and 7 mm at the level of the contact points when a missing central incisor is being restored, for instance.

The clinician should compensate for the difference in the diameter of the implant and the cervical dimension of the missing tooth to obtain natural biological contours of implant supported restorations. (See Figures 4.7A–B.) This is accomplished by soft tissue expansion procedures through the provisional prosthesis to allow a smooth transition from the implant head diameter to that of the natural diameter. Selecting an implant diameter that is wider than or similar to the tooth to be replaced results in an incorrectly sized crown that does not biologically fit with the surrounding tissues.

Recent implant design (Wohrle 2003) in which the collar design follows the natural proximal osseous level at a distance of about 1.5 mm above the bone level, i.e. the scalloped implant, minimizes bone loss in the inter-implant area (papillary area). Long-term results prove that the bone between two adjacent scalloped implants placed at a distance of 3 mm or less will be maintained

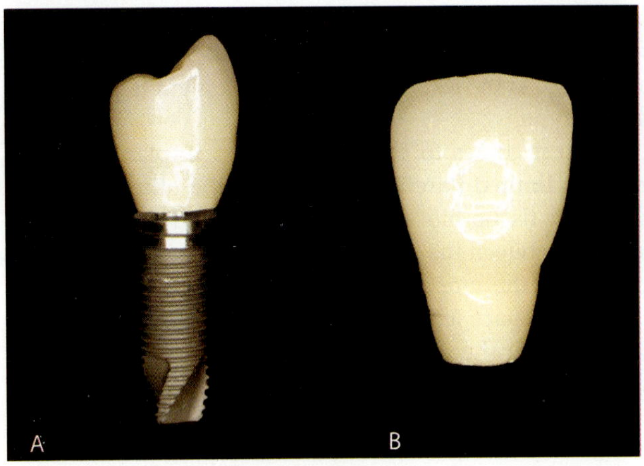

Figure 4.7. **A.** An implant with its prosthetic component. Note the difference between the size of the final crown and the cervical implant dimension. **B.** An implant-supported restoration that has the transition from the cross section of the implant diameter to the original natural crown size diameter.

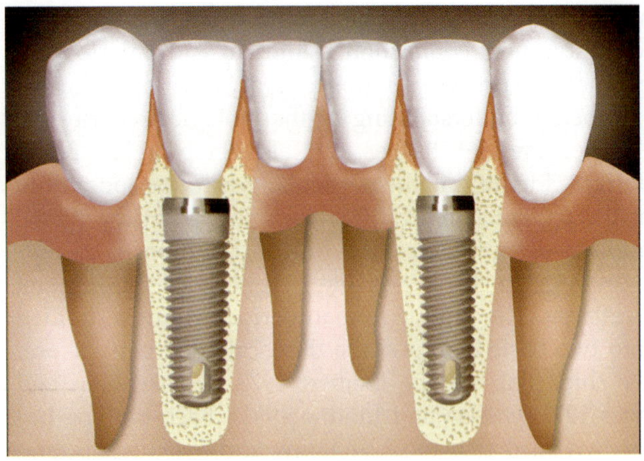

Figure 4.8. An implant replacing the mandibular lateral incisor with a discrepancy in the diameter of the original missing tooth dimension at the crestal bone level. This leads to a bulky restoration at the emergence level compared with its adjacent natural tooth.

for a long time, however exposure of the implant collar is possible if bone resorption occurs. Platform switching, yet another type of implant design, seems to be more promising. This is based on the observation that bone resorption does not occur or is highly minimized when the interface between the implant collar and abutment is moved medially away from the bone. This might be the result of distancing the contaminated microgap away from the bone.

A recent study by Nebot and others (2006) evaluated the implant platform modification, shifting the implant-abutment interface medially to minimize invasion of the biologic width. The study assessed 30 control cases and 30 study cases using the platform-modification technique. Interproximal bone resorption on the medial and distal of each implant was assessed using digital radiography at one, four, and six months. The mean value of bone resorption observed in the mesial measurement for the control group was 2.53 mm, whereas it was .76 mm for those patients in the study group. The mean value of bone resorption observed in the distal measurement for patients in the control group was 2.56 mm, whereas it was .77 mm for those in the study group. The study group had a significant reduction of bone loss in comparison to the control group ($p < 0.0005$), which indicated the clinical usefulness of the platform switching technique.

The implant diameter is directly related to the root diameter at the crest of the alveolar ridge. For example, if a missing maxillary central incisor to be replaced with a dental implant has a diameter that ranges between 7 mm and 8.5 mm at the CEJ level and between 5 mm and 6 mm at the bone level, the diameter of the implant to be used may vary from 4 mm to 6 mm, and so forth (Wheeler 1950). Therefore, the diameter of the implant should be related to the diameter of the root at the bone emergence level and not the CEJ level, because if the diameter of the implant exceeds the diameter of the root at the bone level, it will eventually cause crestal bone resorption. The diameter of the missing tooth can be verified by measuring the dimensions of the same tooth on the contralateral side, or by verifying it on a study cast. The width of the implant dictates its position within the alveolar ridge; wider implants are less apically positioned while narrow diameter implants are more apically placed to allow for "running room" to stack the prosthetic components in it. (See Figure 4.8.)

The use of a specific formula for selecting a particular implant diameter for a specific tooth might not be ideal, because there are many other variables that must be considered in the implant diameter selection process. Some of these include variations in the tissue biotype, differences in the size of the same tooth's diameter among different individuals, changes that occur to the remaining bone after extraction, the altered soft tissue contours, and the variation in implant diameters. Thus, the clinician's personal evaluation is the best method for selecting the proper implant size, and an individualized treatment approach is better than applying a generalized rule to different clinical situations.

Implant Positioning Rational

Placing an implant in the esthetic zone requires accurate attention to all treatment details not only to achieve clinically accepted results but also to preserve the existing natural details. An optimum osseous dimension and restorative dimension should be key in any accurate 3-D positioning procedure. The natural balance between these two dimensions should be preserved in implant therapy. It contributes to the complete biological integration of the dental implant within its housing (Jansen and Weisgold 1995). Certain guidelines to assist in placing the implant in a 3-D fashion—the interproximal dimension, which represents the relationship antroposteriorly between the implant and the natural teeth mesiodistally, and the labiopalatal dimension, which relates to the mediolateral axis and the sagittal dimensional axis, which is the apicoincisal dimension.

Mesiodistal Position

The mesiodistal position of the implant in relation to the adjacent teeth or between adjacent implants has a direct impact on the esthetic outcome and the interproximal marginal integrity of the future restorative contours. It directly affects hygiene maintenance around the implant-supported restorations and its adjacent natural components. In ideal soft and hard tissue conditions, the implant should be positioned midway in the center of the available mesiodistal space to obtain a centrally positioned prothesis. The potential risk of improper mesiodistal positioning of the implant is the approximation to the interdental papilla or, worse, impinging on it. This can cause blunting of the papilla and possible damage to the periodontium of the adjacent tooth to the implant site by compromising the blood supply, which could lead to external root resorption, as shown in Figure 4.9. External root resportion highlights the importance of not using parallel walled roots for dental implants. The use of a tapered implant design may reduce the chance of adjacent root approximation, especially when restoring areas with limited mesiodistal space or with curved roots. (See Figure 4.10.)

Grunder and others (2005) noted that the optimal distance between an implant and a natural tooth should not be less than 1.5 mm. The tooth attachment will be in jeopardy if this minimum distance is not maintained; in turn, this will cause a reduction or loss of the interproximal papilla. If the distance between two implants is less than 3 mm, the interproximal bone level is expected to be more apical to the implant shoulder and therefore

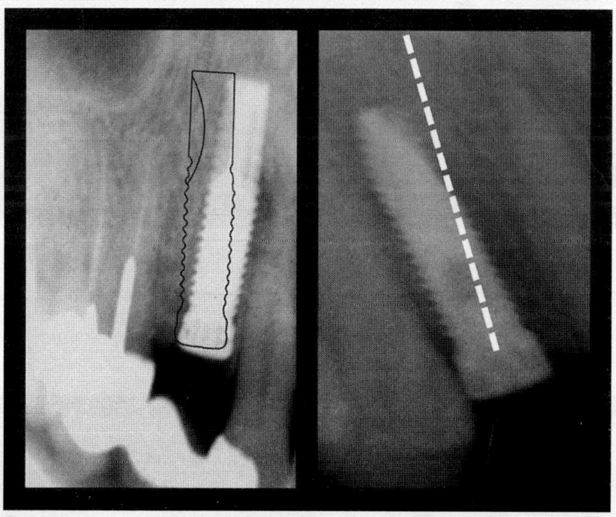

Figure 4.9. (left) Improper mesiodistal positioning of an implant that leads to disruption of the periodontal membrane integrity. The black sketch of the implant represents the optimal position. (right) Improper implant orientation in terms of interproximal position. The white interrupted line represents the optimal implant position.

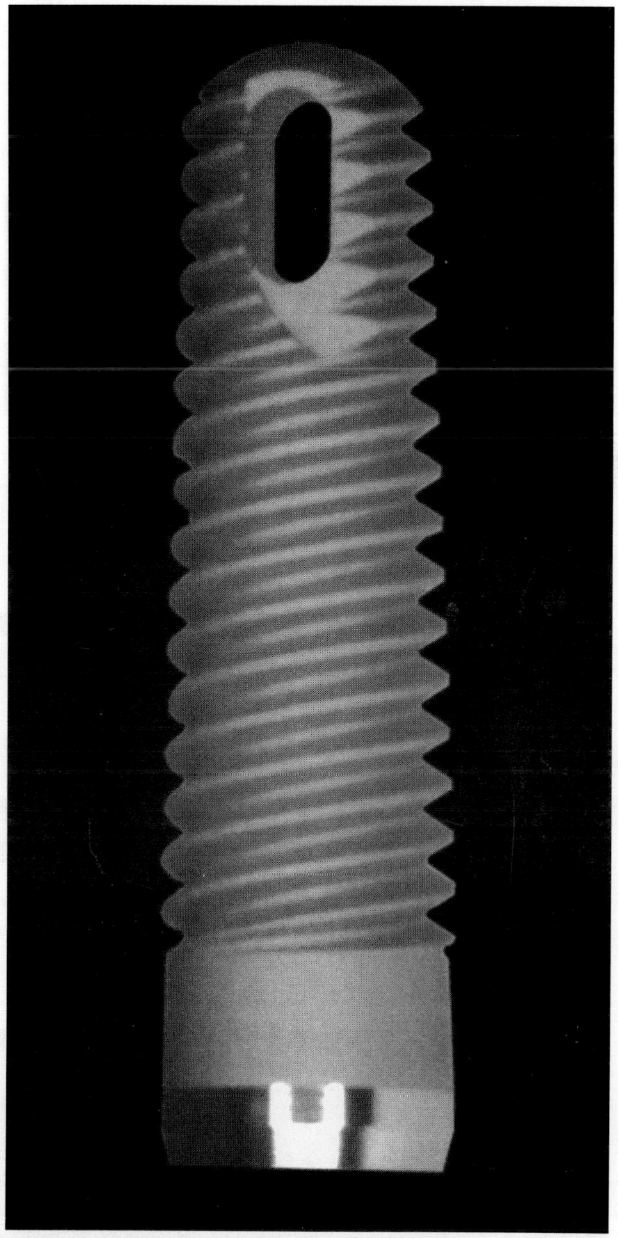

Figure 4.10. Tapered screw vent implant design (Zimmer Dental, Carlsbad, CA, USA).

exhibit a reduced or absent papilla. This situation is even more critical in thin scalloped tissue biotypes because in these cases, the implant head is usually positioned more apical than the bone attachment of the adjacent teeth. Only if the implant-to-implant distance is greater than 3 mm can the interproximal bone peak be maintained above the implant head. In cases where the interimplant distance cannot be optimized, the future restoration will slow many clinical discrepancies.

The presence of diastemas demands more careful mesiodistal positioning of dental implants. With diastemas, the available interproximal space is larger than the original missing tooth size, as shown in Figures 4.11A–B. In these cases, precise surgical templates ensure optimal implant positioning (Kennedy et al. 1998) to determine the exact position of the missing tooth, and at the same time preserve the original size of the diastema prior to tooth loss.

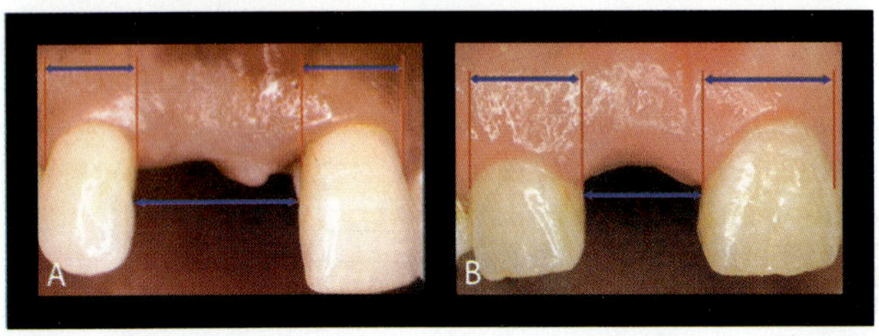

Figure 4.11. **A.** Preoperative view of a missing left maxillary central incisor with preexisting median diastema that mandates accurate mesiodistal positioning of the implant. **B.** Preoperative view of a missing right maxillary central incisor. Note the need to optimize the available space.

In cases of multiple missing teeth with a larger space, the clinician has the freedom to design the shape of the diastema according to some guiding factors such as the pre-planned teeth size, the patient's desire, and the midline position. Optimized clinical results can be obtained via a thorough fabrication of a wax-up and careful presurgical planning, as shown in Figures 4.12A–F. For single-tooth replacements, the method for calculating the minimum space required for the optimal mesiodistal positioning of the implant should include the width of the periodontal ligament (average 0.25 mm), and a minimum of 1 mm of sound bone should be kept between the implant and the periodontal ligament of the adjacent natural tooth (Ohenell et al. 1992). The measurements accounting for the periodontal ligament and sound bone should be doubled to calculate both the mesial and distal aspects of the implant. Simply stated, the required distance for placing a 4 mm-diameter implant between two teeth would be calculated by adding 1 mm + 0.25 mm + 4 mm + 0.25 mm + 1 mm. The resulting sum of 6.5 mm is the minimum space needed to position the implant mesiodistally. When multiple implants are used, the previous equation may be used by adding a distance of 2 mm to 3 mm between each implant (El Askary et al. 1999a).

These measurements are only a guideline; every case should be approached on an individual basis. The mesiodistal position of an implant depends on the

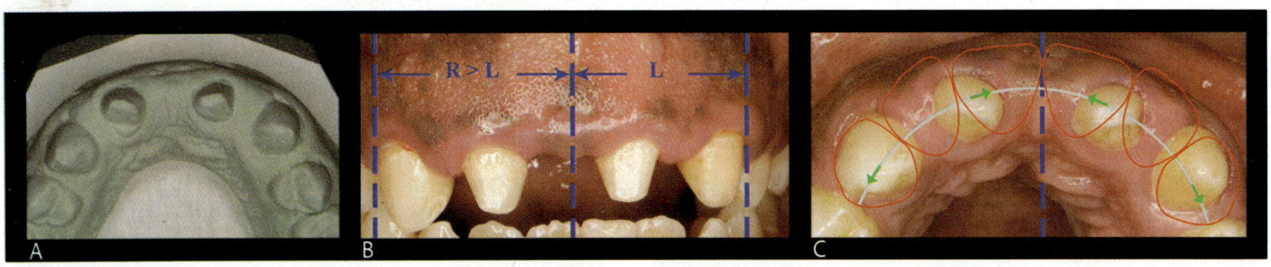

Figure 4.12. **A.** Insufficient interproximal restorative space for the anterior maxillary areas, with two retained deciduous central incisors. **B.** Primary measurements showed misbalance between the right and the left side. **C.** The red lines represent the original position of the natural teeth in relation to the misaligned situation. Note the deviation of the existing natural teeth position.

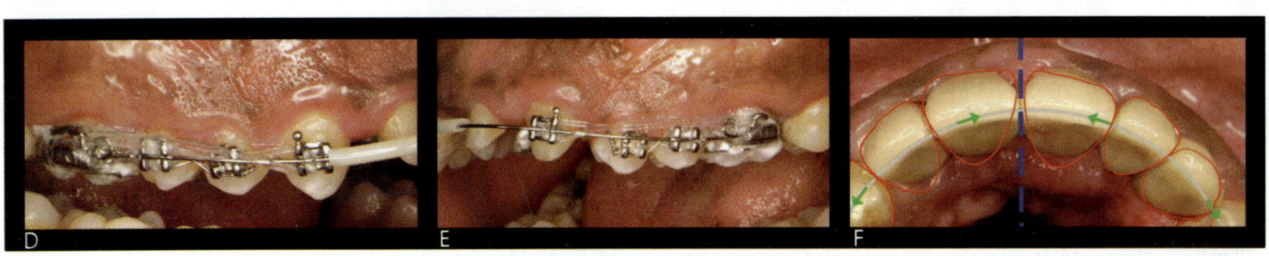

Figure 4.12. **D, E.** Orthodontic treatment made to allow space optimization. **F.** The final case restored showing the mesiodistal space optimization.

mesiodistal dimension of the available edentulous space, the presence or absence of diastemas, the size of the missing teeth (if a record exists), the type of the abutment to be used, and the adjacent root proximity.

Implant Angulation Rationale

The labiopalatal position of the implant within the alveolar ridge influences the emergence point of the implant-supported restoration as well as its contagious marginal contours and the profile of the final restoration. Generally, a proper emergence profile is desirable, for both esthetic and hygienic reasons. Therefore, the labial contour of the implant head has to emerge, as do adjacent natural teeth.

The labiopalatal position of the implant body within the alveolar ridge depends to a great extent on the accuracy of the surgical template and the clinician's stable grasp of the hand piece. Accurate labiopalatal placement can be achieved by leaving 1 mm of intact labial bone covering the implant surface (Grunder et al. 2005). The bone on top of the implant should be almost equal to that of the adjacent natural component (in cases of a single missing tooth). (See Figures 4.13A–C.)

In perfect bone situations, the implant should be placed as close to the buccal contour as the volume of the available bone permits, leaving 1.5 mm from the buccal edge of the bone (Potashnick 1998). For example, in 6 mm of bone width, a 3.75-mm-diameter implant should be placed labiopalatally to leave sufficient bone on the labial aspect of the implant body to maintain an optimal osseointegration. If the labiopalatal dimension of bone is less than 6 mm, a smaller diameter implant may be used. Several methods can treat a deficient bone width; bone dilators and bone splitting methods can be used to increase or expand the amount of available bone accordingly (Jansen and Weisgold 1995).

The placement of the implant in this dimension is critical. A misplaced implant can violate the integrity of the labial plate of bone with subsequent bone fenestration or dehiscence, leading to a final implant-supported restoration with bulky, overcontoured margins. This situation is clinically impossible to correct, even with the use of angulated abutments. In fact, angulated abutments might further complicate the situation because their metallic gingival collar can potentially displace the soft tissue in a more labial direction, resulting in soft tissue recession or grayish, discolored gingiva at the emergence level, as shown in Figures 4.14A–C and 4.15A–C.

There is a direct relationship between the labial edge of the implant interface and the highest point of the future crown contour. When the distance of the labial edge of the implant interface and the highest point of the future crown contour at the emergence level increases,

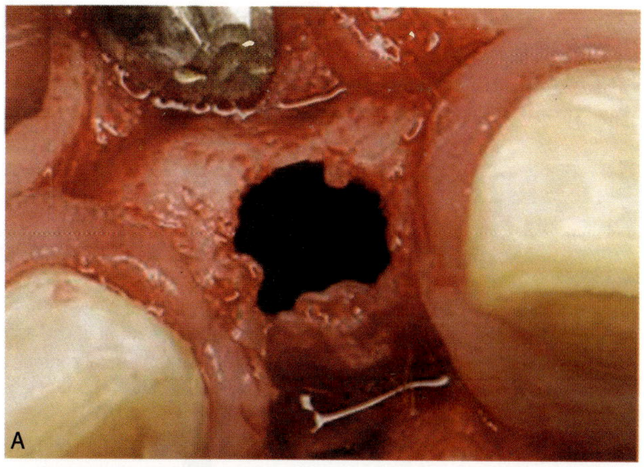

Figure 4.13A. An implant installation osteotomy that leaves 1 mm of buccal bone intact.

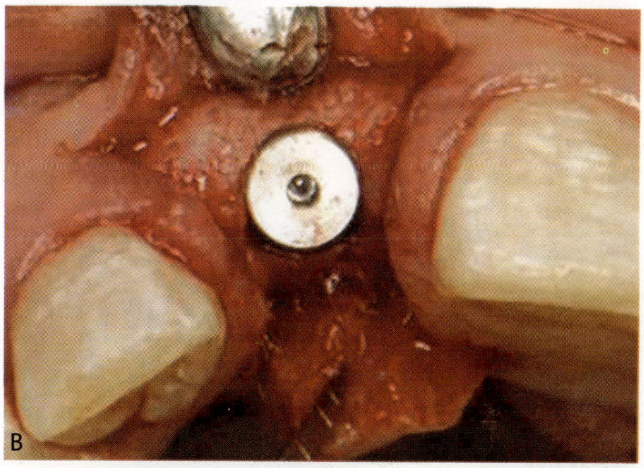

Figure 4.13B. The implant is placed in an optimal buccolingual position.

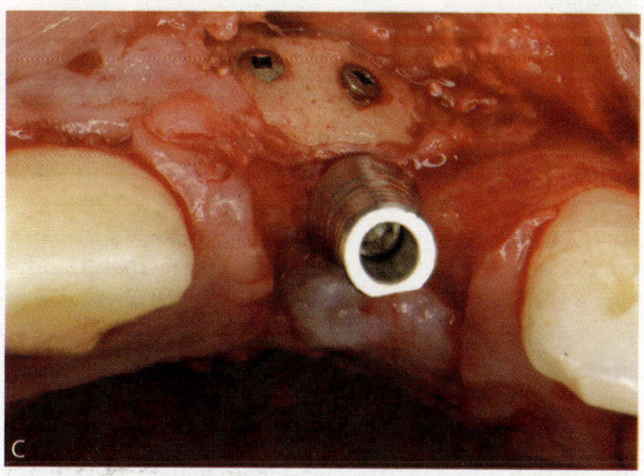

Figure 4.13C. Bone grafting made in order to allow a minimum of 1.5 mm above the implant head.

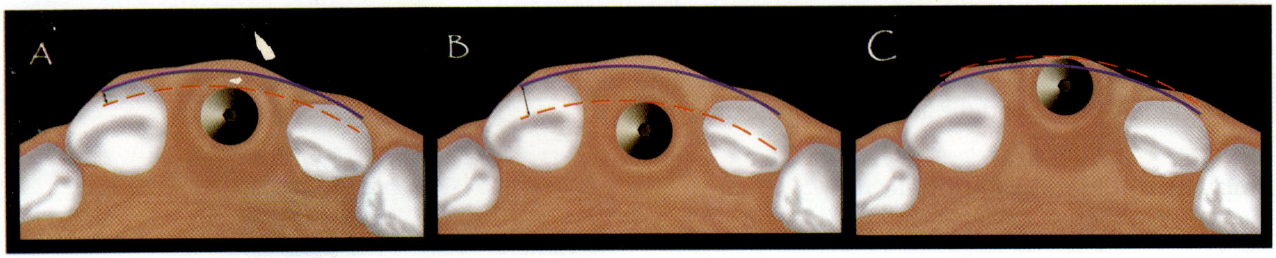

Figure 4.14A, B, C. An illustration showing the different situations of the buccolingual levels of the implant placement. The red line represents the implant head level, and the blue line represents the natural teeth natural buccal contour. In A, an optimal space between the implant head and the natural teeth buccal contours, while in B, the distance is too far from the natural buccal contour, and in C, the implant head is placed at a very close distance from the natural buccal contour, which makes it difficult to restore.

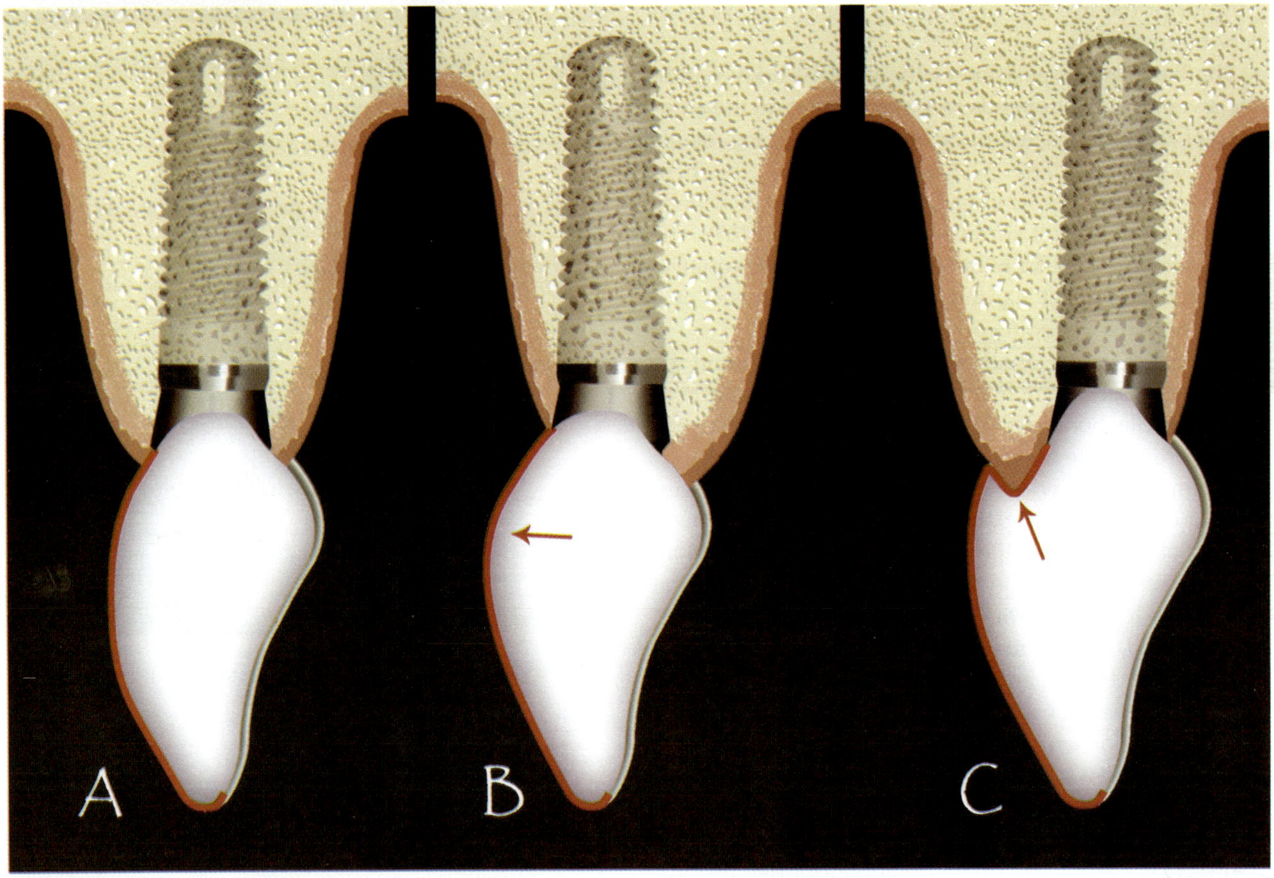

Figure 4.15. **A.** Illustration of the ideal labiopalatal positioning of the implant fixture in relation to the natural teeth buccal contour. **B.** Further buccal placement of the implant fixture that led to an overcontoured crown. **C.** Further palatal placement of the implant head that led to a modified lab ridge design.

there are more restorative complications in the implant-supported prosthesis. In the worst cases, when the distance is too large, the final restoration will appear to be severely "ditched-in" when viewed sagittally. Consequently, fabrication of a restoration with a ridge-lap design at its labial margin to be aligned with the adjacent natural teeth might be the only solution. A ridge-lap design hinders hygiene maintenance around the restoration labial contour, thereby facilitating plaque accumulation and leading to possible inflammation and apical migration of the gingival margin. This may be a potential threat to the implant's very existence, because pocket formation may ensue, resulting in implant failure. As a result of the modified ridge-lap design, there will be an increased strain on the implant surface due to an off-axis loading (Parel and Sullivan 1989), as shown in Figure 4.16.

Many factors control the implant angulation: the available alveolar process angulation, the existing occlusion, the precision of the surgical template, and the mode of implant placement protocol, whether immediate or delayed. Some authors classify implant angulation according to its relation to the occlusal plane (Daftary 1995). The implant may be inserted perpendicular to the occlusal plane, which provides a far more palatal positioning of the final restoration, resulting in a ridge-lap design of the restoration. An angulation of approximately 65 degrees, or 45 degrees to the occlusal plane, results in the most labial positioning of the implant head with optimal esthetic results. This placement often requires using an angulated abutment. (See Figures 4.17A–C and 4.18A–C.)

Usually when an immediate implant is placed, the angulation of the implant does not alter much from the existing natural tooth root angulation. By using the same alveolar socket space as a guide when selecting a delayed method of implantation, an altered or shifted angulation is made due to postextraction alveolar bone loss as well as the loss of the root place reference. The use of angulated abutments in both scenarios does not affect the implant survival. The angulation of the implant within the alveolar ridge is not restricted only to the labiopalatal dimension but also can be in a mesiodistal direction (i.e., moving the implant from one axis to a mesial or mesial angulation). (See Figures 4.19A–C.)

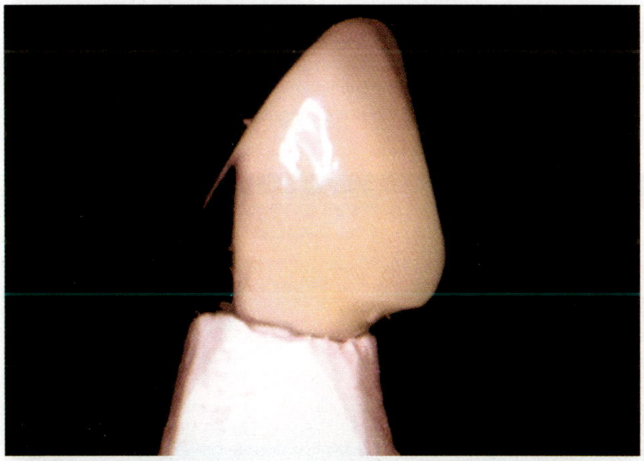

Figure 4.16. A modified ridge-lap design of the crown to compensate for the too far palatal placement of the implant.

A recently developed technique (Koyanagi 2002) to optimize the implant angulation within the alveolar ridge guides the head of the contra-angle hand piece with the surgical guide rather than guiding the drill itself through a guide hole or tube placed into a surgical template. This method is designed to prevent the drill from contacting the template, tube, or other material. The surgical guide should enable the operator, equipped with all of the information gained from preoperative examinations, to prepare the surgical site in the predetermined direction without being influenced by the clinician's visual or tactile senses. Preparation of the planned implant bed is thereby facilitated and the implant angulation is optimized. The described technique allows objective assessment and determination of implant location, inclination, and depth for individual treatment situations.

Final abutment might influence the labiopalatal positioning of the implant as well as its angulation. The final abutment and the final restoration should be determined before starting implant placement. There are two main types of final abutments—screw-retained abutments

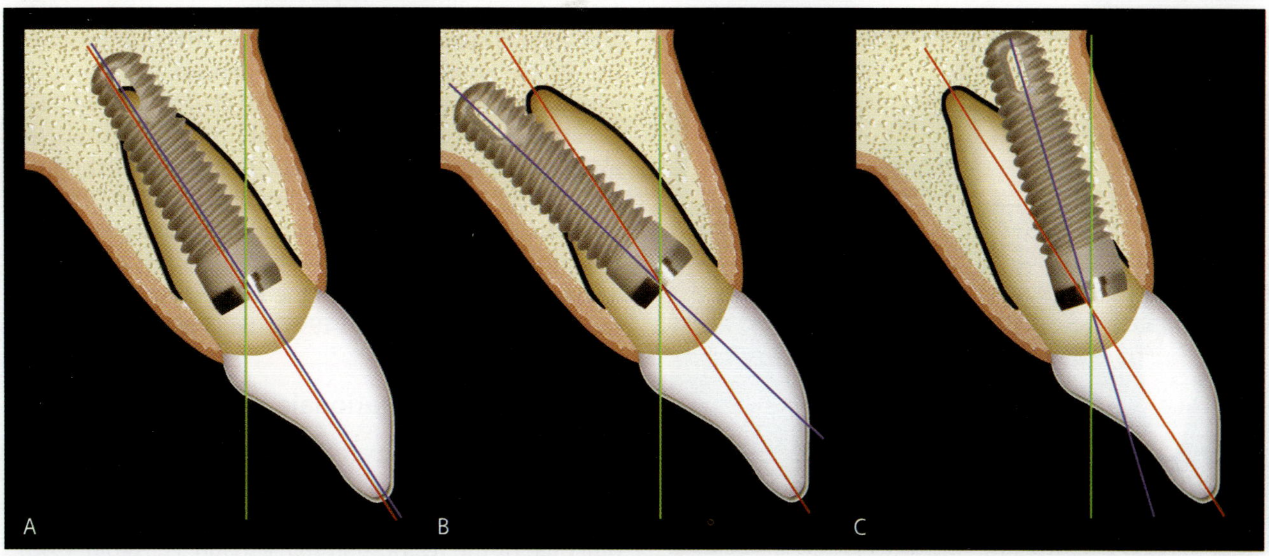

Figure 4.17A, B, C. The red line represents the original natural tooth axis, the blue line represents the implant fixture axis, and the green line represents the sagittal axis of the patient. In A, the implant fixture is coinciding with the natural tooth root position. In B, the implant is slightly palatal to the sagittal plane. In C, the implant is placed in a labial position at a 45-degree angle to the sagittal axis.

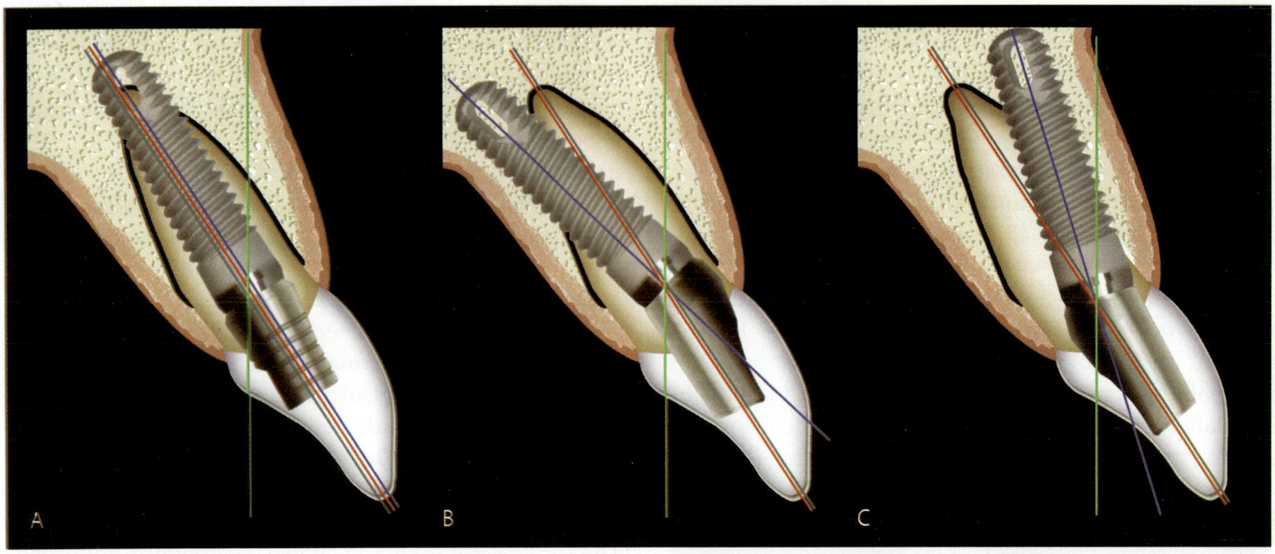

Figure 4.18A, B, C. In A, when the implant fixture is placed in the same tooth position, the abutment used is at the same plane of the implant fixture. However, in B and C, the slight implant fixture angulation to the labial or the lingual from the natural tooth axis dictated the use of angulated abutments.

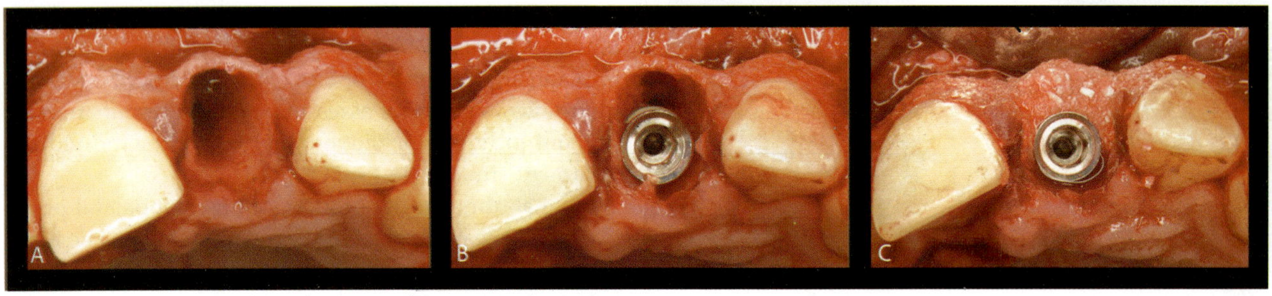

Figure 4.19. **A.** An extraction socket condition. **B.** The implant head is placed in the optimal buccolingual position. Note the space left for natural emergence between the implant and the crest of the bone. **C.** The space is filled with bone-grafting material.

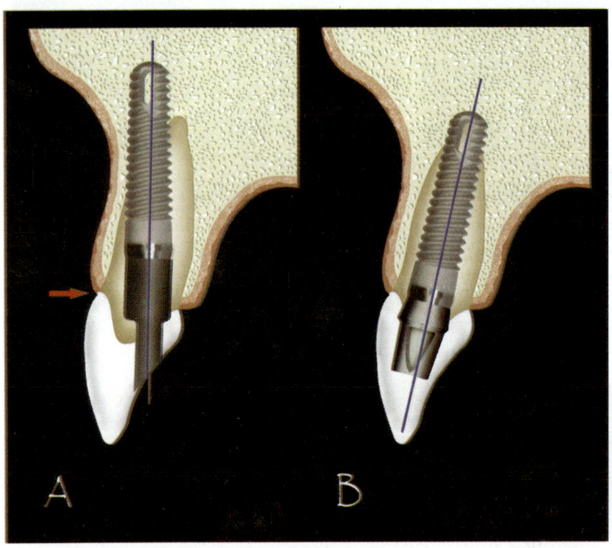

Figure 4.20. **A.** Illustration showing the long-axis positioning of the implant fixture when using a cement-retained abutment. **B.** Illustration showing the long-axis positioning of the implant when using a screw-retained abutment.

and cement-retained abutments. The choice of positioning of the implant fixture will depend on the space needed to gain accessibility to the abutment. For example, when cement-retained abutments are used, the implant is positioned exactly in the center of the long axis of the future implant-supported crown. On the other hand, when screw-retained abutments are used, the implant should be placed slightly palatal to the long axis of the crown to access the connecting screw from the palatal side (Davidoff 1996). (See Figures 4.20A–B.)

Axial Positioning Rationale

Implant positioning in relation to its axial level influences the amount of exposure the final restoration will receive, which in turn dramatically affects the esthetic outcome of the restoration (Jansen and Weisgold 1995). Apicoincisal positioning is no less important than the mesiodistal and labiopalatal positioning aspects of the implant. Unfortunately, surgical templates that offer apicoincisal positioning guidance for functional or esthetic implant placement are few. They are often difficult to fabricate and they are not cost effective. Most of the recent computer-generated templates have a metallic stop to control the apical extent of the drill. The optimal axial positioning of the implant head allows the final restoration to emerge naturally through the marginal gingival tissues with no violation to the gingival sulcus (Wheeler 1974), allowing the contours of the restoration to develop in a progressive manner within the peri-implant soft tissue housing. As a result, the final prosthetic result appears as if it emerges naturally.

Several factors control the location of the implant head in an axial dimension, including (1) the amount of space available for restoration, (2) the topography of the remaining bone, (3) the marginal gingival location of the adjacent natural teeth, and (4) the selected implant diameter. The optimal axial location of the implant head is necessary due to the anatomical difference between the fixture morphology and that of the natural tooth at the cervical level. A morphological transition from the narrow circular implant neck from the implant head to that of the natural tooth form is naturally required.

The reference location of all axial implant positioning is an imaginary line connecting the gingival zeniths of the adjacent natural teeth. There is a greater urgency for restoring natural gingival contours surrounding the new restorations when a natural tooth reference is missing and multiple adjacent implants are to be used. These implants should be placed at the alveolar crest within the circumference of the missing teeth to be restored. This enables the clinician to develop appropriate natural embrasures on both sides adjoining the restorations and duplicate a natural gingival profile (Potashnick 1998). The ideal apicoincisal implant positioning places the implant head 2 mm to 3 mm apical to the line connecting the gingival zeniths of the adjacent natural teeth. This subsequently allows "running room" throughout the biological width of the implant when it is correctly positioned in an apicoincisal plane (Parel and Sullivan 1989), as shown in Figure 4.21.

The "running room" is a space of 2 mm to 3 mm in depth and it surrounds the implant head circumferentially, as shown in Figure 4.22. This room allows for stacking or building up of prosthetic components to create the natural gingival emergence of the final restoration. If any modification or expansion of the gingival tissues to match the original crown size takes place in this particular space, the progressive use of the provisional restoration will develop the original cross-sectional shape of the missing natural tooth. The use of anatomical abutments has not proven to be more effective than the progressive use of the provisional restoration. Because the gingival tissue does not have a memory to keep its original dimensions without existing support, the peri-implant soft tissue tends to collapse and regain its original circular shape (due to the pressure from the circular collagen fibers surrounding the biological seal) upon its removal from the gingival sulcus. Clinically speaking, natural biological contours could be replicated without the need for anatomical abutments. Provisional prostheses have proven to give an optimal gingival influence with great clinical predictability. (See Figure 4.23.)

Implant diameter has an inverse relationship to the amount of subgingival sinking. It influences the amount

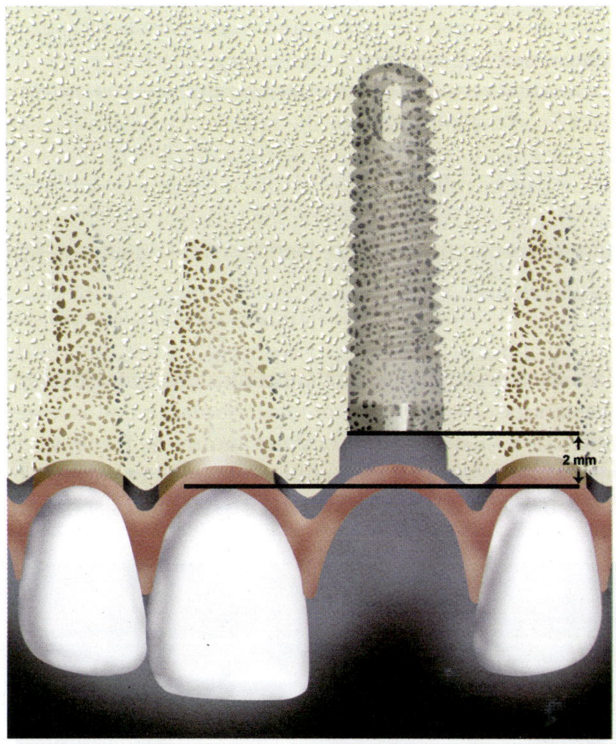

Figure 4.21. An illustration showing the ideal axial positioning of the implant, 2–3 mm from the line connecting the gingival zenith of the natural teeth.

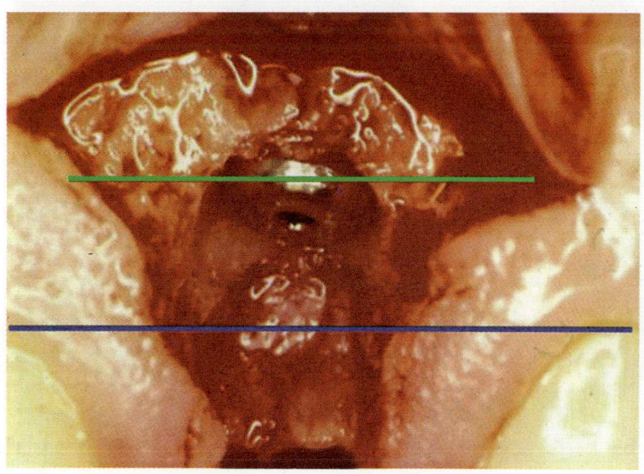

Figure 4.22. The ideal distance from the gingival zenith to the implant head. The blue line represents the gingival zenith, and the green line represents the optimal implant axial position.

of axial sinking of the implant head, because implants with wide diameters eventually require less space for making the transition into a natural tooth form than narrow-diameter implants. Bear in mind that not all the biological concepts are violated. The screw design implant ranks first to allow a more precise axial placement than the cylindrical designs. Its mechanical characters allow control of the depth while threading the fixture in the bone. The cylinder design, on the other hand, requires the use of an implant retrieval tool to adjust the implant's optimal vertical position, which makes the procedure difficult to control. (See Figure 4.24.)

Gingival zenith of the adjacent natural teeth is considered to be the landmark or the reference in apico-incisal implant positioning. Therefore, for a number of reasons, it is recommended that the location of the implant head be related to a line connecting the gingival zenith of the adjacent remaining natural dentition rather than to a line connecting the CEJ or the crest of the ridge. For instance, the gingival zenith is not a static landmark; it sometimes moves apically, such as in the case of gingival recession, because it represents the actual clinical marginal level of the soft tissue at the time of implant placement. In contrast, the CEJ is a constantly static landmark. It follows a uniformly fixed scalloped path along the root surface. It also pursues a wavy course that has a rise and fall on both buccolingual and interproximal margins. This scalloped line does not move when gingival recession occurs, thus it does not allow for optimal apicoincisal positioning in the case of gingival recession and in cases of placing an implant in unbalanced soft tissue margins. (See Figure 4.25.) Also, the wavy course of the CEJ does not give a stable reference with which to measure. The use of the deepest part of the gingival zenith allows the final implant-supported restoration to attain the same marginal level as those existing around natural dentition, as shown in Figure 4.26.

The crest of the ridge is a less than ideal reference point for making a measurement to relate the implant head because the nature of bone resorption sometimes makes it variable in its levels. In other words, in many instances the osseous housing is not the optimal landmark. Soft tissue thickness on top of it can be variable as well, which might lead to unpredictable variable measurements, as shown in Figure 4.27. For example, when the alveolar ridge has undergone a process of vertical osseous resorption, the implant head will eventually be situated above the bone level. Therefore, the osseous crest should not be taken as a reference measuring point. (See Figure 4.28.)

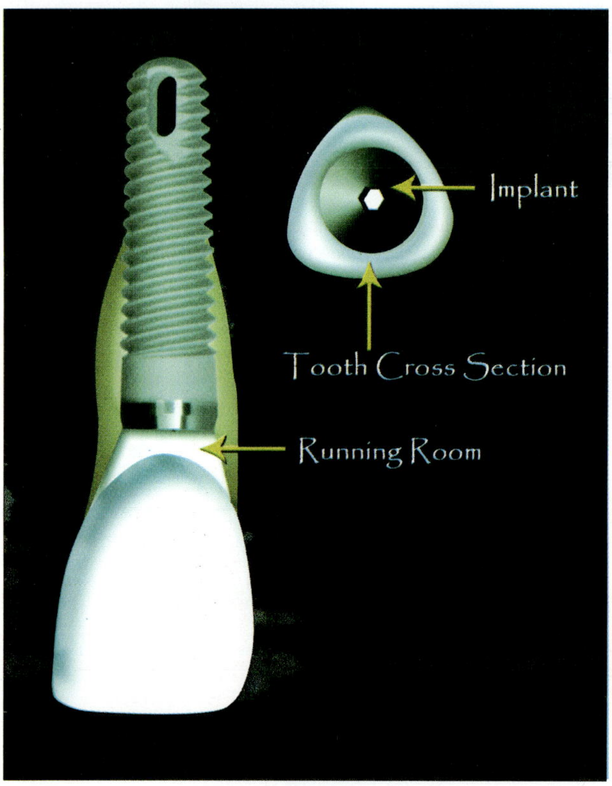

Figure 4.23. An illustration showing the difference in cross section between implant and natural tooth and the running room.

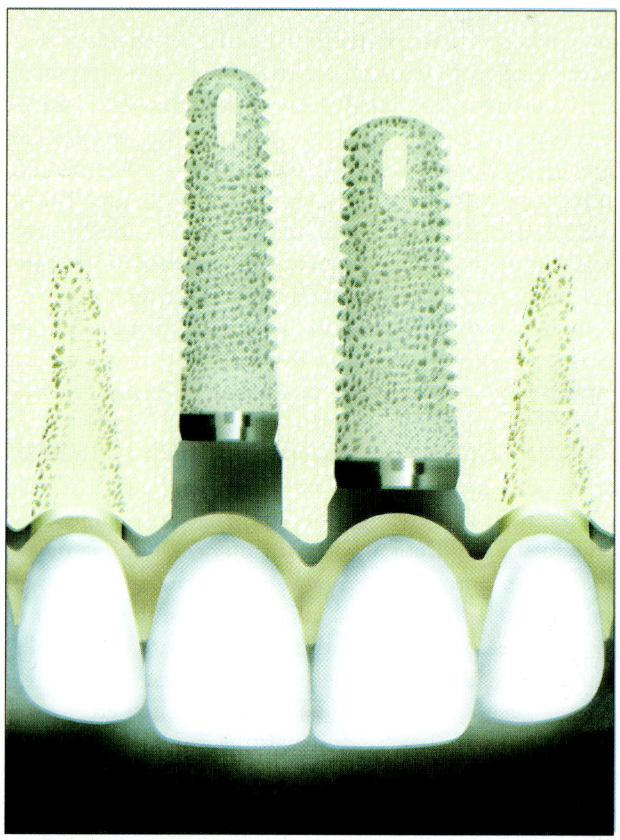

Figure 4.24. An illustration showing that wider implants require less apical positioning.

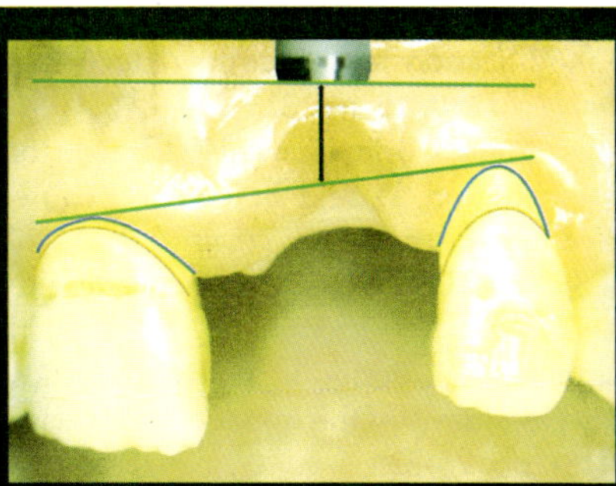

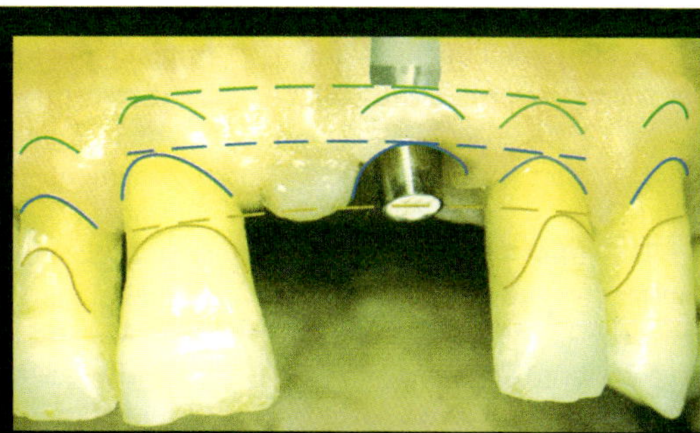

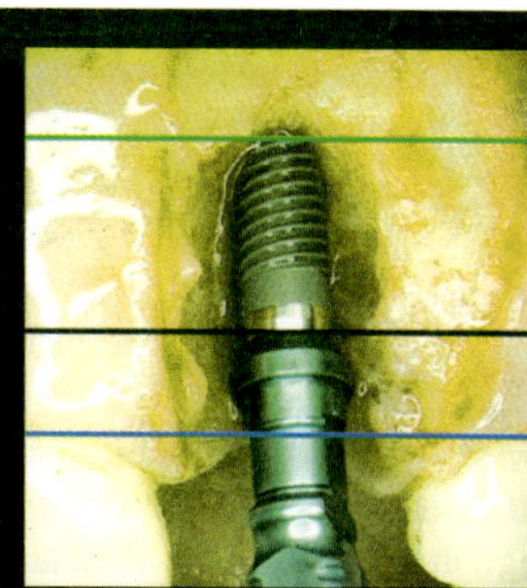

Figure 4.25. Two unsymmetrical gingival margins: the blue line represents the actual gingival zenith, the red line represents the CEJ, and the green lines show the calculation of the distance form the deepest point of the gingival zenith to the implant head represented in the black line.

Figure 4.26. In the case of gingival recession, it is impossible to relate the axial positioning to the CEJ. The red line represents the CEJ, the blue line represents the actual gingival marginal position, and the green line represents the osseous crest levels.

Figure 4.27. In cases of vertical bone resorption, the implant head can be located over the osseous crest, which proves the fact that the implant head should be related to the line connecting the gingival zenith. The green line represents that osseous crest, the black line represents the implant head level, and the blue line represents the gingival zeniths.

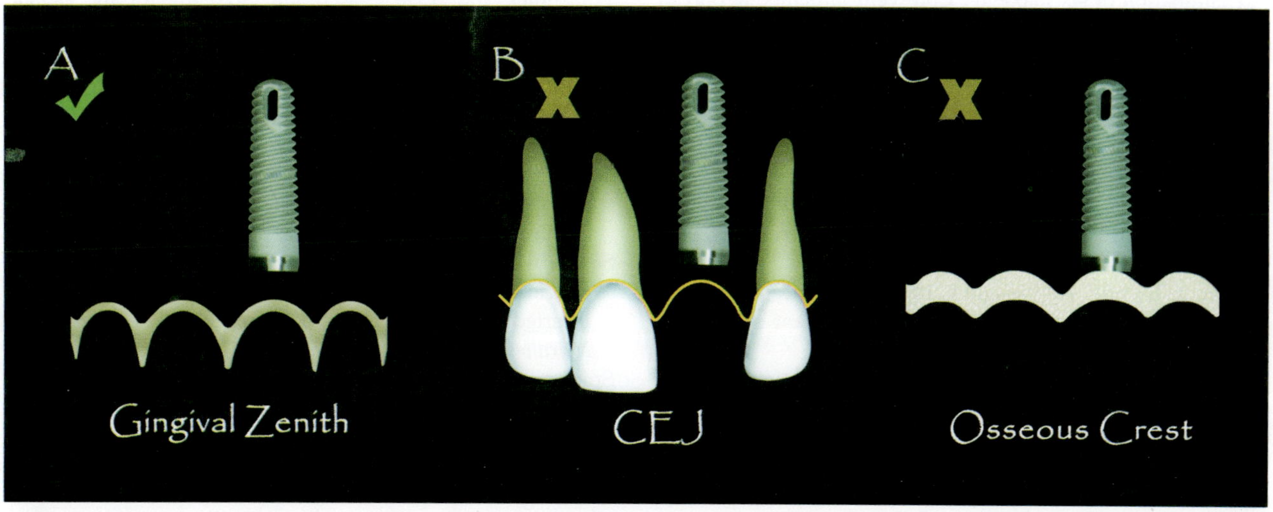

Figure 4.28. An illustration showing the three different positioning possibilities.

References

Atwood, D.A., and D.A. Coy. 1971. Clinical, cephalometric and densitometric study of reduction of residual ridge. *J Prosthet Dent*, (26), pp. 280–293.

Block, M.S., J.N. Kent, and L.R. Guerra. 1997. *Implants in Dentistry*. Philadelphia: W.B. Saunders Co.

Brunski, J.B., D.A. Puleo, and A. Nanci. 2000. Biomaterials and biomechanics of oral and maxillofacial implants: Current status and future developments. *Int J Oral Maxillofac Implants*, (15), pp. 15–46.

Burger, E.H., and J. Klein-Nulend. 1999. Responses of bone cells to biomechanical forces in vitro. *Ady Dent Res*, (13), pp. 93–98.

Buser, D., R. Mericske-Stern, K. Dula, and N.P. Lang. 1999. Clinical experience with one-stage, non-submerged dental implants. *Adv Dent Res*, (13), pp. 153–161.

Carlsson, G.E., B. Bergman, and B. Headegard. 1967. Changes in contour of the maxillary alveolar process under immediate dentures. A longitudinal clinical and X-ray cephalometric study covering 5 years. *Acta Odontol Scand*, (25), pp. 45–75.

Carlsson, L., T. Rostlund, B. Albrektsson, et al. 1988. Removal torques for polished and rough titanium implants. *Int J Oral Maxillofac Implants*, 3, (1), pp. 21–24.

Casap, N., E. Tarazi, A. Wexeler, et al. 2005. Intraoperative Computerized Navigation for Flapless Implant Surgery and Immediate Loading in the Edentulous Mandible. *Int j Oral Maxillofac Implants*, 20, pp. 92–98.

Chiche, G.J., and H. Aoshima. 1997. Functional versus aesthetic articulation of maxillary anterior restorations. *Pract Periodont Aesthet Dent*, 90, pp. 335–342.

Daftary, F. 1995. Natural esthetics with implant prosthesis. *J Esthet Dent*, (7), pp. 9–17.

Davidoff, D. 1996. Developing soft tissue contours for implant supported restorations: A simplified method for enhanced aesthetics. *Pract Periodont Aesthet Dent*, (8), pp. 507–513.

El Askary, A.S., R.M. Meffert, and T. Griffin. 1999a. Why do dental implants fail? Part I. *Implant Dent*, (8), pp. 173–185.

El Askary, A.S., R.M. Meffert, and T. Griffin. 1999b. Why do Dental Implants Fail? Part II. *Implant Dent*, (8), pp. 265–277.

El Askary, A.S. 2000. Multi faceted aspects of Implant esthetics: The anterior maxilla. *Implant Dent*, 10, pp. 182–191.

English, C.E. 1993. Biomechanical concerns with fixed partial dentures involving implants. *Implant Dent*, (2), pp. 221–242.

Esposito, M., A. Ekestubbe, and K. Grondahl. 1993. Radiological evaluation of marginal bone loss at tooth surfaces facing single Branemark implants. *Clin Oral Impl Res*, 4, (3), pp. 151–157.

Garber, D.A. 1995. The esthetic dental implant: Letting the restoration be the guide. *J Am Dent Assoc*, (126), pp. 319–325.

Glickman, I. 1972. *Clinical Periodontology*, 4th ed. Philadelphia: W.B. Saunders Co., p. 21.

Gores, R.J., C.K. Hayes, and K.K. Unni. 1989. Post mortem examination of six maxillary Core-Vent implants. Report of a case. *J Oral Maxillofac Surg*, 47(3), pp. 302–306.

Grunder, U., S. Gracis, and M. Capelli. 2005. Influence of the 3-D Bone-to-Implant Relationship on Esthetics. *Int J Periodontics Restorative Dent*, 25, pp. 113–119.

Herrmann, G. 2000. Primary stability of oral implants. *Int Mag Oral Implantol*, (1), pp. 22–24.

Iglhaut, M. 2003. Implant Surgical Guide and Positioning System—A Case Report. *Int Magazine Oral Implantol.*, (1), pp. 389–391.

Jansen, C.E., and A. Weisgold. 1995. Presurgical treatment planning for the anterior single-tooth implant restoration *Compendium*, (16), pp. 746–763.

Johansson, C., and T. Albrektsson. 1987. Integration of screw implants in the rabbit: A 1-yr follow-up of removal torque of titanium implants. *Int J Oral Maxillofac Implants*, 2, (2), pp. 69–75.

Johnson, K. 1963. A study of the dimensional changes occurring in the maxilla after tooth extraction. Part I: Normal healing. *Aust Dent J*, (8), pp. 428–433.

Kennedy, B.D., T.A. Collins, and P.C. Kline. 1998. Simplified guide for precise implant placement: A technical note. *Int J Oral Maxillofac Implants*, (13), pp. 684–688.

Koyanagi, K. 2002. Development and clinical application of a surgical guide for optimal implant placement. *J Prosthet Dent*, 88, pp. 548–52.

Meffert, R.M. 1992. Treatment of failing dental implants. *Curr Opin Dent*, (2), pp. 109–144.

Misch, C.E. 1995. The maxillary anterior single tooth implant aesthetic health compromise. *Int J Dent Symp*, (1), pp. 4–9.

Misch, C.E, H.L. Wang, C.M. Misch, et al. 2004. Rationale for the Application of Immediate Load In Implant Dentistry: Part II. *Implant Dent*, 13, pp. 310–321.

Morris, M.L. 1958. The position of the margin of the gingival. *Oral Surg Oral Med Oral Pathol*, (11), pp. 722–734.

Nebot, V.X., R. Ciurana, and C. Alfonso. 2006. Benefits of an implant platform modification technique to reduce crestal bone resorption. *Implant Dent*, 15, pp. 313–320.

Ohenell, L., J. Palmquist, and P.I. Branemark. 1992. Single tooth replacement. In: Worthington, P., and Branemark, P.I., eds. *Advanced Osseointegration Surgery Applications in the Maxillofacial Region*. Carol Stream, IL: Quintessence Publishing CO., pp. 211–132.

Olsson, M., and J. Lindhe. 1991. Periodontal characteristics in individuals with varying forms of the upper central incisors. *J Clin Periodontol*, (18), pp. 78–82.

Oschsenbein, C., and S. Ross. 1973. A concept of osseous surgery and its clinical applications. In: Ward, H.L., and Chas, C., eds. *A Periodontal Point of View*. Springfield, IL: Charles C. Thomas.

Palacci, P. 2001. Optimal implant positioning. In: Palacci, P., and Ericsson, I. *Esthetic Implant Dentistry. Soft and Hard Tissue Management*. Berlin: Quintessence Publishing Co., pp. 101–135.

Parel, S.M., and D.Y. Sullivan. 1989. *Esthetics and Osseointegration*. Dallas, TX: Taylor Publishing.

Potashnick, S.R. 1998. Soft tissue modeling for the esthetic single-tooth implant restoration. *J Esthet Dent*, (10), pp. 121–131.

Seibert, J. 1973. Surgical management of osseous defects. In: Gorman, H.M., and Cohen, D.W., eds. *Periodontal Therapy*, 5th ed. St. Louis: C.V. Mosby Co., pp. 765–766.

Seibert, J., and J. Lindhe. 1988. Esthetics and periodontal therapy. Lindhe, J., ed. *Text Book of Clinical Periodontology*, 2nd ed. Copenhagen: Munksgaard.

Sennerby, L., P. Thomsen, and L.E. Ericson. 1992. A morphometric and biomechanic comparison of titanium implants inserted in rabbit corical and cancellous bone. *Int J Oral Maxillofac Implants*, 7, pp. 62–71.

Spiekerman, H.S. 1995. Special diagnostic methods for implant patients. In: *Implantology*. Stuttgart: Thieme Verlag, pp. 91–124.

Szmukler-Moncler, S., H. Salama, Y. Reingewirtz, et al. 1998. Timing of loading and effect of micromotion on bone-dental implant interface: Review of experimental literature. *J Biomed Mater Res*, (43), pp. 192–203.

Tardieu, P., L. Vrielinck, and E. Escolano. 2003. Computer-assisted implant placement. A case report: treatment of the mandible. *Int J Oral Maxillofac Implants*, 18, pp. 599–604.

Wheeler, R.C. 1950. *A Text Book of Dental Anatomy and Physiology*, 2nd ed. Philadelphia: W.B. Saunders Co.

Wheeler, R.C. 1961. Complete crown form and the periodontium. *J Prosthet Dent*, (11), pp. 722–734.

Wheeler, R.C. 1974. *Dental Anatomy, Physiology and Occlusion*. 5th ed. Philadelphia: W.B Saunders Co.

Wohrle, P.S. 2003. Nobel Perfect esthetic scalloped implant: Rationale for a new design. *Clin Implant Dent Relat Res*, 5 (supp) (1), pp. 64–73.

Yousef, H., A. Luke, J. Ricci, et al. 2005. Analysis of Changes in Implant Screws Subject to Occlusal Loading: A Preliminary Analysis. *Implant Dent*, 14, pp. 378–385.

Chapter 5

Intraoral Plastic Soft Tissue Surgery

Abd El Salam El Askary

The unique oral mucosa that invests the alveolar structure is composed of keratinized and nonkeratinized components. Each of the two components possesses its own morphological characteristics and physiological behavior toward trauma and surgical handling. The nonkeratinized, or vestibular mucosa, is more elastic and richer in blood supply; however, it is thin and fragile. The keratinized mucosa has a more sturdy nature, is stable, and voids elasticity. With the evolution of implant plastic reconstructive therapy, oral mucosa has received more attention from clinicians as new tissue preservation procedures and versatile clinical-surgical options have been introduced. The soft tissue in the oral cavity complements the color, contrast, and luster of the natural teeth and subsequently implant-supported restorations.

The soft tissue constitutes the outer frame that also complements the beauty and attractiveness of the mouth. This explains the importance of the peri-implant soft tissue in achieving natural tissue contours and pleasant smiles. Contrary to many clinical opinions, soft tissue can play an important role in the success of dental implantology procedures. It is considered to be the gate for bacterial invasion and microorganisms to the implant fixture, as well as the outer shield to underlying structures.

The proper understanding of the nature of the peri-implant soft tissue that physically surrounds dental implant fixtures warrants using the most suitable methods for tissue handling. The delicate nature and the compromised blood supply in certain sites dictate careful tissue handling. Understandably, it is impossible to achieve satisfactory esthetic results without peri-implant soft tissue that is harmonious with the adjacent tissues in color, form, and contour (El Askary 2002).

Peri-implant architecture thus takes a major share in the esthetic setup of any implant-supported restoration (Croll 1989, Alberktsson and Hansson 1986, Buser et al. 1991, Sennerby et al. 1993, Strid 1985). Most of the current peri-implant soft tissue methods can solve a number of minor clinical dilemmas; for example, connective tissue grafts can amend minor alveolar ridge defects and restore original contours by increasing the soft tissue height or width (Seibert 1993, Garber 1981, Wennstrom 1996).

Soft tissue expansion by means of a provisional restoration is yet another modern application in soft tissue management. It is used to enhance the esthetic outcome or help solve an existing soft tissue clinical problem (Chee et al. 1997, Chee and Donovan 1995, El Askary 1999, Stauts 1991, Neale and Chee 1994). Unlike the natural dentition, a dental implant is a metallic body with a collar that does not receive any blood supply from a surrounding periodontal ligament or any other vessels. Rather, it acquires a fibrous connective tissue band around its collar that is more dense and acellular (Berman et al. 1993, Abrahamsson et al. 1998, Akagawa et al. 1989, Berglundh et al. 1991, Egelberg 1966). In addition, the fragile nature of peri-implant mucosa makes its ability to withstand excessive clinical manipulations unpredictable (Potashnick 1998), especially in thin scalloped tissue biotypes. Generally speaking, the adherence to the basic standard operative principles should be considered in any treatment plan; therefore, clinicians must seek atraumatic tissue handling, impeccable periosteal reflection, and tension-free closure. These guidelines can be vital to the functional and esthetic results of implant therapy.

Several treatment factors can be directly related to the condition of the peri-implant soft tissue health:

1. Esthetic implant positioning has a direct influence on the soft profile and final soft tissue appearance (Palacci 1996). The more precisely the implant is positioned, the easier it will be to obtain a natural-looking implant-supported restoration in its soft tissue housing. This can help minimize the need for further corrective surgeries and soft tissue reconstruction.
2. Accurate diagnosis and treatment planning directly impact the precision of the work and the predictability of the final results by helping to determine the

optimal timing and sequence of the surgical events, leading to optimal soft tissue contours.
3. Complete understanding of oral tissue behavior.
4. Complete understanding of the effect of stystematic aspects to the tissue healing response.

Because proactive soft tissue management must occur in a proper or optimal sequence, management of the soft tissues around dental implants in the esthetic zone has been classified into four categories according to the timing of clinical intervention: (1) before implant placement, (2) during implant placement, (3) at the time of abutment connection, and (4) at postabutment connection (El Askary 2000). Mucogingival surgical corrections can be used prior to implant surgery to enhance a preexisting condition or after implant placement to reconstruct the missing esthetic biological contours as a result of tissue mishandling (Carlsson et al. 1967). This can help improve esthetics, phonetics, and oral hygiene maintenance of the implant-supported prostheses.

Soft tissue management at the time of tooth extraction can affect the final esthetic outcome as well. The method used can be selected from soft tissue management procedures to noninvasive procedures (flapless methods). Soft tissue refining and profiling, on the other hand, are intermediate clinical procedures in implant treatment that can be executed after the abutment connection or at the time of the second-stage surgery. It all depends on the decision of the clinician according to the specific existing clinical situation.

Lazara (1993) noted that ample time for soft tissue to heal and mend is important for achieving optimal results. A stable soft tissue clinical condition must be reached after the surgical interference before continuing with other clinical procedures. Small and Tarnow (2000) reaffirmed this, recommending a three-month waiting period for the soft tissue to stabilize before selecting the final abutment or making the final impression after the second-stage surgery. They evaluated 63 implants in 11 patients, measuring the soft tissue level around dental implants following surgery to determine if a predictable pattern of soft tissue changes could be identified. Baseline measurements were recorded at the second-stage surgery in two different submerged implant systems. Subsequent measurements were recorded at one week, one month, three months, six months, nine months, and one year after baseline measurements. The majority of the recession occurred within the first three months, and 80% of all sites exhibited recession on the buccal surface. Thus, three months' time is recommended to allow the tissue to stabilize and mature before either selecting a final abutment or making a final impression.

Another study that evaluated the incidence of gingival recession around implants in a one-year prospective study included 63 implants. The soft tissue height was measured around implants following surgery to determine whether a predictable pattern of soft tissue changes could be identified. Eighty percent of all sites exhibited recession on the buccal aspect, and the majority of the recession occurred within the first three months. The authors stated that, as a general rule, one can expect approximately 1 mm of gingival recession postabutment connection surgery (Moberg et al. 1999).

Healing time influences soft tissue procedures because peri-implant soft tissue requires longer healing periods to reach a stable condition after remodeling.

Classifying the existing hard and/or soft tissue defects allows the clinician to consider surgical reconstruction from the outset, and allows better communication among the dental team. It not only facilitates the assessment of any given clinically compromised situation, but also helps the dental team identify the existing soft tissue status and describe it in a more specific and scientific manner.

Ridge defects have a wide range of descriptions with numerous variations in size, severity, and extent. Allen and others (1985) identified three categories of ridge defects in relation to the healthy soft tissue margins: (a) mild, a defect of less than 3 mm; (b) moderate, a defect of 3–6 mm; and (c) severe, a defect greater than 6 mm. Seibert and Salama (1996), on the other hand, classified volumetric deformity changes of the edentulous ridge into three general categories: Class I, buccolingual loss of tissue with normal ridge height in an apicocoronal dimension; Class II, apicocoronal loss of tissue with normal ridge width in a buccolingual dimension; and Class III, combination buccolingual and apicocoronal loss of tissue, resulting in loss of normal ridge height and width.

Intraoral Soft Tissue Healing Response

Wound healing can be influential to peri-implant soft tissue health; it is directly related to the prognoses of implant-supported restorations from functional and esthetic aspects. Among the factors—systemic and local—that influence wound healing around dental implants are (1) any existing superficial or deep infection, (2) preoperative wound contamination, (3) the pressure from an existing prostheses, (4) lack of preoperative antibiotics administration, (5) retained sutures, (6) dehydration that causes electrolyte imbalance that can affect cardiac function, (7) kidney dysfunction, (8) cellular metabolism, (9) poor nutrition that is essential to support cellular activity and collagen synthesis at the wound site, (10) poor oxygenation of the blood, (11) low serum protein and vitamin C, A, and K deficiency, or (12) any other hidden systemic pathologic conditions (Sadig and Almas 2004).

Body wounds heal in three different ways: primary, secondary, or tertiary intention. The primary intention healing starts immediately after surgery by attracting undifferentiated mesenchymal cells, fibroblasts, plasma portions, and leukocytes. Upon the completion of this procedure, a total seal of the wound occurs within 24 hours postsurgery; then a local inflammatory process occurs, which results from the leukocytic migration to the area. It produces photolytic enzymes to dissolve and remove damaged tissue debris that is characterized by pain, swelling, and edema (Schultze-Mosgau et al. 2005).

During the first week, fibroblasts start the reconstruction of all nonepithelial tissues, forming collagen fibers along the sides of the wound. This is what gives tensile strength to the wound edges, and helps the wound withstand reinjury after closure. The fibroblasts contain myofibroblasts, which have smooth muscle characteristics that contribute to wound contraction (van Beurden et al. 2005). This procedure is accompanied by a lymphatic drainage and vascularization at the wound area. In time, tensile strength of the wound increases due to the cross-linking process of collagen fibers, and then the further deposition of fibrous connective tissue results in a scar formation.

The secondary intention type of healing, such as in cases of tooth extraction, is the granulation tissue that results from the extraction process. This tissue forms and contains myofibroblasts along the sides of the wound. This type of healing starts from the bottom of the socket and progresses until it reaches the top of it. This type is characterized by its longer healing period and the tendency for infection.

The third type of soft tissue healing involves necrotic tissues that are to be removed and that bring clean nonnecrotic tissues together.

In the presence of implanted graft material, the repair process undergoes a different tissue reaction that deviates from the normal healing process, especially in its intensity and duration (Williamas 1987). An accumulation of extracellular fluid that contains proteins and inflammatory cells surrounds the implanted material. The proteins are absorbed at the surface of the implanted graft and undergo a variation of their configuration to an extent that they condition the functional response of the peri-implant cells (Kenley et al. 1994). The inflammatory cells can then modify the structure (the physical and chemical properties) of the surface of the graft material, usually causing a foreign body giant cell reaction. This activates the macrophages and leads to the production of cytokines that stimulate the production of collagen and bone tissue (Bao 1997). A layer of fibrous tissue will surround the graft material as it will do with any other device that remains for a certain time in the body. The surrounding fibrous tissue layer attains different thicknesses and shapes depending on its location, the mechanical stimuli, and the chemical characteristics of the graft interface. If the implanted graft material is biocompatible, the alterations in the repair process are limited, and the presence of fibrosis (which typically characterizes the final phase) is minimal. Biocompatibility can be defined as the capacity of a material to function in a specific application and provoke an appropriate reaction by the host. Therefore, biocompatibility should involve the chemical and physical characteristics of the bone grafting material to avoid systemic or local toxicity and carcinogenic or genotoxic reactions (Kenley et al. 1994).

Body wounds are classified into four categories: clean, clean-contaminated, contaminated, and infected (Cruse and Foorde 1980). The type of wound that is common in the oral cavity is the clean-contaminated wound, because oral wounds are potentially contaminated with bacterial flora. In intraoral wounds (clean-contaminated), certain precautions should be undertaken to reduce the chance of uneventful healing or an interrupted healing process:

1. Using sterile instrumentation
2. Using aseptic surgical techniques
3. Making sharp and stable incisions that allow enough tissue exposure and visibility, with minimum trauma
4. Applying gentle flap dissection that preserves the underlying periosteum
5. Atraumatic wound handling that allows minimal tension and pressure to the flap because increased flap tension will lead to impaired blood and interrupt lymph flow, thus altering the local physiological state of the wound
6. Controlling intraoperative bleeding to avoid the possibility of hematoma formation that can interfere with wound healing
7. Keeping the flap moisturized and clean at all times
8. Eliminating the possibility of the formation of any dead space that fluids might collect in it after closure
9. Using optimal suture material
10. Providing tension-free soft tissue closure
11. Eliminating any local or external pressure on the wound.

Exceptional care must be given to handling peri-implant soft tissues because of their delicate nature. In an attempt to achieve a less traumatic surgical intervention and precise tissue handling, a microsurgical kit—the El Askary Microsurgery Kit (Storz am Markt GMBH, Emmingen-Liptingen, Germany)—has been introduced to the field of intraoral plastic surgery. The instruments were designed to achieve maximum comfort for grasping, thus allowing better tissue access and less tissue trauma. The kit consists of the following items (see Figure 5.1):

- Microblade handle (or holder) used for precise microincisions next to the interdental papilla
- Microperiosteal elevator (Mini-Buser)
- Tissue forceps 1:2 teeth, straight and curved
- Dressing pliers TC 0.8 mm straight with carbide tips for membrane handling
- Micro-scissors, curved Gomel 16 cm
- Micro needle holder Barraquer TC, 0.8 mm with smooth carbide tips for microsuturing (5/0–8/0).

New and sharp scalpel blades and well-designed instruments should be used for making incisions and reflection to preserve the vitality of the mucosa. Incisions should be made at a right angle to the tissues, and tissues should be stable during the incision. In case the full thickness flap is to be used, periosteum should be reflected with caution to avoid any lacerations. Cases in which spilt thickness dissection is selected, care should be exercised to avoid piercing the flap. In case of long-term edentulism, periosteum can be strongly adherent to the underlying bone; therefore, sharp dissection should be allowed with a scalpel, with its cutting edge moved gently in a direction parallel with the bone. Incisions should be planned on the study cast prior to surgery. When performing surgery in the esthetic zone, the interproximal papilla should never be incised or excised in any case. It can be spared or included along with the flap reflection, and small periosteal elevators should be used to reflect the papilla to avoid tearing it. (See Figures 5.2A–B.) The flapped tissues should be kept hydrated at all times during the surgery; this may be achieved by using wet gauze or sponge or saline spray.

Care should be used when holding the flap with toothed-type forceps to avoid piercing the fragile thin soft tissues and causing further postoperative complications. Palatal flaps should be approached with caution because they lack elasticity, and profuse bleeding is a common surgical event. The clinician should know how to control bleeding because intraoral implantology procedures involve three main arteries: inferior alveolar, facial, and lingual. Intraoral bleeding may result in hypotension or airway obstruction and can be life-threatening if not treated. Intraoral bleeding can be controlled best by first applying digital palpation at the source of the hemorrhage to detect the bleeding source. The next step to controlling intraoral bleeding is head elevation. Head elevation can decrease nasal mucosal blood flow to a great extent by applying pressure, because pressure can be considered to be an effective method for homeostasis, cauterization, ligation, or endoscopic ligation of the artery. Bone wax application to block bleeding osseous channels and intravenous injection of vitamin K also can be used to control bleeding.

Careful periosteal reflection should be undertaken. Round-edged retractors should be used to protect the tissues from being lacerated, or a suture may be taken to keep the flap elevated at all times. Tension-free closure of the soft tissue should be performed, because tissue closure can be vital to the success of the implant therapy as well as tissue esthetics. A strict protocol should be used to close the soft tissue either in grafting or non-grafting procedures. Mastering peri-implant soft tissue procedures becomes vital not only to achieve optimal tissue architecture, but also to avoid undesirable post-operative results.

Tooth extraction prior to or in conjunction with implant therapy should be approached with caution. Atraumatic extraction of a tooth requires patience and

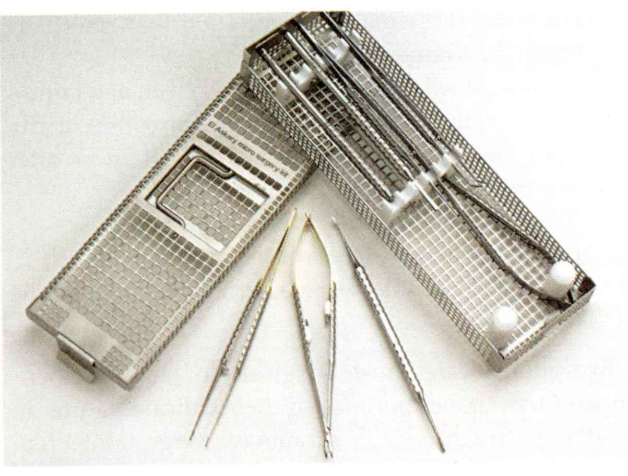

Figure 5.1. El Askary Micro-surgery Kit (Storz am Markt GMBH, Emmingen-Liptingen, Germany).

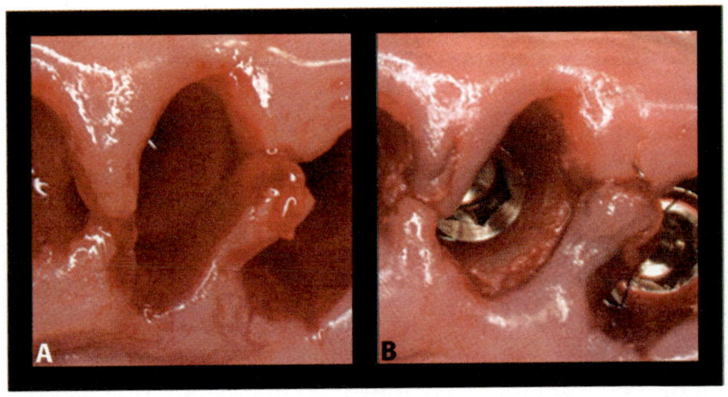

Figure 5.2. **A.** Lacerated interdental papilla postextraction. **B.** The microsuturing to hold the pieces together.

careful attention. Every attempt should be made to minimize trauma to the alveolar bone plate during the extraction. Cases in which immediate implant placement is being undertaken, an incision is made with a blade to separate the periodontal ligament that might help to loosen the tooth. To preserve the buccal plate during tooth extraction, the periodontal ligament fibers can be further separated with the use of a periotome (Storz am Markt GMBH, Emmingen-Liptingen, Germany). Small elevators can be used, but luxation should be in a mesiodistal direction. Consider using tapered forceps that better adapt to the tooth than standard extraction forceps. If there is inadequate tooth structure and the tooth cannot be extracted with the forceps, the tooth can be carefully sectioned so the remaining root fragments can be extracted without placing pressure on the alveolus.

Suturing is yet another critical treatment step in soft tissue management. The optimal suture material has the following characteristics:

1. Attain the minimal size that holds the wound edges together to minimize the tissue trauma and piercing. The tensile strength of the suture need never exceed the tensile strength of the tissue.
2. Pass through tissue readily with minimal drag.
3. Facilitate easy tissue passage.
4. Allow precise knot placement.
5. Allow smooth tie down and a decreased tendency to incarcerate tissue (Van Winkle and Hastings 1972).

The main requirements for any optimal suture material are (1) sterility, (2) nonelectrolytic, (3) noncapillary, (4) nonallergenic, (5) noncarcinogenic, (6) nonferromagnetic, (7) minimally reactive to the tissues, (8) high tensile strength to secure wound edges with no cutting nor tearing, (9) shrinkage resistance, (10) pliability for ease of handling, and (11) consistent uniform diameter.

Sutures need to be either resorbable or nonresorbable or monofilament or multifilament. The monofilament sutures pass through tissue easier than multifilament sutures and do not attract microorganisms that may cause suture line infection (Dineen 1997). They are also tied down easily. On the other hand, multifilament sutures attain greater tensile strength and flexibility, but are liable to attract bacteria.

Resorbable sutures might be naturally or synthetically absorbed by hydrolysis, which offers minimal tissue reaction. During the first stage of the absorption process, tensile strength diminishes in a gradual, almost linear fashion. The second stage often follows with considerable overlap, characterized by loss of suture mass. Both stages exhibit leukocytic cellular responses that serve to remove cellular debris and suture material from the line of tissue approximation, as shown in Figure 5.2A–B. Drawbacks of resorbable sutures are infection and premature absorption due to the exposure to the tissue fluids as in the oral cavity; nonresorbable sutures offer more tensile strength and less tissue reaction. Good examples of nonresorbable sutures are black silk and nylon. Nylon is a very inert suturing material because it causes minimum tissue reaction and provides the least inflammatory response around it. Even if it is left for a longer time in the oral wounds, it does not seem to cause any bacterial aggregation around it. However, its sharp edges can cause oral ulcers when it is located at the site of a moving organ such as the tongue or the lips, as shown in Figure 5.3.

Needles should cause the least trauma to the tissues and should be as small as possible to minimize tissue piercing. They should be sharp, rigid, and corrosion resistant. Sutures should be removed using aseptic and sterile techniques. The steps for suture removal follow:

- Clean with antiseptic solution or swabbing material.
- Pick up one end of the suture with thumb forceps, and cut as close to the skin as possible where the suture enters the skin.
- Gently pull the suture strand out though the side opposite the knot with the forceps.

Recently studies have linked soft tissue healing response to some medications. A recent study (Braganza et al. 2005) related the intake of nonsteroidal anti-inflammatory drugs (NSAID) with possible bleeding problems during periodontal surgery. This study measured the effect of ibuprofen at peak plasma levels on intraoperative bleeding. Fifteen medically healthy subjects (seven males and eight females), each with two sites requiring periodontal surgery of similar complexity, type, and duration, were selected for the study. The subjects were instructed to take ibuprofen prior to one of

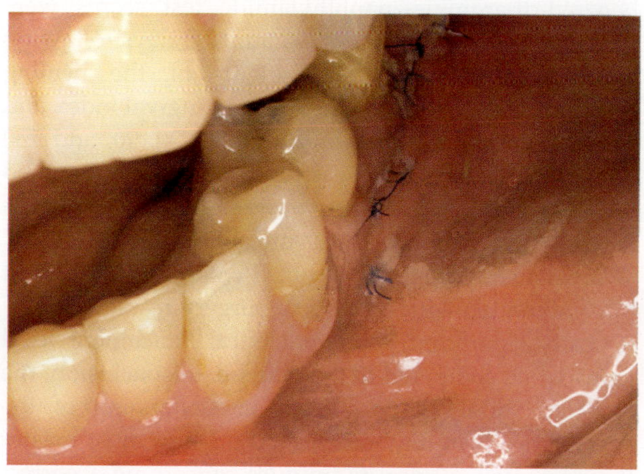

Figure 5.3. Oral traumatic ulcer due to the sharp edges friction of the nylon sutures.

the surgeries. A standard bleeding time and papillary bleeding index score were recorded at initial consultation and prior to the first and second surgeries. The volume of aspirated blood was measured during each surgery by subtracting the amount of water used for irrigation from the total volume of fluid (blood plus irrigation water) collected at 15-minute intervals during the surgery.

Results showed an increase in intraoperative bleeding when ibuprofen was taken prior to surgery (31.93 ± 15.72 versus 17.80 ± 9.57 mL; $P < 0.01$). Ibuprofen appeared to have its greatest effect on bleeding midsurgery. The average bleeding time also increased significantly ($P < 0.01$) when ibuprofen was preadministered (4.17 ± 0.96 versus 3.8 ± 0.92 minutes), although the bleeding remained within the normal range. Papillary bleeding did not show a significant difference between the two surgeries. However, surgeries involving osseous resection showed a significant increase in bleeding when ibuprofen was preadministered. The study concluded that the intraoperative blood loss in patients is almost two times that of those who did not take ibuprofen.

Another study (Nyeiva et al. 2005) was performed to determine if healing capacity and vitamin B complex intake can positively affect wound healing processes. The study gathered a total of 30 patients (13 males, 17 females) with generalized moderate to severe chronic periodontitis. All subjects had more than two teeth in the same sextant with probing depth ≥5 mm and bleeding upon probing and who were in need of access flap surgery. This study was a randomized, double-masked, placebo-controlled clinical trial. Subjects were instructed to take one 50-mg capsule of vitamin B daily in the following form: thiamine HCI, riboflavin, niacinamide, d-Calcium Pantothenate, and pyridoxine HCI; as well as 50 µg each of d-biotin and cyanocobalamin; and 400 µg of folate; or a placebo for 30 days following access flap surgery (AFS). Clinical attachment levels and 1'l-benzoyl-dl-arginine-2naphthylamide test scores were measured at baseline and at 90 and 180 days following surgical intervention. Assessments of the healing response were also performed using gingival index and plaque index at baseline and at 7, 14, 30, 90, and 180 days. The mean results of each parameter were averaged within a group. Differences between groups were analyzed by using repeated measure analysis of variance.

Results showed that vitamin B complex supplement in combination with access flap surgery resulted in statistically significant superior clinical attachment level gains when compared to the placebo. In conclusion, the clinician should have a clear understanding of the specific needs in any given situation, and must master the necessary surgical techniques concerning a correct implant placement and a correct soft tissue handling to achieve the treatment objectives (Nyeiva et al. 2005).

Optimizing Peri-implant Tissues Status

Modern peri-implant soft tissue therapy has evolved with numerous methods to enhance the esthetic results of implant therapy. Those methods are used to improve the soft tissue status prior to therapy, as a precautionary measure to avoid any postoperative complication or to correct an existing poor esthetic situation. Today, it is possible to minimize the alveolar ridge deficiency in height and width by preserving the bone volume at the time of tooth extraction. This provides an ideal condition for the placement of dental implants with greater implant-to-bone contact and allows the placement of longer, wider implants. This enhances the esthetics of the final restoration with better emergence profiles and harmonious gingival architecture. The numerous methods that are now available to preserve the socket condition—either by soft tissue augmentation, bone augmentation, or a combination of the two—help to optimize the socket condition for predictable esthetic and functional implant therapy.

The most popular peri-implant soft tissue techniques include: (1) alveolar socket therapy to preserve natural architecture, (2) minimally invasive procedures that provide less tissue trauma, (3) flap designs that favor esthetics, (4) innovative techniques to close soft tissues, (5) innovative surgical techniques for the second-stage surgery that allows better visualization with less tendency for scar formation, (6) inlay connective tissue grafts that constitute much of the modern implant therapy, and (7) onlay grafting procedures to increase the zone of keratinized band or prevent further soft tissue recession.

Future peri-implant tissues should be carefully examined prior to implant therapy to identify any defects or discrepancies in the keratinized band and to avoid undesirable results during the therapy. The biological nature of the oral mucosa should be kept in mind when performing any preimplant therapy. Any corrective soft tissue surgery (if needed) should be performed two to four months before the first-stage implant placement surgery to allow ample time for the soft tissue to reach a stable remodeling state (Tarnow et al. 1996).

Soft tissue therapy prior to implant placement uses various techniques to enhance the quantity or the quality of the soft tissue or to eliminate any existing soft tissue pathology at the area of interest. Free gingival grafting (Seibert 1983), connective tissue grafting (Langer and Langer 1985), or a combination of the two can also be used at this stage to enhance the final esthetic outcome and minimize potential complications during the first- and second-stage surgeries (Hurzeler and Dietmar 1996). After tooth extraction, alveolar ridge resorption with subsequent soft tissue recession can disturb the harmonious pre-existing dentoalveolar complex to a great extent, and possibly compromise esthetic restorative results because the labial alveolar plate and its corresponding soft tissue usually begin to resorb and recede soon after tooth extraction. Although bone-grafting procedures can improve the osseous and gingival topography postresorption, results sometimes are unpredictable and usually add time and high costs. This is especially critical in the maxillary anterior region, where the condition of the soft tissue complex and its relationship to the implant restoration and its adjacent dentition often determines the implant's success (Kan et al. 2000).

Improving the Alveolar Socket Condition

Improving the socket condition prior to implant surgery can be a safeguard for the future health of the implant and its surrounding tissues because a sufficient zone of keratinized mucosa can minimize soft tissue complications (especially in immediate implant placements) and stabilize the peri-implant tissue margins. Many clinicians have noted that immediate implant placement into a freshly extracted socket might present an especially difficult challenge to achieving soft tissue coverage, especially with patients that have the thin scalloped tissue biotype.

Achieving primary flap closure has been regarded as one of the most challenging aspects of immediate implant placement (Becker et al. 1994). The success rates of immediate implant placement have not been shown to differ between closure and nonclosure, and in many cases the mucogingival conditions around extraction sockets may become unfavorable for primary closure (Becker et al. 1994). Periosteal-releasing incisions as well as palatal rotational flaps have been introduced for complete flap closure. Nonetheless, these procedures may alter the continuity of the keratinized tissue band. Furthermore, the possible tension created by primary flap closure may increase the chance of eventual bone graft or membrane exposure, leading to bone loss, infection, and even loss of implants.

To overcome these clinical difficulties, a technique for developing keratinized tissues on top of the socket orifice has been introduced. (See Figures 5.4A–L.) Langer (1994) suggested using the body's regenerative capacity to produce extra tissue around the root of a tooth that is scheduled for extraction. This provides sufficient keratinized mucosa for a soft tissue closure procedure over the implant. This new tissue subsequently minimizes surgical trauma that results from primary closure in immediate implant placement. In addition, the regenerated tissue restores the anatomical

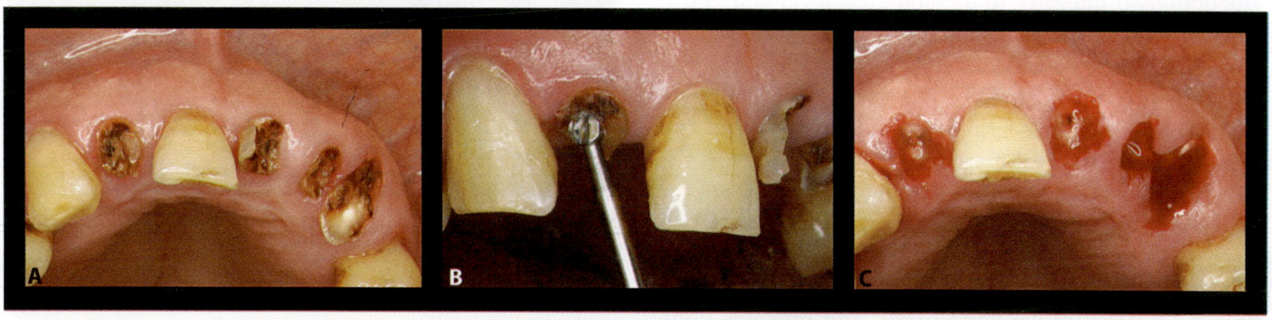

Figure 5.4. A. Intraoral condition for multiple remaining roots scheduled for extraction. **B.** Reducing the level of the roots to the bone level. **C.** The clinical picture postroot reduction.

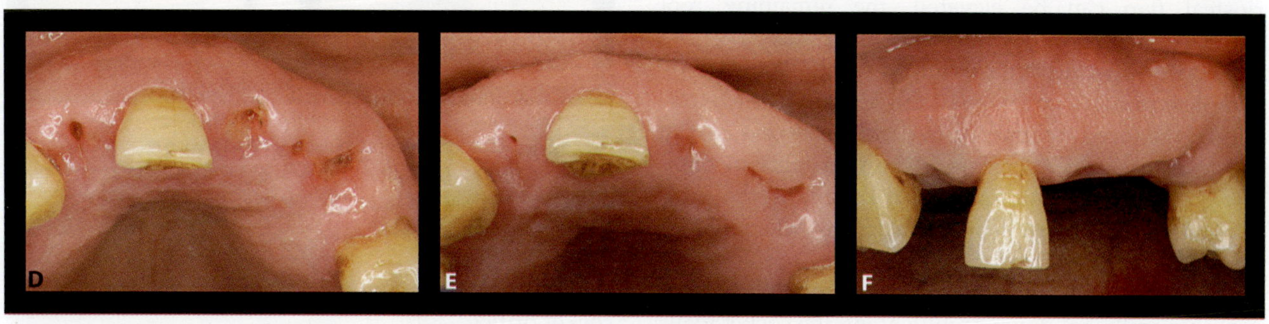

Figure 5.4. D. Two weeks postroot reduction. Note the amount of new regenerated keratinized tissue. **E.** Five weeks postroot reduction (occlusal view). **F.** Five weeks postroot reduction (labial view).

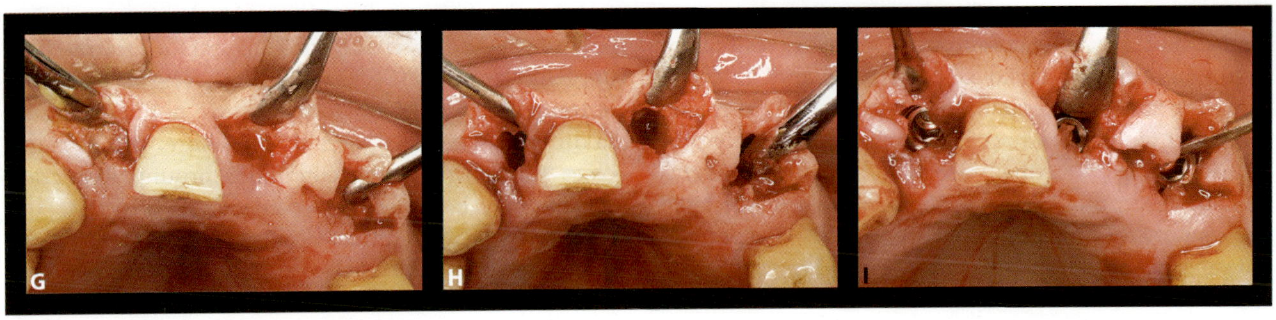

Figure 5.4. **G.** Conservative flap is reflected revealing the remaining roots. **H.** Roots after atraumatic removal. **I.** Three implants (TSV, Zimmer Dental, USA) in place.

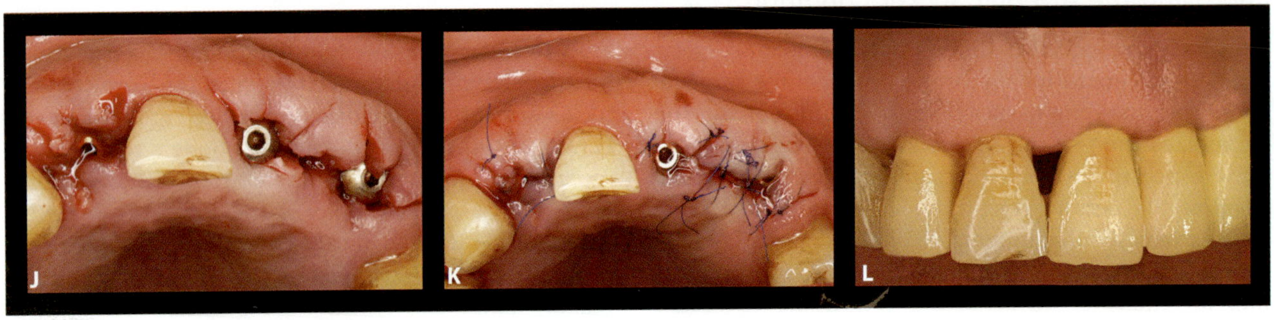

Figure 5.4. **J.** Healing abutments are connected. **K.** The area sutured and wound closure attempted. **L.** Postrestorative view.

mucogingival integrity to its biological level and eliminates the chance for postextraction alveolar bone resorption (Pietrokovski and Massler 1967, Lam 1960, Atwood 1963). (See Figures 5.5A–D.)

This method entails grinding the failing tooth 2 mm below the free gingival margin to make it level with the alveolar bone crest, and then leaving it in the socket for two to four weeks so the surrounding gingival tissue can proliferate over the remaining root. This procedure allows ridge preservation, facilitates complete tissue closure over the implant and grafts, and prevents bone resorption because the root remains in its housing. The gingival tissues proliferate, covering the remaining tooth root with keratinized gingiva. Next, a mucoperiosteal flap can be elevated, the remaining root extracted, and an implant immediately placed.

Some distinct advantages of this technique include complete primary coverage of the implant at stage-one surgery, reduced treatment time, and decreased cost to the patient. Drawbacks include the possibility of damaging the crestal bone during extraction and the presence of fenestration or dehiscence defects, which would necessitate further grafting procedures.

The presence of residual roots of the reduced teeth prevents epithelial down growth along the socket walls and provides scaffolding for the regeneration of keratinized tissues on top of the socket orifice. The soft tissues take only a few weeks to regenerate and fill the socket orifice.

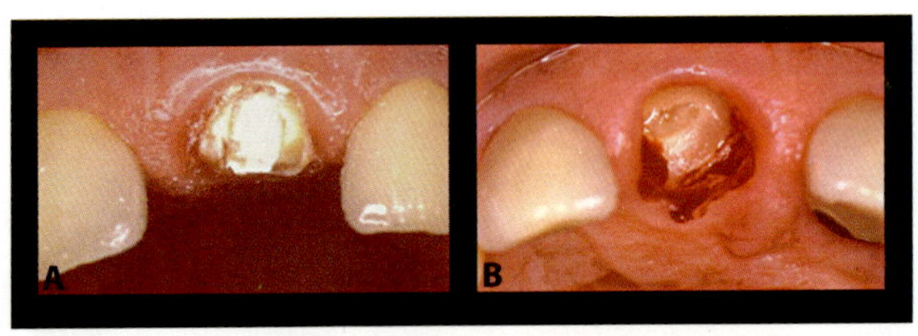

Figure 5.5. **A.** A patient with unsalvageable remaining root of the maxillary left central incisor. **B.** Reduction of the root level below the crest of the alveolar bone.

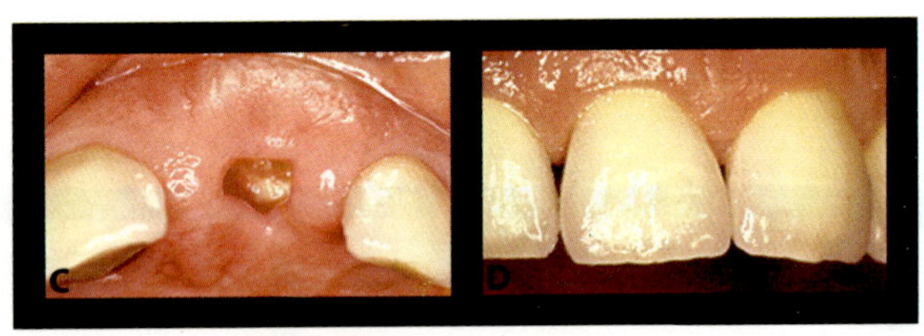

Figure 5.5. **C.** A four-week postoperative view showing regeneration of new keratinized tissues. **D.** Postinsertion view of the final restoration in place, showing an excellent soft tissue condition.

Langer (1994) suggested that pulp extirpation can be performed prior to the procedure to avoid possible pain.

However, complete root canal treatment would ensure absence of infection in the extraction socket during implant placement surgery. With this technique, the degree of tissue closure varies and usually depends on time. The waiting period can last at least three months before complete soft tissue coverage and maturation has occurred. However, some thinning of the soft tissues can be expected over the roots at the time of implant placement, which may necessitate soft tissue manipulations to overcome these possible fenestrations.

Regenerated tissues should exceed that which is required to compensate for ensuing tissue shrinkage or remodeling (Roberts et al. 1987, Garretto et al. 1995). After sufficient healing time has elapsed and a stable tissue contour is established, any excessive tissue can then be trimmed or sculptured to the desired level.

Another technique for improving the soft tissue condition on top of an extraction socket is the socket seal technique. This improves the socket condition prior to implant therapy, reduces the waiting period for developing soft tissues on top of the socket orifice, and augments future peri-implant tissues. Socket sealing blocks the socket orifice of an extracted tooth immediately after unsalvageable tooth extraction. Socket seal surgery was first described by Landsberg (1997a) and Landsberg and Bichacho (1994) as an alternative for preserving the integrity of the alveolar ridge and inhibiting apical epithelial migration into the socket. As a result, the overall socket condition is improved so that it can optimally house an implant body (Dahlin et al. 1988).

The procedure involves atraumatic flapless tooth extraction using the periotomes (Storz am Markt GMBH, Emmingen-Liptingen, Germany). This is followed by debridement and decortication of the socket walls to enhance osteogenic activity by providing a pool of cells into the site through the blood stream. The free gingival margins surrounding the socket orifice should then be circumferentially de-epithelialized—with a water-cooled, round coarse diamond bur or a sharp scalpel—to provide a vascular bed for the future free gingival graft and promote clot formation inside the socket. The socket is then packed with the bone graft of choice; grafting materials can range from allografts to alloplasts with or without growth factors added. A fairly thick free gingival graft is then harvested from the palate to cover the bone-grafting material and protect it from the hostile oral environment. The free gingival graft is then adapted and fitted to the freshly de-epithelialized gingival margins over the bone graft and carefully sutured, to completely seal the socket orifice.

Socket sealing prevents physical, chemical, or bacterial contamination of the organizing blood clot and bone-grafting material until healing occurs (Dahlin et al. 1988). The technique is becoming more popular and considered a simple clinical procedure that can be performed along with tooth extraction in preparation for optimizing a future implant site.

The author's clinical experience has shown that the soft tissue graft lies on the bone graft particles and not on a periosteal or connective tissue bed; therefore, the surrounding gingival tissue located on the rim of the socket becomes the only source of vascularity to the free gingival graft. As a result, the soft tissue graft might be prone to thinning, necrosis, and subsequent infection. Furthermore, if the soft tissue graft survives, it generally does not possess the same texture or color as the surrounding soft tissues. All socket sealing techniques should be approached with caution because the postoperative results have not yet confirmed a highly predictable success rate.

Misch and others (1999) have modified socket sealing in an attempt to improve its clinical outcome and predictability. Their method, called modified socket seal, focuses on providing an excellent source for blood supply to the area.

The modified socket seal surgery can be performed prior to implant placement to improve the quantity and quality of bone and soft tissue and preserve the biological architecture of the alveolar ridge at the tooth extraction site. It is used mainly to optimize the socket condition prior to implant installation. The goal is to place the implant in a completely mature osseous bed and healthy soft tissue contour, which in turn ensures the functional and esthetic success of the overall treatment.

Intact socket walls are a strict clinical condition and an essential requirement for using this technique. A composite graft, consisting of epithelial tissue, connective tissue, periosteum, cortical bone, and cancellous bone, is harvested from the tuberosity area to fill and seal the socket. There are several advantages to using a composite graft. First, the connective tissue portion of the graft has an advantage over the keratinized tissue; it merges and blends with the adjacent keratinized tissues after the healing process, providing keratinized epithelium on top of the socket with a color and texture similar to that of the surrounding original tissues. Also, the use of the autogenous bone is more predictable for bone regenerative procedures (Dahlin et al. 1991, Hammack and Enneking 1960, Male et al. 1983).

Misch and others (1999) have also used platelet-derived growth factor (PDGF) from the patient's own blood to act as a chemoattractant for mesenchymal cells to speed up cartilage and bone formation (Howes et al. 1988). The procedure entails a flapless atraumatic extraction of the unsalvageable tooth, followed by a thorough curettage and decortication of the socket walls. The soft tissue around the rim of the extraction socket is then de-epithelialized with a diamond bur or a sharp scalpel. A wide diameter trephine drill that is larger than the diameter of the socket orifice is used to harvest the composite graft from the tuberosity. A slow-speed, high-torque handpiece with copious internal and external saline irrigation should be used during the harvesting procedure to avoid overheating the graft.

A green stick fracture of the composite graft is performed at its base to separate it from the donor site. Here, caution must be used not to perforate the maxillary sinus; a preoperative X-ray film or digital imaging can help determine the extent of drilling needed. The keratinized layer of the graft core is then peeled with a sharp scalpel to remove only the surface epithelium, leaving almost 3 mm of connective tissue attached to the bone core. If the bone core is found to be larger than the socket orifice, it should be pared so that it will fit snugly in the socket. The apical third of the extraction socket is subsequently filled with demineralized freeze-dried bone and a puffy coat containing PDGF. Afterward, the composite graft is introduced into the socket and tapped gently into place using a mallet and a blunt instrument.

Upon seating, the surface of the composite graft should conform to and be level with the crestal contour of the socket; it may be positioned slightly below the surrounding marginal gingival. This is to allow for epithelial migration from the sides of the socket on top of the connective tissue graft. The connective tissue portion of the graft is then sutured to the surrounding gingival tissues. A provisional removable prosthesis should not be allowed during the first few weeks after surgery when this technique is used, because the composite graft may move upon pressure and become sequestrated due to premature loading of the bone that results from fitting the surface of the prosthesis.

The osteotomy hole of the donor site can be filled with any bone-grafting material or heavily packed with collagen sponge. Primary wound closure can be achieved by undermining the soft tissue edges, or preferably, an acrylic template may be used to seal the area of the defect until it heals by secondary intention.

This technique reduces the risk of morbidity, because the quality of the bone harvested from the tuberosity offers the best environment for blood circulation and bone formation in its wide cancellous compartments. A fair enhancement of the soft tissue quality and quantity over the socket is also offered (it attains the exact color and texture of the surrounding tissues). It also offers faster and more predictable bone regeneration inside the socket, thus improving the overall prognosis for any future implant placement. (See Figures 5.6A–G.)

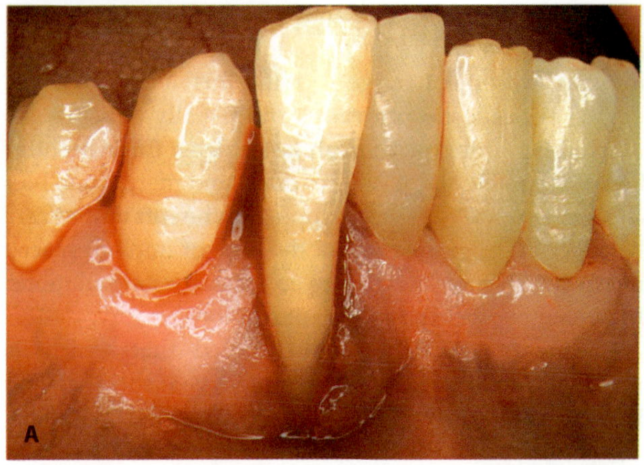

Figure 5.6A. Sever gingival recession with accompanied bone loss that mandates clinical management.

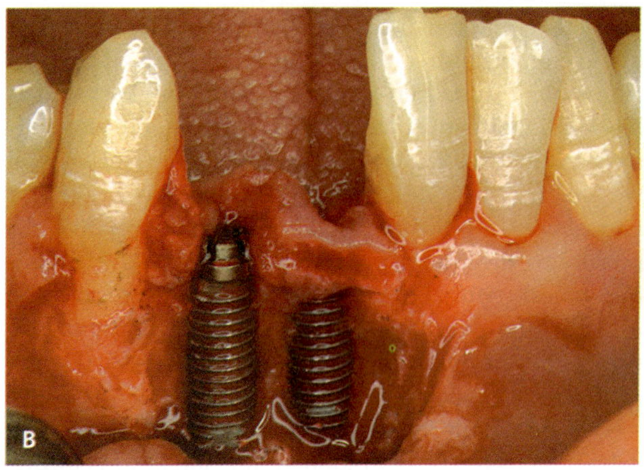

Figure 5.6B. The two involved teeth have been removed and replaced with two dental implants in immediate placement.

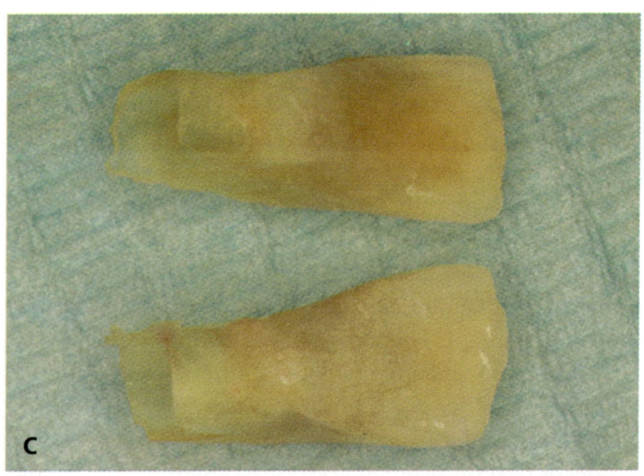

Figure 5.6C. The removed natural crowns have been prepared to act as provisional crowns for the implants (non-functional immediate loading).

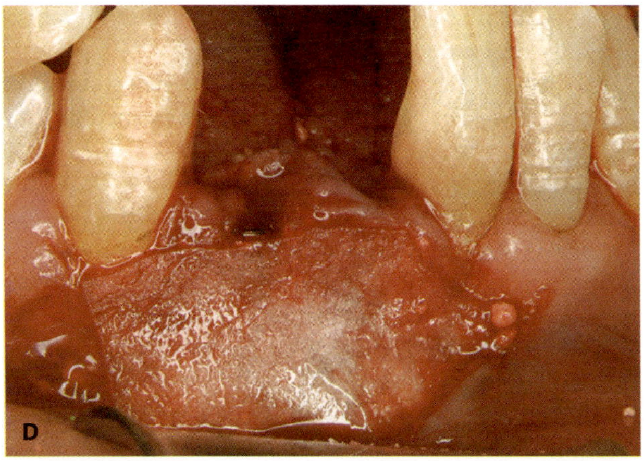

Figure 5.6D. The osseous defect was augmented with particulate bone graft and a resorbable membrane was placed on top.

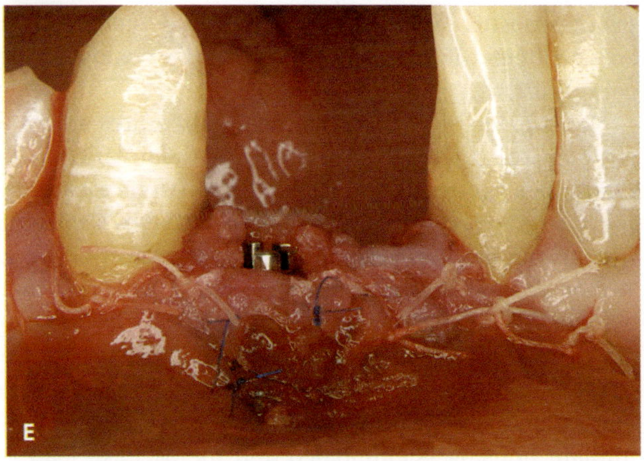

Figure 5.6E. Partial thickness pedicle flap was medially moved along with inlay connective tissue graft to cover the defect.

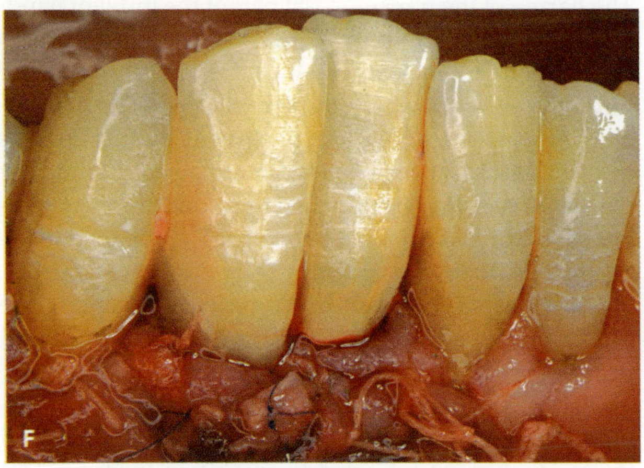

Figure 5.6F. The natural teeth crowns were used as a provisional aid.

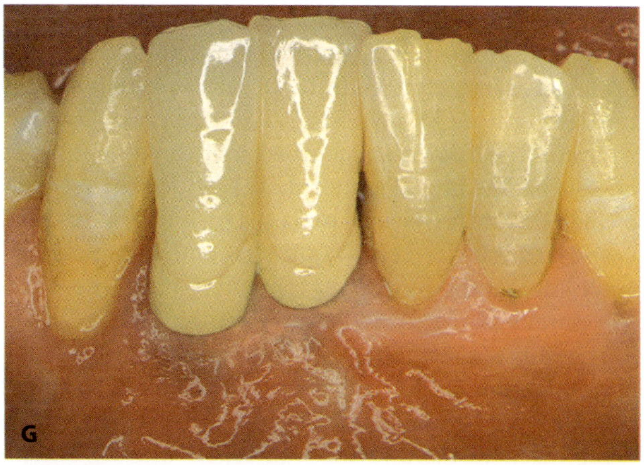

Figure 5.6G. The case finally restored after total soft tissue healing and remodeling.

Innovative Esthetic Incisions

Conservative flap design is becoming a routine treatment discipline in modern esthetic dental implantology. Although it is becoming an integral part of any esthetic treatment plan, it is important to avoid unnecessary tissue reflection when providing sufficient access to the underlying structures during implant surgery. A number of incision designs are used during implant placement at first-stage surgery. Many clinical benefits evolved from these designs that have contributed to today's routine clinical practice (Becker and Becker 1996, Palacci 1995). Most of the currently available techniques aim to preserve natural esthetics and fulfill the standard operative standards for mucoperiosteal flap management. Periosteal integrity and vascularity are considered important elements in wound healing postsurgery, and angiogenesis may be important for designing a flap and a suturing method that gives a stable postoperative result.

Nobuto and others (2005) have monitored the role of the periosteum in tissue healing and postoperative angiogenesis. They investigated the role of the periosteal vascular plexus in the healing process and used 3-D and ultrastructural monitoring of the angiogenic process after elevation of the mucoperiosteal flap. Mucoperiosteal flap surgery was performed on nine adult beagle dogs. The periosteal vascular plexus was observed three, five, and seven days after surgery in histological specimens in which blood vessels were injected with India ink under a light microscope, in ultrathin sections under a transmission electron microscope, and in acryl plastic vascular cast specimens under a scanning electron microscope. On day 3 after surgery, new blood vessels, formed through sprouting, bridging, and intussusceptions, were observed in ultrathin sections and vascular casts. In addition, blood island-like structures consisting of clustered immature endothelial cells were noted in the repaired tissue. On days 5 to 7 after surgery, 3-D observation of vascular casts clarified that these new blood vessels had a sinus-like morphology in the interstitium of the periosteal vascular plexus. These new sinusoidal vessels exhibited a stereoscopic structure with increased continuity as the blood vessels matured and the ultrastructural vascular endothelium was thinned.

The study concluded that after mucoperiosteal flap elevation, the periosteal vascularity exhibited potent blood vessel-forming activity through various angiogenic mechanisms and through repair activity. Therefore, clinicians should minimize periosteal manipulation as much as possible during the surgery to maintain the maximum tissue reparative capacity. Surgical entries to install an implant fixture within the bone have several modalities, and each one offers a clinical benefit and has a clinical indication. The modalities can vary greatly, and include delayed submerged implant placement protocol (crestal and vestibular approaches), flapless nonsubmerged implant placement protocol, delayed nonsubmerged protocol, immediate implant placement protocol with complete soft tissue closure, and immediate implant placement protocol without complete soft tissue closure (Block and Kent 1995, Branemark et al. 1985). (See Figures 5.6H–I.)

The standard protocol for delayed submerged implant installation in the esthetic zone first entails administering local anesthetic solution. Next, a crestal incision is made slightly on the palatal aspect or in the midcrestal position. The incision ends at the distal surface of the adjacent teeth to the buccal and palatal aspect of the alveolar crest. Buccal-relieving incisions are only made when necessary, that is excluding the interproximal papilla. Subsequently, the buccal and palatal mucoperiosteal flaps are then reflected carefully to ensure minimal atraumatic soft tissue handling. The precise position of the implant is then marked with a small round bur through the surgical template. Following

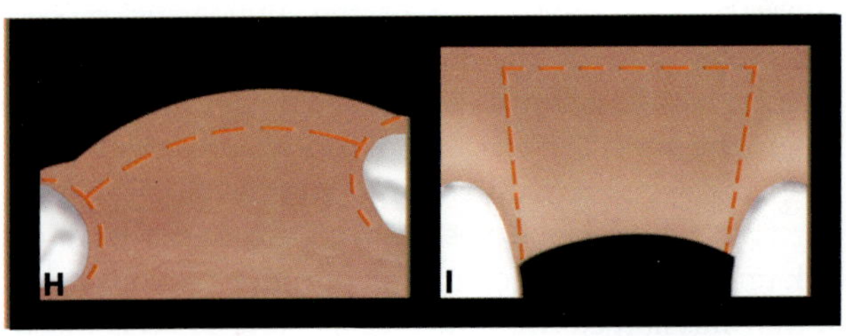

Figure 5.6. **H.** An illustration showing the crestal approach to installing dental implants. **I.** An illustration showing the vestibular approach to installing dental implants.

implant installation, the final position of the implant is carefully checked.

The need to augment the soft tissue with a connective tissue graft might be determined at this particular time to improve the thickness and contour of the buccal mucosa. The buccal flap and the palatal flaps are precisely repositioned and sutured. Selection of the specific incision design depends not only on the mode of implant installation, but also on the surgical procedure that is to be used, whether it is a combined bone-grafting procedure, combined connective tissue-grafting procedure, or a combination.

Surgical procedures that are used to achieve delayed implant installation dramatically differ from those used in immediate placement, and postoperative soft tissue healing differs accordingly in terms of incision design, mucoperiosteal flap handling, soft tissue manipulation, provisionalization, and flap closure. The careful selection of the optimal surgical protocol contributes positively to providing a healthy environment around dental implants and minimizing postoperative complications.

Nonsubmerged implant installation requires a different surgical approach. Nonsubmerged implant placement does not require a second-stage surgery because the access to the implant is maintained above the soft tissue from the time of its placement (Buser et al. 1990, Weber et al. 1996). Buser and others (1990) stated that osseointegration showed high predictability in the one-stage, nonsubmerged surgical protocol. This is because the subgingival implant-abutment connections are eliminated, and thus the bacterial population at the peri-implant housing is eliminated and the occlusal load is located away from the crestal bone level. However, it is now evident that when esthetics is a priority, nonsubmerged (one-stage) implant placement protocol should be restricted due to the inherent character of the design of the one-stage implant system (Bragger et al. 1998). The flaring of the transmucosal part of the implant handicaps the use of the provisional restoration to develop the "running room" within which the natural emergence through the soft tissues can be replicated. The nonsubmerged (two-stage) implant placement protocol entails the attachment of the healing abutment to the implant fixture at the time of implant insertion; the implant is permitted to heal in a nonsubmerged mode to provide greater latitude for proper soft tissue contouring. However, when function is a priority, submerging the implant beneath the soft tissue for a two-stage surgical protocol is still the method most preferred by clinicians, probably because there is extensive long-term documentation in the literature (Branemark et al. 1997) and the implant is not subjected to any biting loads while it is undergoing osseointegration (Misch 1990).

The clinician decides which surgical approach and implant installation to use. The decision should be based on factors such as the implant design to be used, tissue biotype, amount of available bone, quality of bone, type of occlusion, implant-loading protocol, need for esthetics, and other related factors such as finical considerations and the systemic health condition of the patient (Brunski et al. 1979, Boss et al. 1994).

Versatile Esthetic Flap Designs

Esthetic and functional predictability of dental implants require a flap design that provides accessibility, visibility, and workability without violating the harmonious soft tissue health or disturbing soft tissue integrity. The classical mucoperiosteal flap design involves the exposure of the totally edentulous operative site with minimal attention toward the fine esthetic details such as gingival zenith and the interdental papilla. It usually ignores the postoperative healing of minute structures such as the intact gingival contours (Bahat and Handelsman 1991, Dahlberg 1969). All flap designs should allow access and visibility with minimal soft tissue trauma and facilitate maintenance of the attached tissues (Johnson 1976, Corn 1973).

The selection of a specific flap design over another is mainly to achieve optimal wound healing that contributes positively to implant survival and esthetics (McKinney 1991). In fact, the oral cavity is a hostile environment for dental implants, and its wounds are clean-contaminated (Knox et al. 1991). Therefore, placing a dental implant in such an environment warrants special attention. Esposito and others (1998) noted an important link between wound healing and implant survival: clinical signs of oral tissue infection during the postoperative period of a submerged implant insertion can indicate an increased risk of implant failure. Systemic conditions such as uncontrolled diabetes mellitus, severe anemia, uremia, and jaundice can also be considered threats to flap survival and nourishment.

In submerged surgical implant installation, the classic vestibular approach was first described by Branemark and others (1985, 1997). The proposed design mainly provides fully edentulous arches and focuses on allowing optimal access and visualization. The design involves a horizontal incision in the vestibular mucosa parallel to the gingival margin. A lingually or palatally pedicled mucoperiosteal flap is next obtained through two vertical incisions. The objective of this design is to position the incision line away from the head of the implants. It presents a clinical difficulty in patients with shallow vestibules and thin scalloped biotypes. Sometimes postoperative edema accompanied by an inflammatory reaction was noted (which can be a potential risk of infection) (Scharf and Tarnow 1993). The design is called the *vestibular approach*.

Some modifications to this classic design allow partial-thickness dissection at the sides of the crest and full-thickness reflection on the crestal area; however, this approach is becoming less popular. The crestal approach, yet another design to install dental implants in the alveolar ridge, has shown many advantages. It is simple, does not require professional surgical experience, can be easily sutured, offers faster healing, does not compromise the blood supply to the site, and exhibits a mild inflammatory reaction (Scharf and Tarnow 1993, Cranin et al. 1991).

Various studies have judged the efficacy of vestibular versus crestal approaches used for submerged dental implant placement. A study by Casino and others (1997) compared the vestibular and crestal approaches in relation to the success rate of osseointegration. The clinical success of osseointegration was evaluated at the second-stage surgery. In this study, a crestal incision was used for 1,705 implants in 381 patients, and a vestibular approach was used for 593 implants in 141 patients. The outcome showed no statistically significant difference in the clinical success of osseointegration between the two approaches.

A similar retrospective study by Scharf and Tarnow (1993) weighed the clinical success rate of osseointegrated implants at the time of the second-stage surgery using the same two surgical approaches. A total of 360 implants were placed in 92 patients; 265 implants were placed in 60 patients using a vestibular incision and showed a success rate of 98.8%; 121 implants were placed in 32 patients using a crestal incision and showed a success rate of 98.3%. They concluded that there was no statistically significant difference in the success rates of dental implants between the vestibular incision and crestal incision approaches.

Another study by Hunt (1996) attempted to demonstrate which incision, crestal or vestibular, is more suitable for placing dental implants. He found that no single flap design was optimal for implant surgery. More importantly, he recommended that basic factors such as flap design, blood supply, visibility, access, atraumatic handling, and primary tension-free closure on healthy bone be carefully considered in implant placement.

From these valuable studies, it can be concluded that both vestibular and crestal approaches offer the same goal, but can be used only in fully edentulous cases and only when functional results are required. Therefore, the need to develop new surgical approaches or to modify an existing approach to minimize the trauma and preserve the tissues is a priority when esthetics is a concern within the treatment plan.

Fugazzotto (1998) noted the precise flap design should be governed according each individual situation, and not by an overall generic flap design. He categorized implant sites for single-tooth maxillary anterior placement as follows:

- Class I: Minimal or no ridge atrophy buccolingually or apicocoronally; as a result, no hard- or soft-tissue augmentation is necessary following implant placement.
- Class II: Minor buccolingual atrophy with no apicocoronal component and sufficient bone is present buccolingually for ideal implant positioning.
- Class IIA: Both minor buccolingual and apicoocclusal ridge atrophy exist and adequate bone exists for ideal implant positioning.
- Class III: Moderate buccolingual ridge atrophy with no apicocoronal deficiency. Ideal implant positioning will result in a buccal implant dehiscence and/or fenestration.
- Class IIIA: The same as Class III, accompanied by moderate apicocoronal ridge atrophy.
- Class IV: Moderate-to-severe buccolingual ridge atrophy with or without an apicocoronal component; as a result, the hard tissue atrophy precludes ideal implant positioning and necessitates hard tissue augmentation prior to implant placement.

In Class I, which requires nothing more than simple implant placement, the flap design should be devoid of any buccal-releasing incisions. The procedure is described as follows: A horizontal incision is made palatal to the palatal line angles of the adjacent teeth. This tissue is then reflected over the crest of the ridge in a full-thickness manner. The incision extends into the sulci of the adjacent teeth, thus allowing clinicians to reflect the buccal tissue sufficiently to visualize the buccal crest of the ridge. The implant is then placed, the flap is replaced, and sutures are used only on the palatally placed horizontal incision.

In Class II, handling conditions are the same, but the horizontal incision extends further toward the palatal line angles in a split-thickness configuration, approximately 1 mm palatal to the palatal line angle of the teeth. If any bone atrophy is present in those previous classes, the flap design should be placed more toward the buccal aspect with a split thickness dissection and the palatal aspect extended 5 mm. Thus, the flap still may be sutured in a passive manner without performing any buccal-releasing incisions. In case of apicocoronal deficiency, a connective tissue graft is extended over the crest of the ridge to cover the already-placed implant, and a palatally beveled incision begins further toward the palatal aspect, providing more flap lengthening.

In severe Class IV, with extensive buccolingual defect, a more aggressive flap design should be used. The horizontal incision starts approximately 5 mm to 7 mm palatal to the palatal line angles of the adjacent teeth. Long releasing incisions in the buccal fold are placed mesial and distal to the edentulous space. These incisions are highly beveled, and flare away from the edentulous site after they traverse the mucogingival junction. Horizontal extensions approximately 4 mm to 6 mm at the releasing incisions are placed at their apical borders. The handling and closure of this method will be explained extensively in the soft tissue closure section later in this chapter.

Preservative Interproximal Papilla Incision

When operating in the esthetic zone, especially the maxillary anterior area, a conservative approach that preserves the papillary tissues can be used routinely. The extent to which the trauma to the soft and hard tissues created by the surgical flap influences peri-implant bone loss is not known; therefore, it is critical to create a minimally invasive incision design.

The interproximal crestal bone has shown importance and statistically significant healing esthetic values to the overall treatment result. (See Figures 5.7A–B.) To emphasize the value of the interdental papilla preservative incisions, a study (Roman 2001) investigated the interproximal crestal bone loss occurring after placement of single-tooth implants using two different flap designs: a widely mobilized flap design that included papillae, and the preservative interdental papilla flap design. The mean interproximal crestal bone loss was statistically significantly lower when using the preservative interdental papilla incision than with the classic one. At the time of crown placement, the mean interproximal bone loss was 0.29 mm (standard deviation [SD] 0.46) in the preservative interdental papilla sites

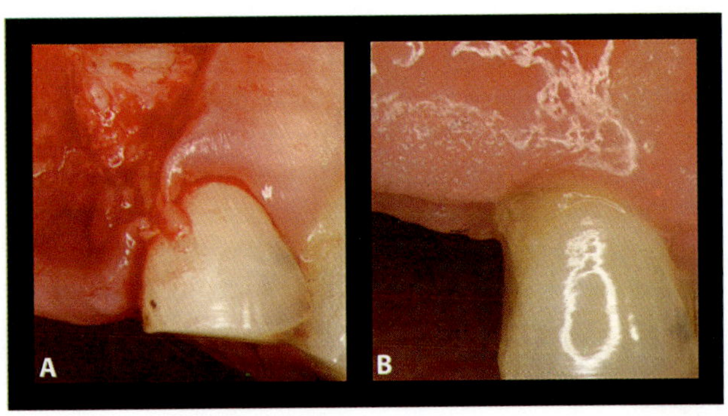

Figure 5.7. **A.** Lacerated interdental papilla during the flap reflection, thus exposing the bone underneath. **B.** Postoperative tissue recession at the site of the interdental papilla due to bone resorption.

and 0.79 mm (SD 0.87) for the classic sites. One year after crown placement, the mean interproximal crestal bone loss in the preservative interdental papilla sites was 0.29 mm (SD 0.38). In the classic sites, the mean bone loss was 1.12 mm (SD 1.14). The mean difference in bone loss one year later was 0.83 mm (SD 1.23) where P = .006.

The higher bone loss rate with the classic incision sites was related to the fact that whenever a papilla is detached from bone, the interdental bone in proximity to the adjacent tooth is denuded from the periosteum, which can affect the bone blood supply. (See Figures 5.8A–B.) Excluding interproximal papillae from the mucoperiosteal flap might help to achieve enhanced esthetic results and stable soft tissue margins.

Some authors stated that raising the interproximal papillae along with the rest of the mucoperiosteal flap might lead to an unpleasant esthetic outcome (Kirkland 1936, Evian et al. 1985). This can be related to the tendency of the soft tissue to shrink or recede after raising a mucoperiosteal flap, based on the fact that a slight amount of bone resorption occurs each time a full mucoperiosteal flap is raised (Wilderman 1964). Using the preservative interproximal papilla approach during the first- and/or second-stage surgery will help preserve the papillae, stabilize the adjacent soft tissue margins of the implant-supported prosthesis, reduce postoperative soft tissue recession, and reduce the tendency for marginal bone loss (Pennel et al. 1967, Bragger et al. 1988).

Because the interproximal papilla is delicate in nature, it is easy to tear or lacerate during the different stages in flap handing; therefore, the preservative interdental papilla incision safeguards the interproximal papilla. The preservative interproximal papilla flap design can be used in several clinical applications: it can be used in placing dental implants routinely, at the second-stage surgery, and in moderate bone-grafting procedures.

The technique entails making a crestal incision through the tissue and periosteum. This, followed by an intercrevicular incision, continues midway around the buccal and lingual sides of the adjacent teeth without including the papilla. Then the tissues are reflected accordingly to allow for optimal site evaluation. Two vertical incisions may be made, passing the keratinized tissue band to allow for more flap mobility (Heller et al. 2000), as shown in Figures 5.9A–B. The preservative interproximal papilla flap design allows better flap adaptation upon closure. In other words, when the preservative design is used, each vertical incision of the mucoperiosteal flap meets with the adjacent tissues in a soft-tissue-to-soft-tissue manner (at the mesiocervical angle of the adjacent natural teeth), while in nonpreservative flap designs, the vertical incision rests on the mesiocervical aspect of the tooth structure. Therefore, the preservative design adapts in a soft-tissue-to-soft-tissue manner, while the nonpreservative design adapts in a soft-tissue-to-tooth manner at the mesiocervical area. The interproximal crestal bone loss was statistically significantly reduced following the use of a limited flap design versus the widely mobilized flap procedure (Roman 2001).

A complete mobilization of the flap is required when major bone-grafting procedures are conducted. Then a mucoperiosteal flap that includes the interproximal papilla might be undertaken to allow for better access, bearing in mind that the vertical incision should be as far as possible from the area of interest to provide a better blood supply to the flap, reduce the tendency for suture rupture, and reduce the tendency for scar tissue formation, as shown in Figures 5.10A–C.

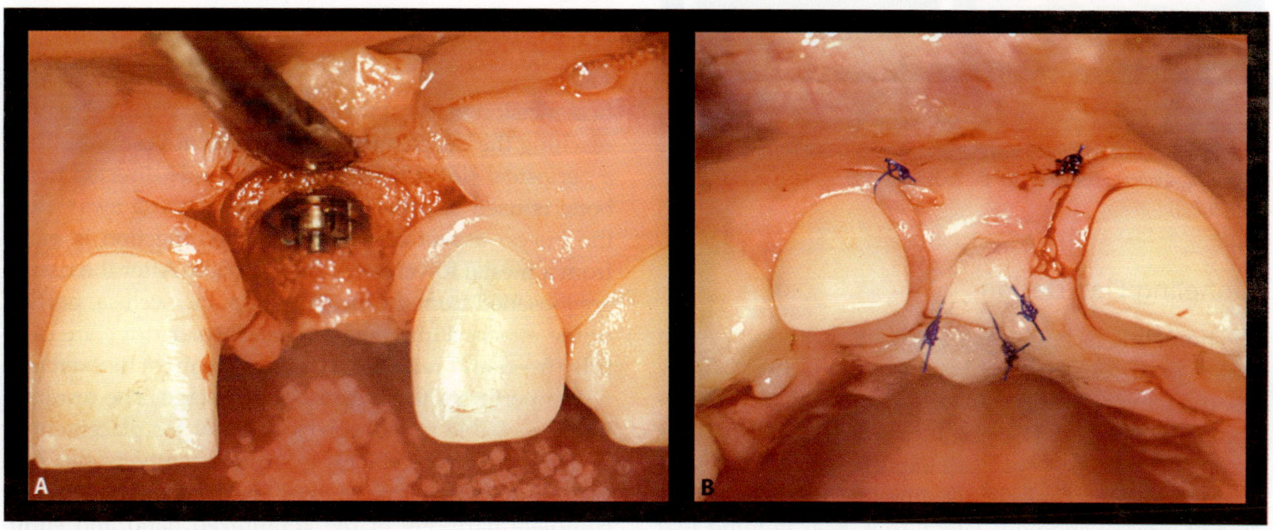

Figure 5.8. **A.** Reflection of a mucoperiosteal flap through a preservative interdental papilla incision. **B.** Closure of the flap showing the intact interdental papillae attachment on both sides.

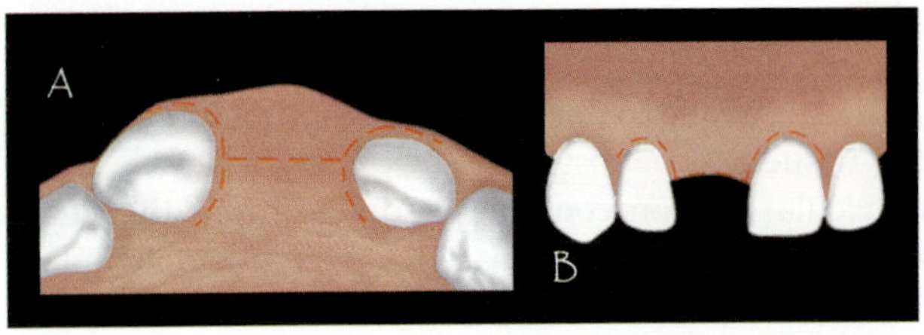

Figure 5.9A, B. An illustration showing the design of the preservative interdental papilla incision from occlusal and buccal views.

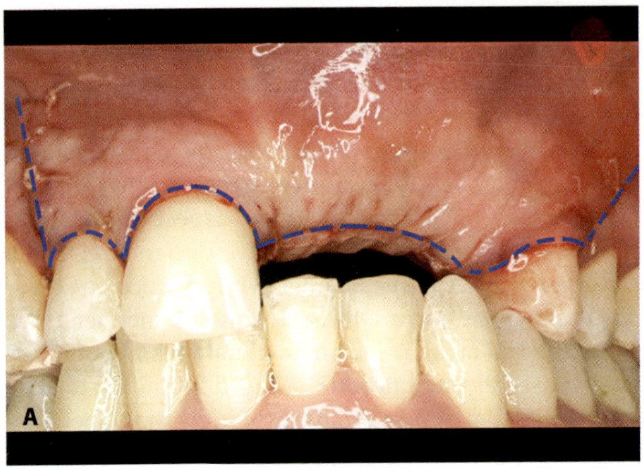

Figure 5.10A. Upon performing major bone reconstructive tasks, the incision might include the interdental papilla along with it and placing the vertical incision as far as possible from the operative site.

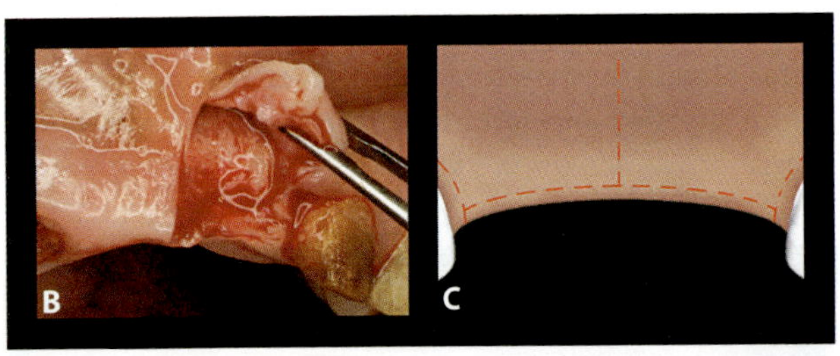

Figure 5.10. **B.** An alternative incision design for accessing the alveolar ridge for miscellaneous procedures that offer more accessibility and less tissue trauma. **C.** Clinical application for the incision design.

Tunneling Flap Design

The tunneling technique is another innovative approach that is used for placing a bone graft on a horizontally resorbed alveolar ridge rather than for implant installation. (See Figure 5.11.) The method does not involve complete reflection of the flap. It provides access throughout a vertical incision line that is medial to the area of interest and ends lateral to it. Bear in mind that the incision should be made at least one tooth away from the area of grafting. The technique starts with a long vertical incision made at the crest of the alveolar ridge until reaching the deepest point in the buccal vestibule. Then a periosteal elevator with its curved side directed to the bone is used to reflect the alveolar mucosa away from the buccal aspect of the ridge. The reflection is made from a mesial toward a distal direction. After the tissues are loosened from the buccal aspect, the occlusal portion of the attached gingivae on the alveolar ridge are carefully freed and reflected as well. Care must be exercised not to perforate the mucosa at this stage. The resultant freely movable tunnel can now allow for placement of grafting materials. Block grafting usually is the best method with this type of flap. The procedure allows for complete harmony of the keratinized band and eliminates the possibility for suture rupture in crestal incision designs. (See Figures 5.12A–K and 5.13A–G.)

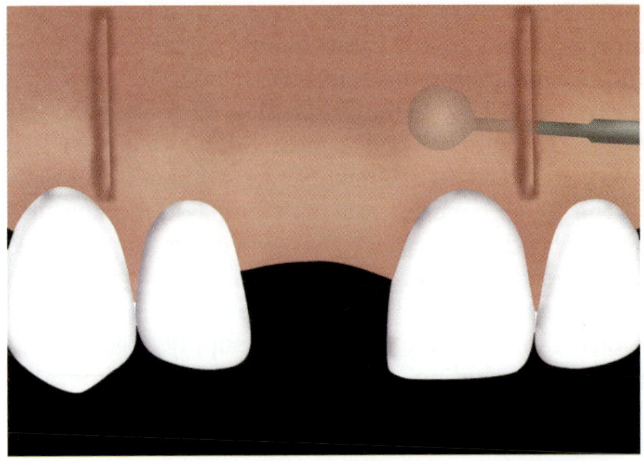

Figure 5.11. An illustration showing the tunnel incision technique.

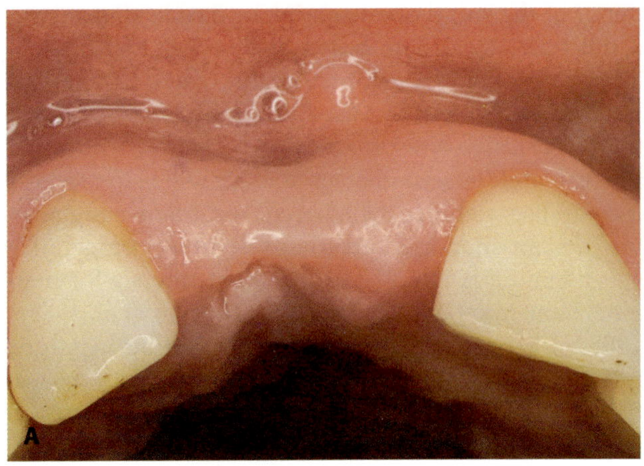

Figure 5.12A. Preoperative incisal view showing horizontal bone defect that warrants atraumatic grafting method due to the fragile nature of the thin mucosa.

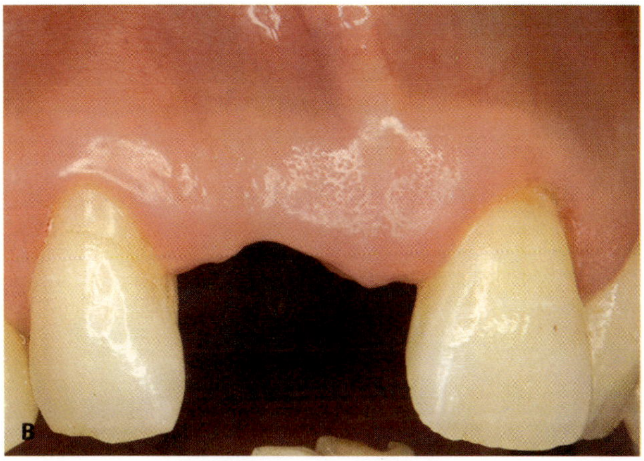

Figure 5.12B. Frontal view of the defect showing the poor soft tissue quality.

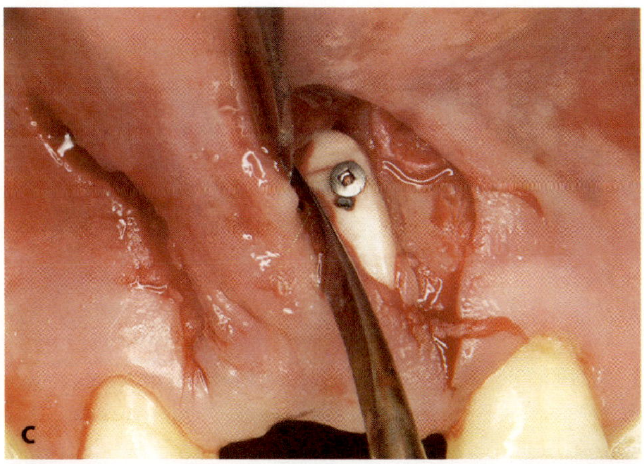

Figure 5.12C. Corticocancellous allograft is being stabilized with a titanium screw at the left side.

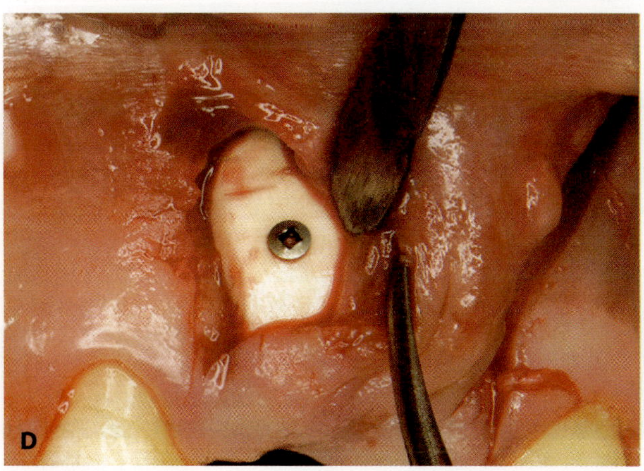

Figure 5.12D. The graft is being stabilized from its right side.

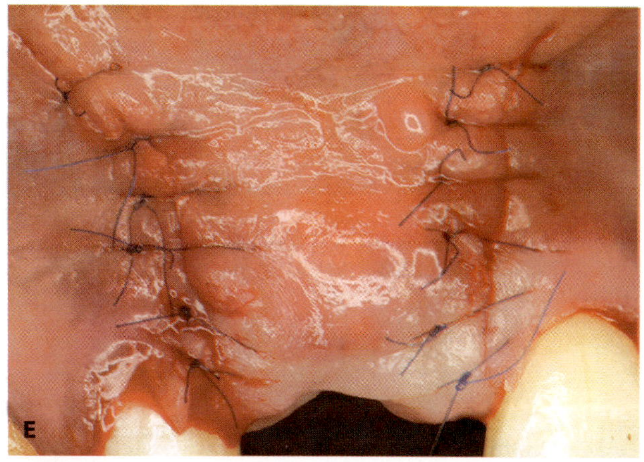

Figure 5.12E. The area sutured.

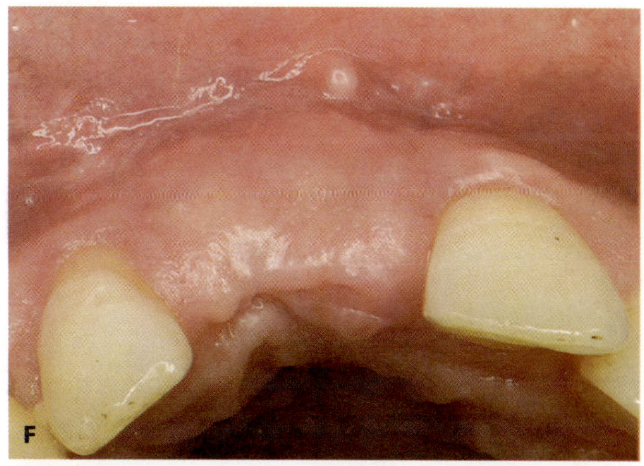

Figure 5.12F. Five months' postsurgical incisal view showing the improvement of tissue profile as a result of grafting procedure.

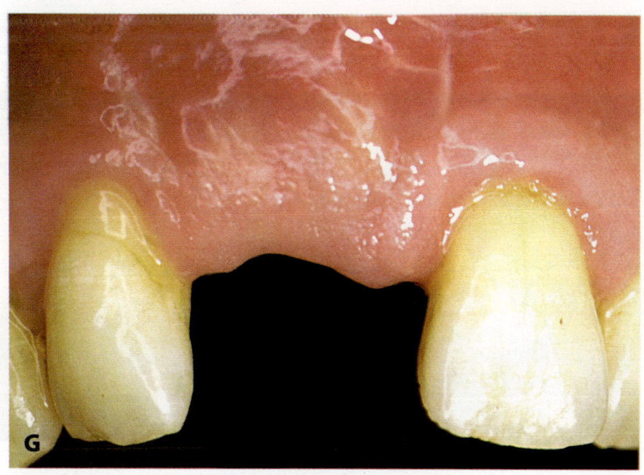

Figure 5.12G. Frontal view of the case prior to implant placement.

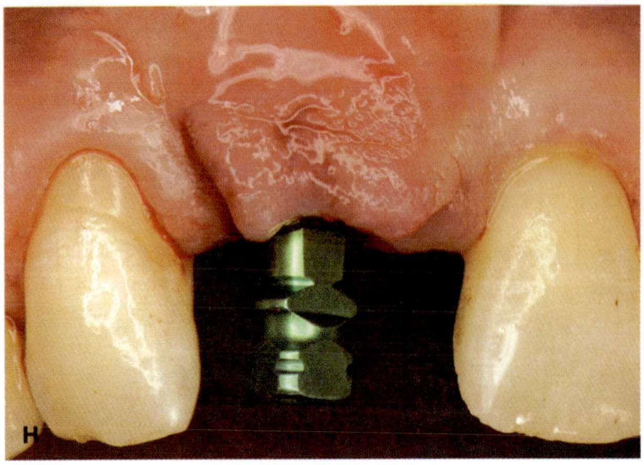

Figure 5.12H. Tapered screw vent implant is being inserted via two minor oblique incisions.

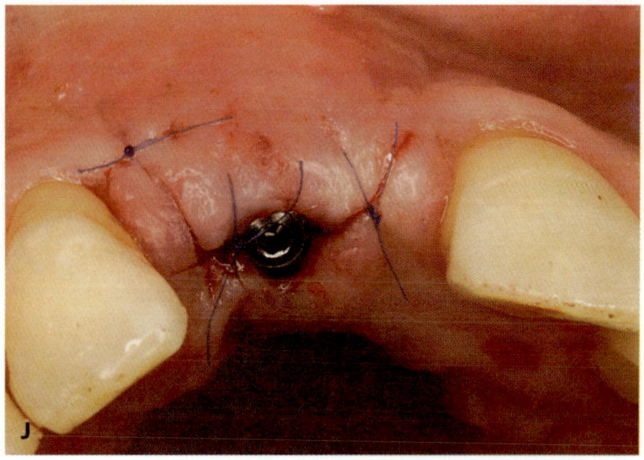

Figure 5.12J. The area sutured around the healing abutment.

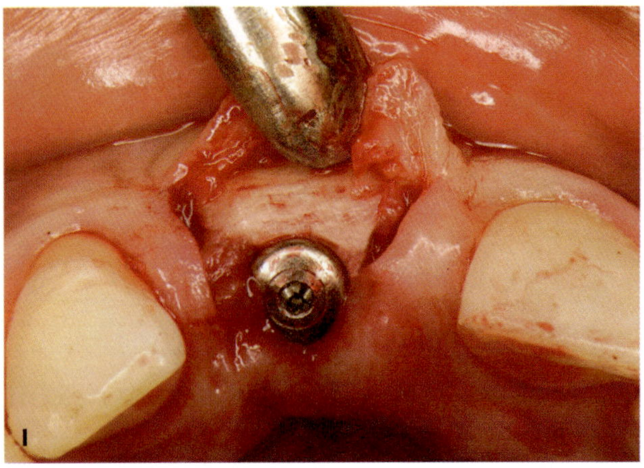

Figure 5.12I. The implant placed in the regenerated bone.

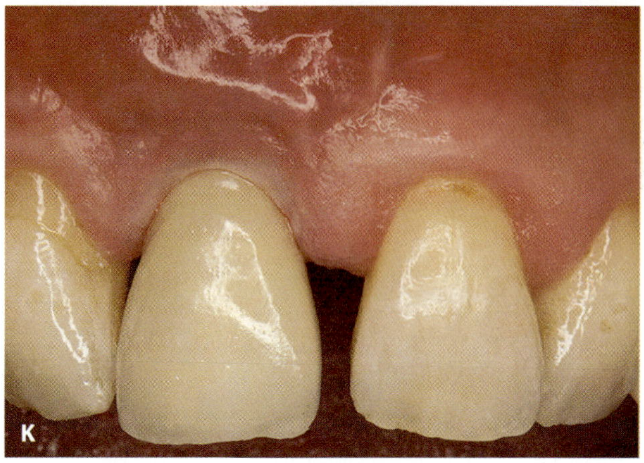

Figure 5.12K. The case finally restored.

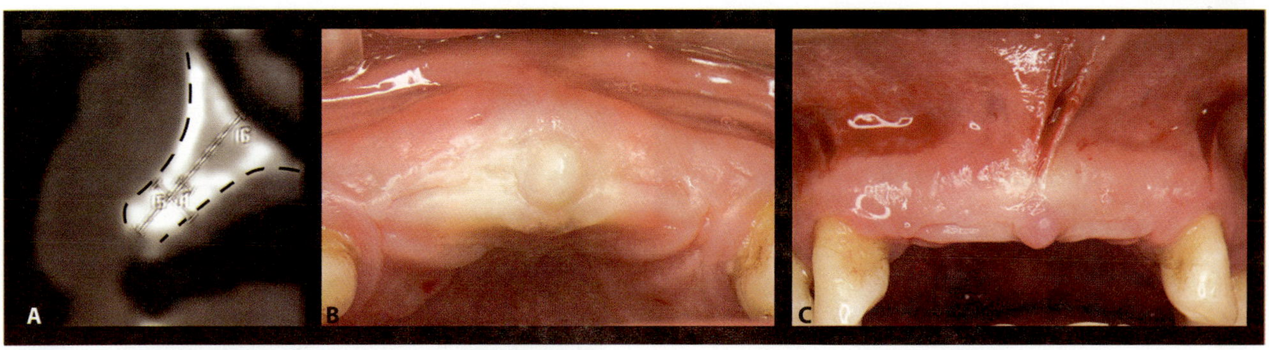

Figure 5.13. A. Preoperative CT for the alveolar ridge prior to grafting. B. Moderate alveolar ridge atrophy (horizontal). C. Tunnel incisions made to place and stabilize an autogeneous corticocancellous graft underneath it.

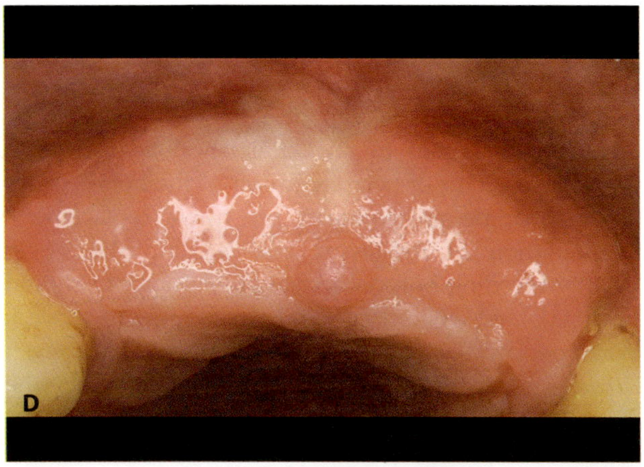

Figure 5.13D. Postoperative complete healing showing remarkable alveolar ridge size improvement.

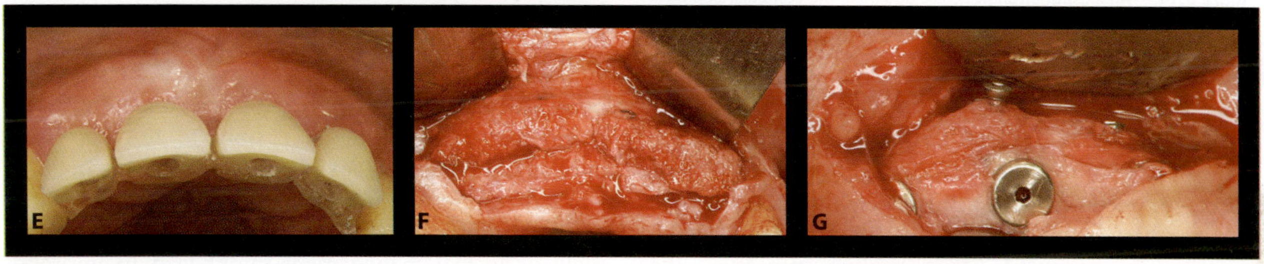

Figure 5.13. **E.** Surgical template in place showing a remarkable improvement of the ridge width. **F.** Six months' postaugmentation showing the amount of bone generated. **G.** The implants placed and the generated bone showed remodeling.

Modified Elden-Mejchar Technique

A modified flap design is an alternative to the classic full-thickness mucoperiosteal design used for submerged implant installation. The modified Elden-Mejchar creates an optimal mucosal condition with maximum stability and reduced pocket depth around dental implants. The original Elden-Mejchar (1963) vestibuloplasty was modified by Hertel and others (1993) and applied to totally edentulous cases receiving dental implants. However, it can be used in partially edentulous patients as well.

The method reduces the thickness of the mucosa at a minimal level around dental implant prosthetic components and preserves the band of keratinized tissues, eliminates the muscle insertion placed close to the future implant site (in the case of totally edentulous patients), and eliminates the need for additional surgical procedures to repair excessive soft issue height. It also allows more interarch space for the implant-supported prosthesis. On the other hand, the procedure poses a greater risk of mucosal perforation during rising of the partial thickness flap, and possible soft tissue sloughing may occur because the absence of the buccal periosteum reduces blood supply to the flap.

The technique entails a shallow incision made approximately 10 mm from the alveolar crest and at least 15 mm distal to the site of the last implant to be placed (in the case of placing implants in totally edentulous areas). Care should be taken to ensure that the incision does not end exactly where the implants will be located. A partial-thickness flap subsequently is reflected toward the crest—leaving the attached fibrous tissue over the periosteum in place, and then dissected with a scalpel to the lingual side to expose the crest of the alveolar bone. The periosteum is incised buccally and lingually next to the fibrous tissue band at the crest of the ridge. The buccal periosteum is again cut approximately 10 mm from the crest of the mandible (at the height of the first incision), and the remaining fibrous tissue at the ridge crest is best removed with a rose-head bur. The implants should be placed under the crestal bone level to avoid perforating the thin remaining attached mucosa. The flap is repositioned and sutured with resorbable suture material to the buccal periosteum at its base. Buccal edges of the incision are then sutured to the adjacent mucosa. (See Figure 5.14.)

Obviously, there is no perfect flap design for all clinical conditions. The optimal flap design is one that is selected according to the clinician's preference. However, the general health condition of the patient, quality and quantity of the keratinized soft tissues, tissue biotype, width of the vestibule, presence of osseous defects, design of the implant, and location of anatomical landmarks are all factors that must be considered during treatment planning.

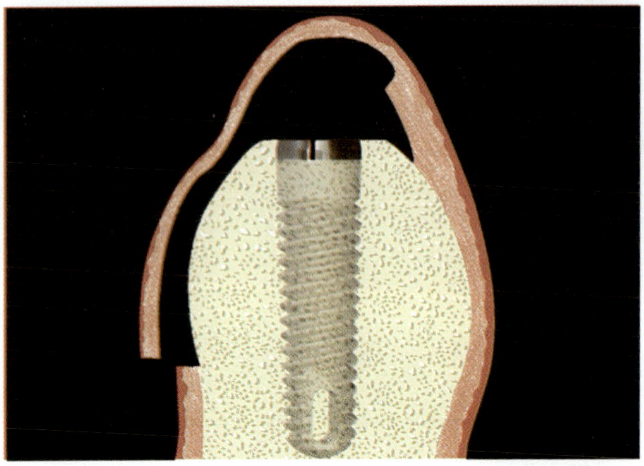

Figure 5.14. An illustration showing the outline of the vestibular approach of the mucoperiosteal flap for the modified Elden and Mejchar technique for implant placement in a partially edentulous case.

Versatile Soft Tissue Closure Techniques

Successful reconstructive esthetic dental implantology is partly achieved via optimal soft tissue closure, which permits uninterrupted tissue healing, preserves the underlying structure from possible exposure to the hostile oral environment, and protects the bone-grafting material from dispersing throughout the wound area. Establishing nontension primary closure over a bone-grafted site is vital to the success of any intraoral reconstructive procedure. Complete and optimal soft tissue closure has certain requirements, including tension-free wound margin approximation, preserving adequate blood supply, and maintaining wound closure using a proven knot-tying technique (Heller et al. 2000, Zola 1972).

Flap design, to a great extent, directly affects the final soft tissue closure because the shape of the base of the flap can help to improve the flexibility and handling characteristics and blood circulation and lymphatic drainage are maintained through this attached tissue base. Failure to achieve a suitable flap design or tension-free closure of the mucoperiosteal flap might negatively affect graft survival or implant osseointegration (Esposito et al. 1998).

Strict emphasis on atraumatic, less-invasive soft tissue closure protocol should be advised at all times because poor soft tissues manipulations can lead to soft tissue trauma, which negatively affects the quantity and quality of regenerated bone (Fugazzotto 1999). Many atraumatic surgical approaches to soft tissue coverage over grafted sites have been developed over the past 20 years to ensure bone graft and dental implant survival (Langer and Langer 1990).

Obtaining adequate tissue closure starts with proper surgical site entry design. Some basic factors should be considered when a mucoperiosteal flap design is to be achieved, including (1) preserving the anatomical landmarks in the proposed surgical site, (2) delicate and knowledgeable handling of the tissues must be exercised during the surgery, and (3) working access should be provided through the flap design itself, because the access can be vital to any clinician during surgery. Careful reflection of periosteum off of the bone creates an appropriate environment for tissue replacement. Readaptation of tissues is best accomplished over healthy bleeding bone. Adequate blood supply should be maintained when tissues are closed without tension. When performing soft tissue closure in the oral cavity, it is preferable to allow the suture needle to penetrate the mucosa on both sides of the incision line equally, and optimal complete flap mobility and flexibility is to be attained to allow tension-free closure. This requires knowledge of the orientation of the muscle fibers and handling skills of the periosteal tissues.

Therefore, there is a delicate balance between the periosteal dissection and stripping from one side and the maintenance of the blood supply to the flap from another side. The excessive periosteal stripping not only jeopardizes the soft tissue flap, but may lead to postoperative necrosis, while the undermanagement or incomplete periosteal management might lead to improper soft tissue closure or a closure under tension. (See Figures 5.15A–B and 5.16A–B.)

Buccal Flap Advancement Closure

One of the most predictable methods of soft tissue closure in esthetic or nonesthetic implant therapy was detailed by Fugazzotto (1999) to overcome the difficulties in major or moderate grafting procedures. The size of the alveolar ridge in such conditions will eventually increase due to the grafting procedure; therefore, the mucoperiosteal flap will not be able to achieve a complete, sealed, edge-to-edge closure. Fugazzotto's method has inspired and assisted many clinicians achieving

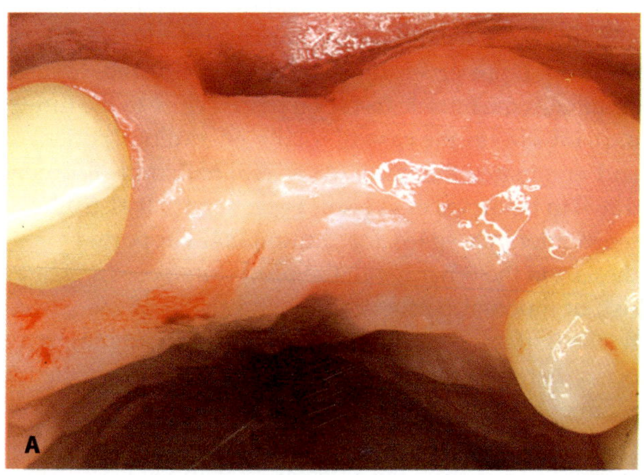

Figure 5.15A. Preoperative view of maxillary horizontal alveolar bone resorption.

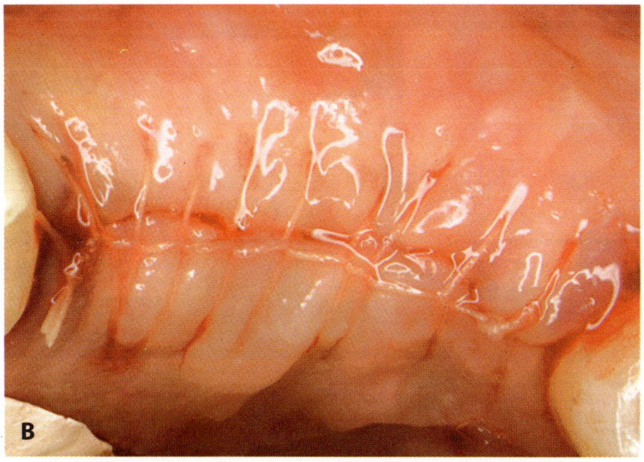

Figure 5.15B. The soft tissue closure after increasing the overall size of the ridge with bone graft.

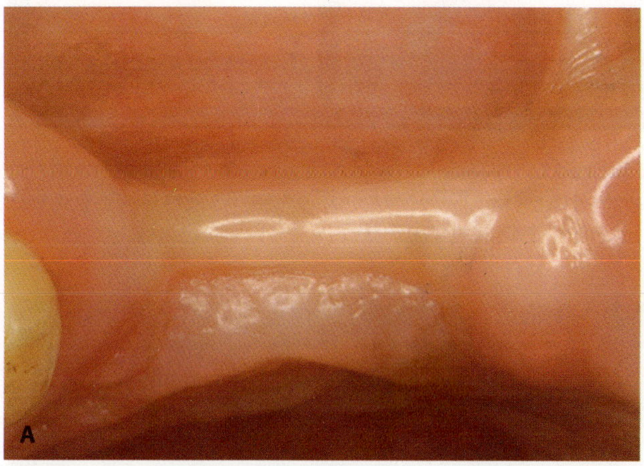

Figure 5.16A. Severe bone resorption in the anterior maxilla that requires grafting.

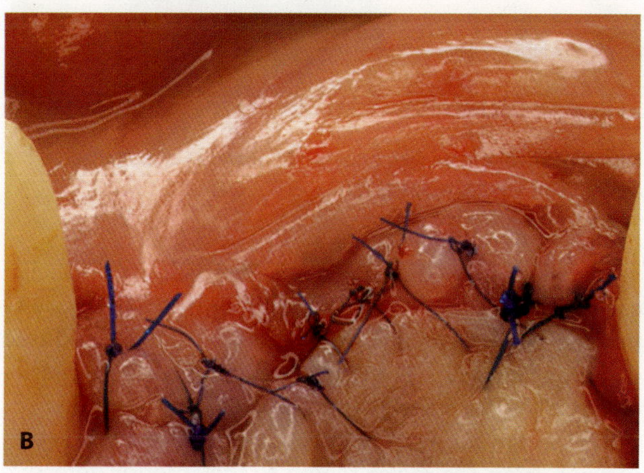

Figure 5.16B. The defect is grafted and the soft tissue closed with no tension. This view shows the importance of the optimal soft tissue closure.

perfect healing results, thanks to the original old soft tissue closure method that dates back to Von Rehrman (1936), who first introduced a method of soft tissue closure to treat oroantral communications.

Fugazzotto (1999) detailed the surgical management and closure of mucoperiosteal flaps on top of grafted sites with guided bone regeneration (GBR) techniques. The surgical protocol of soft tissue closure is considered the most reliable method of achieving primary closure on top of grafted sites. The broad outlines of the clinical procedures follow: (1) extend the vertical incisions from the crest of the ridge to the vestibular mucosa, (2) undermine the flap with two horizontally placed vestibular incisions, and (3) make a deep periosteal slitting incision at the base of the flap, as shown in Figures 5.17A–C.

The Fugazzotto technique entails making a crestal incision that is 1 to 2 mm palatal to the palatal line angle of the ridge. This incision is angled to form a split thickness flap over the crest of the ridge, at the buccal line angle of the crest of the alveolar ridge. The flap is extended to the underlying bone in a full thickness approach. Mesiobuccal and distobuccal releasing incisions extend beyond the turn of the fold in the buccal vestibule, and run perpendicular to the aforementioned crestal incision. Horizontal releasing incisions are then extended from the most apical extent of the vertical releasing incisions, for a distance of 3 to 4 mm. The base of the flap is then undermined with a scalpel. A horizontal slitting incision at the base of the flap is made with caution to allow the mobility and relaxation of the flap. The connective tissue, which remains over the crest of the ridge as a result of the initial split-thickness design of the crestal incision, is reflected as part of the palatal flap.

The flaps are reapproximated following any regenerative procedure, with or without simultaneous implant placement, depending upon the clinical situation. When appropriate passive primary closures are achieved, the flaps are sutured, the needle is pulled completely through the lingual tissue, and is reentered into the buccal tissue corners in a lingual to buccal direction to allow better flap adaptability. An interrupted suture knot is tied next to the proximal tooth. The same type of interrupted suture knot is tied next to the adjacent tooth from the other side to allow for flap stability and security; single interrupted sutures are placed every 1 to 2 mm to close the incision on the crest of the ridge. Vertically incised attached gingival tissue is then sutured immediately after placing the proximal-crestal sutures. Passing the needle through tissue on both sides of the vertical incision line can simultaneously result in torn tissue and compromise esthetics. Therefore, the suture needle should incorporate 2 mm of tissue and is passed through the loose portion of the flap. Then the needle is pulled through the incision line and reinserted into the bound tissue of the adjacent tooth. One interrupted

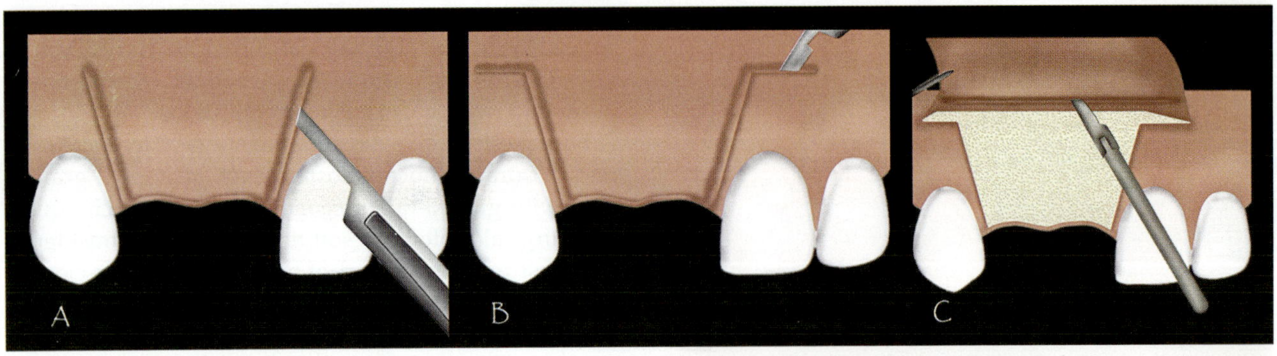

Figure 5.17. **A.** An illustration showing the two vestibular horizontal incisions in Fugazzotto closure protocol. **B.** An illustration showing the two horizontal incisions intraorally according to Fugazzotto closure protocol. **C.** An illustration showing a deep horizontal periosteal slitting incision according to Fugazzotto closure protocol.

suture may be placed to secure the tissue, adjacent to the vertical incision line and next to the tooth, because securing a square knot between two granny knots will prevent unwanted torn tissue adjacent to the vertical incisions. The clinician can determine releasing incision effectiveness by simply pulling the lip in various directions while observing suture line movement. Additional periosteal slitting may be required if suture line movement remains. (See Figures 5.18A–B.)

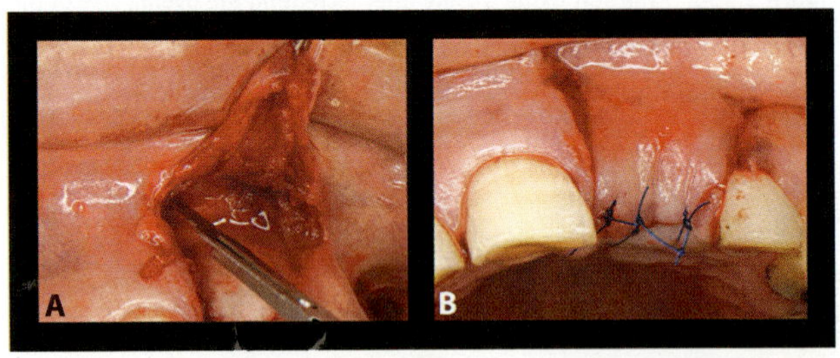

Figure 5.18. **A.** Deep horizontal slitting incision made to release the flap allowing its mobility. **B.** The flap is mobilized and stretched to achieve tension-free primary edge-to-edge closure.

To maintain totally secured suturing for both edges of the mucoperiosteal flap, a suturing method is needed that will prevent the knot from coming loose with swelling tissue or mechanical trauma during the healing period. Heller and others (2000) recommend a four-tie knot tying technique. The first part of the knot includes two forward loops with gentle pulling of the knot to snug close against the tissue with little or no bunching of suture material. The second part is one forward loop, causing a granny knot between the first and second tie. The third part is one reverse loop, causing a square knot with the previous tie. This part of the knot can be pulled with greater force, because all it will do is tighten the square knot and not allow the suture material to bunch up. The fourth part of the knot is a single forward loop, which causes another granny knot with the underlying square knot. This portion can also be pulled tightly, because it will not cause bunching of the suture material since it is protected by the underlying square knot.

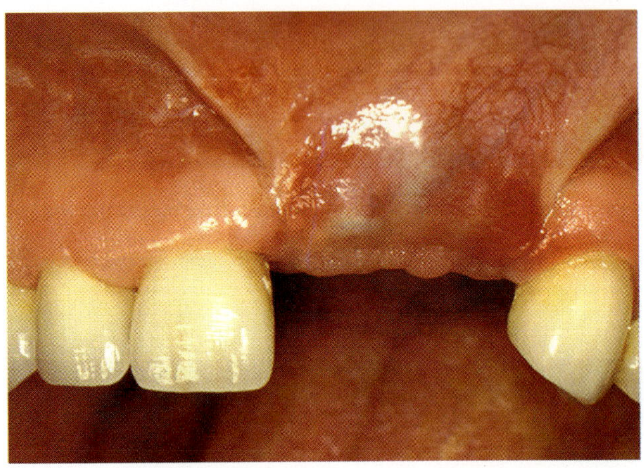

Figure 5.19. The keratinized tissue band is altered as a result of buccal flap advancement soft tissue closure.

Subepithelial Palatal Connective Tissue Flap Closure

The common drawback for the buccal flap closure method is the movement of the keratinized tissue band level from its original position, as shown in Figures 5.19 and 5.20A–E. Several attempts (Langer 1994, Fugazotto et al. 1993, Khoury and Happe 2000, Langer and Calagna 1980, Landsberg 1997b) were introduced to allow tension-free soft tissue closure on top of grafted sites while maintaining the position of the labial mucogingival junction at its original level. A pedicle subepithelial connective tissue flap is prepared from the palatal mucosa near the area to be treated and is displaced into the receptor site. The donor site remains primarily covered (Khoury and Happe 2000).

The technique entails performing a palatal sulcular incision from the molar region to the anterior defective area to be covered. The length of the incision is twice the

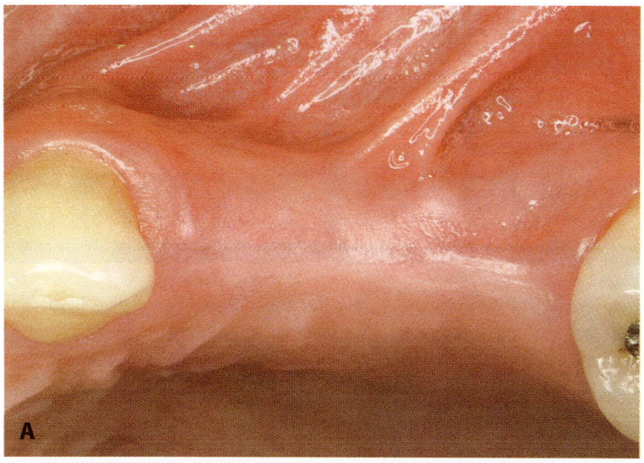

Figure 5.20A. Preoperative view that shows deficient ridge.

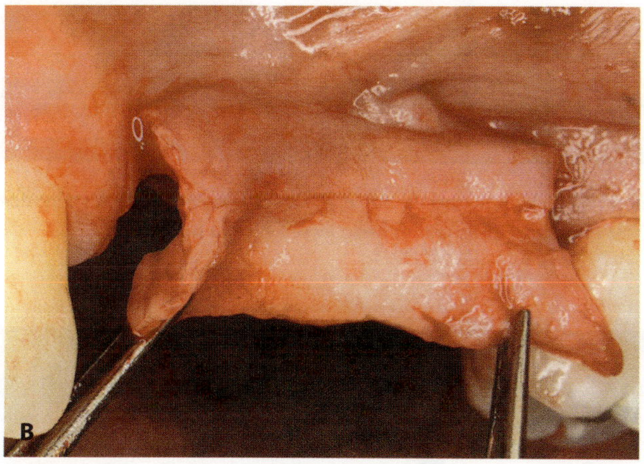

Figure 5.20B. Pedicle connective tissue graft is being reflected from the palate.

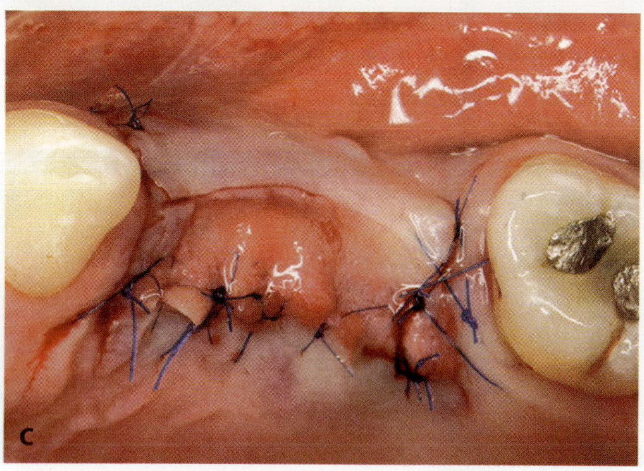

Figure 5.20C. The connective tissue graft is being sutured in place.

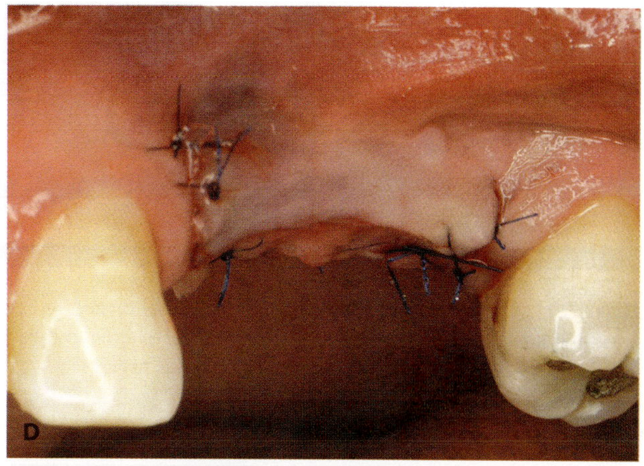

Figure 5.20D. Labial view of the wound showing no alteration of the keratinized tissue band continuity while attempting optimal closure.

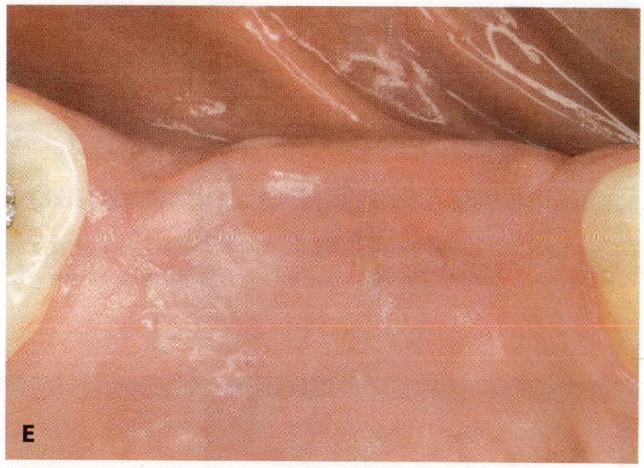

Figure 5.20E. Final complete soft tissue healing showing no alteration of the keratinized tissues.

width of the defect. Dissection of the mucoperiosteal flap and the underlying subepithelial connective tissue flap to a depth of 5 to 8 mm is then performed. A sharp incision of the subepithelial tissue is to be made parallel to the first incision in the same manner to harvest a pedicle connective tissue graft, but it is left attached in the anterior region. The subepithelial connective tissue flap is then elevated and rotated to cover the defect and help achieve tissue coverage. The palatal wound at the donor site can be totally closed and sutured. Patients should rinse with 0.02% chlorhexidine for two weeks. (See Figures 5.21A–D and 5.22A–I.)

The main advantage of this method is that the donor site is covered with the palatal tissues, so it is not left raw, while the keratinized tissue band is kept at its levels with no alteration. However, there may be heavy bleeding with these types of flaps due to the rich blood supply to the palate. This may require further clinical skills on bleeding management.

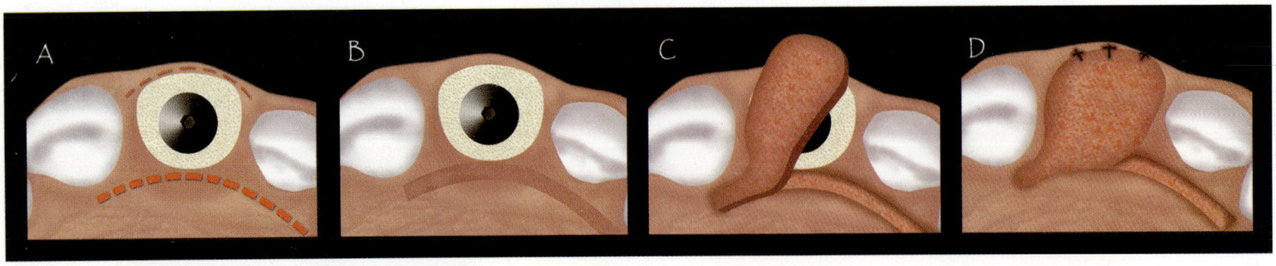

Figure 5.21. **A.** An illustration showing the subepithelial connective tissue flap closure. **B.** An illustration showing the subepithelial connective tissue flap incision in the palate. **C.** An illustration showing the subepithelial pedicle of the palate is rotated to cover the buccal defect. **D.** An illustration showing the suturing of the palatal connective tissue flap to the buccal tissues.

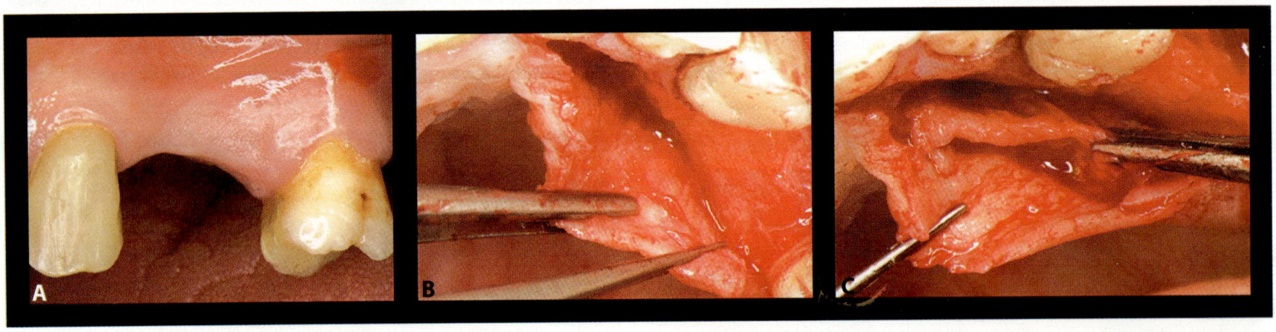

Figure 5.22. **A.** Buccal defect in the maxillary premolar area that warrants bone grafting and increasing the size of the alveolar bone. **B.** Horizontal incision in the palate is made to allow for mobilization of the palatal connective tissue. **C.** The connective tissue graft is being moved from its place.

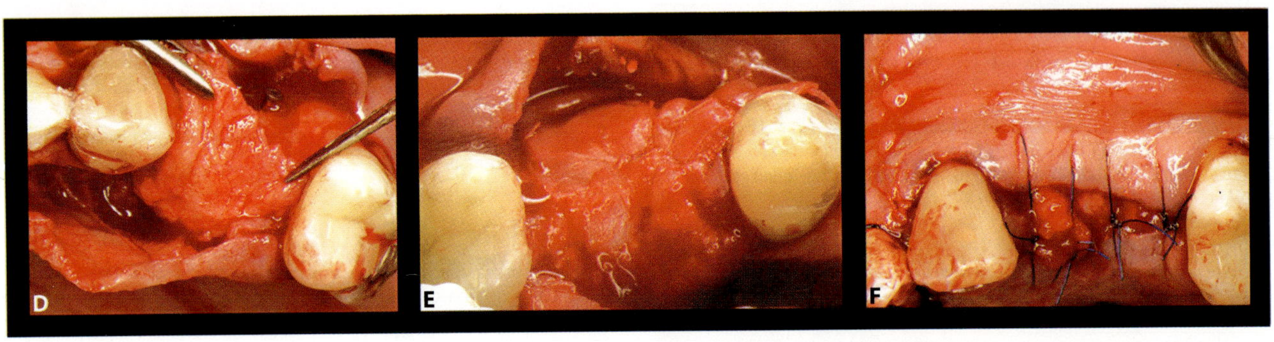

Figure 5.22. **D.** The connective tissue pedicle is moved to the buccal side. **E.** The palatal pedicle is sutured to the buccal tissues. **F.** Final closure is made.

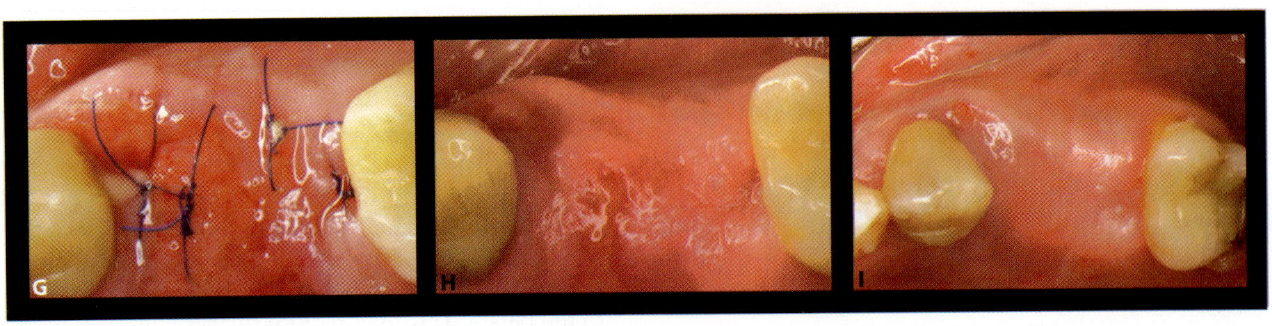

Figure 5.22. **G.** Five days' postoperative view. **H.** Fifteen days' postoperative view. **I.** Four weeks' postoperative result.

The subepithelial palatal flap (Langer 1994) is also prescribed to cover a defective area on the alveolar ridge. The method describes an elongated palatal flap via a split thickness dissection of its inner connective tissue side as a result of the split thickness incision. A connective tissue extension is then reflected with the palatal flap laid over the crest of the ridge. The flap with the connective tissue pedicle is then slid in a labial direction to cover the augmented area without interrupting the continuity of the labial keratinized tissue band. The palatal connective tissue extension is then sutured to the labial soft tissue margin. This procedure has limitations when thin palatal tissue exists, which complicates the partial-thickness reflection procedure. Additionally, the amount of tissue gained from the palatal lengthening might not always be sufficient. Finally, mucoperiosteal soft tissue flap closure is considered to be a critical procedure that involves microvascular anastomosis and re-epithelialization in its mechanism, and when it occurs in such a hostile environment such as the oral cavity, it must be performed accurately to complement the success of the implant therapy on both levels, functionally and esthetically.

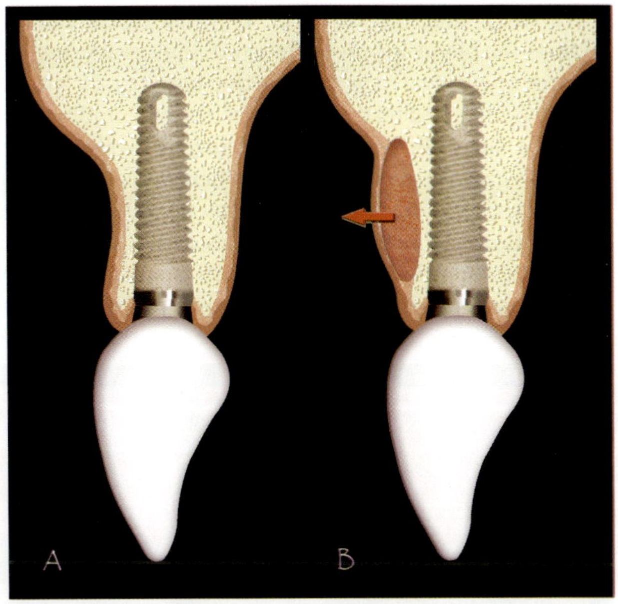

Figure 5.23. **A.** An illustration showing minor labial defect related to the implant. **B.** An illustration showing the use of connective tissue graft to improve the labial contour.

Inlay Tissue Grafting

Minor- to moderate-size edentulous alveolar ridge defects can lead to critical esthetic problems when an anterior fixed prosthesis is to be fabricated, particularly with esthetically conscious patients. In the case of alveolar ridge deformity, the standard pontic size and shape will not maintain a normal and harmonious relationship with the underlying environment, so modifications are necessary. The most common causes of alveolar ridge deformities include developmental defects, advanced periodontal disease, postextraction bone resorption, traumatic removal of teeth, and surgical injury. Reconstructive periodontal procedures permit the restoration of the hard and soft tissues of the alveolar ridge to their former dimensions and allow the clinician to provide improved esthetic results. These procedures can be applied with dental implant treatment with predictable results.

The use of connective tissue grafts in modern esthetic implant therapy is considered to be one of the most predictable basic methods to improve tissue height and topography, treat minor ridge defects, assist in flap closure, and mask any metallic discoloration around abutments collars. (See Figures 5.23A–B.) Connective tissue grafts offer an alternative way to compensate for the fragility and thinning of the oral epithelial tissues. Most of the current technological advancements date back to the work of Langer and Calagna (1982, 1985), who were the first to outline the clinical indications and descriptions for subepithelial connective tissue grafts to cover a denuded root surface or augment the alveolar ridge for esthetic reasons. The technique was later modified and improved by others (Langer and Calagna 1982, Miller 1988). The technique showed greater success and predictability in treating one-, two-, and three-dimensional (3-D) soft tissue defects around natural teeth and dental implants. Interestingly, 2 to 6 mm of root coverage has been documented in cases in which subepithelial grafts were used to treat denuded root surfaces (Langer and Calagna 1982).

This technique is now used routinely by many clinicians to enhance the soft tissue profile with implant-supported dental restorations. Connective tissue grafts can be pedicled or nonpedicled. A graft that has a pedicle at its base is limited to use in the area adjacent to the donor site, but it possesses a higher rate of revascularization, while nonpedicle grafts can be harvested and used in a remote area from the donor site. Connective tissue grafts are applied clinically in two different forms: (1) a graft composed solely of connective tissue or (2) a graft composed of connective tissue that has an epithelial rim (a composite graft). The connective tissue grafts are used for esthetic ridge augmentation procedures, while the composite grafts are used for treating denuded root surfaces and masking gingival discoloration around dental implants.

Connective tissue grafts combine the characters of the soft tissue autograft and the pedicle flap procedure

(Silverstein and Lefkove 1994). This combination doubles the blood supply to the graft, thus increasing its chances of survival. Also, connective tissue grafts attain the same color and texture of the tissues surrounding the recipient site after healing has occurred. A nonpedicle gingival graft is recommended when the anticipated perimucosal tissue abutment will emerge into a zone of nonkeratinized mucosa. This graft should be completed before the second-stage surgery. Thin mucosal alveolar tissues might affect the esthetic outcome of the implant-supported prostheses negatively, especially in patients with a high smile line.

Connective tissue inlay grafts can treat the condition successfully, because the inlay graft masks gingival discoloration by increasing the thickness of the peri-implant soft tissue. In this particular case, the graft should be extended proximally farther from the implant site to compensate for the reduced blood supply to the graft, thereby allowing peripheral anastomosis from the adjacent tissue. (See Figures 5.24A–L.)

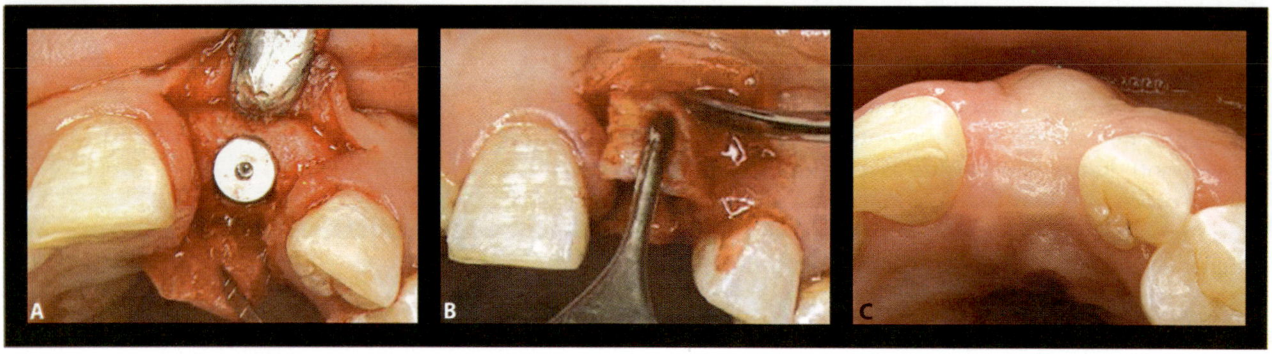

Figure 5.24. **A.** Clinical view showing minor labial defect around an implant fixture. **B.** A nonpedicled connective tissue graft is being introduced to the site. **C.** The effect of the connective tissue graft on the labial contour of the edentulous area. The effect simulates the natural root imminence.

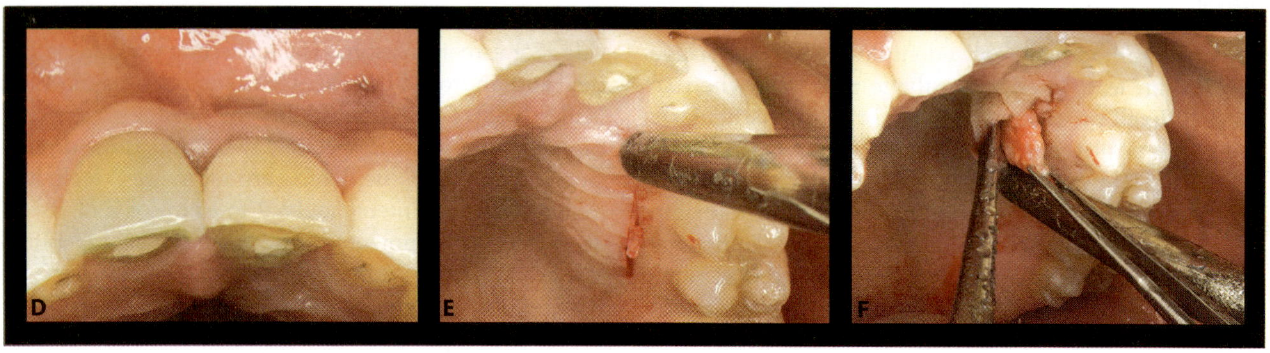

Figure 5.24. **D.** Implant-supported crown restoring the missing maxillary left central incisor showing deficient labial gingival contour. **E.** Palatal one line incision approach to harvest a connective tissue graft. **F.** The connective tissue graft is being dissected from the palate.

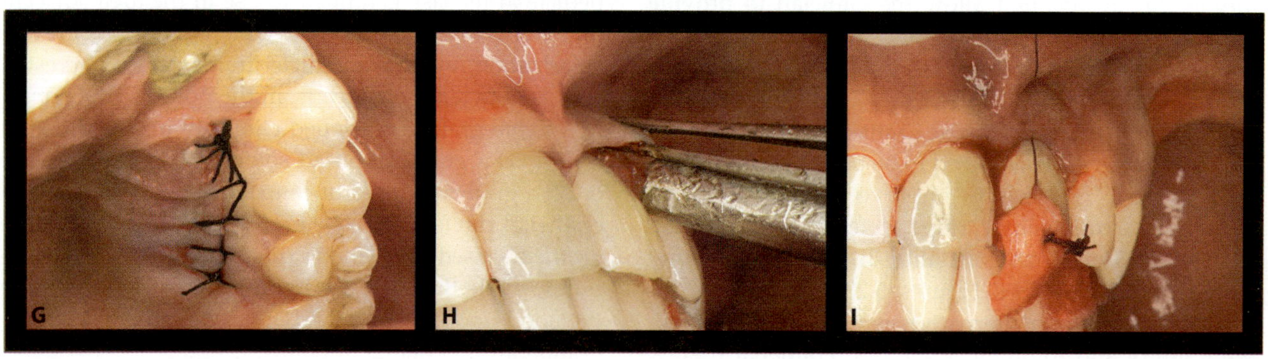

Figure 5.24. **G.** The palatal incision sutured. **H.** A marginal supraperiosteal incision is made opposite to the implant-supported crown and dissected apically. **I.** The connective tissue graft is being pulled inside the pouch.

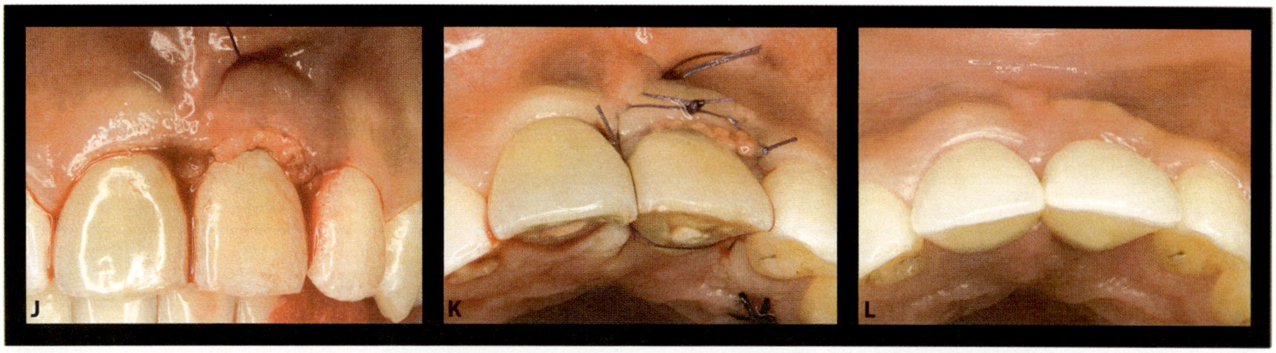

Figure 5.24. **J.** The connective tissue in place. **K.** Wound closure. **L.** Postaugmenting result showing improved tissue topography.

The inlay connective tissue grafting procedure involves two main clinical steps: (1) preparation of the recipient site and (2) harvesting the graft. A horizontal intrasulcular incision is made on the marginal gingiva with the scalpel angle parallel to the tooth long axis. Two vertical incisions are made to facilitate mucoperiosteal flap release. A partial thickness flap is then raised by blunt dissection until it reaches the vestibule. Care must be exercised not to perforate the flap during dissection and thus jeopardize the overall blood supply.

The connective tissue graft can be harvested from the palate or from the tuberosity. A straight, horizontal incision parallel to the alveolar ridge starts posteriorly approximately 5 to 6 mm from the free gingival margin and is extended anteriorly. A second, more coronally positioned, parallel incision is made approximately 3 mm from the free gingival margin and is continued to the same distance as the first incision. Then two small vertical incisions are made mesially and distally to connect the two horizontal incisions. Another horizontal incision is made at the apical border of the graft to completely separate the graft from the underlying bone. This will finally provide a 2-mm to 3 mm-wide connective tissue wedge with an epithelial rim. Finally, the palate is sutured with continuous basting sutures. The graft is then trimmed and introduced into the recipient site, drawn underneath the partial thickness flap, and secured with a sling suture to the labial mucosa.

In esthetically demanding areas where only increased tissue height is required, no vertical relaxing incisions should be made at the recipient site to avoid any possibility of future scar tissue formation. Connective tissue grafts can be applied to the recipient site in a pouch-like shape. These are used to correct confined minor ridge deficiencies, where the color and surface characteristics of the area after grafting should not differ from the original tissue character (Allen et al. 1985, Seibert and Salama 1996, Langer and Calagna 1982, Seibert 1990). The procedure is indicated only in minor ridge deficiencies that do not jeopardize the function of the implant. (See Figure 5.25.)

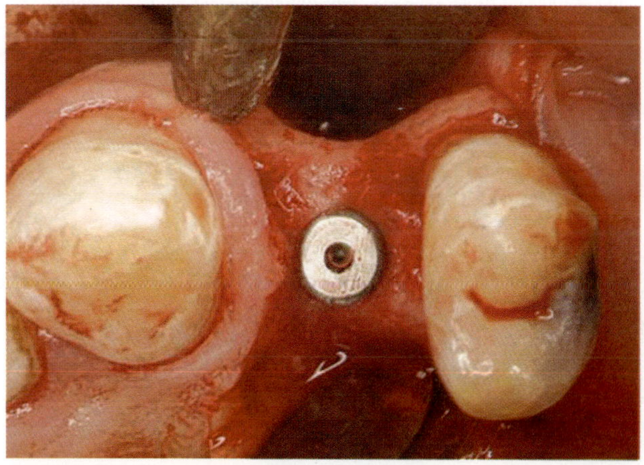

Figure 5.25. A bone defect that does not affect the implant bone contact, which might be indicated for the treatment with a connective tissue graft.

The long-term clinical results of the graft are still questionable. Initially, this procedure exhibits remarkable postoperative results, but graft shrinkage as a result of postoperative tissue remodeling has a tendency to occur over time. The procedure can also be called a "closed connective tissue grafting procedure" because the graft is totally embedded under the soft tissues, thus providing more predictable graft survival, as shown in Figures 5.26A–C.

The procedure involves making a supraperiosteal pouch at the deficient area. A one-line vertical incision, extending apically and bypassing the deformity through the attached gingival and the mucogingival junction, is made. Blunt dissection is used to extend the pouch. The

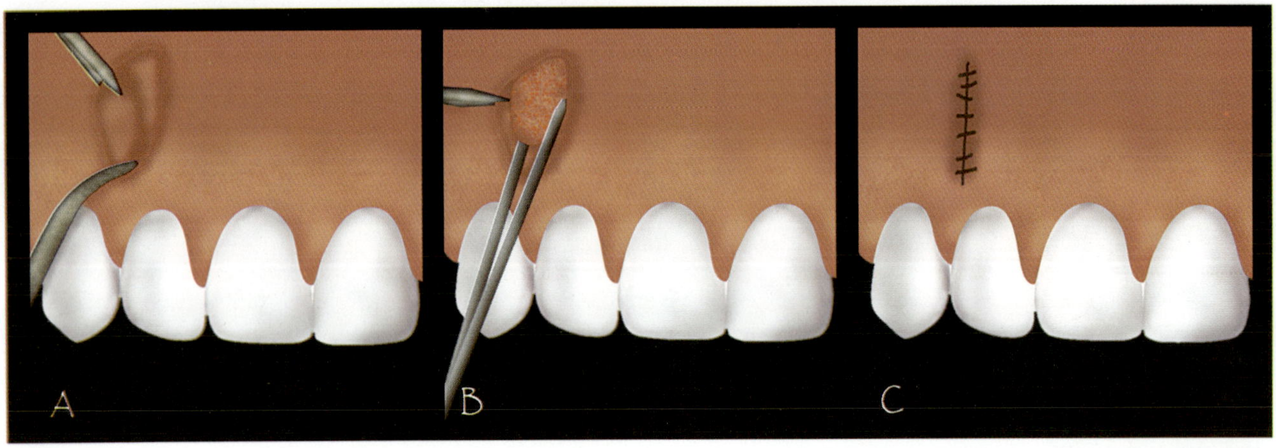

Figure 5.26. **A.** Illustration showing the pouch created in the labial mucosa with a one-line vertical incision. **B.** Illustration showing the connective tissue graft being introduced to the pouch. **C.** Illustration showing the final closure.

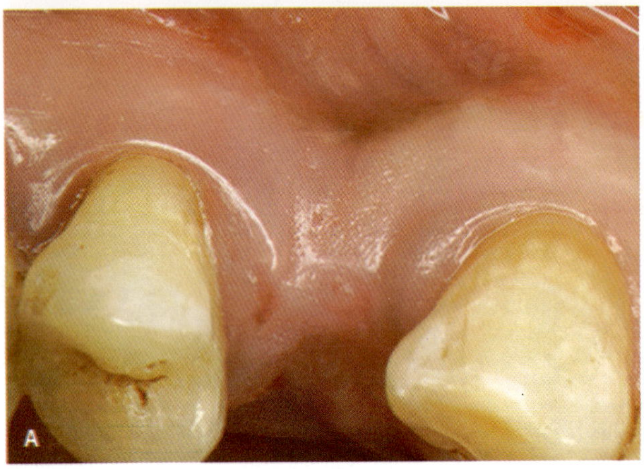

Figure 5.27A. Clinical view showing labial defect related to an implant site.

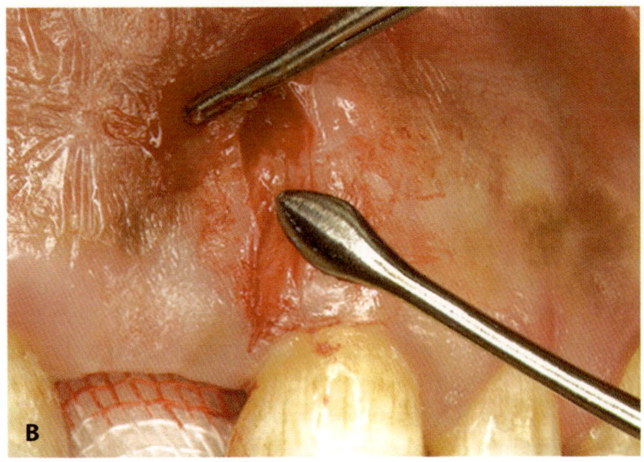

Figure 5.27B. The pouch is created through a one-line vertical incision.

maxillary tuberosity and the palate are readily accessible donor sites for harvesting the connective tissue graft to repair the alveolar defect. A 2-mm to 3 mm-thick connective tissue graft is carefully dissected, de-epithelialized, introduced to the pouch, and placed underneath the flap. The graft is then stabilized with resorbable sutures. A suture is first passed through the base of the pouch to the end of the graft, then another suture is made in the middle of the graft, which helps stabilize the graft to the underlying periosteum. The pouch is then closed with interrupted sutures. (See Figures 5.27A–I.)

In the case of moderate to severely compromised defects in which bone grafts are not indicated, a connective tissue graft can be used in combination with bone grafts to increase the soft tissue quality and quantity (Allen 1993). The connective tissue graft is placed over the bone graft to enhance tissue volume, as shown in Figures 5.28A–C. Combining two types

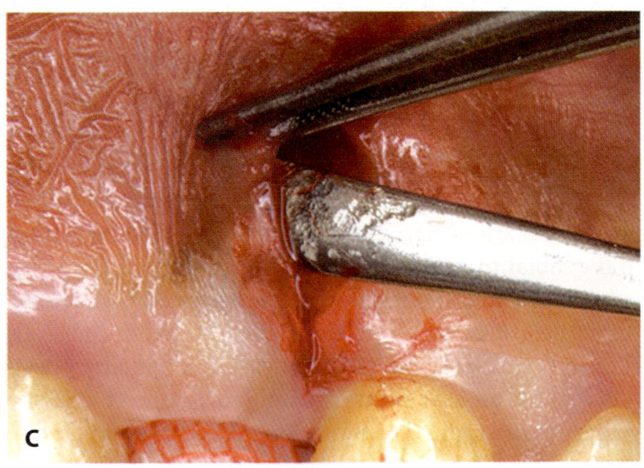

Figure 5.27C. The pouch is being dissected via a curved periosteal elevator.

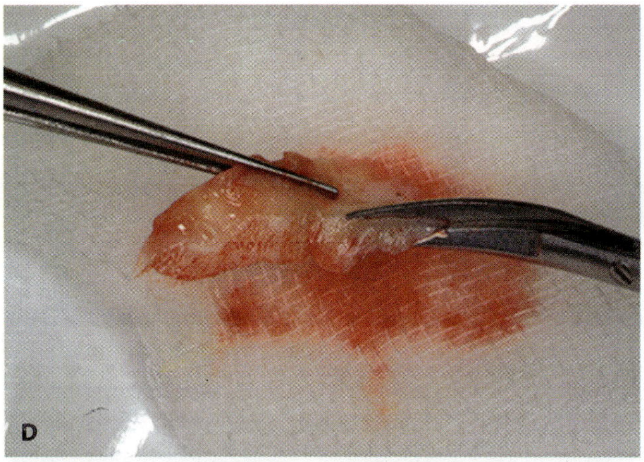

Figure 5.27D. The connective tissue graft is harvested and prepared.

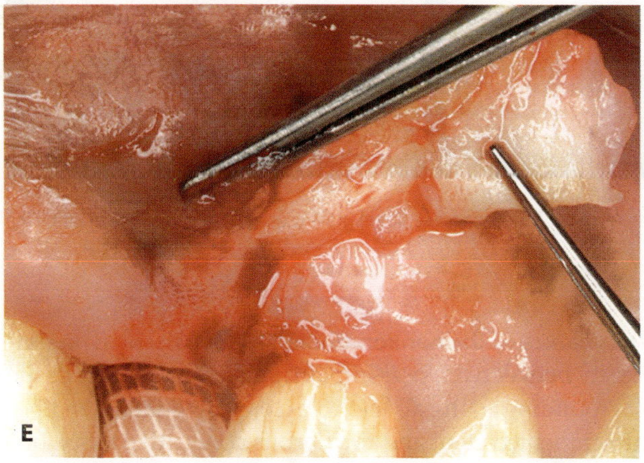

Figure 5.27E. The connective tissue graft is introduced into the pouch.

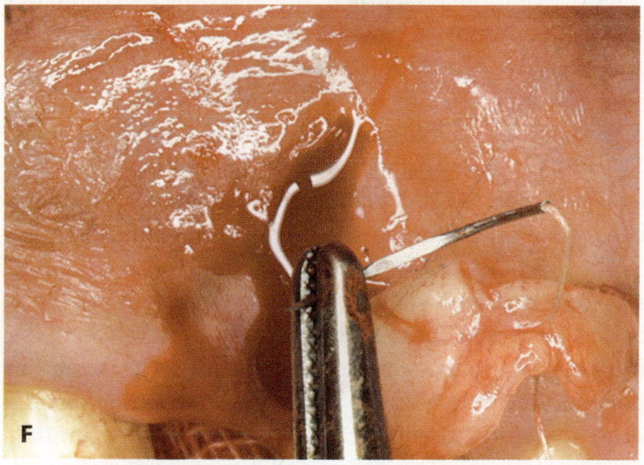

Figure 5.27F. The graft is being stabilized with a securing suture in its place.

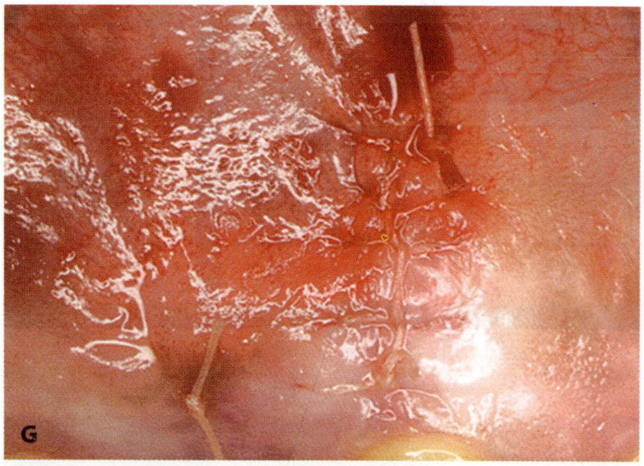

Figure 5.27G. The pouch is closed and sutured.

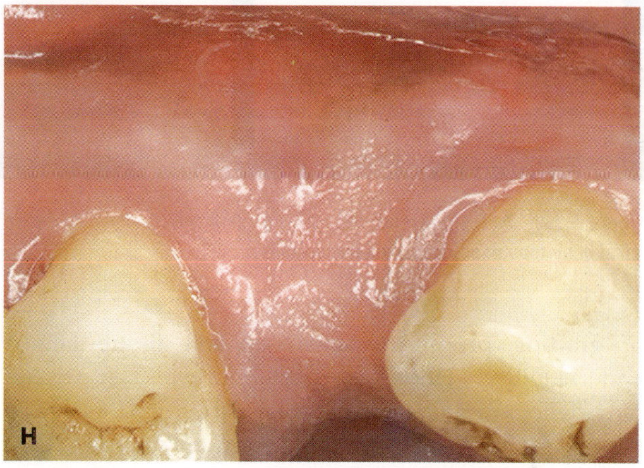

Figure 5.27H. Incisal view showing the profile improvement.

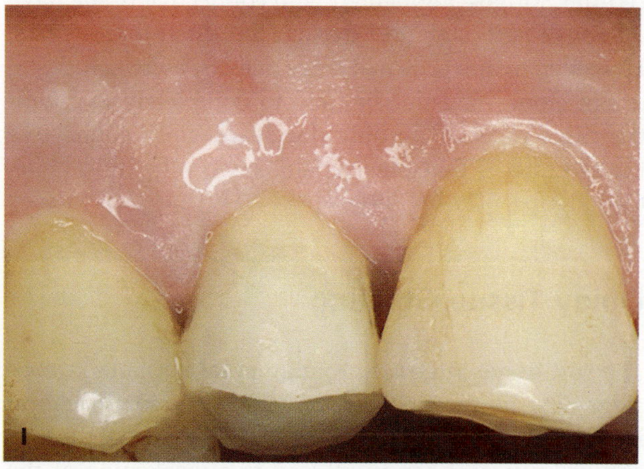

Figure 5.27I. Labial view showing the final case restored.

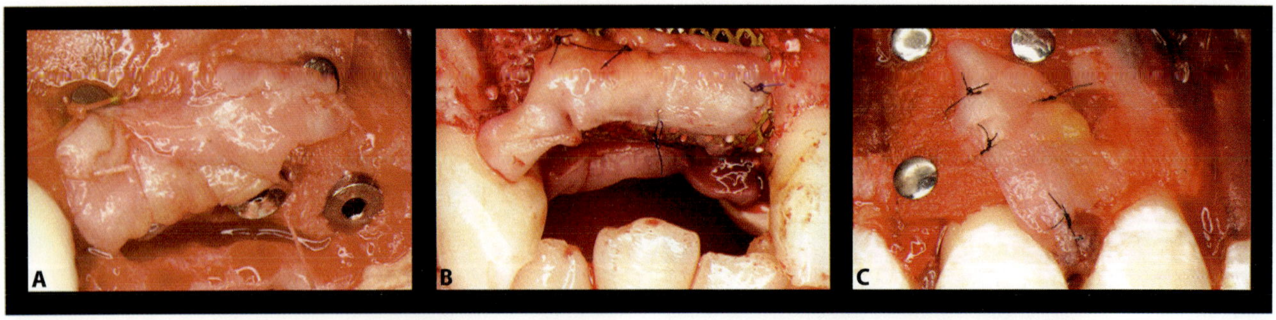

Figure 5.28A, B, C. The use of the connective tissue graft in conjunction with bone-grafting procedure in different clinical applications.

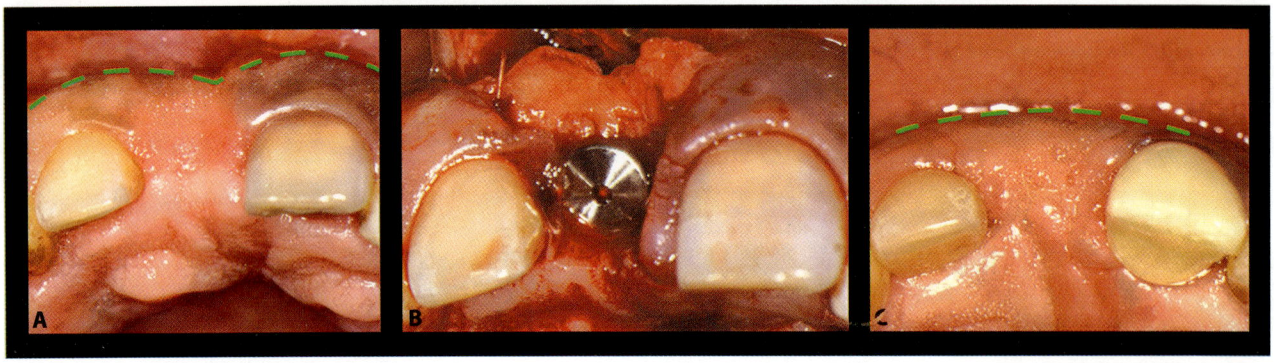

Figure 5.29. **A.** The green line represents a labial defect related to the dental implant site. **B.** A connective tissue graft is used to augment the area. **C.** The labial bone topography improved postoperative.

of grafting procedures increases soft tissue height and stability. However, postoperative soft tissue remodeling remains an issue of concern. Connective tissue grafts used for ridge augmentation have been shown to preserve the original characteristics of the overlying mucosa, resulting in a better esthetic blend in potential highly visible areas. As a result, the natural color and texture that is maintained by connective tissue grafts may reduce the need for secondary procedures. Ridges augmented with connective tissue have demonstrated stability during the first three years. However, in apicocoronal ridge defects, inlay soft tissue grafts alone may not be able to completely augment the ridge defect. The only disadvantage of connective tissue grafts is that they require a second surgical site. (See Figures 5.29A–C.)

Onlay Tissue Grafting

The soft tissue interface around dental implants is considered to be the first line of defense against bacterial invasion. In many instances, reducing the size of the keratinized mucosal band will lead to a weakening of the peri-implant soft tissue interface, probably due to the thin nature of the nonkeratinized mobile tissue. The similarity between the peri-implant soft tissue and the tissue surrounding natural teeth (except in Sharpey's fiber attachment system and the fibrous connective tissue orientation) has led the way to applying the same methods for reconstruction and treatment with some minor modifications. Hence, the peri-implant soft tissue interface does not possess a biologic seal, but rather depends on the tonus of the parallel oriented tissue fibers. The integrity of these attachment fibers is directly correlated with the amount of possible inflammation present. In addition, the condition of the host immune system, as well as the patient's oral hygiene status, affect the inflammatory condition of the peri-implant tissues. Therefore, the importance of maintaining a healthy and resistant soft tissue band around dental implants becomes a vital prerequisite (Silverstein et al. 1994).

The peri-implant soft tissues should be resistant to abrasion and well stabilized to the underlying osseous bed. This helps form a tight adaptation between the implant components and the soft tissues. However, the peri-implant soft tissue is not always in optimal condition; therefore, tissue deficiency might be a limiting treatment factor. The onlay soft tissue grafting procedure can help to regain the deficient soft tissue volume, and it can be performed at any time of the treatment, either prior to implant therapy or at the time of the abutment connection. (See Figures 5.30 and 5.31A–F.)

Onlay grafts are thick, free gingival grafts derived from partial- or total-thickness palatal grafts. They might be used to gain ridge height, and can be useful in eliminating gingival amalgam tattoos as well as treating weakened gingival tissues due to previous trauma. The onlay graft procedure was designed to augment soft tissue ridge defects. The major disadvantage is that the colors do not match, which presents an esthetic challenge. Depending upon the thickness, onlay grafts undergo moderate to severe postsurgical shrinkage. Onlay grafts also require an abundant blood supply and rapid capillary proliferation to heal and mend. Therefore, it is important to note that this technique is

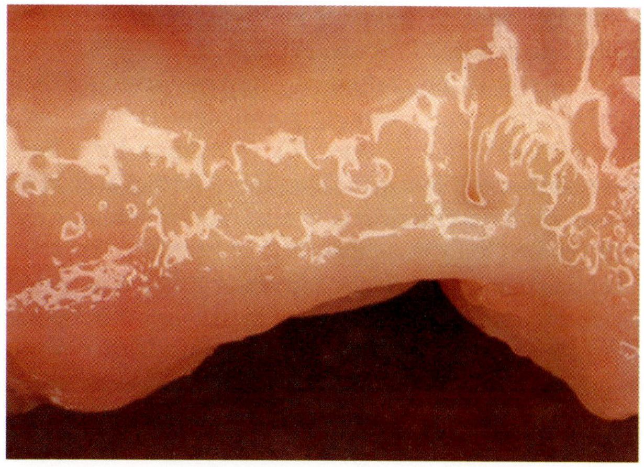

Figure 5.30. Pontic area defect.

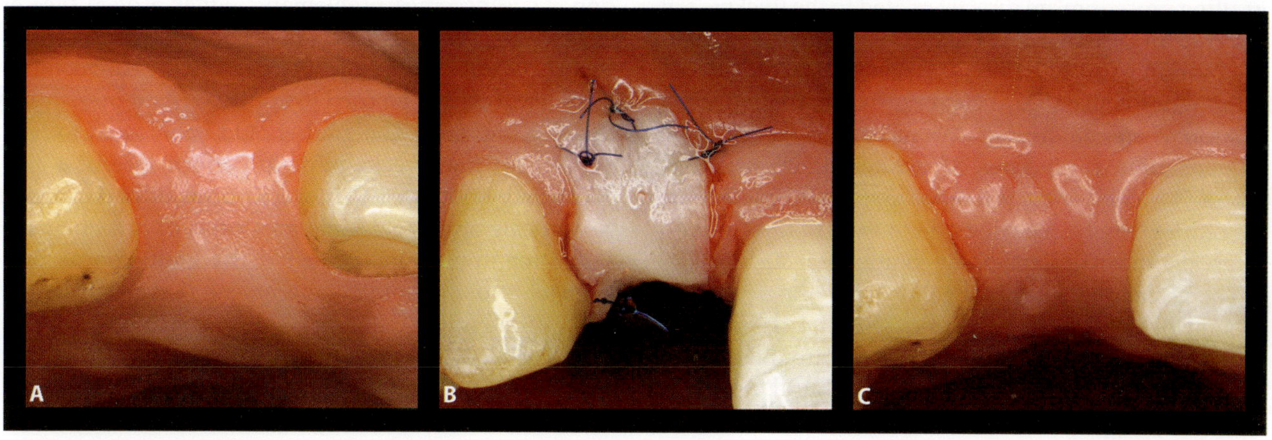

Figure 5.31. **A.** Preoperative view of minor soft tissue defect. **B.** Onlay grafting procedure took place. **C.** One month postsurgical result that shows improvement in the soft tissue profile.

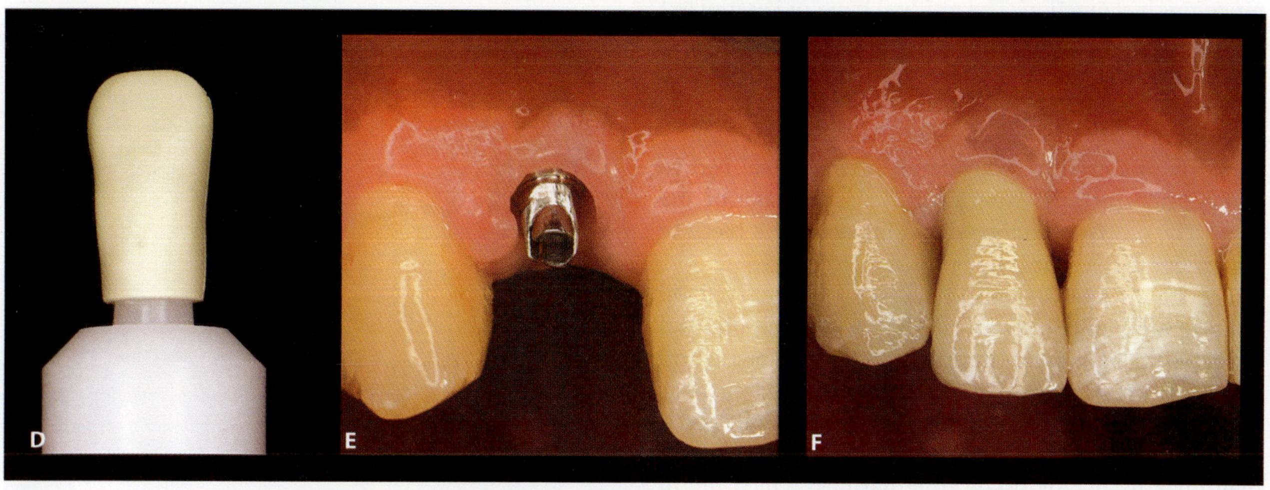

Figure 5.31. **D.** Alumina-Zirconium coping used for esthetic abutment. **E.** The underlying metal connection being used. **F.** The case finally restored.

contraindicated in areas of previous surgical trauma with compromised vascular support.

Onlay soft tissue grafting techniques, including their modifications, are becoming popular for treating peri-implant soft tissue defects. The techniques have been extensively described in the literature (Dordick et al. 1976, Cohen 1994, Haeri and Serio 1999). These techniques originally aimed to increase the width of keratinized tissues, treat mucogingival defects, and arrest gingival recession around natural teeth. Adherence to the basic intraoperative principles of soft tissue grafting—such as determining the amount of soft tissue required to cover the defect, the clinical condition of the recipient site, the availability of donor tissue, detecting the location of any anatomical landmark in the area of grafting, and assessing the patient's oral hygiene condition—are important steps that favor the final clinical results (Dordick et al. 1976). The final soft tissue dimensions gained from any onlay grafting procedure are directly related to the thickness of the graft and the amount of tissue that survives the grafting procedure (Cohen 1994). It is generally accepted that a thin graft is used for increasing the zone of attached tissues, whereas a thick graft is recommended for ridge augmentation procedures. If greater tissue height is required from an onlay soft tissue grafting procedure, the procedure may be repeated after a two- to three-month interval until an optimal tissue contour is achieved.

The technique for placing an onlay gingival graft around dental implants is identical to the classic technique used to augment the soft tissue around natural teeth. The procedure involves two surgical sites: the recipient site and the donor site. The recipient site is prepared by making an incision, with the blade held parallel to the alveolar process, that starts at the distal end of the defect; then the blade is drawn in a mesial direction to the end of the defect. Another horizontal incision (equal in length to the first) is made just below the mucogingival junction. The residual band of keratinized tissue will be removed to allow for epithelial denudation, which can be achieved with a scalpel or high-speed bur. A sharp dissection is performed apically to separate the alveolar mucosa and muscle fibers from the periosteum, and it is preferred to overextend the periosteal bed to compensate for any expected future shrinkage of the graft. The graft size is then determined using a piece of tin foil cut to the exact size of the recipient bed.

The donor site (usually the palate) is prepared by making a beveled incision, starting along the occlusal aspect of the palate and continuing apically, while lifting and separating the graft as it moves. A tissue forceps is used to retract the graft distally until it is finally separated. The graft should be trimmed to remove any fatty glandular tissues or tissue irregularities, which might inhibit the graft's take.

After the graft is prepared, it is adapted and fitted to the underlying periosteum and sutured. Five minutes of pressure with a saline-wetted gauze permits fibrin clot formation and prevents postoperative bleeding. Coverage of the grafted area with rubber dam material (to prevent the sutures from adhering to the dressing) followed by a surgical dressing on top may be recommended. Coverage of the raw area of the donor site relieves the patient's postoperative discomfort and can be achieved by fitting a previously fabricated acrylic template to the palate.

The free gingival graft can be sutured with either resorbable or nonresorbable sutures. Once sutured, the grafted tissue should be stable and immobile to have intimate contact with the periosteal bed; usually a 5-0 tapered reverse cutting needle is recommended for suturing because it penetrates the grafted tissue and periosteum atraumatically. If hemorrhage from the donor site becomes problematic, either a deep (vessel clamping) suture can be placed in the palate or an absorbable hemostatic agent covered by a clear vacuum-form template can be used to apply constant pressure to the bleeding area. The graft should be allowed to heal for at least four weeks prior to performance of a gingivoplasty and at least six weeks prior to performance to fabricate any provisional prosthesis or reflecting the tissue for implant placement if the grafting was performed prior to implant placement (Silverstein et al. 1994). (See Figures 5.32A–F.)

The clinical drawbacks and complications encountered with onlay grafts include the color and texture mismatch between the graft and the surrounding tissues (tire patch appearance), the difficulty of graft adaptation to the recipient site, graft mobility due to hematoma formation, graft shrinkage (approximately 30%) from its original size after healing is complete (Nabers 1966), and the difficulty of achieving proper

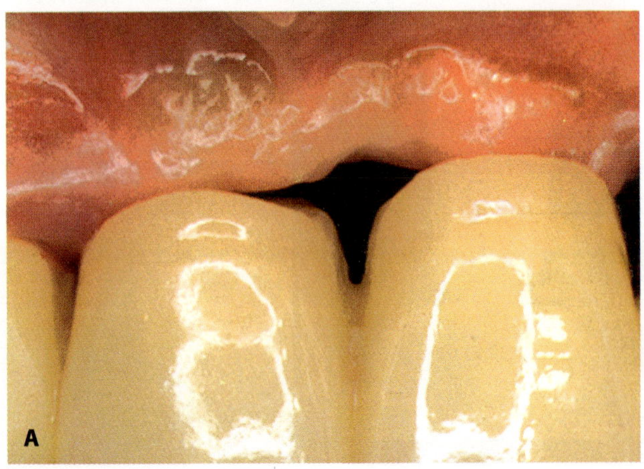

Figure 5.32A. Alveolar ridge defect underneath the pontic area.

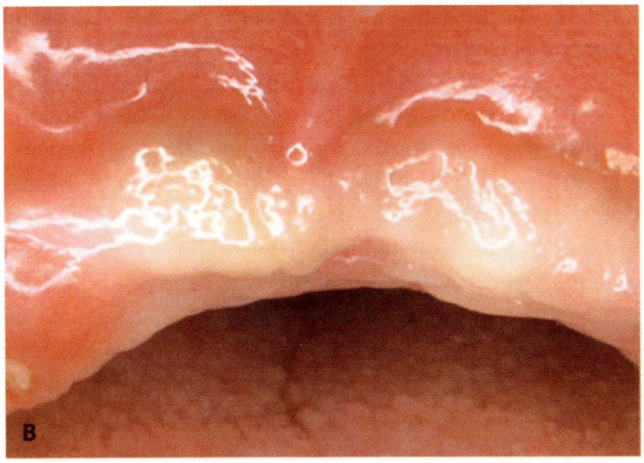

Figure 5.32B. The implant-supported restoration is removed revealing the deficient ridge.

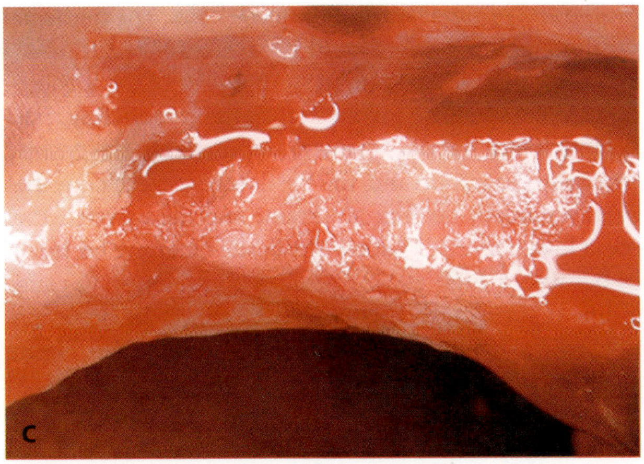

Figure 5.32C. The recipient bed is prepared.

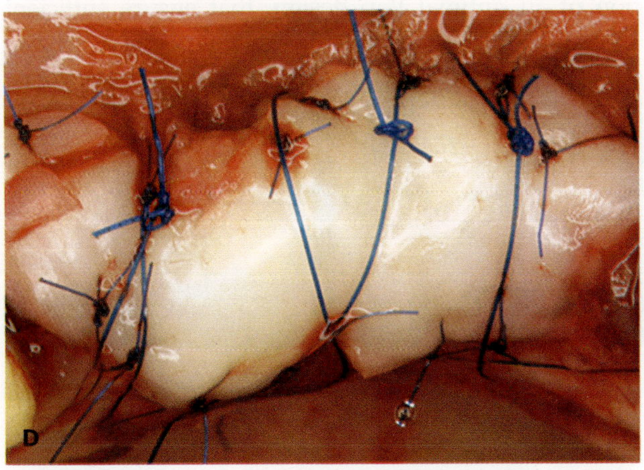

Figure 5.32D. Onlay graft is used to improve the pontic ridge relation.

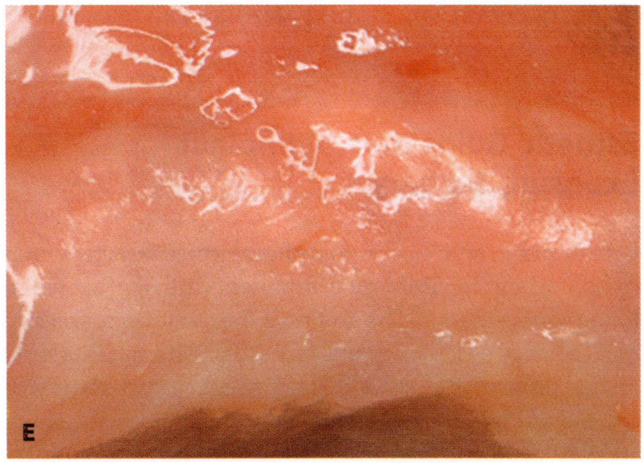

Figure 5.32E. Postoperative view showing the healing of the graft.

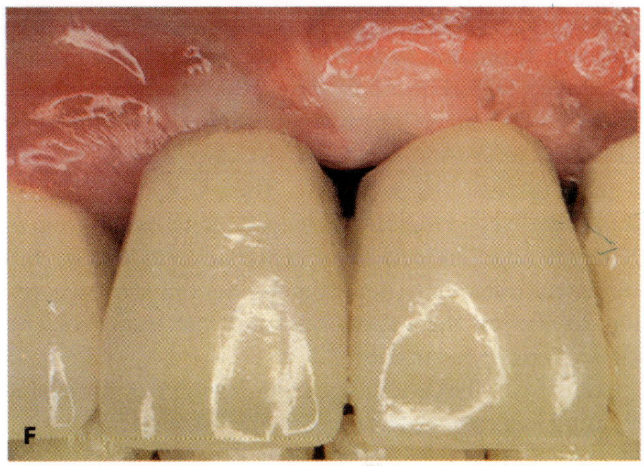

Figure 5.32F. Final case restored.

adherence of the graft to titanium abutments, which has caused some clinicians to abandon this grafting procedure after the abutment connection (James and McFall 1978).

A recent development in onlay grafting procedures is the introduction of the acellular dermal matrix (Alloderm, Biohorizon, USA). Grafting with autogenous tissue or freeze-dried skin can be an accepted method for increasing and/or restoring the width of attached gingiva. The method was originally used to treat burn patients. When used as a gingival graft, it possesses major potential advantages over the traditional onlay grafts, including improved color and contour match to the original tissues, elimination of donor site surgery, and unlimited availability (Shulman 1996). Soft-tissue augmentation around dental implants using the onlay gingival soft tissue technique is an important facet that should be considered prior to any implant placement. The clinician should be able to determine the optimal timing of performing such a procedure (Silverstein et al. 1994).

Esthetic Guidelines of Implant Exposure Surgery

Peri-implant soft tissue morphological characters that closely adjoin the implant components are of great value to implant esthetics. The ability of the clinician to modify and enhance soft tissue contours around dental implants at the time of the second-stage surgery can influence the overall restorative result. An excellent second-stage surgery protocol might help to restore missing biological tissue profile and/or restore any related soft tissue contours. Therefore, numerous flap designs have been introduced to achieve an esthetic soft tissue margin adjacent to the implant-supported restoration, which in turn helps to overcome several esthetic difficulties encountered with dental implants. The soft tissue management at the second-stage surgery is highly critical and technique-sensitive. A minor fault in tissue manipulation can lead to undesirable sequences. Therefore, conceptually individualized surgical protocols along with clinical recommendations can be of great value to the overall treatment outcome. The recommendations vary according to the vision, experience, and preference of the clinician prior to surgery.

Some treatment goals should be considered when performing a second-stage surgery in the esthetic zone:

1. To preserve the keratinized tissue band continuity
2. To avoid creating any defective tissue margins
3. To avoid creating an implant-supported restoration that has asymmetrical contours
4. To have a stable soft tissue condition postoperatively
5. To accomplish natural soft tissue dimensions
6. To avoid the formation of any scar tissue on the labial gingival interface
7. To preserve natural adjacent structures (i.e., the interproximal papillae)

The exposure of the implant body should be accomplished with the soft tissue final architecture in mind. To achieve the proper soft tissue architecture, several clinical options are available; they may be classified as subtractive, additive, or a combination of each (Bichacho and Landsberg 1997). When the soft tissue along the edentulous crest is at its optimal levels and volume, a subtraction technique such as gingivoplasty might be undertaken; however, this method is not recommended in the esthetic zone. The subtraction approach begins with the palpation of the soft tissue until the cover screw is felt with an explorer. Then, using a gum punch with a probe in the middle, the center of the cover screw is located. The punch is then pressed, and the soft tissue covering is excised.

The classic protocol for performing the second-stage surgery starts with a long incision over the crest of bone or midway buccolingual through the gingiva from the site of the most distal implant to the most mesial location. Then, either full- or split-thickness buccal and lingual flaps are elevated to establish access. Any osseous overgrowth over the cover screws should be removed, and the coronal aspect of the fixtures is cleaned. Any osseous recontouring may take place at this time. The healing abutments are then placed and the flaps sutured. However, the major disadvantage of this method is that because more tissue manipulation and trauma are involved, it is a long incision technique that exposes a large area of bone; therefore, several conservative approaches have been introduced.

When esthetics is a prime concern, an additive type of surgery is performed to gain tissue thickness. In this method the gingiva is contoured to create a healthy profile and optimal surrounding contours. The midfacial position of the tissue should be overcorrected to allow an excess of at least 1 mm in the contour of the adjacent teeth to compensate for the soft tissue remodeling, post healing. Once the tissues are manipulated to the desired emergence contour and the first-stage cover screw has been removed, healing abutment may be inserted that has a lower profile to allow for tissue creeping on top of it, because a high profile healing abutment may cause gingival shrinkage. This procedure might be accompanied with or without impression making. (See Figure 5.33A–B.)

The goal of second-stage surgery in the esthetic zone is not only to expose the implant interface for performing the required restorative procedures, but also to create a healthy marginal attached mucosa around the implant components (Hertel et al. 1994). Therefore, all of the basic intraoperative precautions, including the selection of an optimal flap design, that ensure sufficient

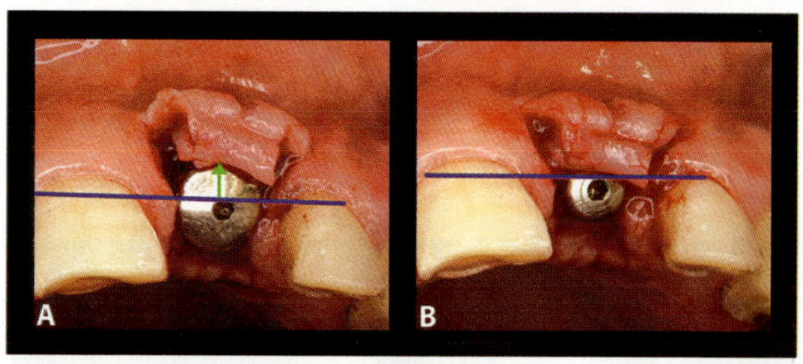

Figure 5.33. **A.** The blue line represents the natural teeth labial contour. The picture shows that when using a high profile abutment, the body of the abutment itself violates the soft tissue natural contours, and then pushes the soft tissue in a far labial position. **B.** Note the harmonious soft tissue profile condition when using a low profile abutment.

blood supply and allow for better access and visibility must be strictly regarded to maintain uneventful healing. The use of cosmetic incisions can improve the esthetic outcome of the second-stage surgery.

Cosmetic incisions can be beveled toward the center of the flap at a 45-degree angle, thereby minimizing the chances of postoperative soft tissue scarring. This can be achieved with the use of microscalpel blades and small-diameter suturing materials. Some second-stage surgical guidelines or recommendations are made to reduce postoperative complications and maximize the esthetic outcome around dental implants. They can be used as a guide or a reference for clinicians who desire esthetic surgical results. There is a close relation between implant positioning osseous crest and resultant perio-implant soft tissue contours.

A study (Choquet et al. 2001) was conducted to determine whether the distance from the base of the contact point to crest of the bone would correlate with the presence or absence of interproximal papillae adjacent to single-tooth implants, and whether the surgical technique at uncovering influences the outcome. A clinical and radiographic retrospective evaluation of the papilla level around single dental implants and their adjacent teeth was performed in the anterior maxilla in 26 patients restored with 27 implants. Six months after insertion, 17 implants were uncovered with a standard technique, while 10 implants were uncovered with a technique designed to generate papilla-like formation around dental implants. Fifty-two papillae were available for clinical and radiographic evaluation. The presence or absence of papillae was determined, and the effects of the following variables were analyzed: the influence of the two surgical techniques; the vertical relation between the papilla height and the crest of bone between the implant and adjacent teeth; the vertical relation between the papilla level and the contact point between the crowns of the teeth and the implant; and the distance from the contact point to the crest of bone.

The data showed a positive correlation between the use of the modified surgical technique designed to reconstruct papillae at uncovering and the outcome. The influence of the bone crest on the presence or absence of papillae between implants and adjacent teeth was also shown to be positive. Therefore, some clinical guidelines have been devolved by the author. Those rules are not obligatory, but they are mandatory for achieving enhanced treatment outcome. They are clinical recommendations that can be applied separately in different situations or together in a single surgery. Applying these guidelines as a clinical reference, the clinician should be able to obtain satisfactory esthetic results. The guidelines can be used in a particular clinical situation and will be determined by location, the quantity of soft tissue, severity of bone resorption, and tissue biotype. Therefore, creating natural-looking soft tissue profiles around dental implants may be achieved by adhering to the following "guidelines":

1. **Bulking Keratinized Tissues:** Increasing the soft tissue mass around the labial aspect of dental implants at the second-stage surgery is one of the treatment merits. Keratinized tissues or connective tissues or both together might be used to increase the volume to enhance the overall peri-implant tissue condition. Surgical procedures require the mobilization of a mucoperiosteal flap, which results in many cases in nonkeratinized mobile mucosa ending up on top of the alveolar ridge or potential implant site. Consequently, in an abutment connection procedure, it is necessary to relocate the keratinized mucosa from the palatal aspect to the buccal. This requires the incision for the abutment connection procedure to be performed on the palatal side of the implants and the full mucoperiosteal flap to be advanced to the buccal. Low-profile healing abutments help maintain the flap in a buccal position. This procedure results in keratinized mucosa on the buccal aspect of the fixtures. This procedure can be called profiling peri-implant soft tissues. Bulking the tissues around the buccal side of the prosthetic components will not only improve the emergence profile but also assists in developing the future biological width that is necessary for the stability of the peri-implant tissue condition. The resultant tissue volume will improve the emergence of the future implant-supported restoration, stabilize tissue margins, and help to compensate for any future tissue shrinkage or remodeling. The complete displacement of the soft tissues to the labial aspect of the implant will in turn lead to bulking and overprofiling around the prosthetic components. Technically speaking, this procedure can be described as a reversed Rehrmanplasty. (See Figure 5.34.)

   Marginal soft tissue shrinkage around dental implant restorative components is expected during the first six months following abutment connection. This was confirmed by two important studies that enlightened many clinicians on the behavior of peri-implant soft tissue dental implants. One longitudinal study conducted by Bengazi and others (1996) measured the alterations in the position of peri-implant soft tissue margin on partial and full arch implant-supported prostheses after the second-stage surgery. The study revealed a gingival recession of 0.4 mm on the labial aspect of implant-supported prostheses in the maxilla after six months, and 0.7 mm after 24 months in non-grafted sites. It was proposed that the recession of the peri-implant soft tissue margin may be mainly the result of a remodeling of the soft tissue to establish an appropriate biological dimension. Another confirming study conducted by Grunder (2000) evaluated the soft tissue stability around 10 single-tooth implants. All cases were treated with guided bone regeneration and connective tissue grafting. One year after prosthesis insertion, 0.6 mm of soft tissue shrinkage was recorded on the buccal side of the implant-supported prosthesis. These findings encouraged the concept of bulking the keratinized mucosa as much as possible on the labial aspect at the second-stage surgery to compensate for any future soft issue shrinkage. They also support the use of a provisional prosthesis for six months after abutment connection, until a stable gingival margin is obtained. Following complete maturation of the tissue after the second-stage surgery, the idea is to allow for a resultant excessive tissue volume that can endure the prosthetic manipulations as well as counteract recession when the gingival margins have reached a stable level. Any soft tissue that exceeds the adjacent natural contour can be trimmed off and removed. (See Figures 5.35 and 5.36A–C.)

2. **Using Connective Tissues:** At the time of the second-stage surgery, not only should keratinized tissues be bulked around the abutment, but connective tissue grafts can also be used to improve the overall tissue profile, as shown in Figures 5.37A–E, to treat minor osseous defects around dental implants or to provide a root-eminence-like profile. A connective tissue graft is placed underneath the mucoperiosteal flap and secured with resorbable sutures to improve the soft tissue profile. Many authors have used connective tissue grafts at the

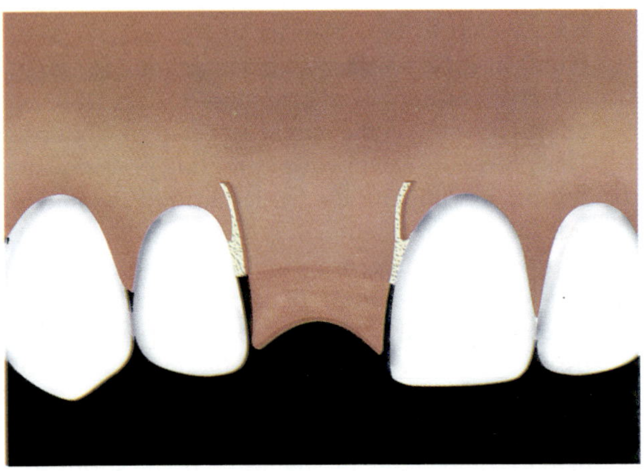

Figure 5.34. An illustration showing the incision design at the second-stage surgery that moves the palatal keratinized mucosa to the labial side (bulking keratinized tissue).

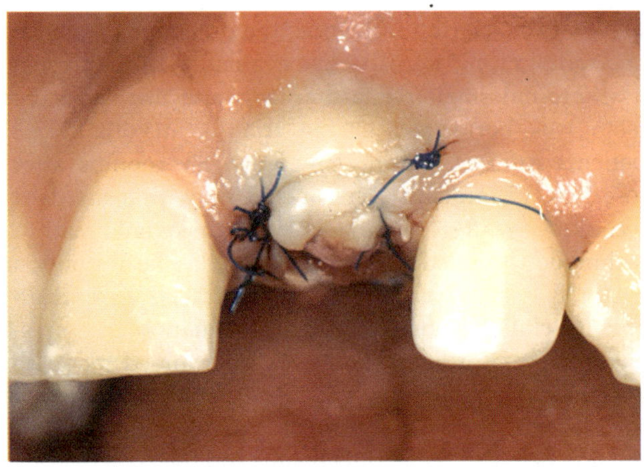

Figure 5.35. Clinical application of bulking the keratinized mucosa labially around healing abutments. Note the amount of keratinized tissues on the labial side.

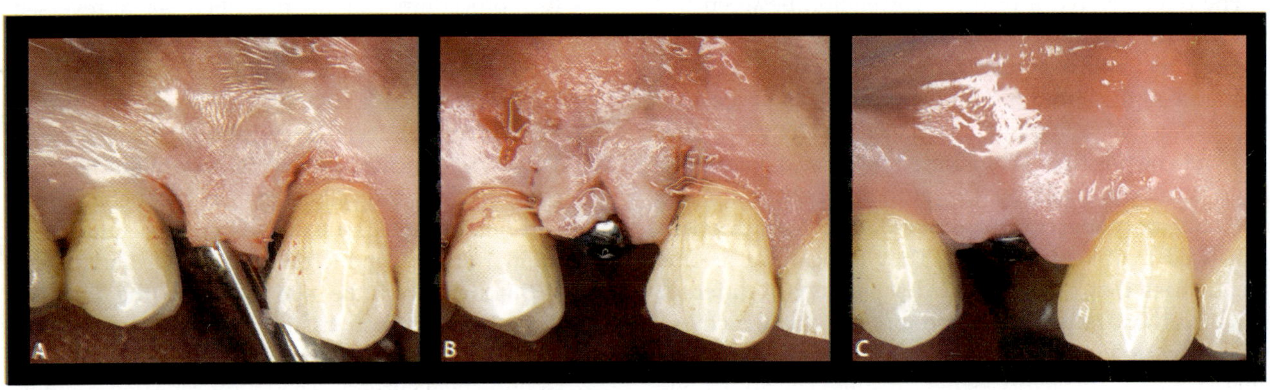

Figure 5.36. **A.** A clinical view at the second-stage surgery showing the mucoperiosteal flap to be stabilized at the labial side. **B.** The flap sutured around the healing abutment via midbuccal releasing incision. **C.** Five weeks' postoperative healing showing excellent labial tissue bulking and stability.

time of the second-stage surgery to treat minor soft tissue deficiencies or simulate a root-like bulging around the neck of the implant-supported prosthesis (Langer and Calagna 1982, Seibert 1990, Abrams 1980). (See Figures 5.38A–C.)

Abrams (1980) introduced an interesting method for augmenting minor edentulous alveolar defects. The technique involved stripping the epithelium from a palatal connective tissue pedicle and rolling it under the buccal mucosa. This procedure has shown high clinical predictability for improving the alveolar ridge topography at the defective area. Scharf and Tarnow (1992) introduced a modification of Abrams' technique. A "trap-door" approach is used to reflect and preserve the epithelium that overlies the connective tissue pedicle. The epithelial pedicle is used to cover the donor site, thus eliminating any raw area. However, the technique that Tarnow offered was limited to use prior to implant therapy, as the use of the modified roll flap technique for soft tissue enhancement therapy prior to implant placement increased the amount of connective tissue at the defective area, which in turn improved peri-implant soft tissue contours and reduced patient discomfort to a great extent by preventing denudation of the palatal bone.

This author (El Askary 2002) introduced the use of the modified roll flap technique at the time of the second-stage surgery along with the healing

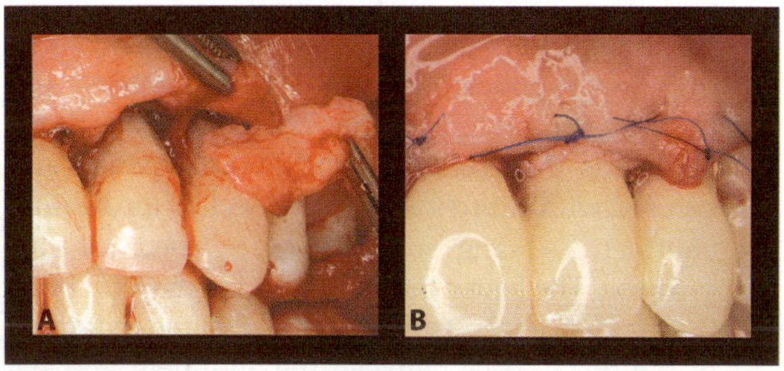

Figure 5.37. **A.** Connective tissue graft is used at the time of the second-surgery to bulk the soft tissue profile. **B.** The flap sutured on the connective tissue graft.

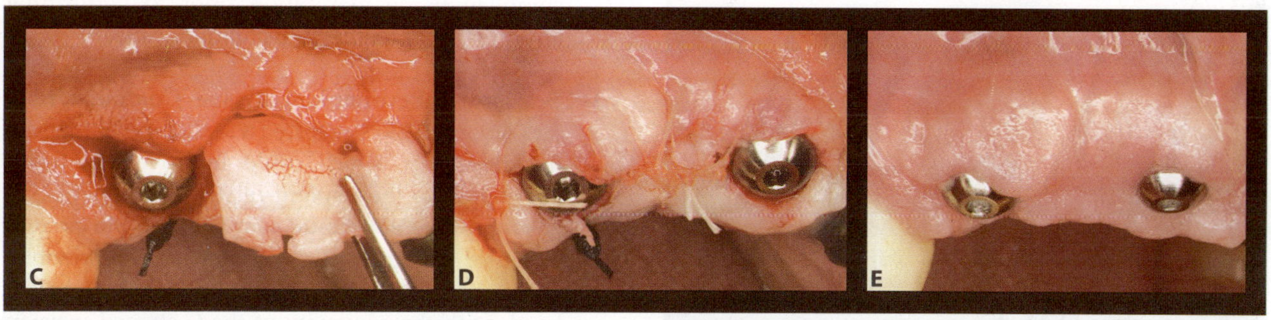

Figure 5.37. **C.** Direct use of the connective tissues on the provisional restoration to improve the buccal contour. **D.** The flap sutured. **E.** Postoperative healing, showing enhancement of the labial tissue quantity and quality.

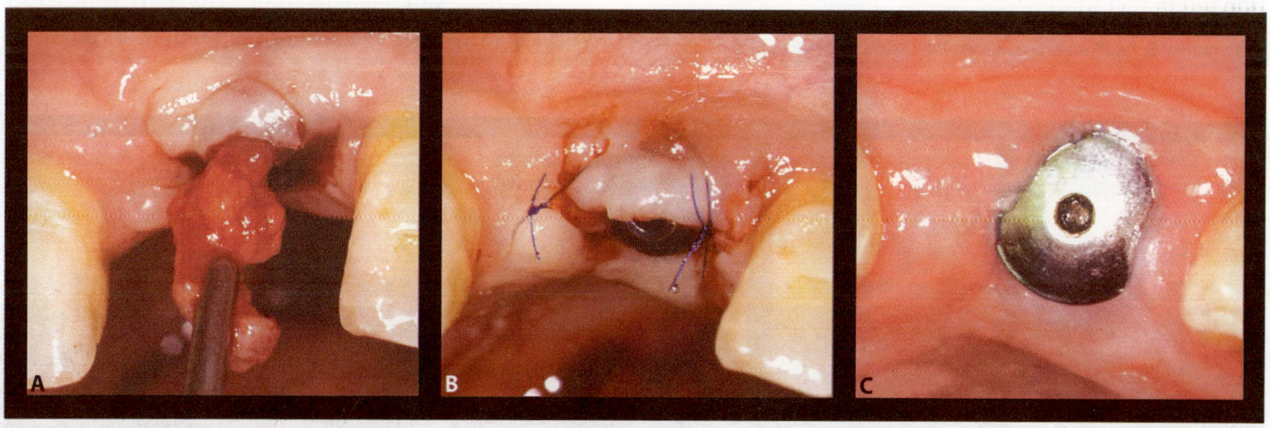

Figure 5.38. **A.** Minor alveolar ridge deficiency around an implant replacing a maxillary left central incisor, and a connective tissue graft is being used to enhance the buccal contour. **B.** The flap sutured securing the graft underneath. **C.** The peri-implant soft tissue contour imitating the bulging root-like shape, which gives a natural appearance to the implant-supported prosthesis.

abutment connection, as shown in Figures 5.39A–B. It is proposed that healing abutments can provide support for the rolled connective tissue pedicle, which in turn improves the final soft tissue profile and simulates forming the root-like eminence. Using the modified roll flap at the time of the second-stage surgery is indicated only when minor defects exist. Larger defects mandate surgical corrective procedures before starting the implant therapy.

The technique requires reflecting an epithelial flap with a connective tissue extension or pedicle from the palate and moving it to the site to be augmented labially. Two full thickness vertical parallel releasing incisions are made from the crest of the ridge toward the palate to outline the pedicle, preserving the papillae in both sides of the defect as much as possible. The length of the incisions depends on the length of connective tissue required. The two vertical incisions are joined with a shallow horizontal incision along the crest of the ridge to be a starting point for the partial thickness reflection of the epithelial flap. Once the epithelial flap is reflected, an incision is made along the connective tissue pedicle, down to the bone. The connective tissue pedicle is now bounded laterally by the two vertical incisions made initially for the epithelial pedicle and apically at its base by another horizontal incision to separate it. The connective tissue pedicle is then reflected in an apicocoronal direction. A pouch between the buccal mucosa and the alveolar ridge is made. The connective tissue pedicle is then rolled into the buccal pouch and secured with sutures around the neck of the healing abutment; a sling suture may be used for this purpose. The better the adaptation of the labial flap the better the results obtained due to the reduction of the dead space between the abutment and the flap. The epithelial pedicle is then replaced over the bone and secured. This method should allow four weeks to obtain satisfactory tissue healing. An ample amount of time should be allowed to offer complete tissue maturation prior to performing any further prosthetic techniques. (See Figures 5.40A–E.)

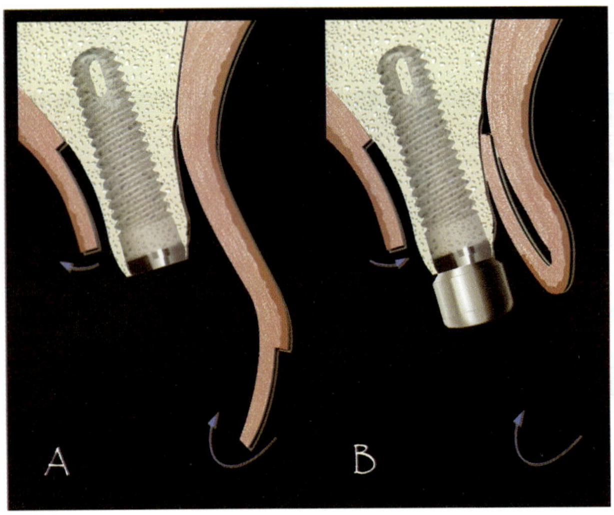

Figure 5.39. **A.** An illustration showing the modified roll flap before rolling and suturing. **B.** An illustration showing the closure and rolling of the flap.

3. **Scalloping Peri-implant Tissue Contours:** Moy and others (1989) suggested a scalloping of the full-thickness flap, which could improve soft tissue adaptation to the implant-related components. To ensure proper soft tissue adaptation to the circular shape of the prosthetic components, a horizontal C-shaped incision is made palatal to the implant head, with the convexity of the C-shaped incision directed buccally, during the second-stage surgery. At the end of the C scallop, two small (1–2 mm) vertical relieving incisions are made to allow for flap reflection and visualization. The flap is pushed backward until the scallop is adapted to embrace

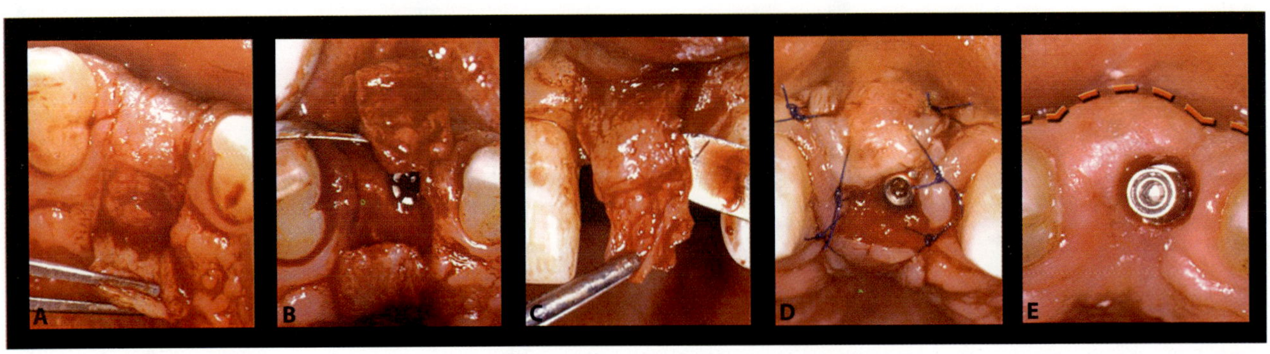

Figure 5.40. **A.** The use of the modified roll flap clinically starting with two vertical incisions. **B.** The buccal flap along with the palatal extension is reflected. **C.** Mobilization of the connective tissue pedicle. **D.** The flap sutured. **E.** Four weeks' postoperative result showing the remarkable buccal contour enhancement.

the facial aspect of the healing abutment collar. This method ensures tighter adaptation of the soft tissue to the abutment, thus reducing the tendency for developing a dead space and minimizing any possible soft tissue marginal discrepancy around the abutment. Hertel and others (1994) described another procedure that serves a similar purpose, the cervical folding technique. This technique achieves an intimate flap-abutment adaptation around the prosthetic components. (See Figures 5.41A–B.)

4. **Using Conserative Incisions and Applying Minimal Tissue Reflection:** Generally, using conservative flap designs to expose the minimal amount of tissues to allow sufficient access will improve the healing result. Hertel and others (1994) described a second-stage surgery protocol with a flap design and an incision that is limited to only the keratinized mucosa to maintain a proper amount of keratinized tissue around the implant collar. Extending the vertical relieving incisions to the vestibular tissues should be avoided at the second stage to avoid any possible postoperative soft tissue scarring or excessive tissue tags. The merit of this technique is minimal tissue refection with maximum tissue adaptation to the titanium surface of the abutments. This will eventually lead to stabilized tissue margins and natural tissue contours. Limiting the incisions to the attached tissues in the second-stage surgery minimizes flap mobility as much as possible, which allows for better healing. (See Figures 5.42A–B.)
5. **Keeping Intact Interroximal Papillae:** Preserving the interproximal papillae in the second-stage surgery or keeping them intact is strict recommended for preventing further drop-down or recession of the adjacent marginal soft tissues, as shown in Figures 5.43A and 5.43B, as recommended in

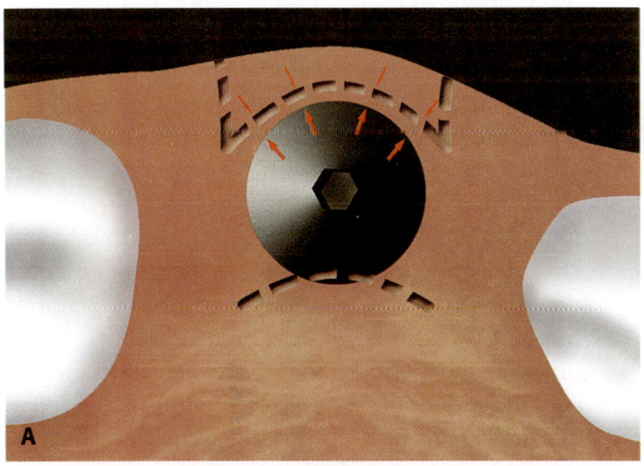

Figure 5.41A. An Illustration showing the scalloped flap effect around healing collars.

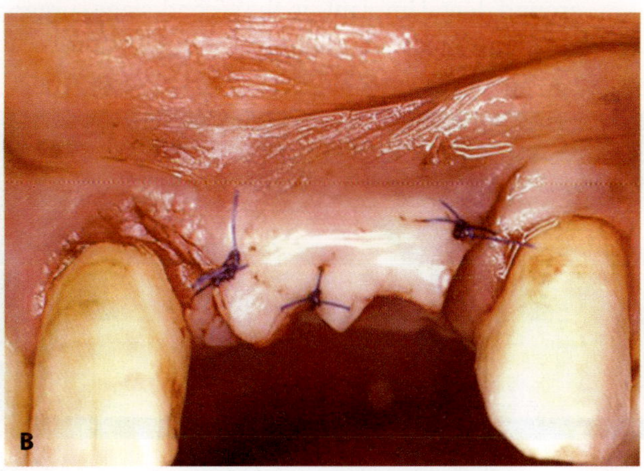

Figure 5.41B. Scalloping soft tissues clinically.

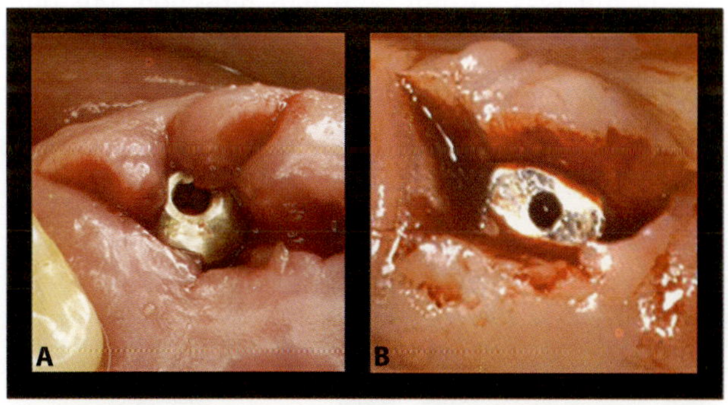

Figure 5.42. **A.** Clinical view of using limited incisions within the keratinized tissues. **B.** Limited incisions are used to expose the implants. Note the oblique direction of the incisions.

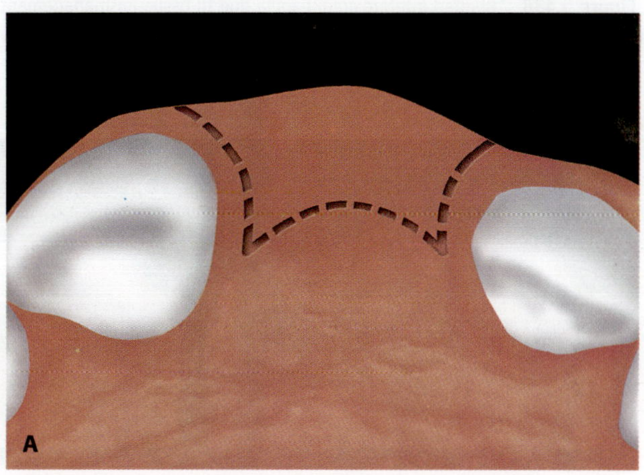

Figure 5.43A. An illustration showing the intact interproximal papilla incision.

cosmetic periodontal surgeries (Abrams 1980, Scharf and Tarnow 1992). Therefore, the recommendation not to displace the papillae from their original location is conceivable and will contribute positively to the stability of the soft-tissue margins. This approach averts postoperative soft tissue shrinkage around natural dentition as well as the implant prosthetic components. Preserving the interproximal papillae might also reduce soft tissue trauma during the surgery.

This was confirmed by an interesting work (Douglass 2005) that studied the effect of mucoperiosteal flap reflection on the condition of the inert dental papilla height. A total of 35 single-tooth extractions of maxillary anterior teeth with flap elevation were compared to 38 consecutive extractions of maxillary anterior teeth without flap elevation. The height of the mesial and distal papillae was measured from the incisal edge before extraction and at six weeks after. The average loss of papillae height was 1.6 mm with flap reflection, but only 0.85 mm without flap reflection. Thus, the importance of preserving or sparing the papilla during the surgery is a valid clinical option.

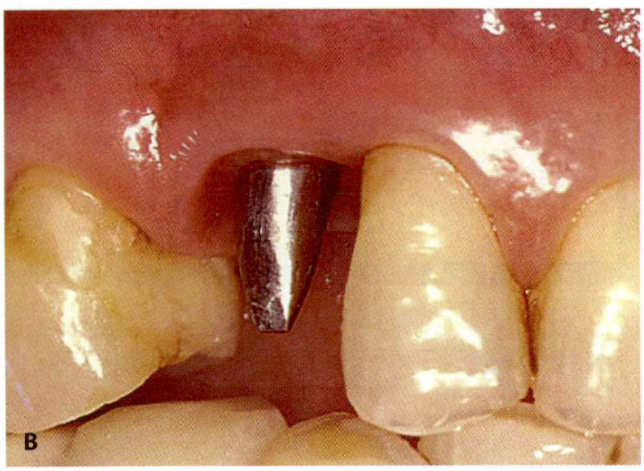

Figure 5.43B. Blunted interproximal papilla due to tissue mismanagement in the second-stage surgery, which warrants the importance of the papilla preservation.

Misch and others (2004) have introduced the split-finger technique to bulk the soft tissue around a peri-implant papilla. The method has shown predictability and clinical efficiency. (See Figures 5.44A–C.) A sulcular incision is made 2 to 3 mm to the palatal side from each tooth with a loop design (at least 2 to 2.5 mm) adjacent to the implant location. The incisions are then joined facially with a semicircular incision at the preplanned free tissue margin of the implant crown. The facial "fingers" are elevated to the desired interimplant height for the papillae. The middle "palatal finger" is then split and is reflected to the respective mesial and distal sides (each is at least 2 to 2.5 mm wide). The soft tissue maintains its elevated position on the healing abutment.

The split-finger papillae approach can also be used for two or more adjacent implants. In this case, a modified vertical mattress suture is used to suture each papilla using 4-0 or 5-0 sutures. One interrupted suture at the base of the papilla is suggested when the interproximal tissue is thin. The authors evaluated 21 patients with 39 implants consecutively placed in the maxillary anterior region. The implants were evaluated at six months to one year after prosthodontic restoration. The implants evaluated included 16 single-tooth implants, 12-unit implant prosthesis, 24-unit tooth implants, one 6-unit prosthesis, and one 7-unit restoration. Results concluded the efficacy of the technique provided an alternate procedure to promote/augment papillae formation around dental implants. (See Figures 5.45A–D.)

Adriaenssens and others (1999) described a similar approach to enhance the papilla formation around dental implants in the second-stage surgery, either in single or multiple teeth situations. The

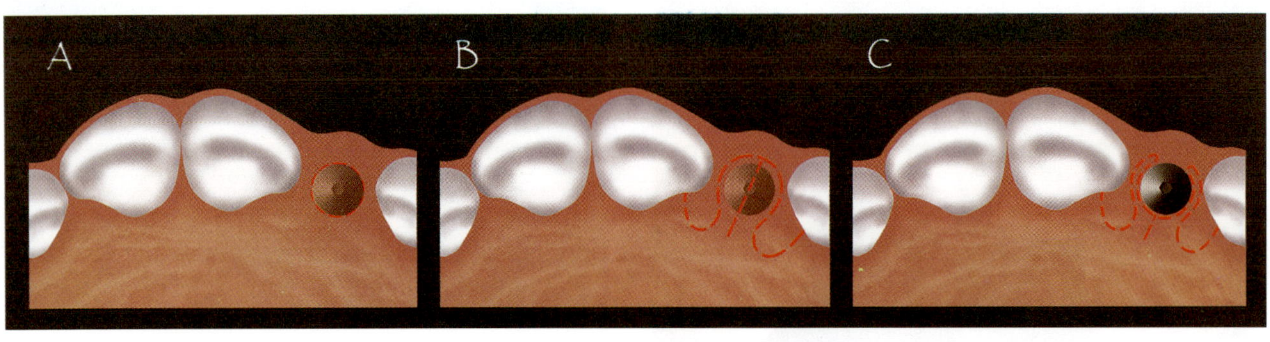

Figure 5.44. **A.** An illustration showing the use of the split-finger method. **B.** An illustration showing the incision design of the split-finger method. **C.** An illustration showing the suturing of the tissues around the healing collars.

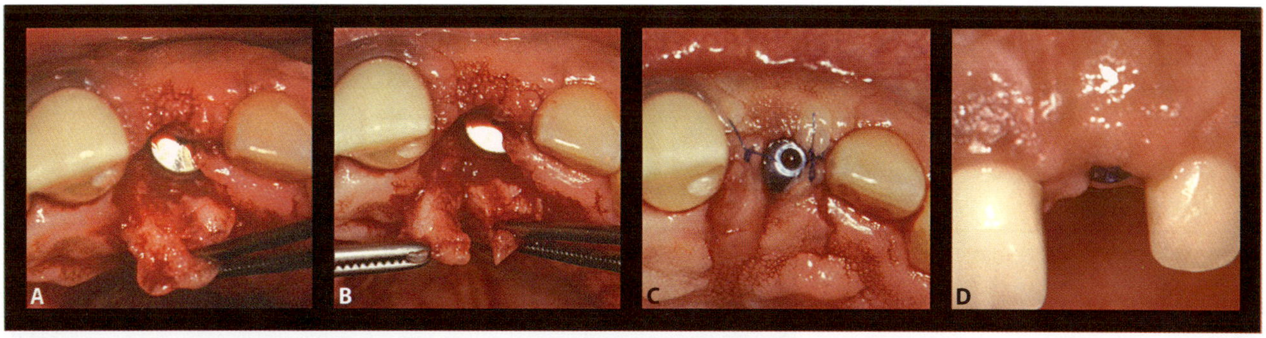

Figure 5.45. **A.** Clinical view of performing the split finger method. Note the palatal finger reflection. **B.** Dividing the palatal finger with a scissor. **C.** The two splits being sutured. **D.** Three weeks' postoperative healing.

method is called palatal sliding strip flap. This flap design helps form the papillae between implants and between natural teeth in the anterior area of the maxilla. The flap is designed and managed so that the palatal-attached mucosa slides in a labial direction to create papillae and at the same time augment the labial ridge.

The procedure entails an incision that allows the dissection of the masticatory mucosa from the underlying bone with a full-thickness sulcular approach in a labiopalatal direction perpendicular to the ridge crest, both on the mesial and distal aspects of the implant. A full thickness horizontal incision is extended from the distal to the mesial on the palatal side comprising approximately two-thirds of the distance between the two teeth. Two incisions, which are parallel to each other, are then made in a labiopalatal direction to create a partial-thickness flap extending in the palate, leaving the periosteum intact. This extension portion is designed into a strip to be located at the mesial aspect of the implant. A partial-thickness horizontal dissection is made to connect the two parallel incisions to form the sliding palatal strip. A final incision dissects the masticatory mucosa from the bone and incorporates the partial-thickness incision into a full-thickness incision in a labial direction.

Once the incisions are made, the partial- and full-thickness flaps are prepared for flap elevation. The partial-full–thickness flap with a strip is raised to uncover the implant. The healing abutment is connected and a semilunar incision is made to the distal, away from the side of the strip. Care must be taken that the semilunar incision is coronal to the cementoenamel junction (CEJ) or the gingival line of the adjacent teeth; otherwise, the healing abutment will displace the flap apically and the final gingival margin will heal apical to the gingival line of the adjacent teeth. The semilunar incision will provide a second strip, which gives two pedicles. The distal pedicle created by the semilunar bevel incision will be rotated 90 degrees in the palatal direction around the healing abutment. The mesial pedicle with the partial-thickness component from the palate will fill the interproximal space. This flap manipulation between the teeth and the healing abutment will allow the reconstruction of two papillae at one time. The buccal soft tissue augmentation is related to the support by the healing abutment and the buccal repositioning of the flap. Simple sutures are used around each newly formed papilla to maintain the flap in position.

In the case of two adjacent implants, the flap design for multiple restorations in the anterior maxilla follows the general principle of a palatal strip of split-thickness tail harvested from the palate, combined with a full-thickness flap displaced in the midpalate toward the sulcus of the adjacent tooth. The difference is the location of the palatal strip and the semilunar incisions. The palatal strip of split-thickness connective tissue tail harvested from the palate must be made between the implants. A full-thickness incision displaced in the midpalatal area dissects the masticatory mucosa toward each adjacent tooth. A final incision dissects the masticatory mucosa from the bone over the ridge crest, creating a full-thickness sulcular incision.

Once the incisions are made, the partial- and full-thickness flaps are prepared for elevation. (See Figures 5.45E–F.) The partial-/full–thickness flap with a strip adjacent to the distal tooth is raised to uncover the implants and their cover screws. The healing abutments are connected, allowing the flap to be sustained on the buccal side. Two semilunar incisions are made toward the contralateral side of the strip. Care must be taken that the semilunar incision is coronal to the CEJ; otherwise, the healing

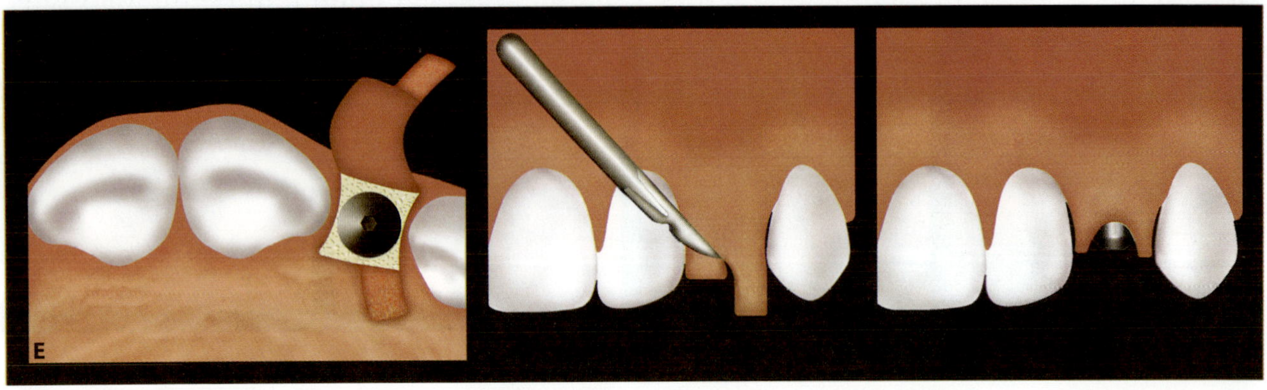

Figure 5.45E. An illustration showing the Adriaenssens technique for second-stage surgery for single-tooth situation.

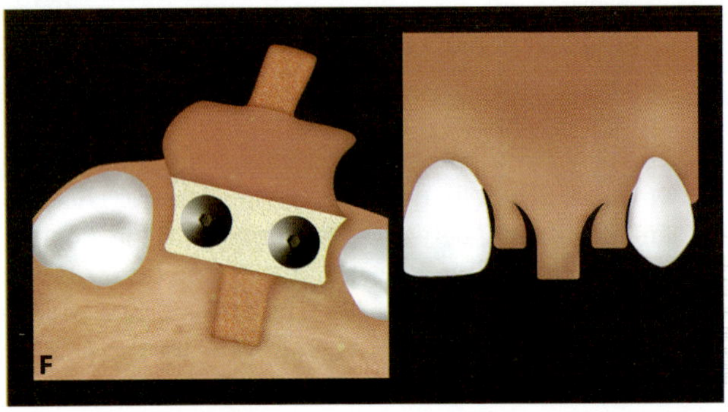

Figure 5.45F. An illustration showing the Adriaenssens technique for second-stage surgery for adjacent multiple teeth situation.

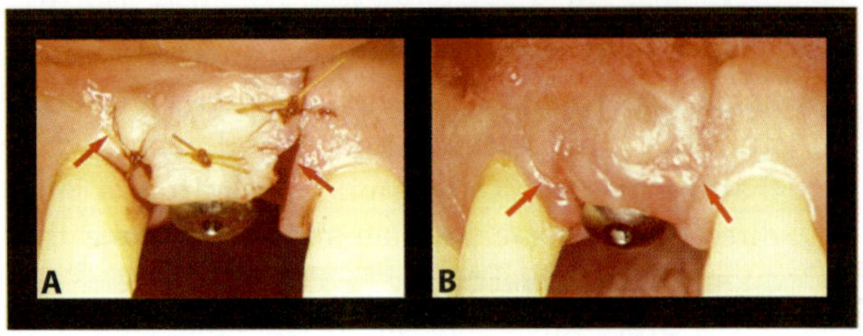

Figure 5.46. **A.** The gap formed between the flap and the wound edges is due to the poor flexibility of the keratinized tissues. **B.** The red arrows pointing at the tissue scar and tag formation due to the improper tissue edges adaptation.

abutment will displace the flap apically. The two semilunar incisions will provide two small pedicles. They are rotated in the palatal direction, each one creating a tissue augmentation in the interproximal space between the tooth and the implant. The palatal strip of partial thickness will be foiled to fill the interproximal space between the two implants. The soft tissues are repositioned and sutured within the pedicles using simple sutures.

The author claimed that the technique appears to have several advantages: (1) minimal surgical trauma; (2) flap nutrition preservation; (3) soft tissue augmentation; (4) formation of papilla-like tissue; and (5) avoidance of a donor site with a second surgical area or multiple surgeries. The residual palatal wounds have healed uneventfully by secondary intention. This modification of the Abrams technique (Becker et al. 1994) has the benefit of increased blood supply, lack of donor site, ability to achieve primary closure, and greater soft tissue thickness in the anterior region of the palate.

6. **Midbuccal Tissue Release:** Because keratinized mucosa lacks elasticity, the adaptation of the mucoperiosteal flap to the sides of the wound edges can be a difficult task. When the tissues are moved from the palatal to the buccal side to allow for tissue bulking, they should be adapted to the wound edges and sutured to the adjacent papillae bilaterally, which is sometimes a difficult task to achieve. (See Figures 5.46A–B.) To allow for bilateral tension-free suturing to the adjacent interproximal papillae, a midbuccal vertical incision might be made in the mucoperiosteal flap of the second-stage surgery. To facilitate suturing to the adjacent papillae, the incision should be as small as possible (i.e., does not exceed 1 mm), and it should be restricted to the keratinized band and not involve any vestibular tissues. The releasing incision allows flexibility of the flap and eliminates the dead space or tissue ledges between the edge of the flap and the adjacent papillary tissues. (See Figures 5.47A–F.) The method has shown highly predictable success rates in stabilizing tissue contours and achieving harmonious margins. (See Figures 5.48A–F and 5.49A–C.)
7. **Using Cosmetic Incisions:** The second-stage surgery is considered the most delicate and influential surgery to the overall esthetic success of implant therapy. Therefore, use maximum care and

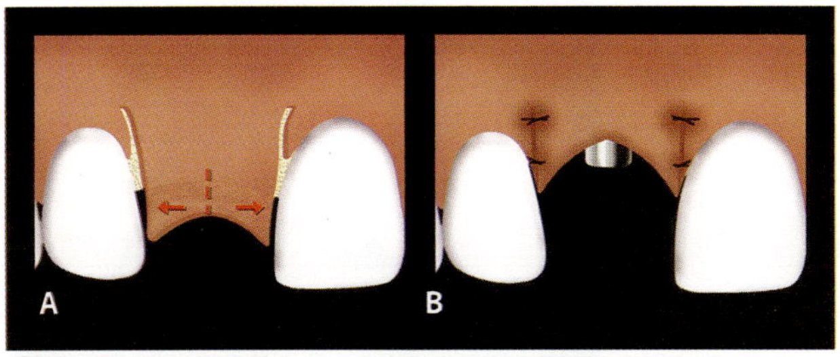

Figure 5.47. **A.** An illustration showing the incision design of the midbuccal release of flap. **B.** An illustration showing the flap suturing.

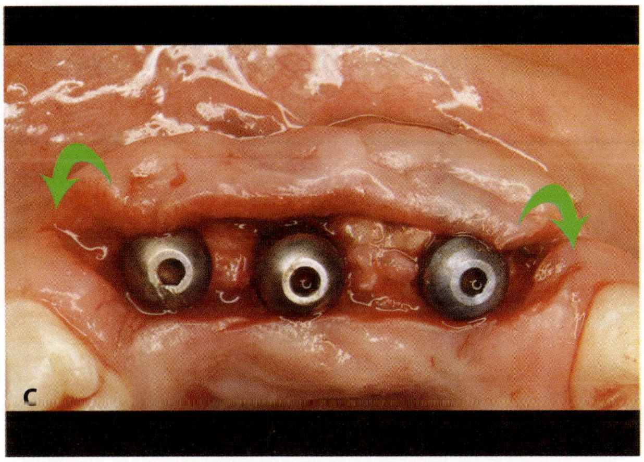

Figure 5.47C. Three implants with the healing collars connected. The soft tissue flap could not be fully adapted to the collars. The green arrows represent the direction of the flaps to be released and sutured.

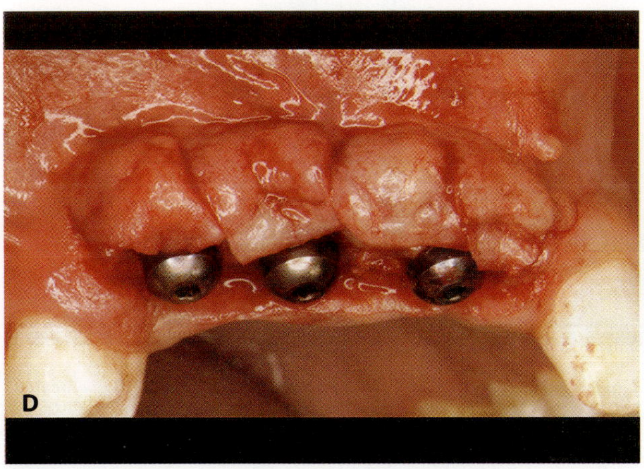

Figure 5.47D. Midbuccal releasing incisions were made.

caution when handling peri-implant soft tissues. When performing only the second-stage surgery, conservative atraumatic cosmetic incisions should be made to achieve optimal healing. It is preferable

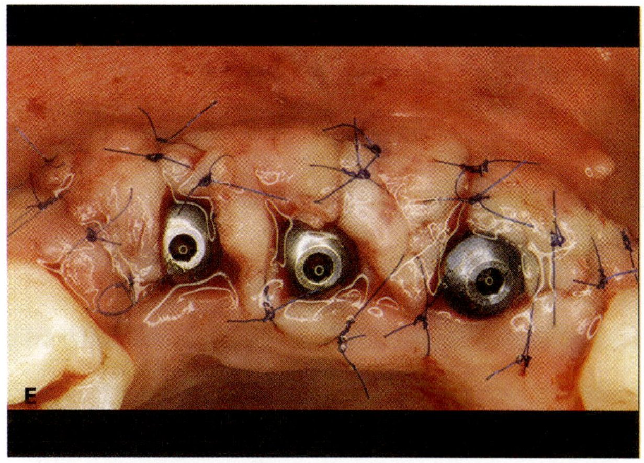

Figure 5.47E. Flap adapted and sutured properly after the midbuccal release.

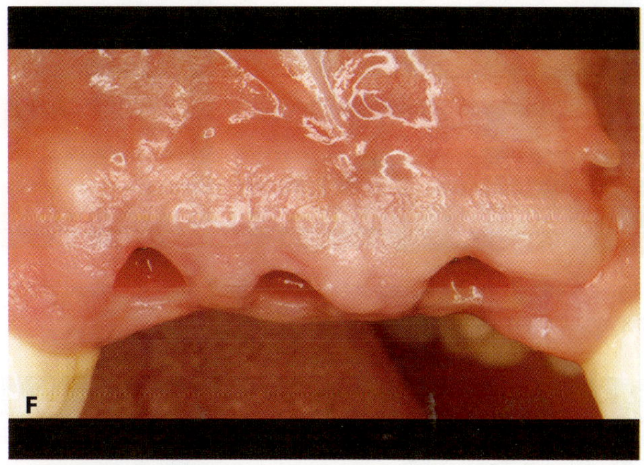

Figure 5.47F. Three weeks' posthealing showing tissue response.

to avoid using perpendicular incisions to the bone; more oblique or horizontal incisions are suggested. Also, 45-degree beveled incisions allow more tissue contact and adaptation between the flap and the adjacent nonflapped tissues, thus reducing the tendency for soft tissue ledge, scar tissues, or tag formation. Using scalpel microblades can provide the clinician with the maximum benefits, and using miniperiosteal elevators elevates the thin tissues with minimal trauma. (See Figure 5.50.)

8. **Overcorrection:** In the science of regenerative implantology, the current conceptual thinking is overdoing, or overcorrection. This means that tissues should be regenerated in excess, to overcome the behavior of the oral tissues whether bone or soft tissue volume is increased. The tissues tend to remodel; or in clinical terms, they shrink. From this perspective, during the second-stage surgery,

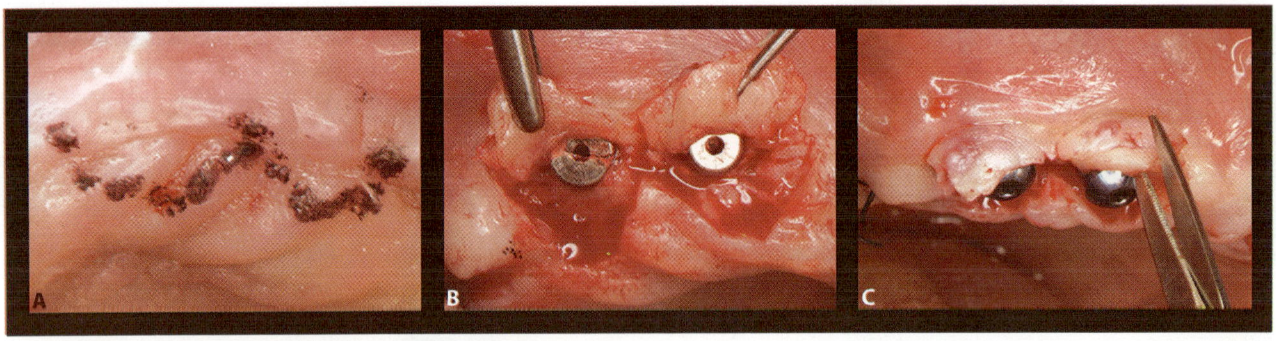

Figure 5.48. **A.** Intraoral view showing the outlines of the second-stage surgical entry in black dots. **B.** Implants exposed. Note the amount of palatal tissue to be moved. **C.** The midbuccal incision release is performed with a scissor.

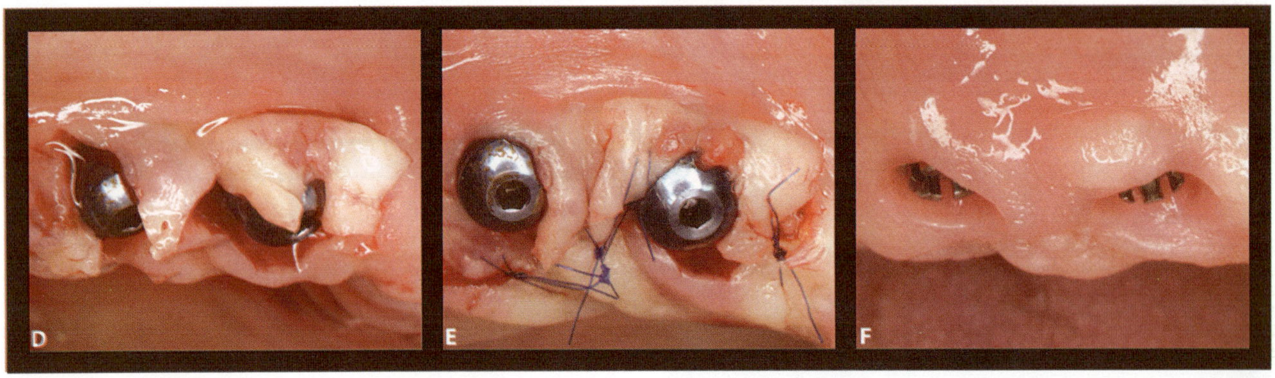

Figure 5.48. **D.** The midbuccal-releasing incisions. **E.** The flap sutured and the papillae are being sutured to the sides of the wound. **F.** Three weeks' post healing showing improved healing result.

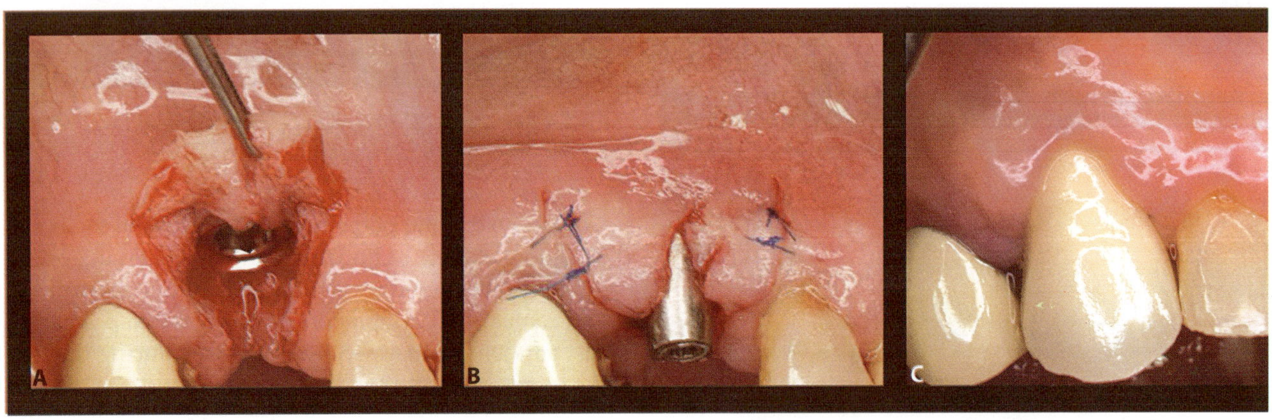

Figure 5.49. **A.** A mucoperiosteal flap is being used to expose the implant. **B.** The midbuccal incision is used and the flap sutured bilaterally. **C.** Three months' postrestorative showing the efficacy of the midbuccal release technique.

any flap design should allow for excess tissue formation. The overcorrection of the soft tissue in the second-stage surgery can be performed via the use of connective tissue grafts, sliding flaps, and rotational flaps. After enough time to allow complete tissue remodeling and stabilization, the undesirable tissue can be excised or trimmed to its optimal size. (See Figure 5.51A.)

9. **Soft Tissue Refining and Profiling:** As a result of the second-stage surgery, soft tissue healing might not be optimized due to numerous reasons, either systemic or local. Even when the previous steps have been taken into consideration, there are other contributing factors to healing, such as the patient's oral habits. The resulting poor healing might be manifested as tissue tags, dimples, roughness,

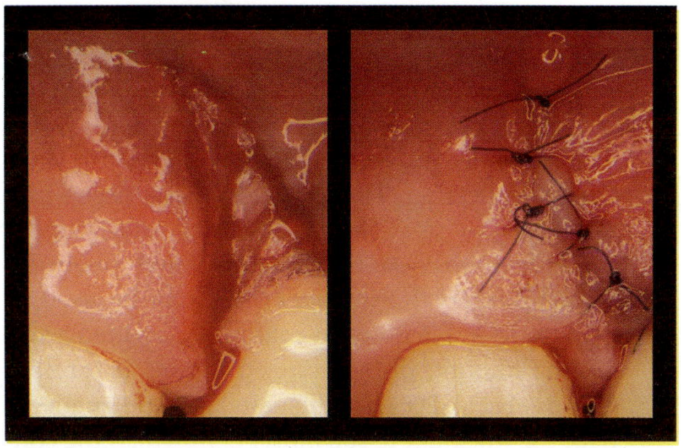

Figure 5.50. A 45-degree beveled incision.

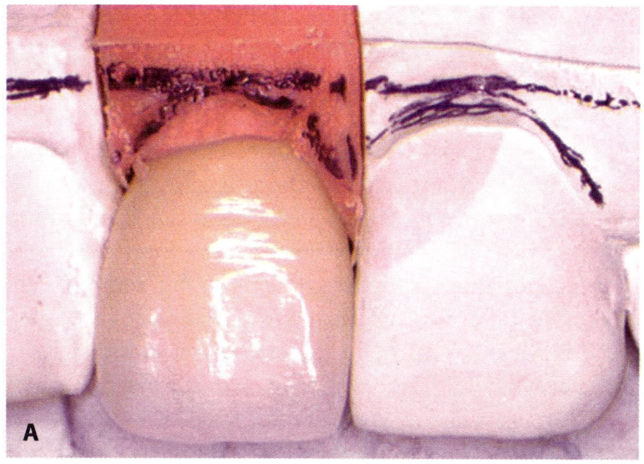

Figure 5.51A. A soft tissue mask on the cast to detect the amount of excess tissue to be removed.

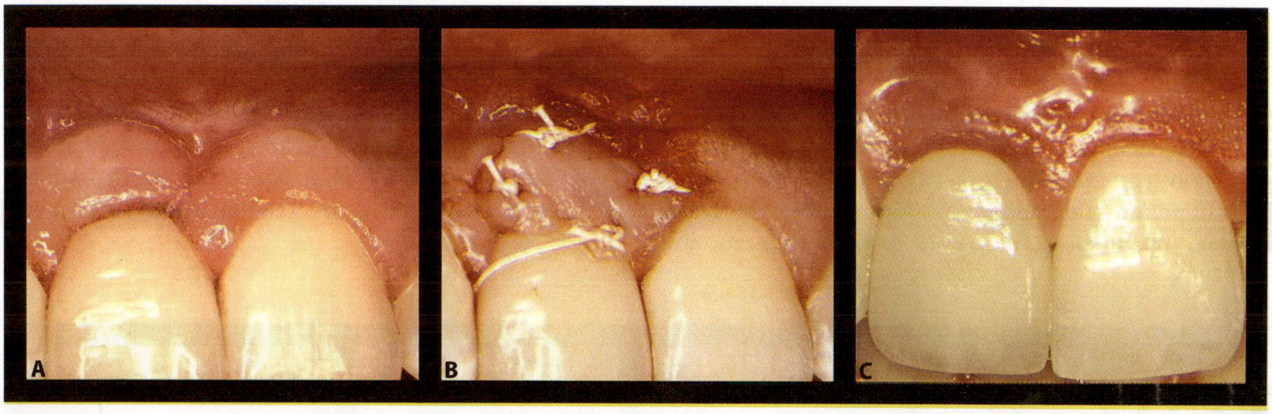

Figure 5.52. **A.** Scar tissue postsecond-stage surgery related to the place of the maxillary right central incisor. **B.** Mini onlay soft tissue graft is used to treat the deficiency. **C.** Three months' postcorrective surgery.

recession, ledges, or scars. Therefore, there is a demand to refine the tissue and eliminate any existing tissue tags or scars that result from the surgical manipulations to achieve a natural looking implant-supported restoration. This treatment step can be called peri-implant tissue refining and profiling.

To overcome any deficiency, and/or to treat some tissue deformity, intraoral plastic periodontal soft tissue surgery is the method of choice when such events occur. The basis of plastic intraoral soft tissue surgery was originally described by Miller (1988) and he was the first to introduce mucogingival surgery, or periodontal plastic surgery. Such surgical procedures are used to correct or eliminate anatomic, developmental, and/or traumatic deformities of the gingival and alveolar mucosa. These surgical procedures are currently applied in conjunction with implant therapy to help achieve an enhanced peri-implant soft tissue appearance. Corrective procedures may involve one or more of the following treatment options:

- Gingival recontouring techniques
- Mini soft tissue grafting to treat soft tissue grooves or deficiencies, as shown in Figures 5.52A–C
- Modifying and expanding the gingival margin with a provisional restoration

Gingival recontouring techniques (Bichacho and Landsberg 1997) require a favorable keratinized tissue condition, in terms of quality and quantity. The techniques include cosmetic laser resurfacing, which is currently used in many of soft tissue procedures to attain a bactericidal effect. It has demonstrated improved homeostasis intraoperatively. This procedure does not induce any postoperative patient discomfort; thus it reduces the need for postoperative medications when compared to procedures performed with a scalpel alone.

Cosmetic laser soft tissue resurfacing is widely used by plastic surgeons because it has been shown to control the depth of tissue removal better than any other traditional method. It allows for precise tissue trimming, offers a bloodless field, and emits less heat to the underlying tissues than do rotary instruments. Troughing or tissue tag removal via laser therapy, provides the minimal removal of gingival tissues during a given therapy. Another laser application, tissue welding, is very useful when primary closure is desirable, such as with grafts. The laser is used at a very low setting and the result is a nearly watertight tissue bond that resists the intrusion of epithelial cells (Hertel et al. 1994, Neill 1997).

Electrosurgical sculpturing is a minor plastic surgical procedure that helps in performing gingivoplasty procedures. Electrosurgery offers many unique, invaluable advantages. Hemostasis obtained with fully rectified cutting current, scar-free healing of electrosurgical wounds by granulation secondary repair as well as by primary intention, the ability to perform precise tissue cutting without the use of manual pressure, and sterilization of the surgical field are especially noteworthy advantages. Atraumatic tissue cleavage and sterilization of the wound eliminate an unfavorable postoperative sequence common to scalpel surgery and contribute to rapid, uneventful postoperative healing. The ability to incise tissue precisely makes possible sophisticated oral surgery procedures that cannot be duplicated safely by scalpel surgery (Oringer 1982). It can be used to treat undesirable gingival contours, provided a sufficient amount of keratinized tissue is present (Choquet et al. 2001). It is usually limited to patients with the thick flat tissue biotype, in which the condition of the soft tissue can withstand further surgical manipulations. Electrosurgery is used when final maturation of the soft tissue around the implant-supported restoration has occurred. Tissue warming due to the heat emitted from the electrodes sometimes delays healing. If it is used at a very low dosage, it can minimize the bleeding and trauma that accompany regular excision methods. However, this method should be used with caution because there is an increased risk of implant de-integration if the electrode contacts the implant surface for long times. (See Figures 5.53A–D and 5.54A–C.)

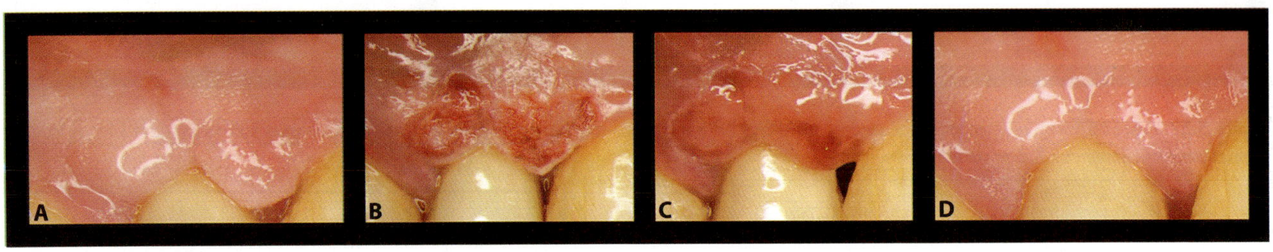

Figure 5.53. **A.** Tissue tags and resultant dimples postsecond-stage surgery. **B.** Surface recontouring using electrosurgery. **C.** Three days' posthealing. **D.** One month posthealing.

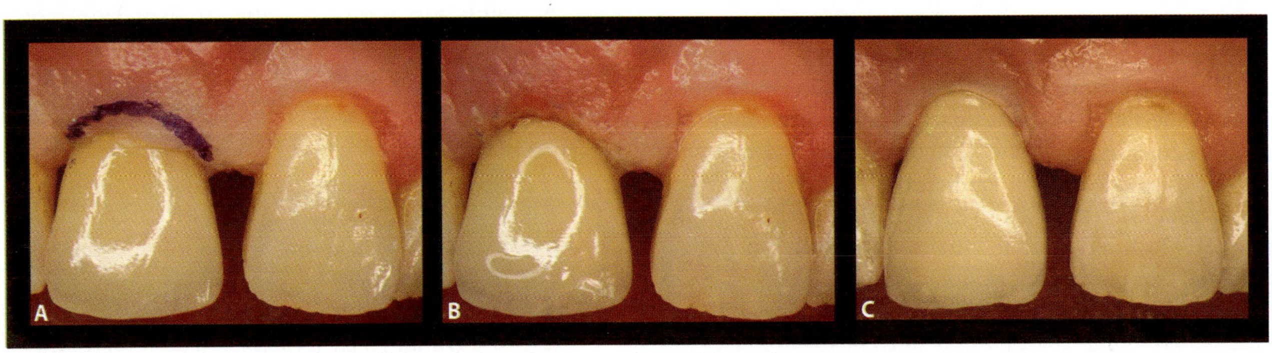

Figure 5.54. **A.** Presurgery clinical picture of excessive tissue margins. **B.** The tissue was excised and trimmed using electrosurgery. **C.** One month posthealing clinical picture.

In gradual tissue expansion, the provisional restoration is considered an important element for reshaping the peri-implant soft tissue after the second-stage surgery. It is considered an important factor responsible for a natural appearance of implant-supported restorations. It stimulates peri-implant tissues to attain the same configuration and dimensions as missing original natural soft tissue contours. After the peri-implant tissues are duplicated on the working cast, envisioned, and carved to the optimal desired configuration, a provisional restoration is fabricated accordingly and transferred to the implant site. The provisional prosthesis is then seated. Digital pressure is exerted to compress the peri-implant tissue in an outward labial direction. Temporary blanching of the soft tissue occurs as a result of the pressure, as shown in Figure 5.55, which changes the soft tissue contours to the future final implant-supported restoration dimension.

10. **Soft Tissue Punching:** Excisional or subtractive soft tissue procedures to uncover the implant fixture were developed for minimally invasive implant installation as well as uncovering in the presence of abundant keratinized gingiva. It maintains the existing soft tissue and its surrounding contours with no flap reflection. The technique entails excising a circular area of the keratinized mucosa on top of the implant cover screw, which makes the technique excisional in nature. The technique has limited indications; it is only indicated when a wide and stable keratinized band is present. It is a simplified clinical technique, less traumatic to the tissues, and does not require an extensive surgical inventory to be applied, as it can be performed with a scalpel, a gum-punching tool, or a diamond bur. Imperfect positioning of the tissue punch may jeopardize the labial tissue contour around the implant fixture, and the attendant subsequent loss of almost 3 to 4 mm of keratinized tissue limits its application in the esthetic zone. Furthermore, tissue punching sometimes involves guesswork in locating the implant head unless the original surgical template is used to locate the implant cover screw. When an implant is placed below the bone crest level, bone contouring may be recommended at the second-stage surgery, because it does not allow complete seating of the prosthetic component. With the punching technique it may be difficult to apply particular bone-contouring concepts. (See Figure 5.56.)

The 10 previous guidelines can be helpful in achieving predictable esthetic results; however the rules cannot be applied in one clinical case. The clinician should be able to select the best of the guidelines to suit the particular clinical situation. For example, in thin-scalloped tissue biotype cases, the bulking of the tissue is valuable in either keratinized or connective tissues. The split-finger method or Adriaenssens and others (1999) method should be used when the papilla is deficient and is to be augmented, while scalloping the tissues can be used only in single-tooth situations. The midbuccal release is very helpful in cases in which the papilla is at its normal level and a well-contoured buccal contour is required; however, an ample amount of keratinized tissue should be available to perform such a method.

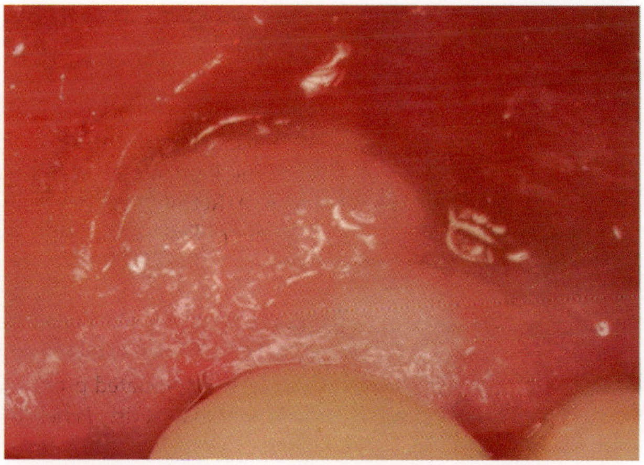

Figure 5.55. Tissue blanching due to the effect of the provisional restoration.

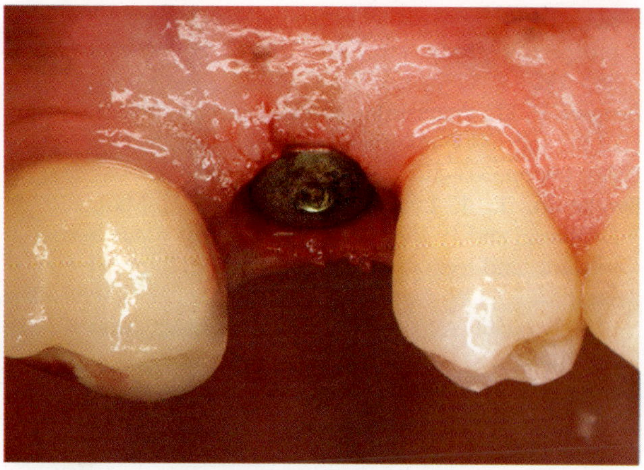

Figure 5.56. The subtractive method of implant exposure.

References

Abrahamsson, I., T. Berglundh, P.O. Glantz, and J. Lindhe. 1998. The mucosal attachment at different abutment: An experimental study in dogs. *J Clin Periodontol*, (25), pp. 721–727.

Abrams, L. 1980. Augmentation of the deformed residual edentulous ridge for fixed prosthesis. *Compend Cont Educ Dept*, (1), pp. 205–213.

Adriaenssens, P., M. Hermans, A. Ingber, et al. 1999. Palatal Sliding Strip Flap: Soft Tissue Management to Restore Maxillary Anterior Esthetics at Stage 2 Surgery: A Clinical Report. *Int J Oral Maxillofac Implants*, 14, pp. 30–36.

Akagawa, Y., T. Takata, T. Matsumoto, H. Nikai, and H. Tsuru. 1989. Correlation between clinical and histological evaluations of the peri-implant gingival around single crystal sapphire endosseous implant. *J Oral Rehabil*, (16), pp. 581–587.

Alberktsson, T., and H.A. Hansson. 1986. An ultrastructural characterization of the interface between bone and sputtered titanium or stainless steel surfaces. *Biomaterials*, (7), pp. 201–205.

Allen, E.P. 1993. Pedicle flaps, grafts, and connective tissue grafts in aesthetic treatment of gingival recession. *Pract Periodont Aesthet Dent*, (5), pp. 29–38.

Allen, E.P., C.S. Gainza, G.C. Farthing, and D.A. Newbold. 1985. Improved technique for localized ridge augmentation. A Report of 21 cases. *J Periodontol*, (56), pp. 195–199.

Atwood, D.A. 1963. Postextraction changes in the adult mandible as illustrated by microradiographs of midsagittal sections and serial cephalometric roentgenograms. *J Prosthet Dent*, (13), pp. 810–842.

Bahat, O., and M. Handelsman. 1991. Periodontal reconstructive flaps, Classification and surgical considerations. *Int J Periodontics Restorative Dent*, (11):481–487.

Bao, J.Y. 1997. Comparative bone healing. *J Biomater Sci Polym*, (8), pp. 517–532.

Becker, W., and B. Becker. 1996. Flap designs for minimization of recession adjacent to maxillary anterior sites, a clinical study, *Int J Oral Maxillofac Implants*, (11), pp. 46–54.

Becker, W., B.E. Becker, G. Polizzi, and C. Berstrom. 1994. Autogeneous bone grafting of bone defects adjacent to implants placed into immediate extraction sockets in patients: a prospective study. *Int J Oral Maxillofac Implants*, 9, pp. 389–396.

Bengazi, F., J.L. Wennstrom, and U. Lekholm. 1996. Recession of the soft tissue margin at oral implants. *Clin Oral Implant Res*, (7), pp. 303–310.

Berglundh, T., J. Lindhe, I. Ericsson, C.P. Marinello, B. Lijenberg, and P. Thomsen. 1991. The soft tissue barrier at implants and teeth. *Clin Oral Implant Res*, (2), pp. 81–90.

Berman, G.R., J.W. Rapley, W.W. Hallmonn, et al. 1993. The peri- implant sulcus. *Int J Oral Maxilofac Implants*, (8), pp. 273–280.

Bichacho, N., and C.J. Landsberg. 1997. Single implants restoration prosthetically induced soft tissue topography, *Pract Periodontics Aesthet Dent* 9, pp. 745–752.

Block, M.S., and J.N. Kent. 1995. *Endosseous Implant for Maxillofacial Reconstruction*. Philadelphia: W.B. Saunders.

Boss, J.H., I. Shajrawi, and D.G. Mendes. 1994. The nature of the bone-implant interface. *Med Prog Technol*, (20), pp. 199–142.

Braganza, A., N. Bissada, C. Hatch, et al. 2005. The effect of non-steroidal anti-inflammatory drugs on bleeding during periodontal surgery. *J Periodontol*, 76, pp. 1154–1160.

Bragger, U., L. Pasquali, and K.S. Kornman. 1988. Remodeling of interdental alveolar bone after periodontal flap procedures assessed by means of computer-assisted ensitometric image analysis (CADIA). *J Clin Periodontol*, (15), pp. 558–564.

Bragger, U., U. Hafeli, B. Huber, et al. 1998. Evaluation of post-surgical crestal bone levels adjacent to non-submerged dental implants. *Clinl Oral Implant Res*, (9), pp. 218–224.

Branemark, P.I., G.A. Zarb, and T. Albrektsson, Eds. 1985. Tissue-integrated Prostheses: *Osseointegration in Clinical Dentistry*. Chicago: Quintessence.

Branemark, P.I., B.O. Hansson, R. Adel, et al. 1997. Osseointegrated implants in the treatment of the edentulous Jaw. Experience from the 10-year period. *Scand J Plastic Reconstr Surg*, 11 (Suppl. 16), pp. 1–132.

Brunski, J.B., et al. 1979. The influence of functional use of endosseous dental implants on the tissue-implant interface. II. Clinical aspects. *J Dent Res*, (58), pp. 1970–1980.

Buser, D., H.P. Weber, and N.P. Long. 1990. Tissue integration of non-submerged implants: One-year results of a prospective study with 100 ITI hollow-screw and hollow cylinder implants. *Clin Oral Impl Res*, (1), pp. 33–40.

Buser, D., R.K. Schenk, S. Steinemann, et al. 1991. Influence of surface characteristics on bone integration of titanium implants. A histomorpho metric study in miniature pigs. *J Biomend Mater Res*, (25), pp. 889–902.

Carlsson, G.E., H. Thilander, and G. Hedegard. 1967. Histologic changes in the upper alveolar process after extractions with or without insertion of an immediate full denture. *Acta Odontol Scand*, (25), pp. 1–31.

Casino, A.J., P. Harrison, D.P. Tarnow, et al. 1997. The influence of type of in incision on the success rate of implant integration at stage II uncovering surgery. *J Oral Maxillofac Surg*, (55), pp. 31–37.

Chee, W.W.L., and T.E. Donovan. 1995. Treatment planning and soft tissue management for optimal implant aesthetics, *Ann Acad Med Singapore*, (24), pp. 113–117.

Chee, W.W.L., G.C. Cho, and T.E. Donovan. 1997. Restoration of the anterior edentulous space. *J Calif Dent Assoc*, (25), pp. 381–385.

Choquet, V., M. Hermans, P. Adriaenssens, et al. 2001. Clinical and Radiographic Evaluation of the Papilla Level Adjacent to Single-Tooth Dental Implants. A Retrospective Study in the Maxillary Anterior Region. *J Periodontol*, 72, pp. 1364–1371.

Cohen, E.S. 1994. *Atlas of Cosmetic and Reconstructive Periodontal Surgery, 2nd ed.* Baltimore, MD: Lea and Febiger, pp. 84–98.

Corn, H. 1973. Mucogingival surgery and associated problems. In: Goldman, H.M., and Cohen, D.W., Eds. *Periodontal Therapy, 5th ed.* St Louis: Mosby, pp. 638–751.

Cranin, A.N., M. Klein, A. Sirakian, et al. 1991. Comparison of incisions made for the placement of dental implants. *J Dent Res*, (70), p. 279.

Croll, B.M. 1989. Emergence profiles in natural tooth contour. Part I: Photographic observations. *J Prosthet Dent*, (62), pp. 374–379.

Cruse, P., and R. Foorde. 1980. The epidemiology of wound infection, *Surg Clin NA*, 60, (1), pp. 27–40.

Dahlberg, W.H. 1969. Incisions and suturing. Some basic considerations about each in periodontal flap surgery. *Dent Clin North AM*, (13), p. 149.

Dahlin, C., A. Lindhe, J. Gottlow, and S. Nyman. 1988. Healing of bone defects by guided tissue regeneration. *Plast Reconstr Surg*, (8), 1, p. 672.

Dahlin, C., P. Alberius, and A. Linde. 1991. Osteopromotion for cranioplasty. An experimental study in rats using a membrane technique. *J Neurosurg*, (74), p. 487.

Dineen, P. 1997. The effect of suture material in the development of vascular infection. *Vasc Surg II(I)*, pp. 29–32, January/February.

Dordick, B., J.G. Coslet, and J.S. Seibert. 1976. Clinical evaluation of free autogenous grafts placed on alveolar bone. Part I. Clinical predictability. *J Periodontol*, (47), pp. 559–567.

Douglass, G.L. 2005. Alveolar ridge preservation at tooth extraction. *J Calif Dent Assoc*, 33, pp. 223–223.

Egelberg, J. 1966. The blood vessels of the dento-gingival junction. *J Periodontal Res*, 1 (3), pp. 163–179.

El Askary, A.S. 1999. Esthetic considerations in anterior single tooth replacement. *Implant Dent*, (8), pp. 61–67.

El Askary, A.S. 2000. Multifaceted aspects of esthetic implantology. *Implant Dent*, (10), pp. 182–191.

El Askary, A.S. 2002. The use of connective tissue grafts to enhance esthetics. *J Prosthet Dent*, (87), pp. 129–132.

Elden, A., and B. Mejchar. 1963. Plastic surgery of the vestibulum in periodontal therapy. *Int Dent* J, (13), p. 593.

Esposito, M., J.M. Hirsch, U. Lekholm, et al. 1998. Biological factors contributing to failures of osseointegrated oral implants. I. Success criteria and epidemiology. *Eur J Oral Sci*, (106), pp. 527–551.

Evian, C.I., H. Corn, and E.S. Rosenberg. 1985. Retained interdental procedures for maintaining anterior esthetics. *Compend Contin Educ Dent*, (1), pp. 58–65.

Fugazotto, P.A., S. DePaoli, and S.P. Benefenati. 1993. Flap design considerations in the placement of single maxillary anterior implants: Clinical report. *Implant Dent*, (2), pp. 93–96.

Fugazzotto, P.A. 1998. Flap designs and suturing techniques related to anterior single tooth implant procedures. *Dent Implantol Update*, 9, (2), Feb.

Fugazzotto, P. 1999. Maintenance of soft tissue closure following guided bone regeneration; technical considerations and report of 723 Cases. *J Periodontol*, (70), pp. 1085–1097.

Garber, D.A. 1981. The edentulous ridge and fixed prosthodontics. *Compend Contin Educ Dent*, (2), p. 212.

Garretto, L.P., J. Chen, J.A. Parr, et al. 1995. Remodeling dynamics of bone supporting rigidly fixed titanium implants. A histomorphometric comparison in four species including human, *Implant Dent*, (4), pp. 235–243.

Grunder, U. 2000. Stability of the mucosal topography around single-tooth implants and adjacent teeth: One-year results. *Int J Periodontics Restorative Dent*, (20), pp. 11–17.

Haeri, A, and F.G. Serio. 1999. Mucoginigval surgical procedures: A review of the literature. *Quintessence Int*, (30), pp. 475–483.

Hammack, B.L., and W.F. Enneking. 1960. Comparative vascularization of autogenous and homogenous bone transplants, *J Bone Joint Surg*, (42A), p. 811.

Heller, A.L., R.L. Heller, G. Cook, et al. 2000. Soft tissue management techniques for implant dentistry: a clinical guide. *J Oral Implantol*, 26, pp. 91–103.

Hertel, R.C., P.A. Blijdorp, and D.L. Baker. 1993. A preventive mucosal flap technique for use in implantology. *Int J Oral Maxillofac Implants*, (8), pp. 452–458.

Hertel, R.C., P.A. Blijdorp, W. Kalk, and D.L. Baker. 1994. Stage 2 surgical techniques in Endosseous Implantation. *Int J Oral Maxillofac Implants*, (9), pp. 273–278.

Howes, R., J.M. Bowness, G.R. Grotendorst, G.R. Martin, and A.H. Reddi. 1988. Platelet derived growth factor enhances demineralized bone matrix and induces cartilage and bone formation. *Calcif Tissue Int*, (42), pp. 34–38.

Hunt, B.W. 1996. Effect of flap design on healing and osseointegration of dental implants. *Int J Periodontics Restorative Dent*, (16), pp. 582–593.

Hurzeler, M.B., and W. Dietmar. 1996. Peri-implant tissue management: Optimal timing for an aesthetic result. *Pract Periodont Aesthet Dent*, (8), pp. 857–869.

James, W.C., and W.T. McFall. 1978. Placement of free gingival grafts on denuded alveolar bone. Part I: Clinical evaluations. *J Periodontol*, (49), p. 283.

Johnson, R.H. 1976. Basic flap management, *Dent Clin North Am*, (20), p. 3.

Kan, J.Y., G. Shiotsu, K. Rungcharassaeng, and J.L. Lozada. 2000. Maintaining and attenuating periodontal tissues for aesthetic implant placement. *J Oral Implantol*, 26, pp. 35–41.

Kenley, R., L. Marden, T. Turek, L. Jin, E. Ron, and J.O. Hollinger. 1994. Osseous regeneration. *J Biomend Mater Res*, (28), pp. 1139–1147.

Khoury, F., and A. Happe. 2000. The palatal subepithelial connective tissue flap method for soft tissue management to cover maxillary defects: A clinical report. *Int J Oral Maxillofac Implants*, 15, pp. 415–418.

Kirkland, O. 1936. Surgical flap and semilunar technique in periodontal surgery. *Dent Digest*, (42), p. 125.

Knox, R., R. Caudill, and R. Meffert. 1991. Histologic evaluation of dental endosseous implants placed in surgically created extraction defects. *Int J Periodontics Restorative Dent*, (11), pp. 365–375.

Lam, R.V. 1960. Contour changes of the alveolar process following extraction. *J Prosthet Dent*, (10), pp. 25–32.

Landsberg, C.J. 1997a. Socket seal surgery combined with mediate implant placement: A novel approach for single-tooth replacement. *Int J Periodontics Restorative Dent*, (17), pp. 141–49.

Landsberg, C.J. 1997b. Chirurgischer Verschluss der Alveole mitunmittelbarer Implantation: Ein neuer Ansatz für das Einzelzahnimplantat. *Int J Parodontol Rest Zahnheilkd*, 17, 133–141.

Landsberg, C.J., and N. Bichacho. 1994. A modified surgical/prosthetic approach for optimal single implant supported crown. Part I: The socket seal surgery. *Pract Periodont Aesthet Dent*, (6), pp. 11–17.

Langer, B. 1994. Spontaneous in situ gingival augmentation. *Int J Periodontics Restorative Dent*, (14), pp. 525–535.

Langer, B., and L. Calagna. 1980. Subepithelial connective tissue graft. *J Prosthet Dent*, 44, pp. 363–367.

Langer, B., and L. Calagna. 1982. The subepithelial connective tissue graft. A new approach to the enhancement of anterior cosmetics. *Int J Periodontics Restorative Dent*, (2), pp. 22–33.

Langer, B., and L. Langer. 1985. The subepithelial connective tissue graft technique for root coverage. *J Periodontol*, (56), pp. 715–720.

Langer, B., and L. Langer. 1990. The overlapped flap: A surgical modification for implant fixture installation. *Int J Periodontics Restorative Dent*, (10), pp. 209–216.

Lazara, R.J. 1993. Managing the soft tissue margin: The key to implant aesthetics. *Pract Periodont Aesthet Dent*, (5), pp. 81–87.

Male, A.J., J. Gasser, R.J. Fonseca, et al. 1983. Comparison of only autogenous and allogenic bone grafts to the maxilla in primates, *J Oral Maxillofac Surg*, (42), pp. 487–499.

McKinney, Jr., R.V. 1991. Endosteal Dental Implants. In: Shelton, D.W, Ed. *Basic Surgical Principles for Implantology*. St. Louis: Mosby Yearbook, pp. 75–87.

Miller, P.D. 1988. Regenerative and reconstructive periodontal plastic surgery. *Dent Clin North Am*, (32), pp. 287–306.

Misch, C.E. 1990. Progressive bone loading. *Pract Period Esthet Dent*, 20, pp. 27–30.

Misch, C.E., F.D. Misch, and C.M. Misch. 1999. A modified socket seal surgery with composite graft approach. *J Oral Implantol*, (4), pp. 244–250.

Misch, C.E., K. Al Shammari, and H.L. Wang. 2004. Creation of Inter-implant Papillae Through a Split-Finger Technique. *Implant Dent*, 13, pp. 20–27.

Moberg, L.E., P.A. Kondell, L. Kullman, A. Heimdahl, and G.W. Gyniher. 1999. Evaluation of single-tooth restorations on ITI dental implants. A prospective study of 29 patients. *Clin Oral Implants Res*, 10, pp. 45–53.

Moy, P.K., M. Weinlaendes, and E.B. Kenny. 1989. Soft tissue modifications of surgical techniques for placement and uncovering of osseointegrated implants. *Dent Clin North Am*, 33, pp. 665–681.

Nabers, J. 1966. Free gingival grafts. *Periodontics*, (4), pp. 243–245.

Neale, D., and W.W.L. Chee. 1994. Development of soft tissue emergence profile: A technique. *J Prosthet Dent*, (71), pp. 364–368.

Neill, M.E. 1997. Clinical efficacy of the Nd-YAG laser for combination periodontitis therapy. *Pract Periodont Aesthet Dent*, 9, (Suppl 6), pp. 1–5.

Nobuto, T., F. Suwa, T. Kono, et al. 2005. Microvascular Response in the Periosteum Following Mucoperiosteal Flap Surgery in Dogs: 3-Dimensional Observation of an Angiogenic Process. *J Periodontol*, 76, pp. 1339–1345.

Nyeiva, R., K. Shammari, F. Nociti, et al. 2005. Effects of Vitamin-B Complex Supplementation on Periodontal Wound Healing. *J Periodontol*, 76, pp. 1084–1091.

Oringer, M.J. 1982. Broader horizons and indications for use of electrosurgery in oral surgery. *Dent Clin North Am.*, Oct, 26, (4), pp. 729–44.

Palacci, P. 1995. Peri-implant soft tissue management: Papilla regeneration technique. In: Palacci, P., Ericsson, I., Engstrand, P., et al. Eds. *Optimal Implant Positioning and Soft Tissue Management for the Branemark System*. Chicago: Quintessence, pp. 59–70.

Palacci, P. 1996. Optimal implant positioning and soft-tissue considerations. *Oral Maxillofac Surg Clin North Am*, (8), pp. 445–452.

Pennel, B.M., K.O. King, M.N. Wilderman, and J.M. Barron. 1967. Repair of the alveolar process following osseous surgery. *J Periodontol*, (28), pp. 426–431.

Pietrokovski, J., and M. Massler. 1967. Alveolar ridge resorption following tooth extraction, *J Prosthet Dent*, (17), pp. 21–27.

Potashnick, S.R. 1998. Soft tissue modeling for the esthetic single-tooth implant restoration. *J Esthet Dent*, (10), pp. 121–131.

Roberts, E.W., P.K. Turley, N. Brezneak, et al. 1987. Bone physiology and metabolism. *J Calif Dent Assoc*, (15), pp. 54–61.

Roman, G. 2001. Influence of Flap Design on Peri-implant Interproximal Crestal Bone Loss Around Single-tooth Implants. *Int Oral Maxillofac Implants*, 16, pp. 61–67.

Sadig, W., and K. Almas. 2004. Risk factors and management of dehiscent wounds in implant dentistry. *Implant dent*, 13, pp. 140–147.

Scharf, D.R., and D.P. Tarnow. 1992. Modified roll technique for localized alveolar ridge augmentation. *Int J Periodontics Restorative Dent*, (12), pp. 415–425.

Scharf, D.R., and D.P. Tarnow. 1993. The effect of crestal versus mucobuccal incisions on the success rate of implant osseointegration. *Int J Oral Maxillofac Implants*, (8), pp. 187–190.

Schultze-Mosgau, S., M.B. Blatz, F. Wehrhan, et al. 2005. *Principles and mechanisms of peri-implant soft tissue healing*. Quintessence Int., 36, (10), pp. 759–69.

Seibert, J.S. 1983. Reconstruction of deformed, partially edentulous ridge, using full thickness onlay grafts. Part I. Technique and wound healing. *Compendium*, (4), pp. 437–453.

Seibert, J.S. 1990. Surgical preparation for fixed and removable prosthesis. In: Genco, R.J., Goldman, H.M., and Cohen, D.W., Eds. *Contemporary Periodontics*. St. Louis: Mosby, pp. 637–652.

Seibert, J. 1993. Reconstruction of the partially edentulous ridge: Gateway to improved prosthetics and superior aesthetics. *Peract Periodont Aesthet Dent*, (5), pp. 47–55.

Seibert, J.S., and H. Salama. 1996. Alveolar ridge preservation and reconstruction. *Periodontol 2000*, (6), pp. 69–84.

Sennerby, L., P. Thomsen, and L.E. Ericson. 1993. Early bone tissue response to titanium implant inserted in rabbit cortical bone. I. Light microscopic observations. *J Mat Sci Mat Med*, (4), pp. 240–250.

Shulman, J. 1996. Clinical evaluation of an acellular dermal allograft for increasing the zone of attached gingival. *Pract Periodont Aesthet Dent*, (8), pp. 203–208.

Silverstein, L.H., and M.D. Lefkove. 1994. The use of the subepithelial connective tissue graft to enhance both the aesthetics and periodontal contours surrounding dental implants. *J Oral Implantol*, (2), pp. 135–138.

Silverstein, L., M. Lefkove, and J. Garnick. 1994. The use of free gingival soft tissue to improve the implant/soft-tissue interface. *J Oral Implantol*, 20, (1), pp. 36–40.

Small, P.N., and D.P. Tarnow. 2000. Gingival recession around implants: A 1-year longitudinal prosoective study. *Int J Oral Maxillofac Implants*, (15), pp. 527–532.

Stauts, B. 1991. The anterior single-tooth implant restoration. *J Calif Dent Assoc*, (20), pp. 35–40.

Strid, K.G. 1985. Radiographic procedures. In: Branemark, P.I., Zarb, K.G., and Albrektsson, T., Eds. *Tissue Integrated Prostheses. Osseointegration in Clinical Dentistry*. Chicago: Quintessence.

Tarnow, D.P., R.N. Eskow, and J. Zamok. 1996. Aesthetics and implant dentistry. *Periodontol 2000*, (11), pp. 85–94.

Van Beurden, H.E., P.A. Snoek, J.W. Von den Hoff, et al. 2005. Dynamic protein expression patterns during intraoral wound healing in the rat. *Eur J Oral Sci*, Apr, 113, (2), pp. 153–8.

Van Winkle, Jr., W., and J.C. Hastings. 1972. Considerations in the choice of suture material for various tissues, *Surg Gyn and Obs*, 135, pp. 113–126, July.

Von Rehrman, A. 1936. Eine Methode zur Schliessung von Keiferhohlen Perforationen. *Dtsch Zahnaerzth Wochen-Schr*, (39), p. 1137.

Weber, H.P., D. Buser, K. Donath, et al. 1996. Comparison of healed tissues adjacent to submerged and non-submerged unloaded titanium dental implants. A histometric study in beagle dogs. *Clin Oral Implant Res*, (7), pp. 11–19.

Wennstrom, J.L. 1996. Mucogingival therapy. *Ann Periodontol*, (1), pp. 671–701.

Wilderman, M.N. 1964. Exposure of bone in periodontal surgery. *Dent Clin North Am*, (3), pp. 23–36.

Williamas, D.F. 1987. Bone healing processes. *J Bio Eng*, (1), pp. 231–245.

Zola, M.A. 1972. Methods of designing, elevating and suturing the intra oral flap. *Oral Implantol*, 3, pp. 5–18.

Chapter 6
Immediate Esthetic Implant Therapy

Abd El Salam El Askary

The high clinical success rates that have been reported when implants placed in standard situations have encouraged efforts to improve esthetic success, especially for implants that are placed in more demanding esthetic situations. One of these improvements is the procedure for immediate tooth replacement with dental implants in fresh extraction sockets. Although the first clinical procedures for placing implants immediately following tooth removal were described long ago, it is only recently that the details of such clinical approaches have been studied thoroughly (Hammerle et al. 2004).

Immediate esthetic implant therapy has a highly pronounced value. It has been developed to save time and preserve the condition of the alveolar ridge by avoiding postextraction bone resorption, thus maintaining original alveolar crest width and height, reducing surgical procedures and treatment time, and offering enhanced esthetic results. Paolantonio and others (2001) recently suggested that the placement of implants in fresh extraction sockets would prevent postextraction bone resorption and hence maintain the original shape of the ridge. They stated that early implantation may preserve the alveolar anatomy and that the placement of a fixture in a fresh extraction socket may help to maintain the osseous crest structure. Findings reported from a clinical study by Botticelli and others (2004) failed to support this hypothesis.

An animal study (Araujo et al. 2005) that focused on determining the dimensional alterations of the alveolar ridge following implant placement in fresh extraction sockets using beagle dogs stated that placing an implant in the fresh extraction site obviously failed to prevent the remodeling that occurred in the walls of the socket. The resulting height of the buccal and lingual walls at three months was similar at implant and edentulous sites, and the vertical bone level change was more pronounced at the buccal than the lingual aspect of the ridge. Also, the height of the buccal hard tissue wall was reduced considerably more than that of the lingual wall of the same extraction socket. This was due to either the early disappearance of the bundle bone or the delicate nature of the buccal bone rather than the lingual bone wall of the socket.

Because the implant can be seated according to the existing natural tooth angulation, this minimizes the possibility for injury of the anatomical landmarks. This also limits postdrilling bone resorption, thus reducing heat generation, which in turn favors marginal soft tissue stability around dental implant-supported restorations. The overall procedure has proven to have a positive psychological impact on the patient (Gelb 1993, Cornelini et al. 2000, Kan and Rungcharassaeng 2000).

Immediate implant placement offers success rates that are strongly evidenced in the literature; results are equal to that of the delayed implant placement modes (Becker 2005, Meredith et al. 1996). There are some clinical factors that should be considered prior to selecting an immediate implant placement protocol versus the other clinical approaches, such as: (1) bone topography, (2) level of crestal and interproximal bone, (3) smile line, (4) condition of the gingival tissues, (5) pathological and morphological condition of the alveolar socket, (6) soft tissue biotype, (7) the need for preservation of interdental papilla, (8) the need to prevent alveolar ridge resorption, and (9) patient demands.

However, certain clinical requirements should be fulfilled to attain high success rates for immediate implant therapy, such as: (1) absence of any frank active infection, (2) good mechanical anchorage and primary stability of the implant fixture within the alveolar socket, (3) atraumatic removal of the unsalvageable tooth, (4) preservation of the labial plate of bone, (5) use of the appropriate implant design that corresponds to the socket's configuration, and (6) proper implant position in terms of angulation and position.

These requirements are important not only to achieve functional success, but also esthetic success. This is backed by strong literature support that indicates the high success rate of dental implant placement in the esthetic zone (Hammerle et al. 2004, Gelb 1993, Cornelini et al. 2000, Kan and Rungcharassaeng 2000). The basic therapeutic protocol of immediate implant installation entails careful patient selection, which is a key factor in achieving a successful clinical outcome, depending on individual circumstances such as medical and dental histories. After patient selection, clinical documentation such as photographs, study casts, and periapical and panoramic radiographs (if necessary) might be made; in critical conditions a computerized tomography of the proposed implant sites may be created (Becker 2005).

Reasons for tooth extraction include, but are not limited to, insufficient crown-to-root ratios, remaining root length, periodontal attachment levels, periodontal health of teeth adjacent to the proposed implant sites, severe subgingival caries, root fractures with large endodontic posts, root resorption, teeth with deep furcation involvement that is being considered as an abutment for fixed partial dentures, and questionable teeth in need of endodontic retreatment. Usually teeth requiring root amputations, hemi-sections, or advanced periodontal procedures have questionable prognosis, and patients should be given the implant option and information on long-term success rates before these procedures are implemented. Similarly, nonvital teeth fractured at the gingival margin with roots shorter than 13 mm should be considered for implants. However, clinicians are urged to remember that dental implants are a method for restoring missing teeth, not the teeth that are not yet missing.

Atraumatic extraction of the unsalvageable tooth is intraoperative. The careful removal of the tooth from the alveolar socket is highly important, and preserving the labial plate becomes a priority. Minimized buccolingual luxations, controlled hand motion, and the use of the periotomes to disrupt the periodontal membrane are all precautions that must be taken to remove the tooth while preserving the labial plate of bone. There is a tremendous deference between installing dental implants immediately in a preserved labial plate socket and in a socket that has lost its labial plate. The latter mandates further complicated flap design to perform regenerative bone grafting therapy. (See Figure 6.1.)

After tooth removal, a curette or an explorer is used to explore the location of the buccal plate and confirm its integrity. Socket curettage and cleaning is then followed by drilling to allow the placement of the fixture at a minimum of 3 mm beyond the socket apex to allow for primary stabilization. Implant stability can be verified using resonance frequency analysis. This method requires placing an electronic transducer onto the implant head or prosthetic abutment with a retaining screw, and passing a low-voltage current through the transducer. The current is not detected by the patient. Resistance to vibration of the transducer by the surrounding bone is registered in a computer. The original research measurements were made in hertz. Hertz measurements are calibrated for each transducer and converted to implant stability quotient units by the computer. Measurements then are recorded as implant stability quotient values (Becker 2005, Meredith et al. 1996).

The stability of the implant also can be confirmed by the torque resistance of 30–40 Ncm that is indicative of initial implant stability. Excessive torque should not be applied to the implant because this may strip the implant threads or exert excessive compression on the adjacent bone, which may result in bone necrosis. The resultant gap between the osseous walls of the socket and the implant fixture is then filled with the bone-grafting material of choice and covered with a barrier membrane. Then the soft tissue is approximated and closed with no tension.

Implant morphological characteristics can influence the treatment outcome of immediate implant therapy. Root form tapered implants probably offer better handling and stability than the parallel walled implants because they reduce the possibility of adjacent root injury and labial bone perforation. In the maxillary anterior region, it is important to avoid placing the implant directly into the extraction socket. Placing the implant in this position will invariably cause the implant to perforate the buccal plate and jeopardize the survival of the implant or cause a poor esthetic result. The implant long axis should be shifted to a more palatal position from the long axis of the extracted tooth and slightly palatal to the incisal edges of the adjacent teeth. The palatal placement also allows enough buccal bone on the implant body to counteract against the shear stresses. An accurately fabricated surgical template may be used to ensure the correct angulation and trajectory of the proposed implant (Becker 2005). Impressions can be made

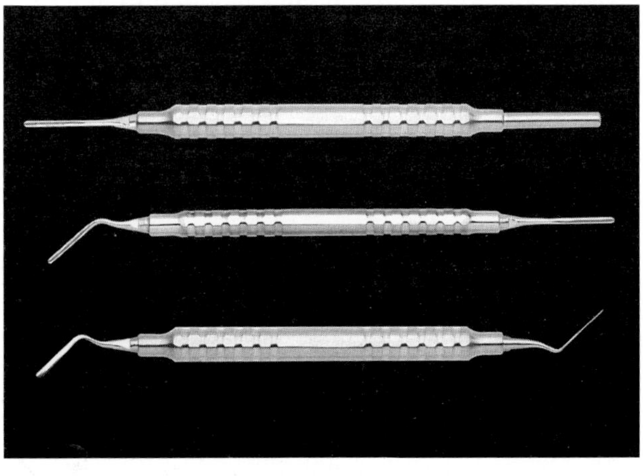

Figure 6.1. Periotome kit to remove teeth atraumatically (Storz am Markt GMBH, Emmingen-Liptingen, Germany).

immediately after implant placement, which facilitates fabrication of prosthetic abutments and provisional restorations. The abutments and provisional restorations can be inserted in place post-healing.

The use of grafting material to fill the peri-implant space within the socket has also been extensively studied. Some authors (Schwartz-Arad and Chaushu 1997) used autogenous bone chips without using barrier membranes to fill the osseous defect with a high survival rate. To enhance the predictability of the bone-grafting procedure around dental implants placed in immediate protocol, Cochran and others (1999) used bone morphogenetic protein (rhBMP-2) with and without PTFE membranes. Histological analysis after four and 12 weeks showed slightly less bone gain in sites treated with barrier membranes than in sites treated without membranes (i.e., with rhBMP-2 alone), which accumulated more bone more quickly. The quality of the new bone was exactly the same in all specimens.

Using recombinant BMP offers some advantages, such as no contaminating proteins and no risk of transmitting infectious disease. Thirteen proteins have already been purified and cloned; they are called BMP-1 through BMP-13. Recombinant human BMP-2 (rhBMP-2) has been assayed in several systems and has been found to have very high osteogenic activity, making it the most promising of the 13 proteins. BMPs induce formation of new bone that has all the characteristics of normal bone, including cartilage formation followed by endochondral ossification. BMPs accelerate the time of implant-bone integration and have excellent therapeutic potential in dental and periodontal attachment complex repair (Branemark et al. 1999). They are all highly active, which leaves the still unanswered question of how to control their activity. The full potential and safety of BMPs will require further clinical studies.

The use of the demineralized, freeze-dried bone allografts (DFDBA) (Pacific Coast Tissue Bank, USA) has been extensively investigated as well (Block and Kent 1991). DFDBA may regenerate bone by osteoinduction, by its effect on the host's undifferentiated mesenchymal cells while blood vessels penetrate the graft. DFDBAs may also regenerate bone by osteoconduction, by serving as a scaffold for the host bone while resorbing. Clinical observations did not find any significant differences between the efficacy of FDBAs and DFDBAs in promoting bone repair of human bone defects. The advantages of allografts include ready availability, elimination of donor site surgery, reduced anesthesia and surgical time, and decreased blood loss (Block and Kent 1991). Disadvantages consist primarily of the history of the obtained grafting material. The quality of the graft material depends mainly on the donor's health condition; for example, no history of infection, cancer, degenerative bone disease, hepatitis B or C, sexually transmitted disease, autoimmune deficiency, or other medical problems that might lead to cross-infection. Therefore, the first priority must be given to thorough donor screening, which involves a traceable medical, demographic, and social history. Other disadvantages of allografts include the risk of rejection, high rate of infection, nonunion, risk of rapid resorption, and problems related to the considerable technical precision required to pack and hold the graft in place in bleeding sites.

Alloplasts have also been used to avoid the previously mentioned complications and drawbacks of allografts and xenografts. Biocompatible synthetic materials have been used over the past two decades. There are high expectations regarding their use in clinical applications, and recent advances have greatly improved their clinical outcome. They can be resorbable or nonresorbable; microporous (less than 350 μ), macroporous (greater than 350 μ), or nonporous; crystalline or amorphous; or granular or molded in form. There is a consensus about their advantages; they are readily available, sterile, easily stored, safe, and well tolerated. But their main advantage is the elimination of the possibility of cross-infection. They are osteoconductive materials, but all differ from each other in some chemical and physical properties. These differing properties will determine which material is best for a specific clinical application.

There is no consensus in literature regarding the regenerative barrier. Some authors (Lazzara 1989, Becker and Becker 1990) used expanded polytetrafluoroethylene (ePTFE) barrier membranes to prevent the connective and epithelial tissue from invading the gap between the implant and surrounding osseous defects. This technology has been termed guided bone regeneration (GBR). The principles of GBR are derived from guided tissue regeneration (GTR). GBR shares with GTR the use of barrier membranes to achieve regeneration of new tissues. But whereas the goal of GTR is to regenerate bone, cementum, new attachment, and periodontal ligament contiguous with root structure(s), the only goal of GBR is to regenerate bone. It seems reasonable to assume that GBR procedures are even more predictable than GTR procedures for osseous regeneration, because the regeneration in GTR occurs in a hostile healing environment due to the proximity of root surfaces contaminated with plaque, calculus, and toxins. This hostile environment is contrary to that in GBR procedures. Additional use of bone-grafting materials for space maintenance tends to improve GBR outcomes (Block and Kent 1991).

Today GBR is a widely accepted regenerative treatment modality in the field of implant dentistry. Guided bone regenerative membranes are used to separate tissue during healing, retard apical migration of epithelium to the site, maintain the necessary space for bone in-growth (tenting), and protect the graft material in the defect. GBR barriers are of two types, nonresorbable and resorbable. However, many authors using ePTFE membranes for regenerative purposes around implants have experienced high percentages (39% to 41%) of membrane exposure and infection, prompting premature removal of the membranes (Becker et al. 1994).

Resorbable membranes also have been used in immediate implant therapy. Collagen membranes have become the subject of research lately, mainly because of their favorable biological properties. Type I collagen is a predominant component found in periodontal connective tissue and forms the main component of this type of membrane. In addition, collagen possesses extra advantages, including weak immunogenicity, hemostasis, and chemotaxis for fibroblasts (Bunyaratavay and Wang 2001).

When implanted into the body, collagen is absorbed at a rate that can be controlled by the degree of chemical treatment or cross-linkage. Various cross-linking techniques have been developed, such as ultraviolet light, hexamethylenediisocyanate (HMDIC), diphenylphosphorylazide (DPPA), and glutaraldehyde (GA) or formaldehyde (FA) plus irradiation (Dreesman 1892, Wang and Carroll 2000). However, cross-linkage seems to inhibit epithelial migration effectively (Lang et al. 1994).

The clinical use of resorbable barriers, without a grafting procedure, interestingly showed a remarkable reduction in alveolar ridge resorption post-tooth extraction (Lekovic et al. 1998), as shown in Figures 6.2A–B. The study involved the elevation of buccal and lingual full-thickness flaps and extraction of teeth, and experimental sites were covered with resorbable membranes. Control sites did not receive any membrane. Flaps were advanced to achieve primary closure of the surgical wound. There was no single membrane exposure during the course of healing. Six months later, the implant was uncovered. Results showed that sites treated with resorbable membranes presented with significantly less loss of alveolar bone height, more internal socket bone fill, and less horizontal resorption of the alveolar bone ridge. The study suggested that the treatment of extraction sockets with restorable membranes is valuable in preserving alveolar bone in extraction sockets and preventing alveolar ridge defects.

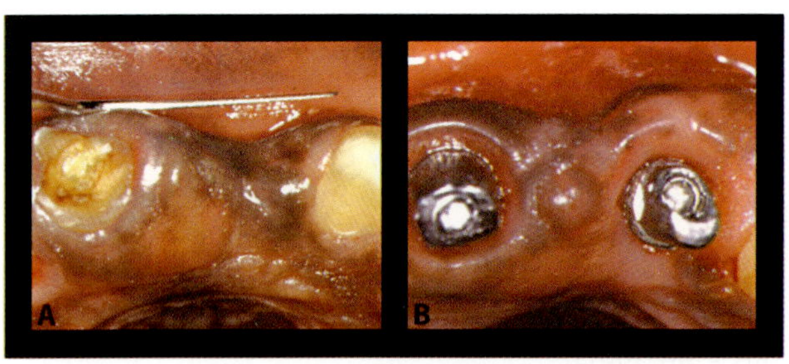

Figure 6.2. **A.** A remarkable postextraction labial bone resorption in the area of the left maxillary central incisor when compared to the right side where the remaining root presence prevents the bone resorption procedure. **B.** The bone defect is corrected via bone-grafting procedure.

On the other hand, the placement of immediate implants with neither bone grafting nor a barrier membrane was also investigated (Covani et al. 2004a). It indicated that circumferential defects could heal clinically without any GBR and that the procedure was virtually free from complications in the postoperative period, probably because of the absence of barrier membranes and/or grafting materials. But histologically, peri-implant defects of more than 1.5 mm heal by connective tissue apposition, rather than by direct bone-to-implant contact, based on the work in a histological study (Wilson et al. 1998) in which immediate implant placement was carried out in humans. The study showed that for small peri-implant defects not exceeding 1.5 mm in horizontal dimension, the use of barrier membranes was not necessary, as long as the socket walls were intact and favorable defect morphology was present. However, the author did not explain the relationship between the gap size and the epithelial down growth along the socket walls.

From another perspective, the use of GTR barriers to close the socket orifice has been said to help eliminate the need for soft tissue closure (Rosenquist and Ahmad 2000). The technique involves a horizontal incision extending along the marginal gingiva of two teeth adjacent to the extraction site from both buccal and lingual sides. The mucoperiosteal flap is then reflected without vertical releasing incisions, and the implant is placed (socket voids may be grafted). A homologous cortical bone membrane (Lambone, Pacific Coast Tissue Bank, Los Angeles, USA) is tucked above the implant head and underneath the flap at least 5–6 mm under the mucoperiosteum, buccally and lingually. This type of membrane is preferred due to its high biocompatibility. The membrane should fit precisely to the bone from each side. The flap is then returned to its place with the membrane, secured, and sutured. The central area of the membrane is left exposed, allowing the tissues to migrate over it and, given ample of time, heal completely.

Using GTR to close freshly extracted sites can be questionable, because this technique is considered highly susceptible to infection due to the hostile environment of the oral cavity that favors bacterial populations on top of or underneath the membrane. Furthermore, the possible formation of granulation tissue underneath the membrane can lead to its loosening, which can compromise the predictability of the bone-grafting procedure or the osseointegration.

A study by Wilson and others (2003) used connective tissue barriers along with immediate implant therapy to improve the bone-to-implant contact and the initial bone-to-implant contact in a vertical dimension. The study used 10 large-grit sandblasted, acid-attacked (SLA) titanium implants that were placed into immediate extraction sites in five patients. Following insertion, the implants were completely covered with a connective tissue membrane. Primary closure of soft tissue flaps was achieved in each case. Six months after placement, seven of the implants were histologically examined. The study confirmed that osseointegration occurred across all defects, with a higher percentage of bone-to-implant contact. It also stated that osseointegration was successful in immediate implant placement sites with horizontal defect dimensions wider than 4 mm in humans when SLA titanium implants were completely covered with connective tissue membranes. It is still undetermined whether the different type of membrane, placement of the membrane, type of implant surface, or a combination of these three factors was responsible for the improved osseointegration in osseous defects.

In a recently published consensus (Hammerle et al. 2004) that concerns the use of dental implants in immediate placement protocol, the authors concluded that radiological and histological studies indicate that bony healing of extraction sites proceeds with external resorption of the original socket walls and a varying degree of bone fill within the socket. They evaluated human and animal implant sites with a horizontal defect dimension (i.e., the peri-implant space) of 2 mm or less, and found that spontaneous bone healing and osseointegration of implants with a rough titanium surface took place. In sites with larger than 2 mm and/or nonintact socket walls, techniques using barrier membranes and/or membrane-supporting materials have been shown to be effective in regenerating bone and allowing osseointegration. The consensus (Hammerle et al. 2004) also concluded that there is evidence to suggest that the survival rate for implants placed immediately following extraction of teeth associated with local pathology is similar to that of implants placed into healed ridges. However, most of the studies did not specify whether thin scalloped or thick flat tissue types were being included in their evaluation.

The consensus recommended that all patients undergoing immediate implant therapy must follow the same diagnostic protocol of delayed standard implant placement. Antibiotics are advantageous when augmentation procedures are performed. Atraumatic tooth extraction should be performed and, in cases in which buccal plate integrity is lost, implant placement should be avoided at the time of tooth removal. Rather, augmentation therapy is performed in thin scalloped tissue patients. Implant primary stability is of great concern to the success of dental implants placed immediately.

Achieving Soft Tissue Closure in Immediate Implant Therapy

Complete soft tissue closure on top of dental implants might present a prerequisite for the overall success of dental implant therapy (Lekholm et al. 1993). Submerging dental implants was originally performed to protect the bone-grafting material from the hostile oral environment and to prevent the migration of epithelial tissues along the socket walls. As a consequence, primary soft tissue closure in immediate implant procedures became a standard clinical routine by many authors (Gelb 1993, Becker and Becker 1990, Rosenquist and Grenthe 1996, Gotfredsen et al. 1993). As a result, many techniques have been introduced to achieve complete soft tissue closure with a variable clinical outcome, either by undermining and releasing the soft tissue margins to approximate the wound edges or by applying a special surgical procedure to achieve the same goal (Gher et al. 1994a, Becker et al. 1998, Artzi and Nemcovsky 1997, Gher et al. 1994b, Edel 1995, Evian and Cutler 1994).

Early exposure of immediately placed implants in fresh sockets was a common event until these new techniques offered predictable soft tissue closure results. This early exposure of dental implants might have a negative impact on osseous regenerative procedures and jeopardize implant survival rates (Becker et al. 1994, Lekholm et al. 1993, Mellonig and Nevins 1995, Simion et al. 1994, Jovanovic et al. 1992). Complete socket closure in immediate implant placement is a technique-sensitive procedure that warrants special attention. It influences the width, position, and configuration of the attached mucosa as well as the future emergence profile (Rosenquist 1997). The most common methods of achieving primary soft tissue closure in immediate implant placement are Rehrmanplasty, palatal rotated flap, buccal rotated flap, pedicle island flap, and the use of GTR barriers.

Rehrmanplasty

Rehrmanplasty is the most common method preferred by clinicians for primary soft tissue closure in the oral cavity. It was originally developed to close oroantral fistulae (Von Rehrman 1936, Kay 1970), as shown in Figures 6.3A–B, and is currently used successfully to achieve primary soft tissue closure in immediate implant placement cases. This method entails raising a full-thickness mucoperiosteal flap through two vertical parallel incisions that are made along both sides of the extraction socket and extended vestibularly. The flap is then reflected and extended farther vestibularly. A periosteal slitting incision is then made horizontally at the base of the flap, after which multiple incisions in the periosteum can be made to lengthen and release the flap if required. The flap is then released and extended to cover the socket and sutured to the palatal or lingual mucosa. This method provides an excellent predictable socket seal, but is not satisfactory from an esthetic point of view because the attached buccal mucosa shifts from its original position to the crest of the ridge, thus losing its continuity. Nevertheless, this mucogingival discontinuity can be corrected during second-stage surgery. This can be achieved by apically repositioning the keratinized tissues from the crest of the ridge to the labial side, thus restoring soft tissue integrity. (See Figures 6.4A–O.)

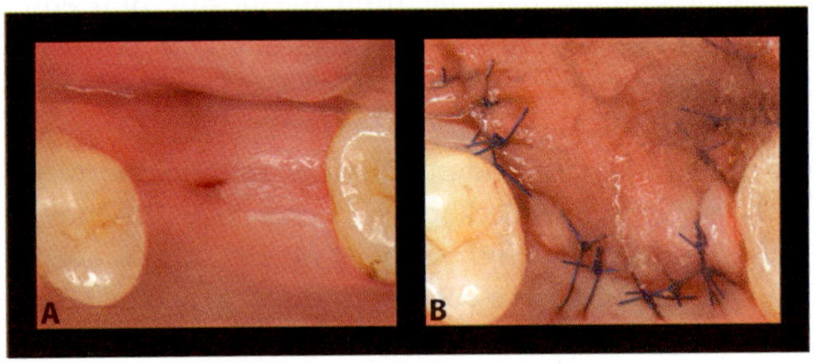

Figure 6.3. **A.** Oroantral communication in the place of a missing maxillary first molar. **B.** The closure of the oroantral communication using Rehermanplasty.

Palatal Rotated Flap

The palatal rotated flap technique was introduced by Nemkovesky and others (2000). The palatal rotated flap can be either a full-thickness or a partial-thickness flap; both originally aimed at achieving primary closure on top of an immediate implant without modifying or altering the buccal contour of keratinized mucosa, which can be vital to the final esthetic outcome of implant-supported prostheses. A palatal pedicle flap is rotated toward the buccal mucosa to cover the socket orifice. In using the partial-thickness rotated palatal flap, an intrasulcular incision is made around the maxillary tooth to be extracted and the proximal palatal aspect. Maximum soft tissue, including interdental papillae, is preserved in the flap design.

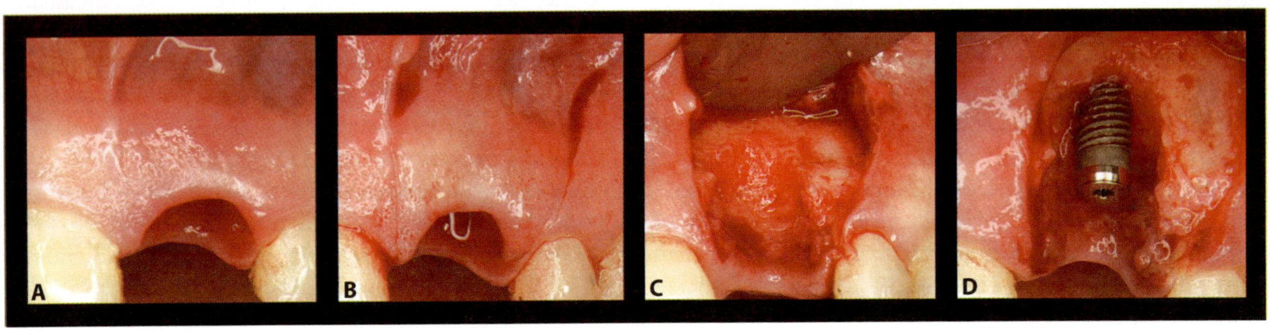

Figure 6.4. **A.** Socket condition post tooth extraction. **B.** A mucoperiosteal flap designed for immediate implant placement. **C.** A mucoperiosteal flap reflection. **D.** Implant installation with an osseous defect.

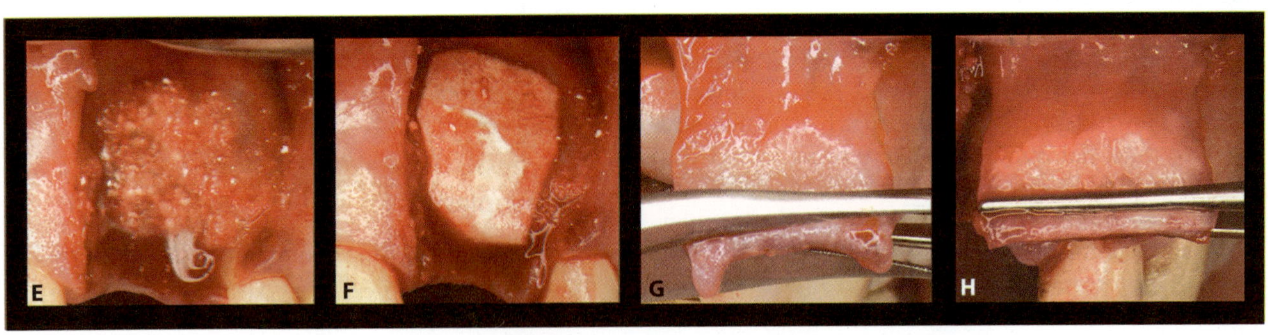

Figure 6.4. **E.** The osseous defect is being grafted. **F.** The bone graft is covered with a resorbable membrane (BioMend, Zimmer Dental, Carlsbad, CA, USA). Complete soft tissue closure. **G.** The scallop of the gingival margin is being trimmed with a scissor in order to adapt to the palatal side. **H.** The gingival scallop after trimming.

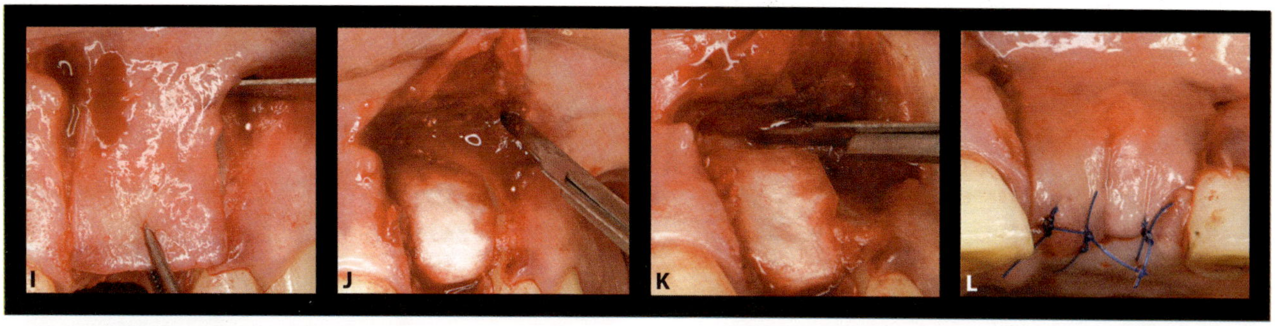

Figure 6.4. **I.** The flap is being tested for edges approximation. **J, K.** Deep basal periosteal slitting incision is being made to release and relax the flap. **L.** The labial and palatal ends are sutured.

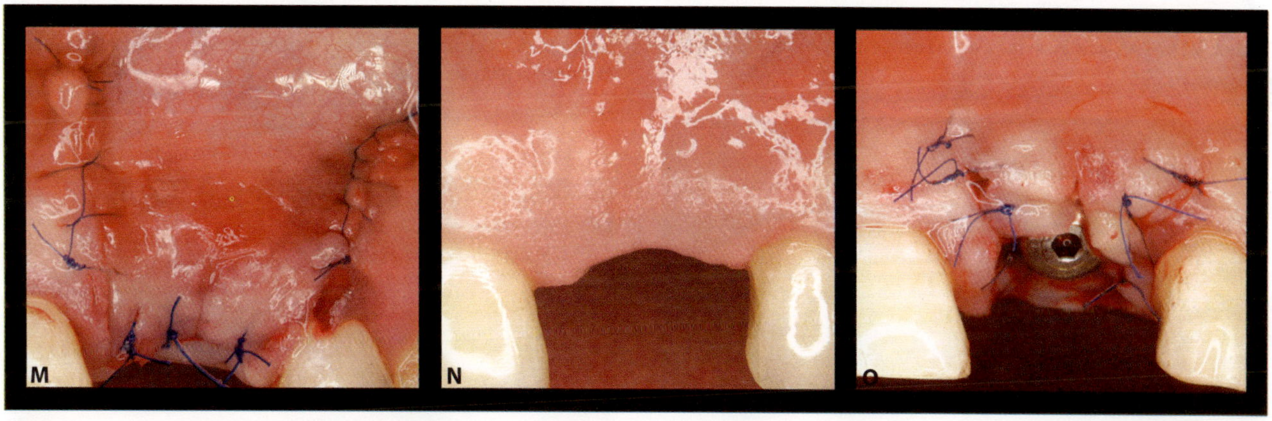

Figure 6.4. **M.** The mucoperiosteal flap being fully closed. **N.** Postoperative healing completed. **O.** The second-stage surgery and abutment connection.

A full-thickness mucoperiosteal palatal flap is raised, extending at least one tooth mesially and distally from the tooth to be extracted. A minimal buccal flap is then reflected, including only interdental papillae and marginal gingiva, exposing the bone crest. The tooth is carefully extracted, and granulation tissue, epithelium, and bone walls are curetted. The receptor site is prepared and the implant is placed. The palatal flap is split in two. The deeper flap contains periosteum and the inner part of the subepithelial connective tissue. The superficial flap contains epithelium and the superficial part of the connective tissue. A second incision, involving only the deeper flap, further disconnects these two flaps. The deeper flap is thus transformed into a pediculated one, becoming mobile and easily rotated under the minimally reflected buccal flap, covering the augmented implant site. The superficial layer of the palatal flap is then repositioned and sutured. Consequently, complete primary soft tissue closure over the implant site is achieved.

The full-thickness palatal rotated flap requires an intrasulcular incision to be made around the maxillary tooth to be extracted and the proximal palatal aspect of the adjacent teeth. A minimal buccal flap, including only interdental papillae and marginal gingiva, exposing the bone crest, is then reflected. The socket is then curetted properly. A sharp internal beveled incision delineating a pediculated full-thickness palatal flap is then made. The extension should be sufficient to allow complete coverage of the alveolus and overlapping of the crestal buccal bone. An oblique proximal incision facilitates rotation of the pedicle, which is wider than 5 mm. Bone-grafting material is used to fill the gap between the implant and the bone wall. The palatal flap is tucked and sutured under the minimally reflected buccal flap covering the grafted implant site, achieving primary soft tissue closure, as shown in Figures 6.5A–B.

The need for coronal repositioning of the marginal gingiva is avoided in this method. The mucogingival junction remains unchanged, vestibular depth is preserved, and potential gingival recession at adjacent donor sites is avoided. When performing palatal rotated flaps to cover immediately placed implants, the palatal incision should be made distal to the midline for better blood supply, bearing in mind that the procedure might exhibit intraoperative bleeding that can be controlled. The use of the rotated palatal flap for socket closure has shown great clinical predictability for the sufficient blood supply to the flap itself, and the thickness of the palatal

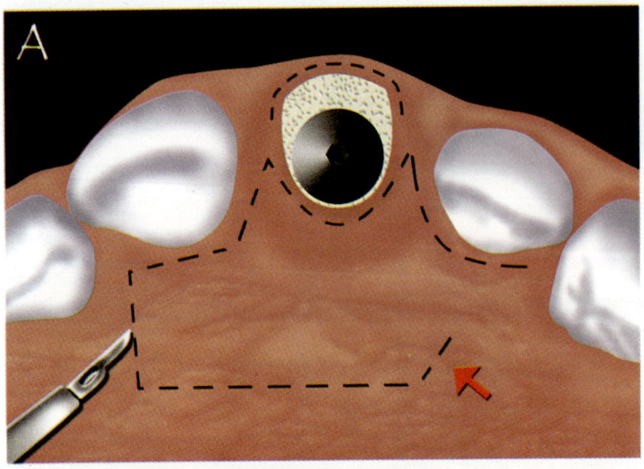

Figure 6.5A. An illustration showing the design of the rotated palatal flap.

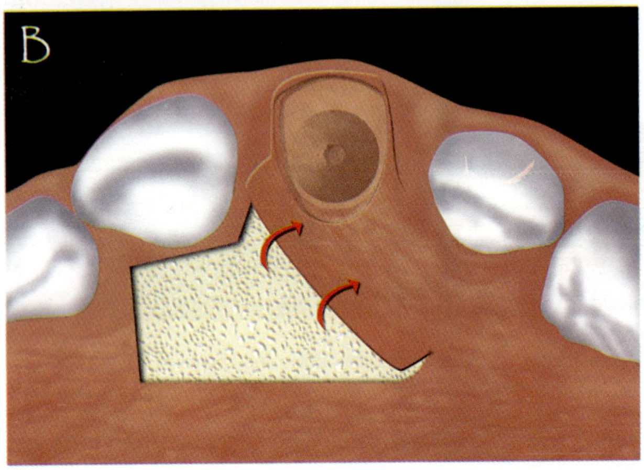

Figure 6.5B. Illustration showing rotation of the flap to the labial side to cover the implant site.

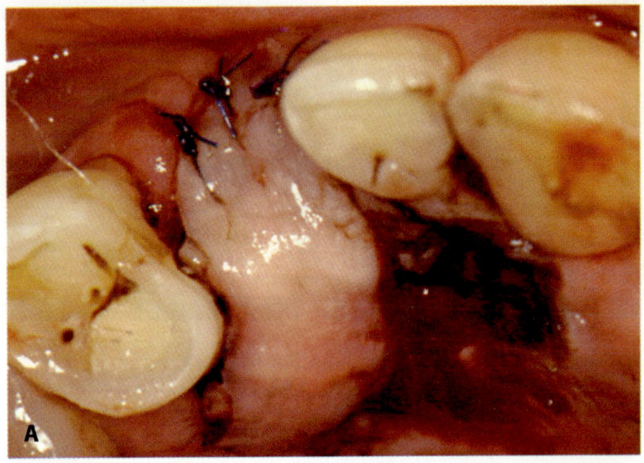

Figure 6.6A. A palatal rotated flap is made to cover the implant and sutured to the labial mucosa.

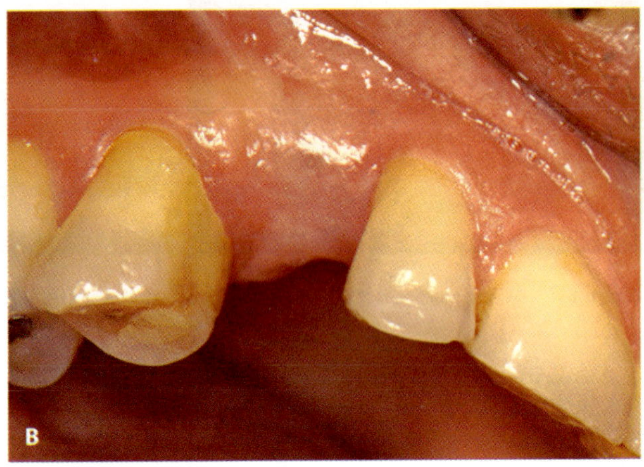

Figure 6.6B. Six weeks after healing.

soft tissue offers a better mechanical barrier against wound sloughing. (See Figures 6.6A–B and 6.7A–B.)

Buccal Rotated Flap

Becker and Becker (1990) developed another clinical solution to achieve soft tissue closure on top of immediately placed implant fixtures. The buccal rotated flap technique was used to obtain a tension-free closure on top of dental implants placed in freshly extracted sockets, thus achieving soft tissue closure without creating any labial mucogingival discrepancies. However, the procedure requires advanced surgical skills in soft tissue handling. The authors recommended a split thickness flap from the tooth adjacent to the donor tooth to cover the exposed bone on the donor tooth itself (Becker et al. 1994). Novaes (1997) modified this technique by incorporating various incisions that improved the clinical outcome and reduced postoperative complications. (See Figures 6.8A–B.)

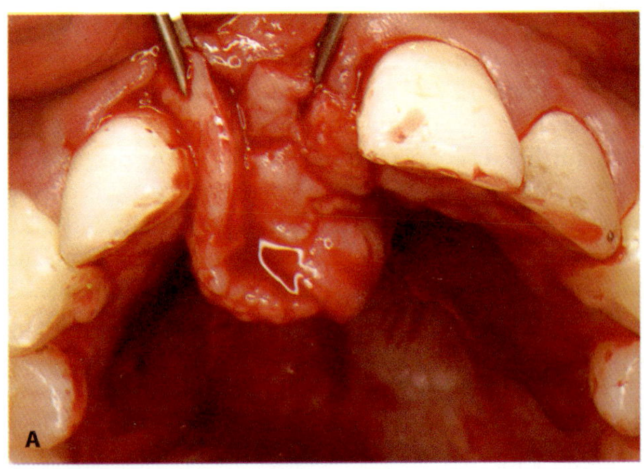

Figure 6.7A. Soft tissue defect corrected using a double palatal tissue rotated flap.

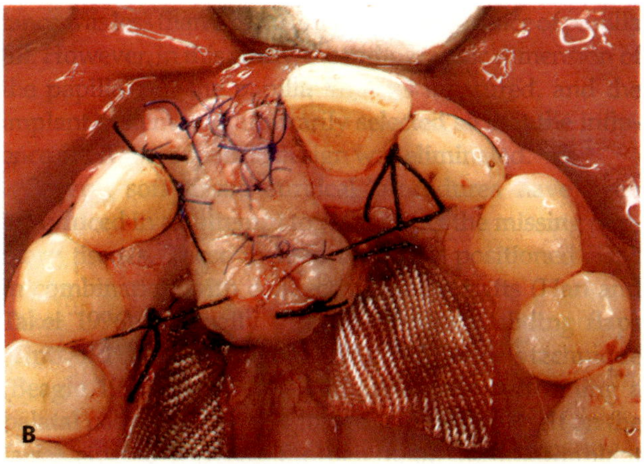

Figure 6.7B. The flap is sutured.

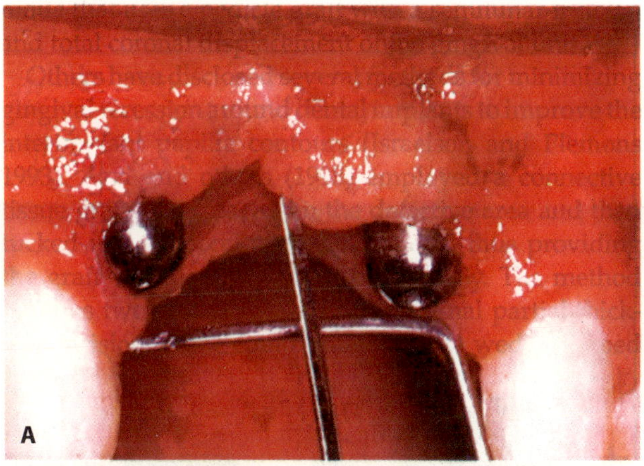

Figure 6.8A. Sever soft tissue defect due to several bone graft procedure failures.

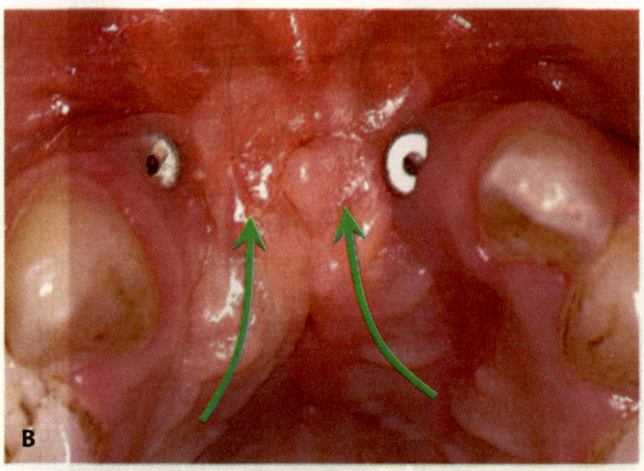

Figure 6.8B. The use of a rotated palatal flap to overcome the situation and to bulk up the palatal tissues labially and on top of the ridge area.

Novaes's technique (Novaes and Novaes 1997) starts by placing a releasing incision on the mesial line angle of the tooth to be extracted followed by a second releasing incision placed on the line angle of the tooth adjacent to the tooth to be extracted. A split-thickness flap is made over the tooth to be extracted, starting at the releasing incision and continuing distally until reaching the distal line angle of the same tooth. At this point, a vertical incision is made in the periosteum down to the bone surface and a combination full-thickness (more coronal portion) and split-thickness (more apical portion) flap is made. The tooth is gently extracted, all granulation tissue curetted, and the alveolus rinsed with sterile saline.

Next, a grafting material is used or a blood clot is allowed to form. The author used a resorbable hydroxyapatite (Bon-Apatite, Bio-Interfaces, San Diego, USA) and covered it using a nonresorbable cellulose membrane (Gengiflex, Bio Fill, Produtos Biotecnologicos, Curitiba, Brazil). The membrane is recommended to impede connective tissue of the inner surface of the flap from invading the socket, which could hamper complete bone formation. Grafting material is used to avoid collapse of the membrane into the socket when bone resorption of one or more walls of the socket has occurred. The flap is then moved distally and coronally and sutured over the membrane to the palatal or lingual tissue. Just prior to suturing, tension on the flap must be tested, and a small horizontal incision may be placed on the mesial and most apical portion of the flap to relieve any tension on the flap. A gingivectomy-type incision is made on the most coronal portion of the palatal or lingual flap to create a beveled surface of exposed connective tissue on which to lay the border of the buccal flap. This connective tissue-to-connective tissue contact is important in the maintenance of the primary soft tissue closure. When the flap is displaced distally from the adjacent tooth, as in this situation, some excessive soft tissue will need to be trimmed on its distal portion to facilitate closure of the distal vertical incision. The excessive tissue is carefully removed to preserve all of the keratinized tissue that was used as a free gingival graft to cover the exposed periosteum on the buccal surface of the donor tooth.

The free gingival graft might lead to the creation of an adequate zone of keratinized tissues on the donor tooth, avoiding the creation of mucogingival problems; however, scar tissue can be noticeable a few months' posthealing. Becker and Becker (1990) have recommended using a split-thickness flap from the tooth adjacent to the donor tooth to cover the exposed bone on the donor tooth, or closing the mesial and the vertical incision the best way possible, and to correct any mucogingival problems at a later date, if they arise. The patient is placed on 500 mg of amoxicillin every 8 hours for 10 days, starting 24 hours before the procedure, and is instructed to rinse twice daily with a solution of 0.12% chlorhexidine for 10 days. (See Figures 6.9A–D.)

Pedicle Island Flap

The pedicle island flap (Rosenquist 1997) is yet another method of achieving a soft tissue seal on top of immediate implant fixtures. It offers a predictable socket closure and achieves an excellent esthetic post-operative result. In this technique, the attached buccal mucosa is not altered or repositioned, and therefore the mucogingival integrity is kept intact. After the implant is placed in the fresh extraction socket, two parallel horizontal incisions are made in the vestibular mucosa, creating a tongue-like extension. The base of the mucosal extension is placed posterior or distal to the socket opening. The flap is made approximately 20 mm long and as wide as the socket width. The surface of the mucosal extension is thereafter de-epithelialized, except for the apical portion that corresponds to the surface of the extraction socket. A subperiosteal tunnel connecting the marginal keratinized mucosa is then made, buccal to the extraction socket and the corresponding site in the vestibule. The flap extension is subsequently pulled through the tunnel until the epithelialized apex of the flap covers the socket and then is sutured to the attached free gingival from the palatal side of the socket. Finally, the vestibular wound is approximated and sutured.

The base of the mucosal extension exhibits a rich blood supply, which enhances the predictability of the technique (Rosenquist 1997). (See Figures 6.10A–F.) It also provides a proper tissue seal on top of the socket. However, the delicate nature of the mobile soft tissue making up the mucosal extension may create difficulty in clinical handling. The mucosa can easily be torn or lacerated, especially during the dissection or de-epithelialization of the tongue-like mucosal extension. The color difference between the extension and the surrounding attached mucosa makes it a distinct island of vestibular tissues to be identified and excised at the second-stage surgery. (See Figures 6.11A–E.) The pedicle island flap technique might provide great assistance in soft tissue closure in critical conditions such as exposed bone grafts or in cases of jeopardized loss of keratinized tissue band. The method offers greater predictability in such conditions because it offers a predictable blood supply to the flap.

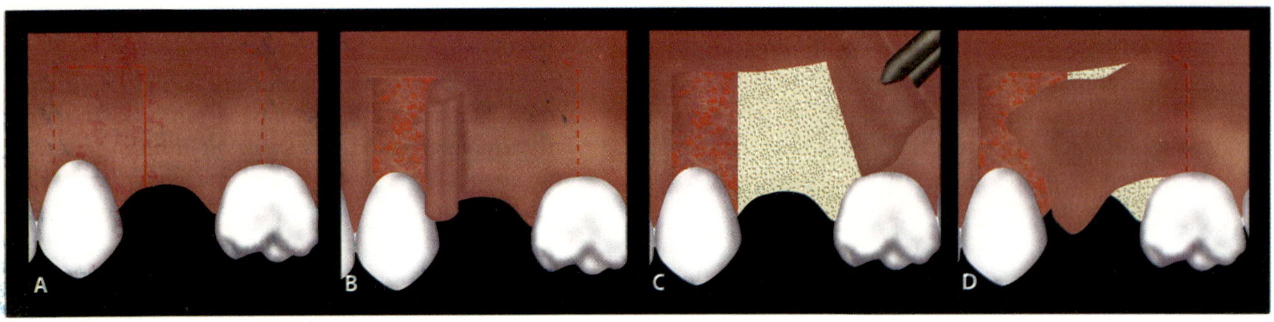

Figure 6.9A, B, C, D. An illustration showing the design of the buccal rotated flap.

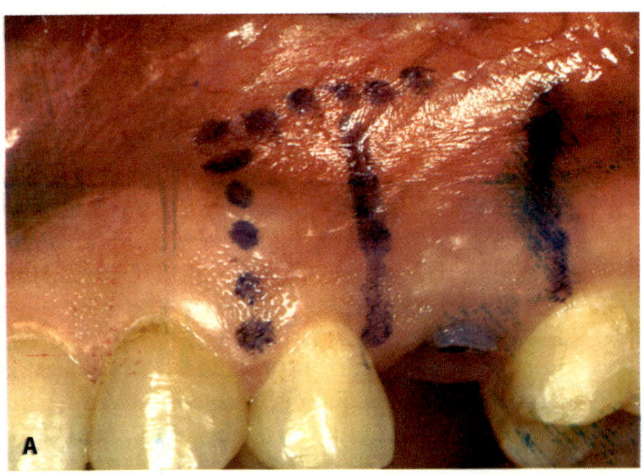

Figure 6.10A. A patient with an unsalvageable remaining root of the maxillary second premolar, with the outlines of the flap marked using a blue marker.

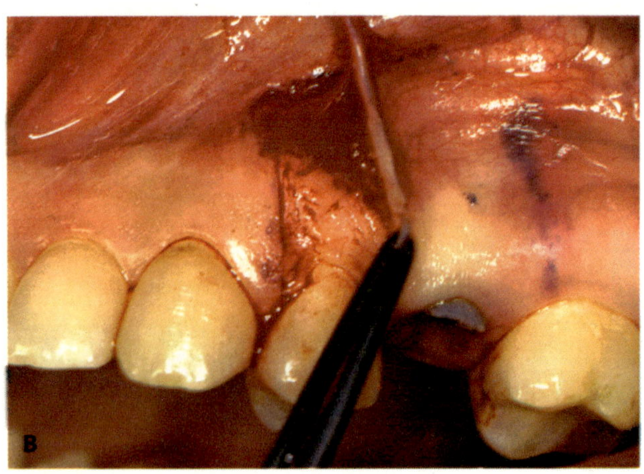

Figure 6.10B. Illustration showing the split thickness flap being dissected.

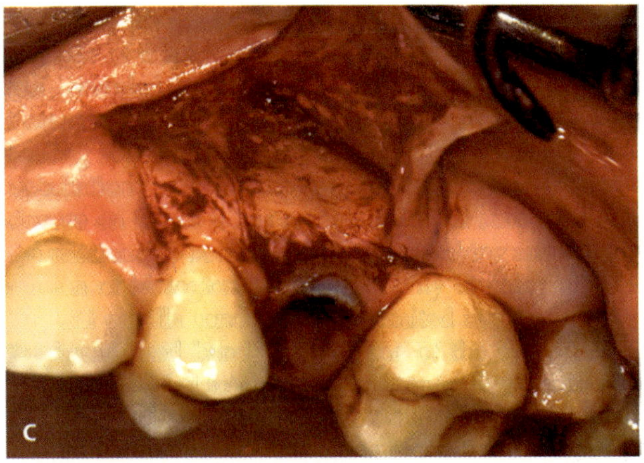

Figure 6.10C. The reflected split thickness flap completed.

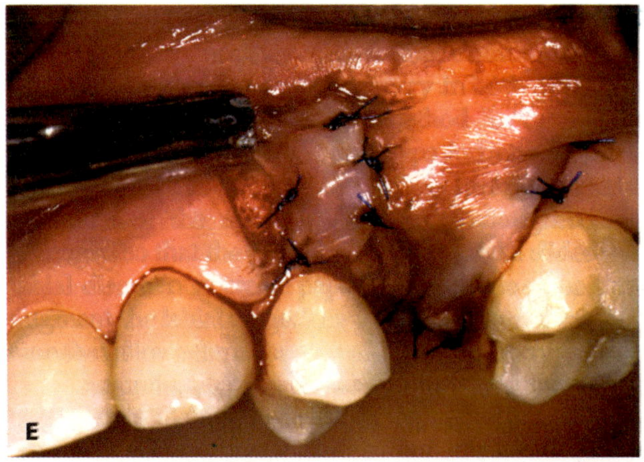

Figure 6.10E. The rotated buccal flap is sutured. A free gingival graft excised from the excessive soft tissue distally covers the exposed periosteum.

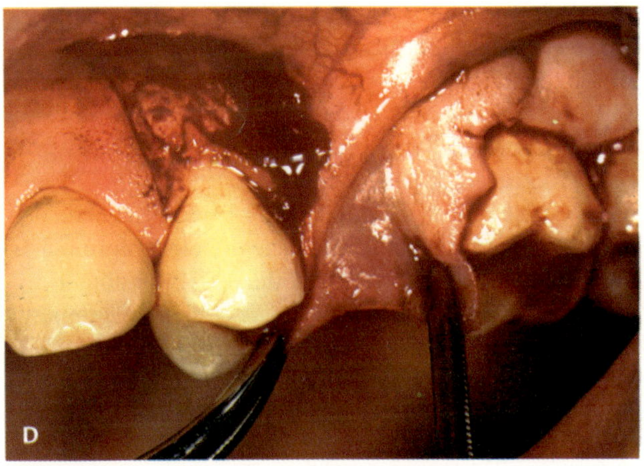

Figure 6.10D. View of the rotation of the buccal flap to cover the implant site.

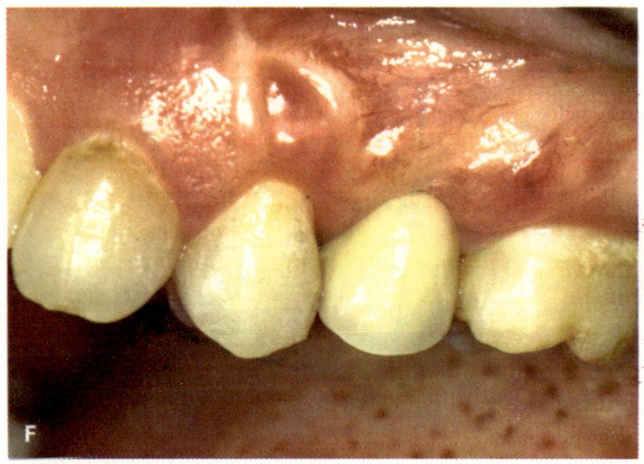

Figure 6.10F. The final healing leaving scar tissue formation and the final restoration in place.

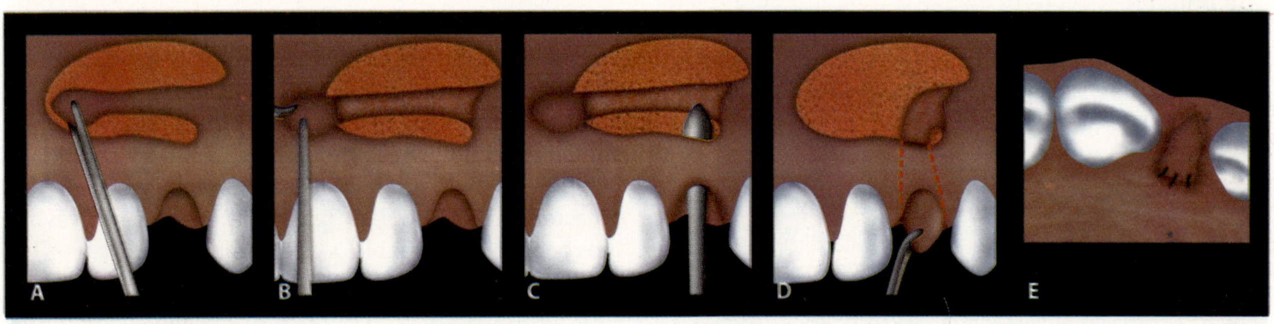

Figure 6.11. **A.** Illustration showing the tongue-like extension dissected from the vestibular mucosa. **B.** Illustration showing the tongue-like extension with its epithelium stripped. **C.** An illustration showing the subperiosteal tunnel created. **D.** An illustration showing the mucosal extension being tucked underneath the tunnel to cover the implant site. **E.** Illustration showing the mucosal extension sutured to the palatal free gingival margins of the socket.

Flapless Implant Installation

Recently the flapless implant placement technique has been increasingly used to offer several clinical advantages; however, the technique requires strict meticulous clinical handling to achieve optimal treatment outcome. Some factors are considered to be detrimental to this treatment modality, including lack of direct visibility because it is considered to be a blind surgical technique, the difficulty in assessing any existing labial osseous defects at the time of implant placement, the absolute necessity for using axial tomography or a CT scan preoperatively to evaluate the osseous topography required in many instances that might be an additional cost to the treatment, and the limited ability to augment implant sites due to lack of visibility. In addition, the potential contamination of the implant surface by the soft tissue surrounding the surgical site might complicate the overall prognosis. These factors are to be regarded when one is to perform a flapless method of implantation.

The literature (al-Ansari and Morris 1998, Landsberg and Bichacho 1998, Landsberg and Bichacho 1999) has reported the use of a flapless approach for immediate and delayed dental implant placement in the alveolar ridge to maintain the natural soft tissue contours, reduce intraoperative bleeding, reduce post-operative patient discomfort, preserve alveolar ridge integrity, and avoid additional soft tissue trauma by raising a mucoperiosteal flap. Preservation of the delicate vascular network adjacent to implant receptor sites may be an important factor in maintaining facial bone height and esthetics. In edentulous regions in which the vascular network is compromised by tooth loss, the associated periosteum and soft tissues may serve as primary blood sources for the area. The soft tissue status and healing capacity with the flapless implant placement method in freshly extracted sites has also been evaluated. Another study (Covani et al. 2004b) evaluated 15 patients (nine men and six women) aged 31 to 54 years old, and each had at least 4 mm of bone beyond the root apex. Teeth with multiple roots were excluded from this study. The second-stage surgical procedure was performed six months after the first procedure. The following clinical parameters were evaluated at the time of implant placement and at second-stage surgery:

- Levels of mesial and distal papillae
- Width of keratinized mucosa
- Position of mucogingival junction relating to the surrounding tissues
- Peri-implant radiolucency and marginal bone loss, which were evaluated radiographically

The postsurgical healing period was uneventful for all patients. Soft tissue closure over the implant sites was achieved in one to three weeks after surgery at all sites. At second-stage surgery, no peri-implant bone defects were observed or detected by probing around all the experimental implants. The soft tissue anatomy was considered clinically acceptable in all patients.

Another study (Schwartz and Chaushu 1998) evaluated the clinical success of osseointegration achieved with nine immediate implants placed without incisions in fresh extraction sites, and without the use of GBR membranes. The only allowed grafting material to fill the socket gaps was autogenous bone chips harvested from the drilling procedure. Interestingly, the results showed high clinical success without soft tissue primary closure. The study was based on the fact that there is no absolute necessity for either bone augmentation or primary flap closure when placing implants in freshly extracted sites. In other words, the absolute need for soft tissue closure for dental implants placed in freshly extracted sites has not yet been confirmed. Auty and Siddiqui (1999) used nonsubmerged implants in healed sites and exposed the alveolar bone with a mucosal punch. The authors stated that placing an implant without raising a mucoperiosteal flap reduces surgical morbidity and post-operative bone resorption. Furthermore, it stabilizes the papillary height after surgery and has an increased patient acceptance.

In the case of immediate implant placement, the clinical procedure for the flapless placement technique starts with an atraumatic extraction of the unsalvageable teeth. Drilling is then performed through a surgical template with the use of a buccally placed guiding finger, to avoid perforating the labial plate of bone. Autogenous bone chips are collected from the drill flutes and packed back into the surgical site around the implant fixture to fill any existing gaps. Finally, the wound edges are approximated and may be sutured.

This approach is used to avoid soft tissue complications, including postoperative recession. It also helps to simplify the implant surgery for both the patient and clinician, because achieving primary closure with immediate implant placement sometimes is considered a difficult task. In the delayed implant placement protocol in which gum punching is used to expose the bone for the drilling procedure and implant placement, the flapless technique may help achieve acceptable esthetic results and reduce postoperative complications. A conservative palatal flap may be reflected during implant placement, which can reveal the condition of the labial plate of bone. It can be viewed through the palatal side at a 45-degree angle to the occlusal plane. This modified palatal approach adds more predictability by helping to detect any labial osseous defect before implant placement. (See Figures 6.12A–M and 6.13A–F.)

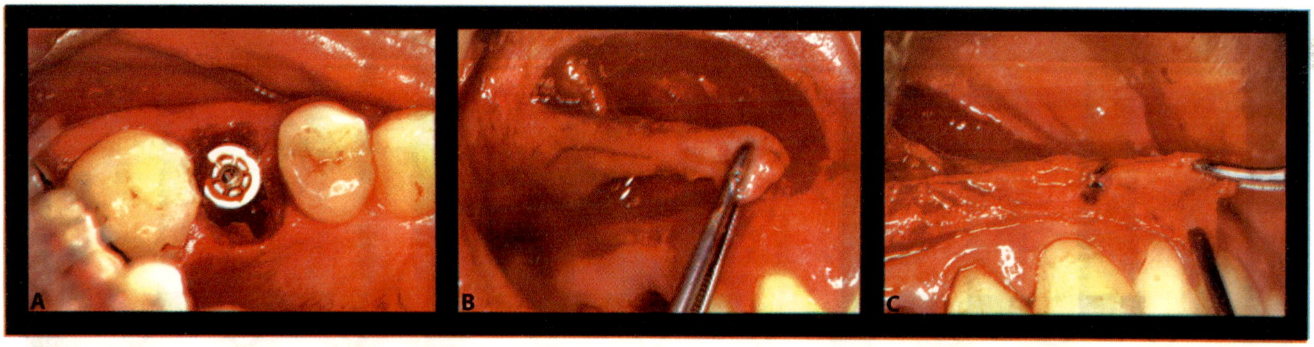

Figure 6.12. **A.** Flapless placement of an implant into the fresh extraction socket. **B.** The tongue-like extension on the buccal side after being released. **C.** The mucosal extension is partially deepithelialized.

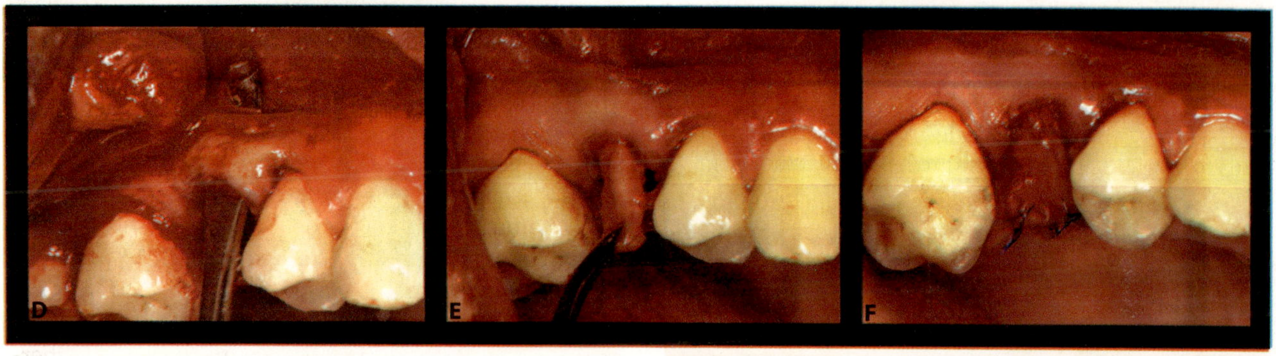

Figure 6.12. **D.** Creation of the subperiosteal tunnel. **E.** The mucosal extension appearing from the tunnel after being pulled. **F.** View of the socket closed.

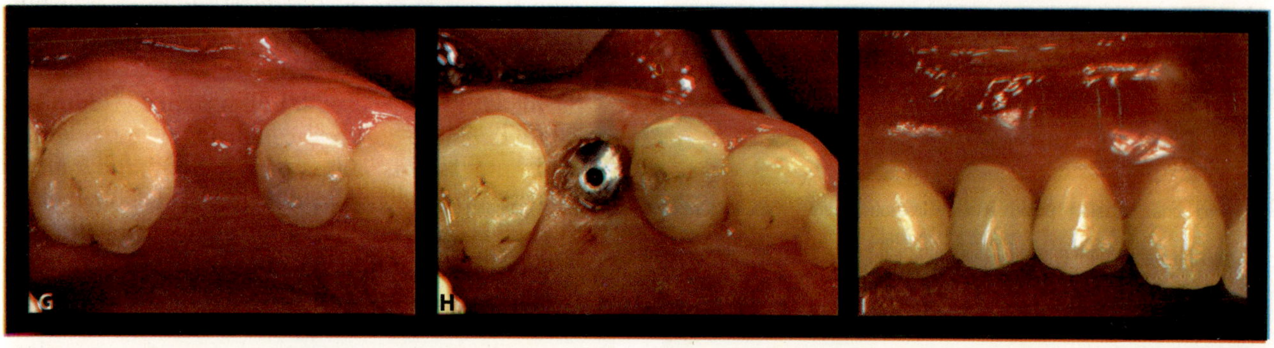

Figure 6.12. **G.** Four weeks after surgery, showing favorable healing; note the color distinction between the tongue-like extension and the surrounding attached tissue that gives the shape of an island. **H.** Second-stage surgery using the punch technique, only removing the soft tissue pedicle island. **I.** The final restoration in place. Note the continuity of the keratinized tissue band.

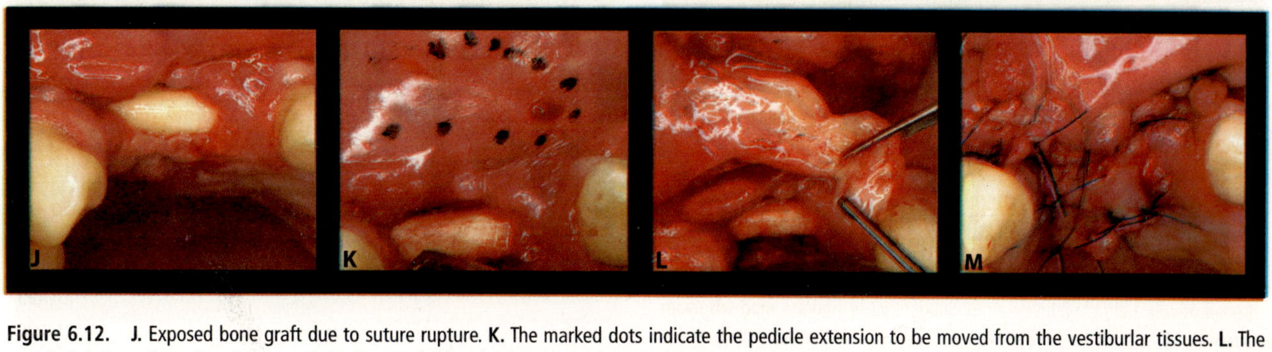

Figure 6.12. **J.** Exposed bone graft due to suture rupture. **K.** The marked dots indicate the pedicle extension to be moved from the vestiburlar tissues. **L.** The pedicle is being released and dissected. **M.** The vestibular island is being rotated and stabilized in its place.

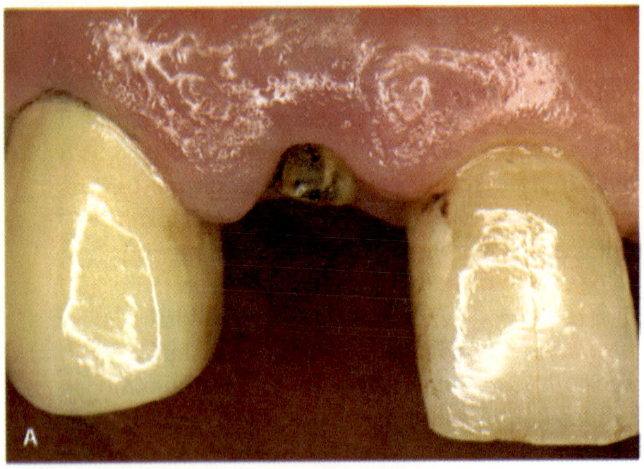

Figure 6.13A. A remaining root that needed to be replaced with implant-supported restoration.

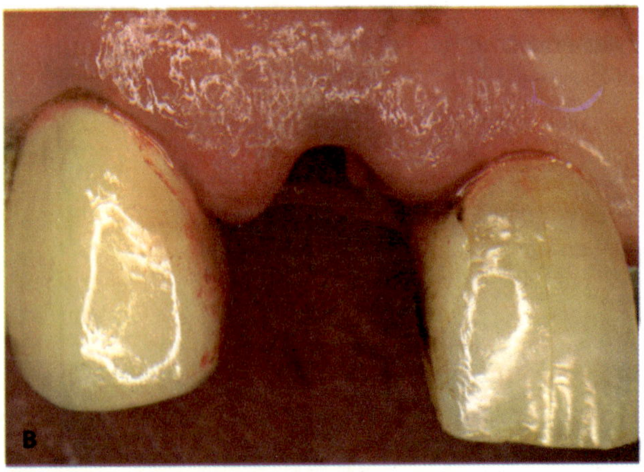

Figure 6.13B. The root has been atraumatically extracted.

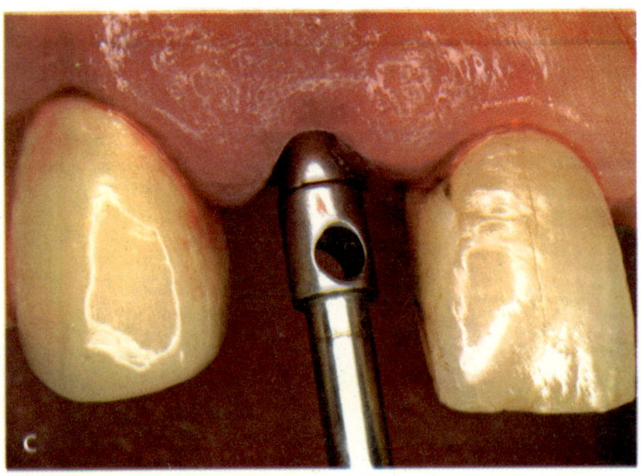

Figure 6.13C. A centralized position of the drill in order not to injure the adjacent teeth.

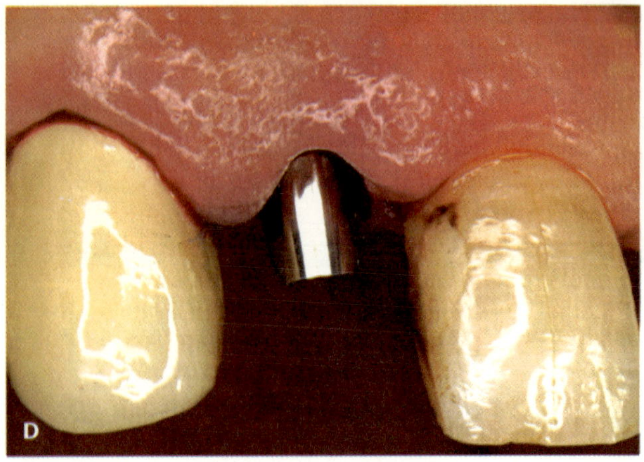

Figure 6.13D. The abutment is being connected for immediate loading protocol.

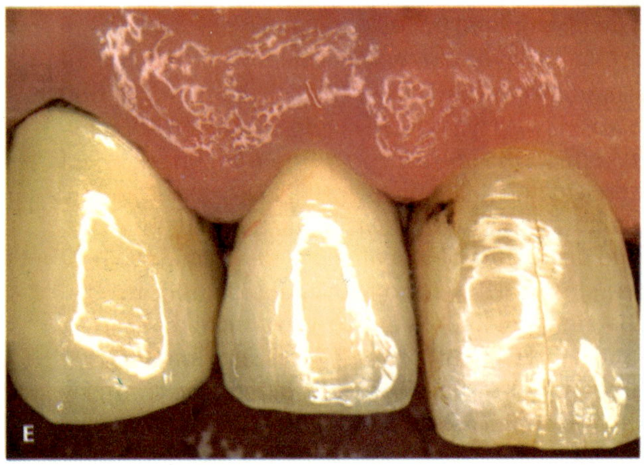

Figure 6.13E. The case restored.

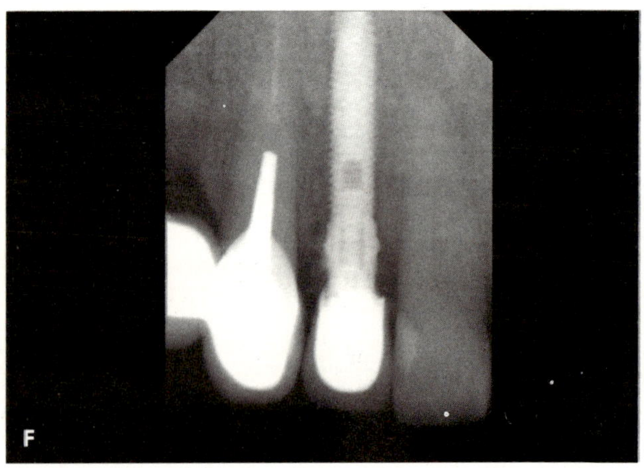

Figure 6.13F. A radiographic view showing the implant fixture in place.

Placing dental implants in delayed protocol or in healed sites using the flapless approach was presented by Campelo and Camara (2002). They placed dental implants in 359 patients to restore both completely edentulous and partially edentulous arches with fixed prostheses or removable complete dentures. Each patient was examined after three months, six months, one year, and then once every year. The cumulative success rate for implants placed using a flapless single-stage surgical technique after a 10-year period varied from 74.1% for implants placed in the year 1990 to 100% for those placed in 2000. However, flapless implant placement is considered a generally "blind" surgical technique, and care must be taken when placing implants.

Angulation of the implants affected by drilling is critical to avoid perforation of the cortical plates, either lingual or buccal, especially on the lingual in the mandibular molar areas and the anterior maxilla. In this technique, a circumferential incision is made in the gingiva at the center of the implant site using a surgical template. The cut is made with a circumferential rotary blade at low speed (100 rpm). The circumferential scalpel should be at least 1 mm wider than the implant to be placed. The incised gingival tissue is removed with a curette or mosquito hemostat. The thickness of the gingiva covering the bone is measured, and the implants are placed as recommended by the manufacturer. Healing abutments are connected to the implants. With the incision of the circumferential scalpel being 1 mm wider than the size of the implant to be placed, closure of the wound generally occurs between three and four days post-surgery. This technique has shown several disadvantages that include the possible perforation of the labial plate of bone without notice; therefore, installing dental implants via the flapless method in delayed healed sites should not be used except in very limited surgical situations that include the patient's acceptance to share the responsibility for the increased failure rate.

In conclusion, the flapless approach is still a blind surgical procedure that should be approached with caution and performed only by skillful experienced clinicians (Landsberg and Bichacho 1999). (See Figures 6.14A–I.)

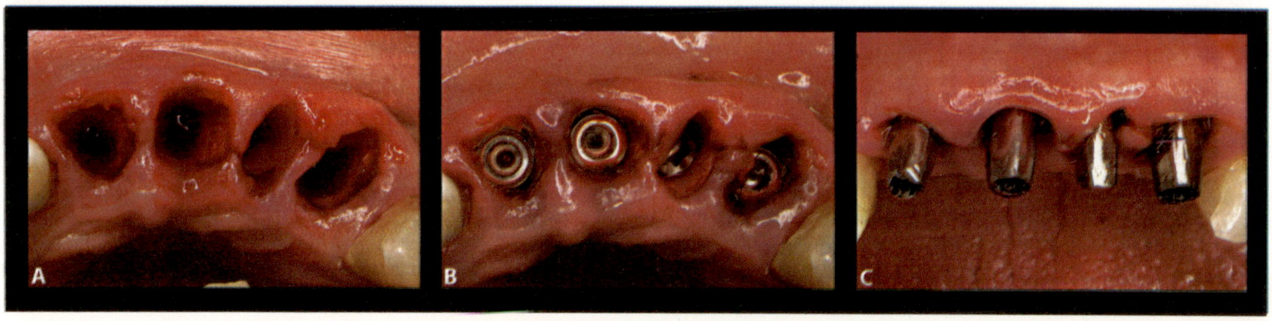

Figure 6.14. **A.** Empty four sockets after teeth extraction. **B.** Four tapered screw vent implants (Zimmer Dental, Carlsbad, CA, USA) after placement in flapless fashion. **C.** Temporary abutments being connected to allow for the use of the provisional prostheses placement.

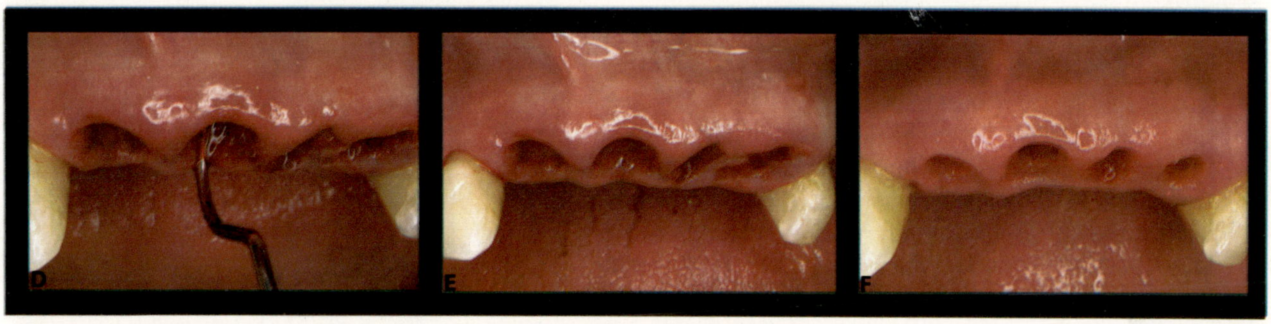

Figure 6.14. **D.** The labial plate is being checked for integrity prior to placing implants. **E, F** The gingival margin condition immediately after teeth extraction and at 10 days and at 20 days. Note the stability of the gingival margins and stabilized papillary height.

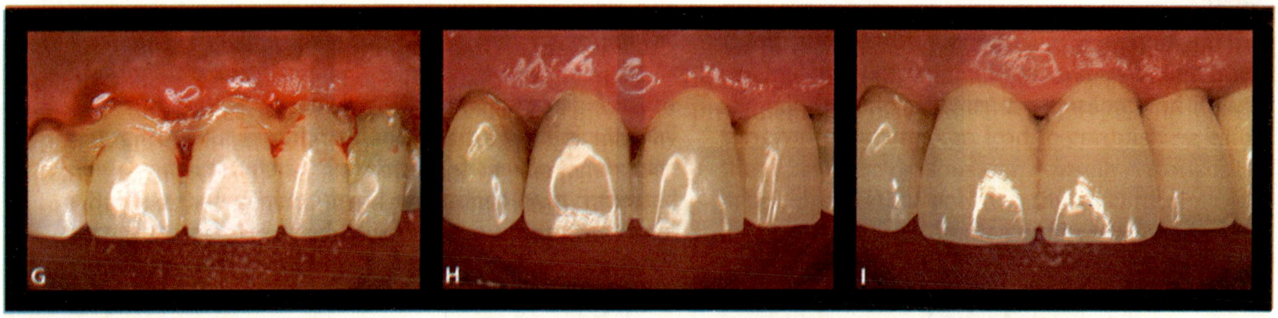

Figure 6.14. **G.** The provisional prostheses in place using corticosteroid ointment to allow for better soft tissue healing. **H.** One week post provisional delivery, note the soft tissue marginal stability. **I.** The final case restored.

Preserving Biological Soft Tissue Contours

Socket Seal Template

Due to the significant advancements in dental implantology, new titanium or ceramic abutments have been developed for esthetic implant restorations. Also, anatomical abutments that replicate tooth morphology have been introduced to create a better emergence profile (Pow and McMillan 2004). This in turn has facilitated impression making and provisional restoration fabrication. Upon the second-stage surgery, conventional healing abutment is installed that is smaller in size, and therefore the soft tissue profile created does not replicate the original tissue profile, which makes it difficult to make an impression and a provisional restoration because of the tight soft tissue cuff. The search for a customized healing abutment with an optimal finishing line to produce an ideal emergence profile is always a concern for many clinicians.

Several methods are used to guide the peri-implant tissues to their optimal contour with a provisional restoration immediately after implant installation or exposure (El Askary 2001). A novel method is used to improve the esthetic outcome of dental implants and to stabilize soft tissue margins. It might also stimulate gingival creeping in an incisal direction, which in turn improves many unfavorable clinical conditions. The method is used when immediate implant therapy is being conducted, by applying an immediate, delayed, or nonfunctional type of loading. This method is aimed at preserving natural tissue contours post-operatively, and was developed to avoid the resultant soft tissue complications from attempting soft tissue closure in the first-stage surgery, after which resultant scar tissue and altered mucosal continuity have been observed (Rosenquist and Grenthe 1996). This is especially true in patients with thin scalloped tissue biotype, which represents the most unpredictable reaction to surgical trauma, and in whom soft tissue shrinkage can be a common postoperative event.

The method preserves the soft and hard tissue architecture (Kan and Rungcharassaeng 2000, Becker et al. 1997). It aims at isolating the implant and possible bone-grafting material in immediate implant placement from the oral environment (Gelb 1993, al-Ansari and Morris 1998, Lazarra 1989), which explains the "socket sealing technique" name. After the atraumatic removal of the unsalvageable tooth, the area is curetted and the labial plate of bone integrity is checked. The implant fixture is then placed according to the esthetic placement protocol of dental implants in the esthetic zone. Then the voids between the implant and the socket walls (if they exist) are filled with the preferred bone-grafting material. A tailored collagen pack (Cola Tape, Zimmer Dental, Carlsbad, California, USA) is placed on top of the graft to prevent loss or contamination of the graft particles during handing; then a temporary abutment (Zimmer Dental, Carlsbad, California, USA) is connected to the implant and trimmed to the required height. (See Figures 6.15 and 6.16A–J.)

Self-cure acrylic resin in its rubbery stage of curing is then introduced to the socket and packed around the temporary abutment. Just before final curing occurs it is withdrawn along with the temporary abutment to prevent tissue exposure to the heat emitted from the polymerization reaction. Once polymerization is completed extraorally, the template is trimmed and polished to remove the excess material so it will snugly fit into the socket, then it is secured in place with the temporary abutment connecting screw. When the template is used in delayed implant loading protocol, the margins of the template should be flush with the gingival marginal level; when used in immediate implant (functional or nonfunctional) loading protocol, a temporary abutment might be fitted to the implant to receive a provisional crown that duplicates the socket dimensions on top of it.

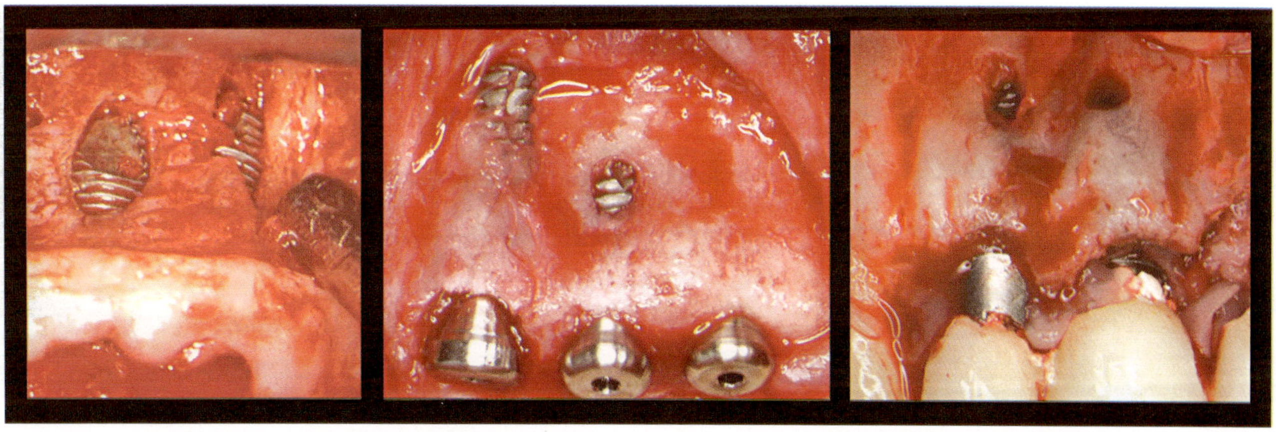

Figure 6.15. Different clinical picture that shows blind placement of dental implants might lead to the buccal fenestration of the labial bone.

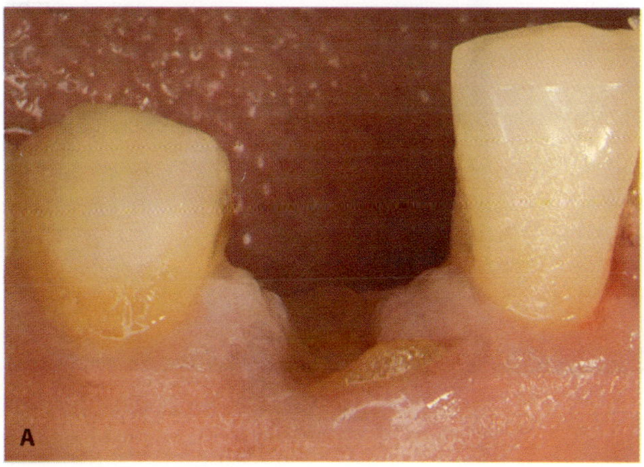

Figure 6.16A. A remaining root of a mandibular canine that needs to be restored.

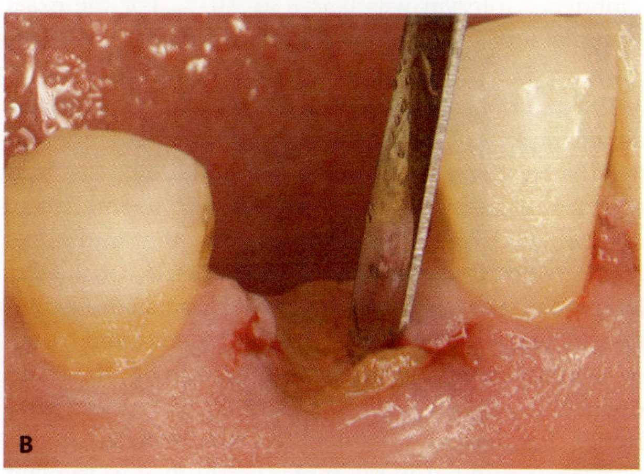

Figure 6.16B. The remaining root is being forced out using the periotome.

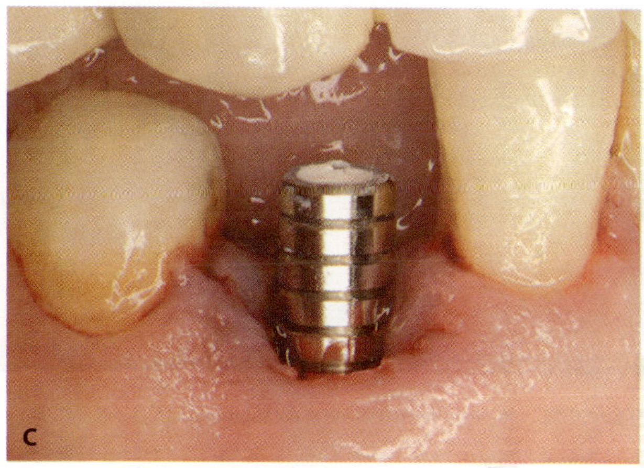

Figure 6.16C. The implant is placed and the abutment is being connected.

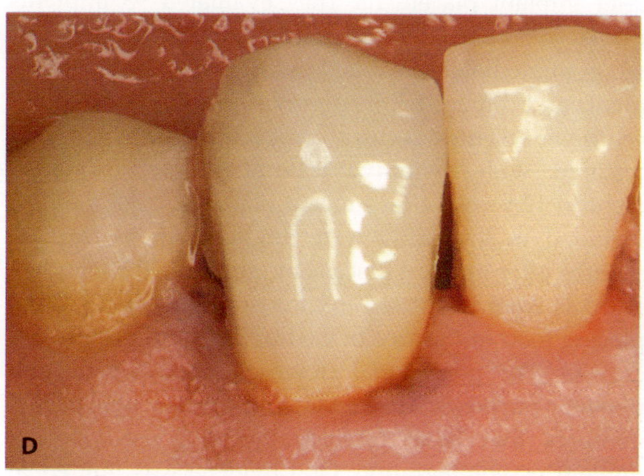

Figure 6.16D. The case is temporarily restored. Note the immediate clinical improvement.

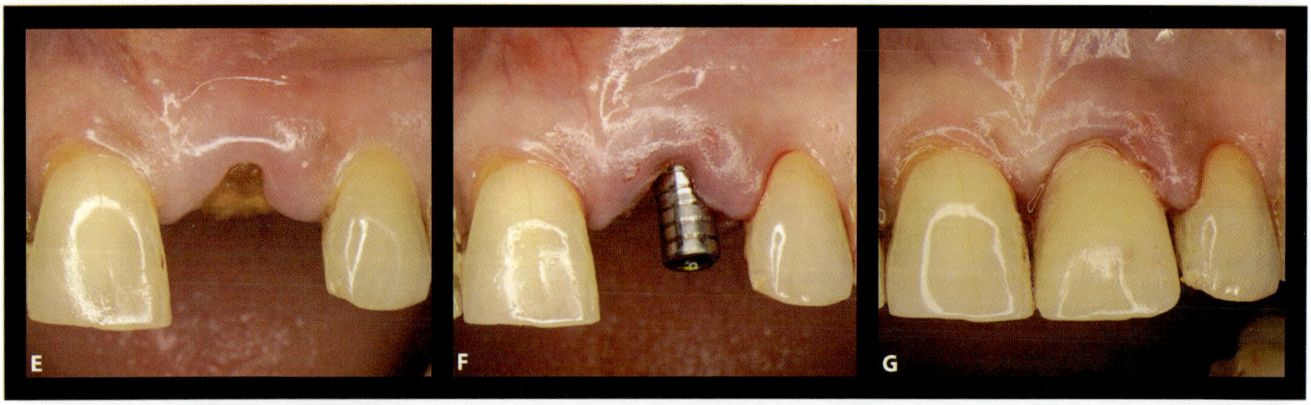

Figure 6.16. **E.** A remaining root of an upper left maxillary central incisor to be restored. **F.** The root was removed and replaced with an implant and the abutment connected. **G.** The provisional crown in place.

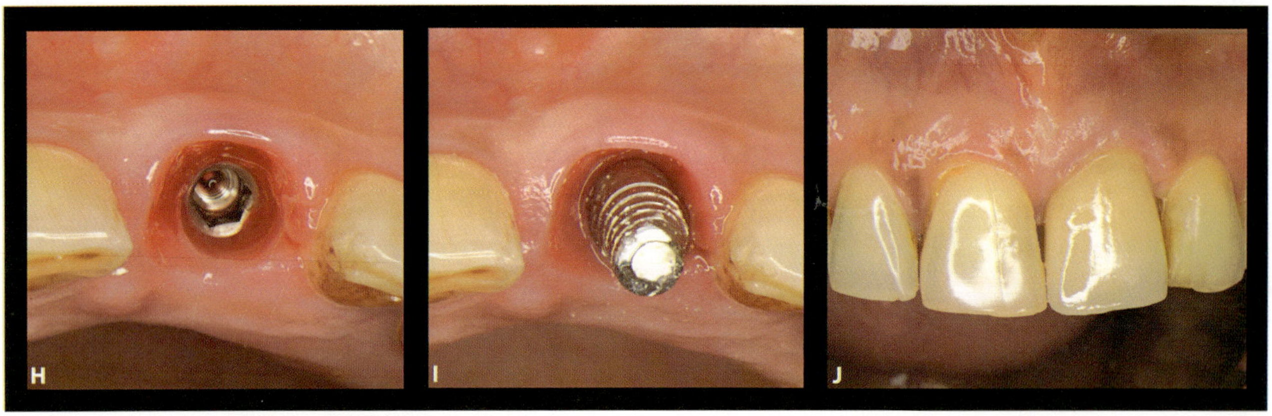

Figure 6.16. **H.** Note the soft tissue maturation around the implant fixture. **I.** The final abetment is being connected. **J.** The final prosthesis in place.

This was confirmed by Drago and Lazzara (2004). They studied the survival rates and interproximal bone levels for Osseotite implants that were restored with fixed provisional crowns without occlusion immediately after implant placement. They evaluated 93 implants placed in 38 partially edentulous patients. All implants were immediately restored with prefabricated abutments and cement-retained provisional crowns without centric or eccentric occlusal contacts. The implants were restored with definitive restorations approximately eight to 12 weeks after implant placement. All patients included in the study were followed for at least 18 months after implant placement (average 20.3 months). Patients were instructed to eat a soft diet and to avoid placing food in the area of the implants and provisional crowns. The provisional crowns served esthetic and phonetic purposes. They replaced the transitional partial dentures that have traditionally been used during implant osseointegration. Oral hygiene was limited to brushing around the implants with a soft toothbrush for the first two weeks. Thereafter, conventional brushing and flossing were permitted. Patients were encouraged to rinse with 0.12% chlorhexidine on a daily basis. The overall survival rate was 97.41. Radiographic bone loss 18 months after implant placement (the mean of both interproximal surfaces) was 0.76 mm. The exact binomial confidence interval was 0.32% to 9.07%. For the exact binomial test with the null hypothesis proportion = .05, P was .3334 and was not statistically significant.

The authors concluded that immediate restoration of dental implants significantly reduces treatment time and may be beneficial in reducing the morbidity associated with loss of teeth, alveolar bone resorption, and loss of interdental papillae associated with the traditional method of treatment following tooth loss. In conclusion, Drago and Lazzara suggested that immediate restoration of Osseotite implants can be accomplished with results that are similar to those obtained with the traditional one- or two-stage surgical, unloaded healing protocols. Parameters identified for the success of this protocol include primary implant stability (i.e., implant placement torque values of at least 30 Ncm), elimination of occlusal contacts prior to osseointegration, dietary modifications during the initial healing period (eight weeks post-placement), and the replacement of teeth with implants appropriate to the clinical situation. Repeated removal and insertion of the template should be avoided unless osseointegration is confirmed. (See Figures 6.17A–E.) After the recommended healing period for the implant and bone graft has elapsed, the template is removed and an impression is made directly or indirectly. Upon the final restorative phase, and upon the template removal, the resultant peri-implant tissues are matured during the healing phase, revealing an exact replica of the soft tissue surrounding the socket at the time of tooth extraction. This represents a major esthetic improvement that saves time and more surgeries.

Using the socket seal template technique has several advantages. It may prevent the apical migration of the gingival epithelium into the socket and the bone graft. Additionally, it favors tissue healing from the

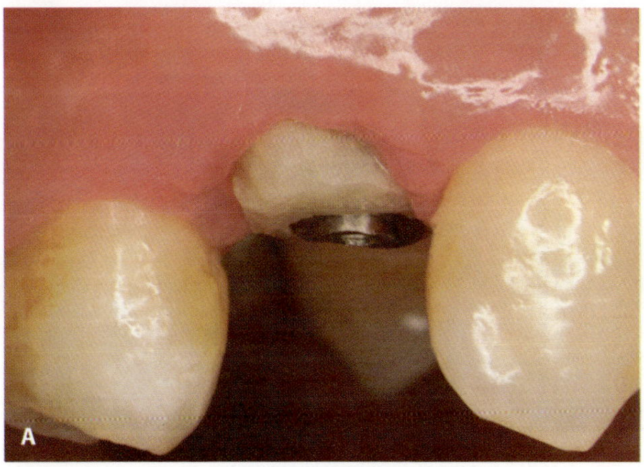

Figure 6.17A. The socket is being sealed with the template on top of the temporary abutment.

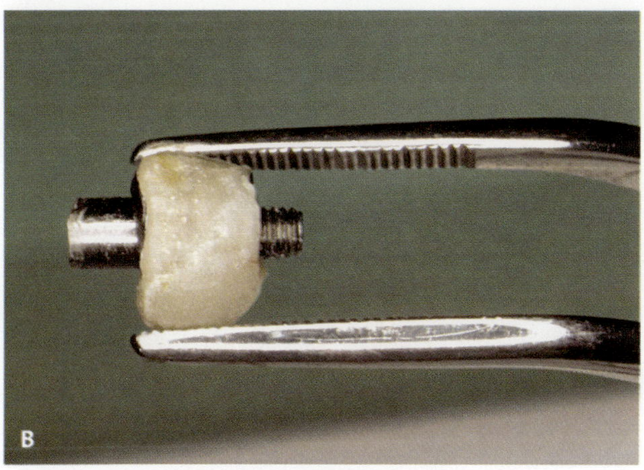

Figure 6.17B. The template after removal.

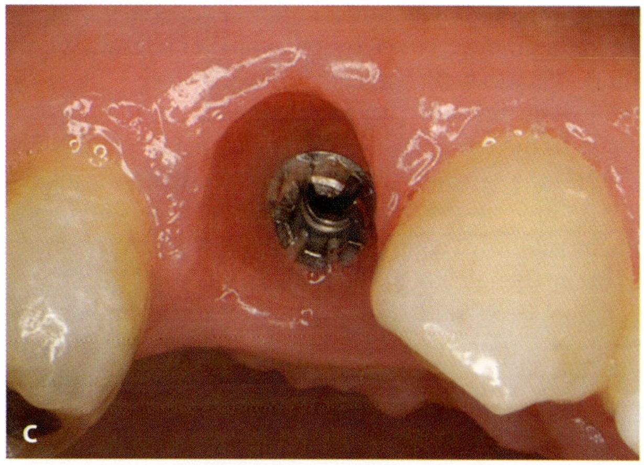

Figure 6.17C. The marginal gingival tissues showing natural contour development.

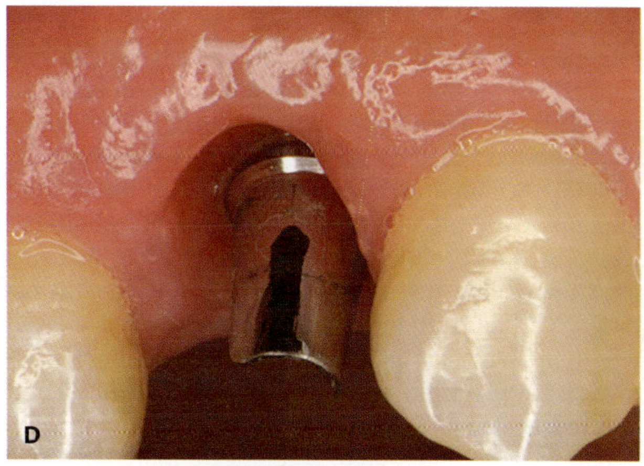

Figure 6.17D. The abutment connected.

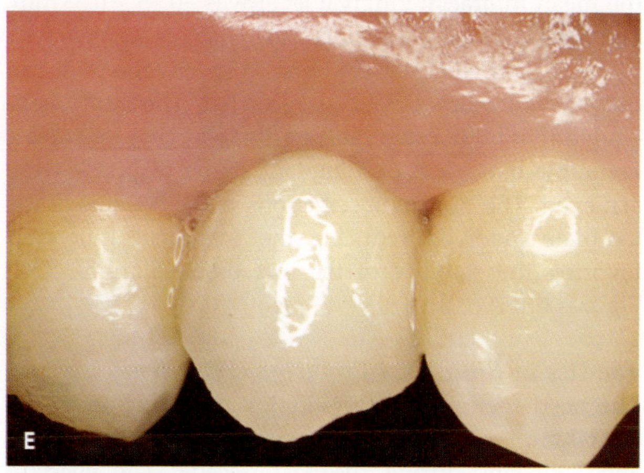

Figure 6.17E. The case finally restored.

periodontal ligament site (Gottlow et al. 1986) because periodontal ligament cells are capable of migrating only short distances (Becker et al. 1988, Minabe 1991). In immediate implant placement, especially in thin scalloped tissue biotypes, the soft tissue manipulations can result in a greater amount of soft tissue shrinkage (Cochran et al. 1997), but with the socket seal template, the possibility of soft tissue shrinkage is much less likely to occur (Bengazi et al. 1996).

It has been said that the socket seal template can provide a function that is similar to GBR membranes. However, the socket seal template technique should be limited to patients with excellent oral hygiene, areas that allow a placement of a minimum 13-mm long implant, a mechanically well stabilized implant in the socket, and only a small osseous defect around the dental implant that does not exceed 1 mm circumferentially. If the void exceeds 1 mm then another surgical approach should be undertaken.

A study (Kan et al. 2003) evaluated the implant success rate, peri-implant tissue response, and the esthetic outcome of implants immediately placed and temporized in the anterior maxilla after a one-year period. Thirty-five patients with a mean age of 36.5 years were selected based on specific inclusion and exclusion criteria. Atraumatic extraction was performed and implants were placed. A metallic temporary abutment was placed and self-cured acrylic resin provisional was used for sealing the socket and as a provisional prosthesis. The fabrication of the final restorations started five months after implant placement. Evaluations were made at implant placement and provisionalization and at three, six, and 12 months. At 12 months, all implants remained osseointegrated. The mean marginal bone change from the time of placement to 12 months was -0.26 ± 0.40 mm mesially and -0.22 ± 0.28 mm distally. The study indicated no significant difference in the plaque index scores. From pretreatment to 12 months, the mean midfacial gingival level was -0.55 ± 0.53 mm, and mesial and distal papilla level changes were -0.53 ± 0.39 mm and -0.39 ± 0.40 mm, respectively. A mean esthetic outcome of 9.9 was recorded. The study concluded that both a favorable implant success rate and a favorable biological peri-implant tissue response were achieved. The clinical observations of the benefits of the template involved reducing the treatment time and favoring the stability of the soft tissue margins. (See Figures 6.18A–C.)

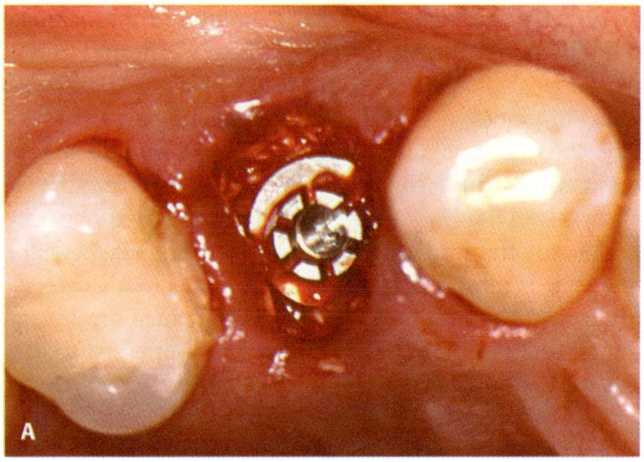

Figure 6.18A. An immediate implant placement with the socket voids filld with bone-grafting material.

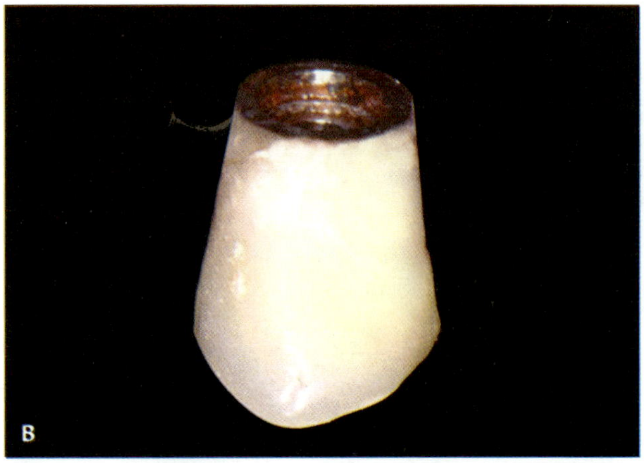

Figure 6.18B. The template is connected to a temporary crown.

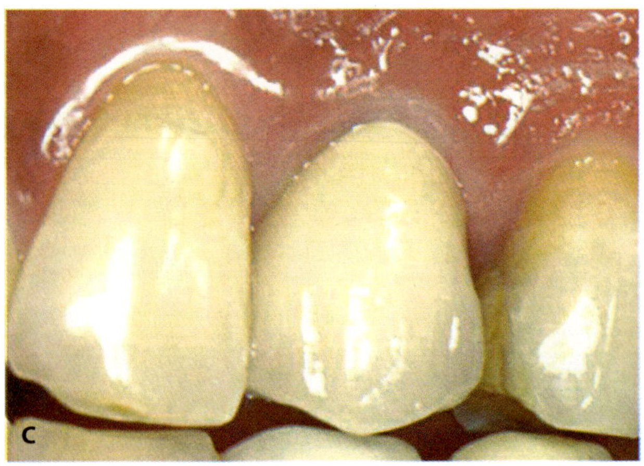

Figure 6.18C. The case finally restored.

The Use of Biological Provisional Barriers

The need for immediate esthetics and function of the dental implants has become a concern for both patients and clinicians during the past decade. The need to provide the patient with a predictable provisional prosthesis immediately after immediate implant installation is becoming a major prerequisite for a successful esthetic implant therapy. In cases of immediate implant therapy, the socket orifice must be sealed to isolate the implant and its related components for the hostile oral environment. The related soft tissue margins of the socket orifice also require support and stabilization until the final prosthesis is inserted; therefore, thought has been given to using the patient's own natural tooth as a provisional prosthesis due to its shade matching and its favorable biological contours. The use of the natural tooth along with immediate implant therapy might be applied in cases of immediate functional and nonfunctional loading protocols; it depends on the clinician's decision prior to the treatment. However, some requirements should be met before making the decision to use this method:

1. The natural tooth that is to be removed and used as a provisional restoration must be sound and free from extensive fillings.
2. The implant must be primary stable and resist torque at 30–40 Ncm.
3. All osseous walls of the socket must be intact.

The technique starts with atraumatic tooth extraction that preserves the labial plate of bone as mentioned previously, and then the tooth is stored in natural saline. (See Figures 6.19A–B.) This is followed by careful socket cleaning and curettage to ensure the complete removal of any remaining soft tissues in the socket. Then the implant is placed according to the 3-D implant positioning esthetic protocol. The abutment height and orientation is then checked and connected to the implant fixture. The extracted tooth is cut at 2 mm below the CEJ and then hollowed out. A self-cured resin material is used to reline the hollowed tooth to the underlying abutment. Note that the resin material should be introduced to the abutment intraorally at the rubbery stage and then withdrawn just prior to final curing. The excess resin is then finished and trimmed, and the tooth is perforated at the palatal surface to make a vent to allow for the excess cement to flow out of the socket and not in the socket itself. Then the tooth is fitted in place and cemented. The occlusion is adjusted according to the loading protocol planned pre-operatively. (See Figures 6.20A–E.)

The use of natural teeth as provisional prostheses in the esthetic zone for nonfunctional loading purposes was confirmed by a study (Tsirlis 2005) that evaluated the methods currently available for the clinical esthetic restoration in the anterior maxilla or in the esthetic zone. Immediately loaded single implants that were loaded in two ways were used: Group A had immediate implant installation, and Group B had delayed implant installation. Forty-three patients were selected using the following criteria:

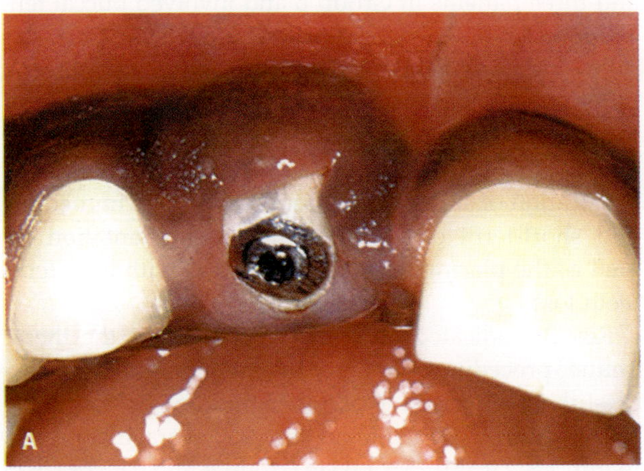

Figure 6.19A. The socket is being sealed with the template on top of the temporary abutment. Note the importance of using this method in order not to interrupt the hyperpigmented tissue band.

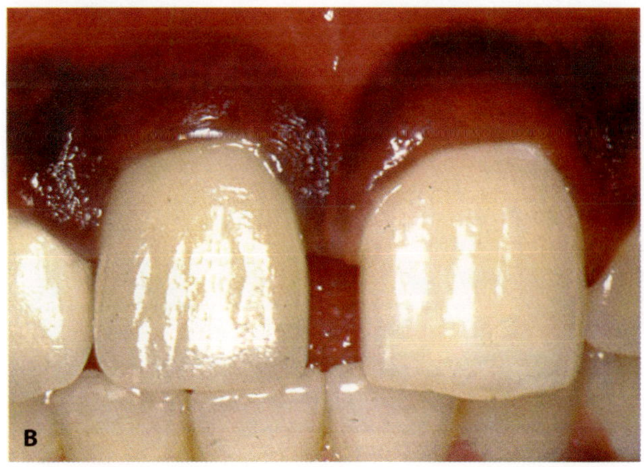

Figure 6.19B. The case restored. Note the preserved continuity of the band.

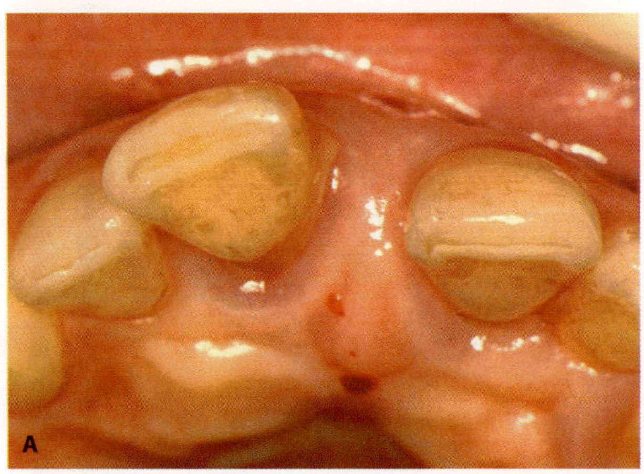

Figure 6.20A. An unsalvageable right central incisor scheduled for extraction and implant placement.

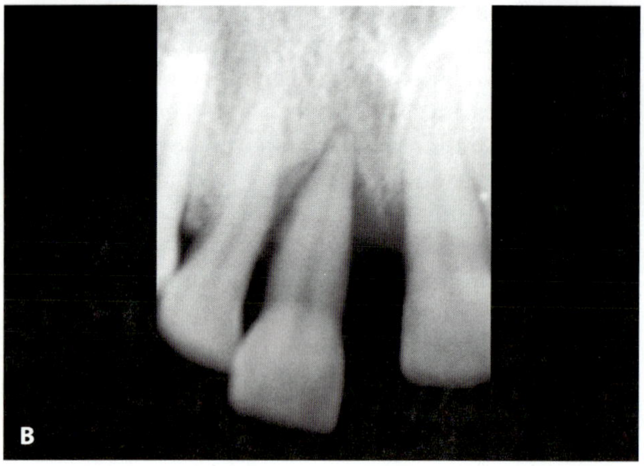

Figure 6.20B. A radiographic view showing the hopeless tooth.

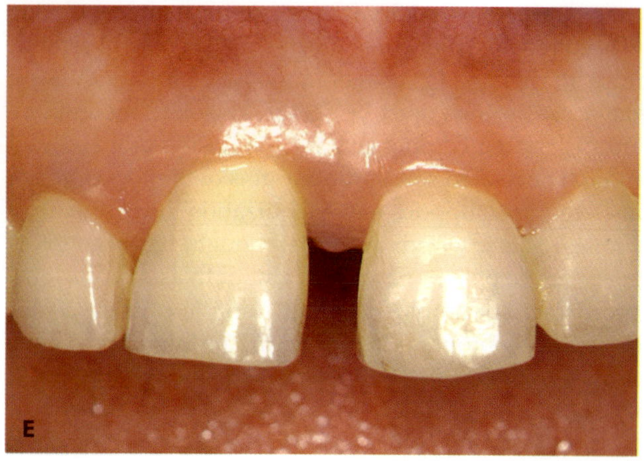

Figure 6.20E. The natural tooth is cemented in place.

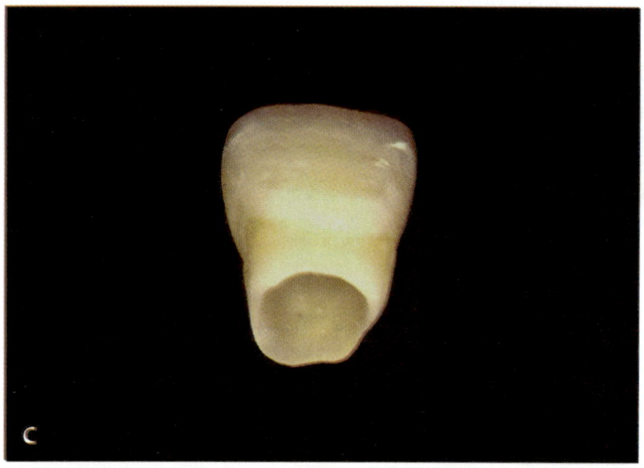

Figure 6.20C. The tooth after extraction and preparation.

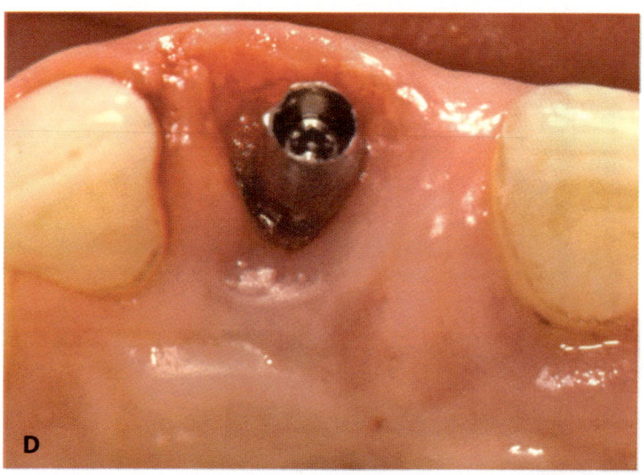

Figure 6.20D. The abutment is connected.

1. No concomitant systemic disease was present.
2. Heavy smokers (≥10 cigarettes per day) were excluded.
3. Acute inflammation related to the natural teeth and the alveolar bone at the surgical sites was not present.
4. There was no extensive bone loss (e.g., the available bone should have been sufficient to ensure the appropriate primary stability during implant installation).
5. The restorations concerned single implants at the anterior maxilla between the left and right premolar regions.

Patients were treated over two years using single implants with immediate nonfunctional loading. GBR techniques were performed in 10 patients in Group A and three patients in Group B and involved buccal fenestrations or buccal dehiscence around the implants. The following parameters were studied: (1) the anatomical requirements necessary in selecting such patients and the limitations that might affect (to a lesser or greater degree) the desired results; and (2) the planning and application of surgical techniques, both with immediate and short-term delay postextraction implantation, as well as the placing of implants in areas with long-term teeth loss.

Results indicated no implant failure, and the therapeutic procedures were considered completely successful in all cases, without significant radiographic peri-implant marginal bone loss (i.e., average bone loss in mm ± SD was 0.75 ± 1.05 in Group A and 0.875 ± 0.625 in Group B) or significant clinical differences in peri-implant sulcus depth (average difference in mm ± SD was 0.3 ± 0.2 in Group A and 0.4 ± 0.375 in Group B). In cases in which GBR techniques were used, the results were considered successful and final, and the esthetic results were deemed more satisfactory than was expected. The procedure was successful in all cases in terms of both osseointegration and esthetics.

The use of dental implants with nonfunctional loading in particularly sensitive esthetic areas is recommended, given the existence of the anatomical requirements, good initial stability, and the absence of extensive bone loss in the area receiving the implant. In addition, application of this treatment method leads to a particularly successful esthetic result, reducing the number of surgeries and the duration of treatment. (See Figures 6.21A–F.) According to the author's experience, the life span and shade stability of the provisional natural teeth are unexpectedly superior and last longer with stable shades. The longest recorded time was five years. The method showed an enhanced soft tissue marginal stability as well as greater patient confidence. Treatment complications were minor and seldom occurred. (See Figures 6.22A–J, 6.23A–F, 6.24A–B, and 6.25.)

Loading Conditions

In flapless implant installation or when the natural tooth is being used as a provisional restoration, immediate function and esthetics may be required in many cases. Therefore, the clinician must have the skills to apply suitable loading protocols that provide an instant improvement as well as ensure long-term success for the dental implants. When it comes to loading dental implants, many factors are to be considered, such as the number of implants used, bone quality and quantity, the position of the implants placed, the type of the future prostheses, the physical design of the implant used, the type of occlusion, the nature of the opposing arch, and finally the decision of the clinician. Some authors (Branemark et al. 1977, Zarb and Schmitt 1994) applied the immediate loading of implants with certain criteria with a high degree of success, whereas others (Balshi and Wolfinger 1997, Tarnow et al. 1997) reported an early failure rate for immediate loaded fixtures seven times higher than that recorded for delayed cases.

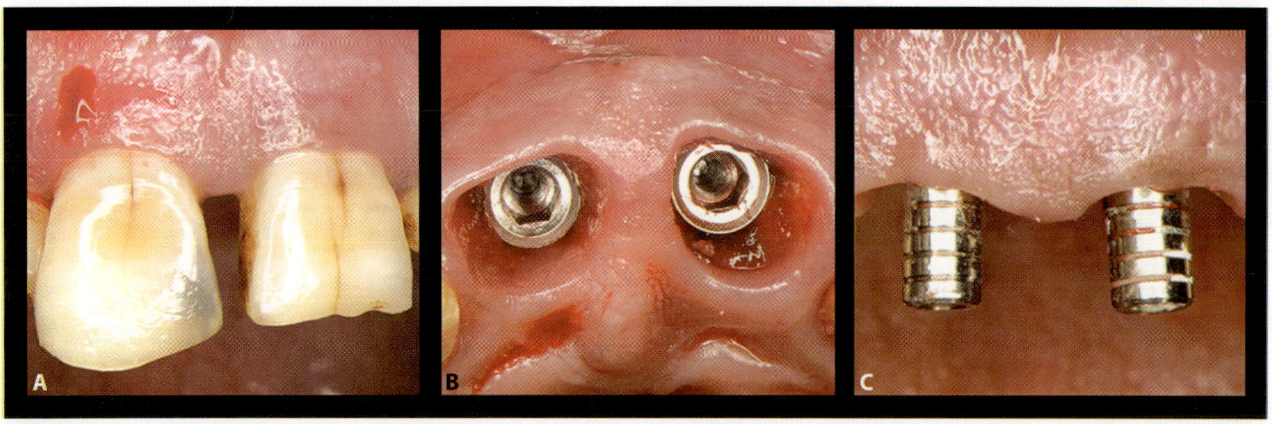

Figure 6.21. **A.** Two central incisors are planned to be removed due to internal root resorption. **B.** Two TSV implants placed in a flapless mode (Zimmer Dental, Carlsbad, CA, USA). **C.** Cement retained abutments connected.

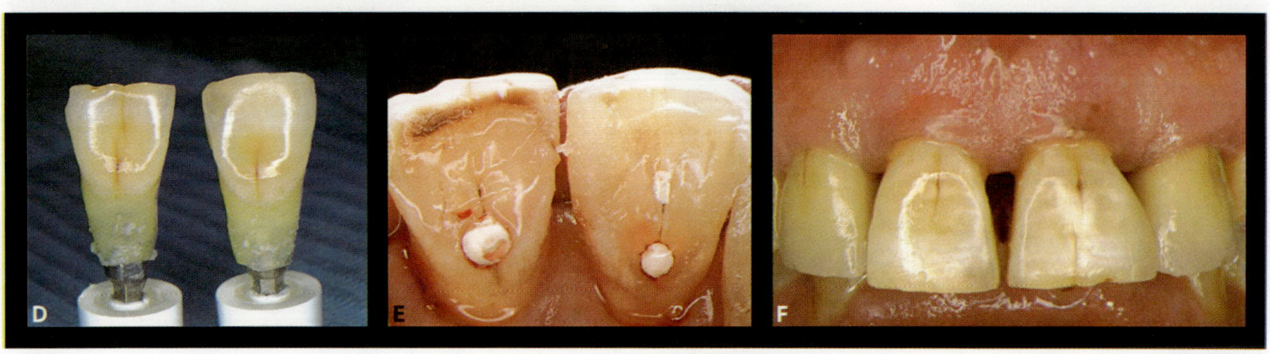

Figure 6.21. **D.** The two extracted central incisors being hollowed and prepared. **E.** Note the palatal vents in order to allow for the escape of the excess cement. **F.** The central incisors are in place, note the natural biological contours.

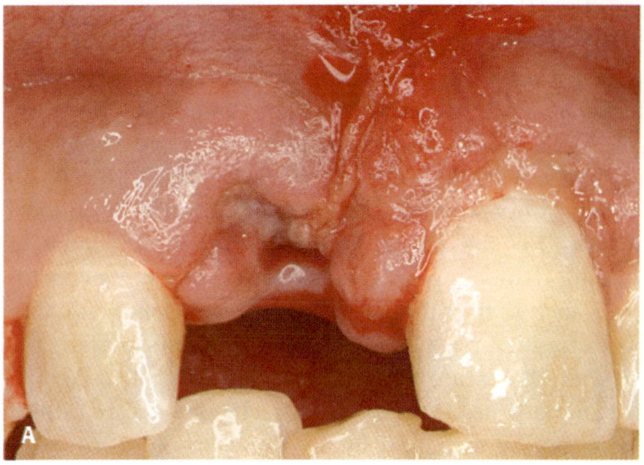

Figure 6.22A. Preoperative view of an avulsion trauma for the maxillary right central incisor.

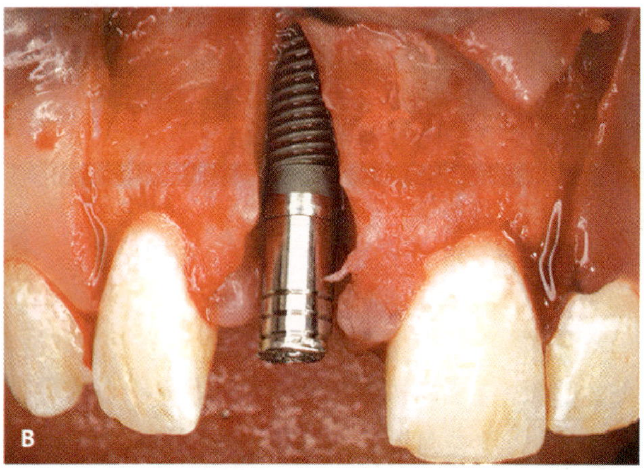

Figure 6.22B. One TSV implant with the abutment connected (Zimmer Dental, Carlsbad, CA, USA) restoring an avulsed central incisor.

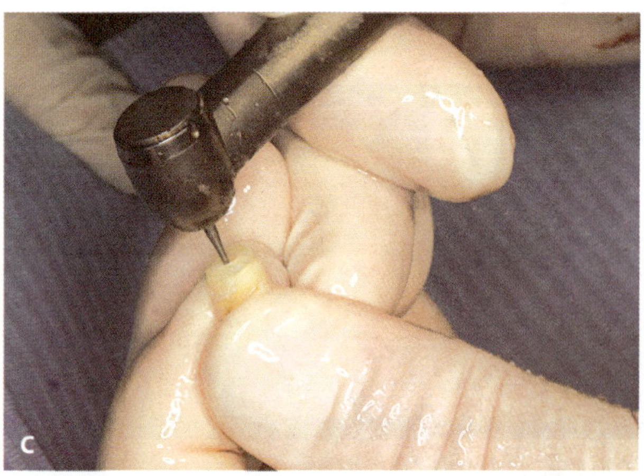

Figure 6.22C. The natural tooth being hollowed from inside.

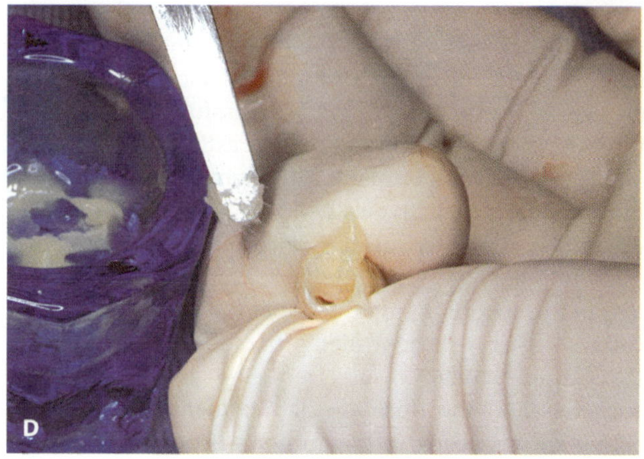

Figure 6.22D. Self-curing resin being added in its fitting surface.

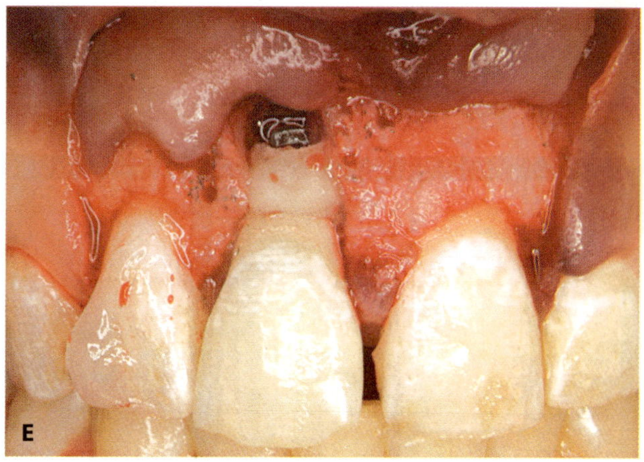

Figure 6.22E. The tooth being adapted and fitted to the abutment.

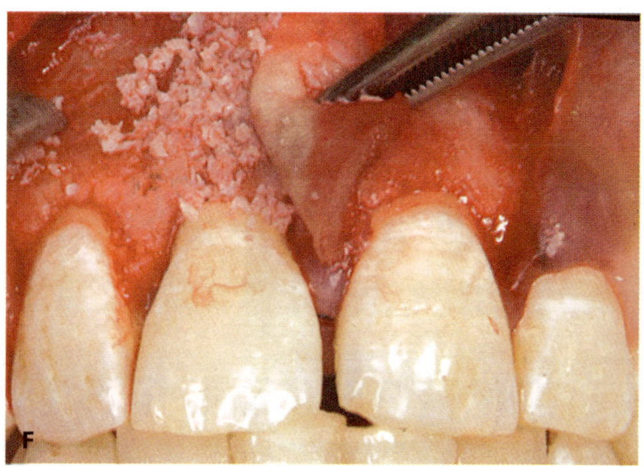

Figure 6.22F. The area is grafted and a BioMend membrane is being stabilized from one end only (Zimmer Dental, Carlsbad, CA, USA).

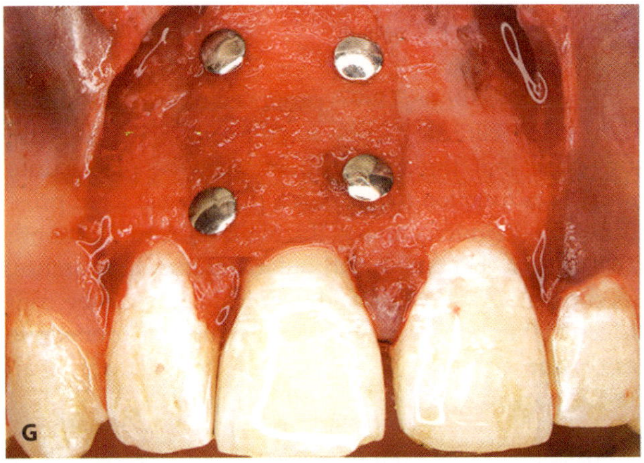

Figure 6.22G. The membrane is being stabilized with four membrane tacks.

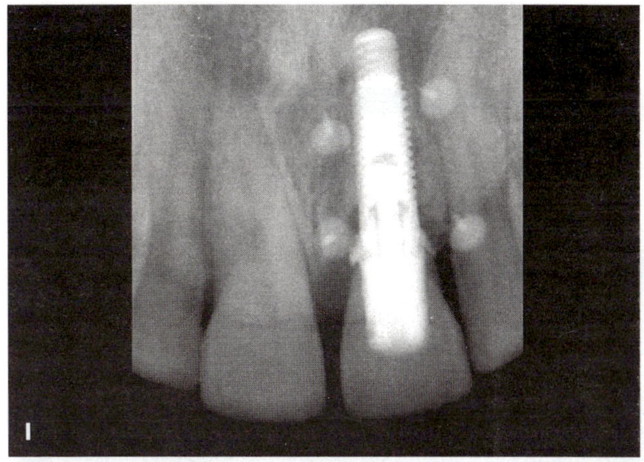

Figure 6.22I. Radiographic view six months post surgery.

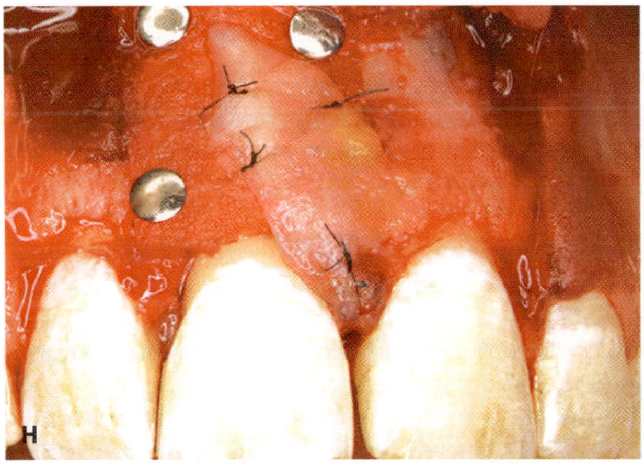

Figure 6.22H. A connective tissue graft is being secured in place to increase the soft tissue thickness.

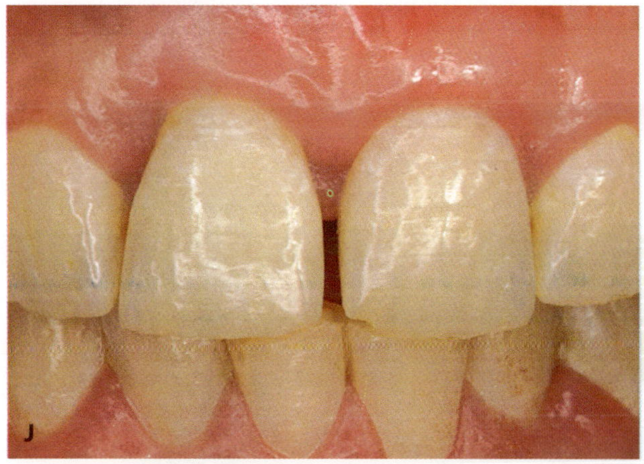

Figure 6.22J. 10 months post restorative result.

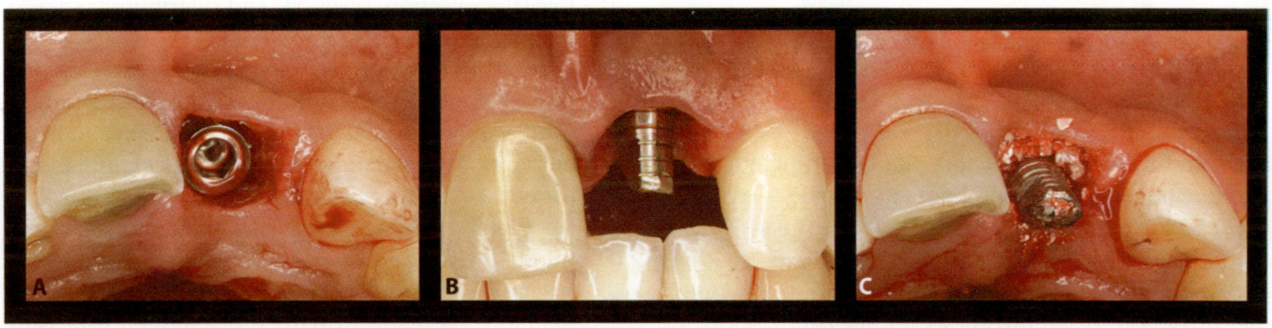

Figure 6.23. **A.** Maxillary left central incisor was extracted and restored with a dental implant in a flapless fashion (Zimmer Dental, Carlsbad, CA, USA). **B.** The abutment connected at the time of the surgery. **C.** The resultant space between the implant fixture and the socket wall is being grafted with an alloplast.

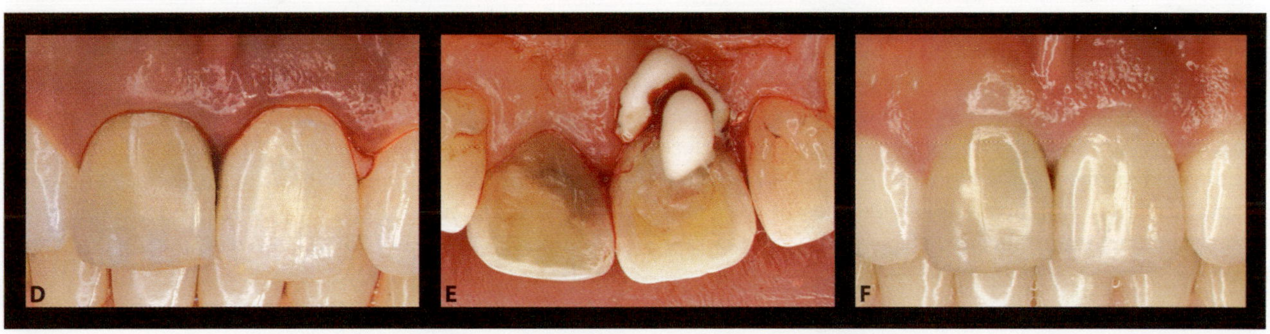

Figure 6.23. **D.** The natural tooth was trimmed and fitted onto the abutment. **E.** Note the excess cement comes out of the palatal vent. **F.** Case finally cemented.

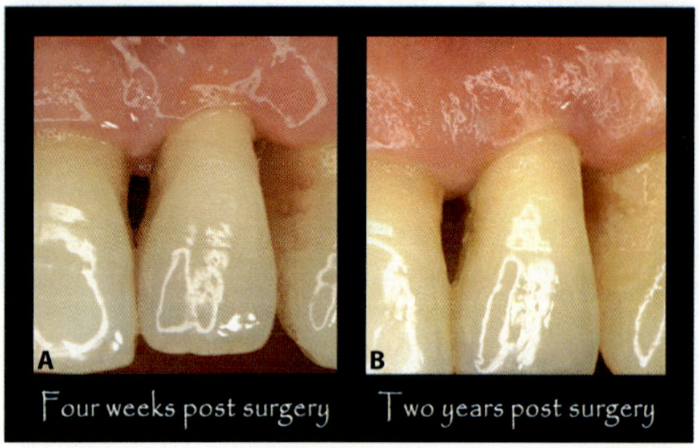

Figure 6.24. **A.** A maxillary left lateral incisor restored with natural tooth at 4 weeks' postsurgery. **B.** Note the improvement in the attachment level.

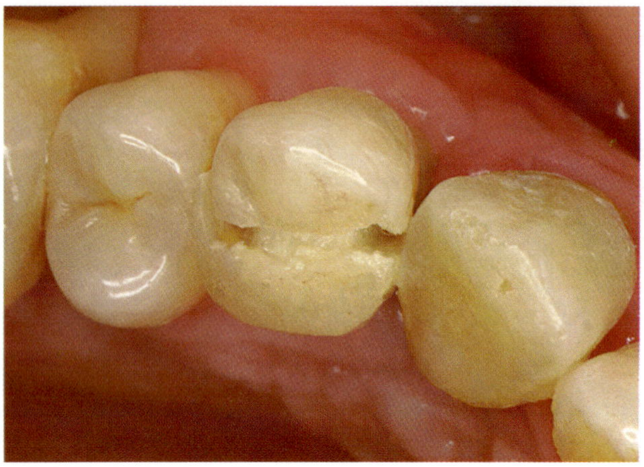

Figure 6.25. post operative complication showing a crack in the natural tooth being used a provisional crown.

Degidi and Piattelli (2003) described differences between functional and nonfunctional loading. Immediate functional loading of implants provides patients with occlusal function on the day of implant placement, whereas nonfunctional immediate loading (termed *immediate restoration* by this group) involved the provision of a prosthesis 1- to 2-mm short of occlusal contact. Early loading of dental implants has been defined as restoration of implants in or out of occlusion at least 48 hours after implant placement (Ganeles and Willsmijer 2004), but at a shorter time interval than conventional healing. Immediate loading or restoration has been defined as the attachment of a restoration in or out of direct occlusal function within 48 hours of surgical placement. Different implant surface characteristics, in particular surface properties (e.g., roughness, bioactive coatings), seem to be of major importance for successful early loading results.

Tarnow and others (1997) proposed nine guidelines to help ensure clinical success for immediate loading and suggested that threaded implants can be placed into immediate function to support a provisional fixed prosthesis in edentulous arches during a four- to six-month healing period in both mandibular and maxillary arches. Several authors have detailed clinical factors to be considered when assessing the applicability of immediate restoration or loading (Tarnow et al. 1997, Ganeles et al. 2001, Aparicio et al. 2003), such as:

1. Primary clinical stability of the implants.
2. Adequate implant splinting where appropriate.
3. Provisional restorations that promote splinting and reduce or control the mechanical load applied to the implants.
4. Prevention of provisional restoration removal during the recommended period of implant healing.
5. Incorporation of the team approach and the use of surgical templates.

In addition, authors have identified risk factors associated with immediate restoration or loading of dental implants. These include (1) the presence of high masticatory or parafunctional forces, (2) poor bone quality or volume, and (3) the presence of infection.

However, a recently published consensus (Morton et al. 2004) offered some clinical recommendations for early and immediate loaded implants for surgical considerations:

1. Implant selection, position, and distribution should be guided by the restorative plan.
2. Diagnostic and surgical templates indicating the prosthodontic plan should be used where possible.
3. Care should be taken to optimize distribution of implants placed in edentulous arches and intended for immediate or early restoration or loading.
4. Minimizing biomechanical risk to implants in edentulous arches and in patients exhibiting extended edentulous regions is recommended. Effort should therefore be made to reduce the influence of cantilevers by using an appropriate number of implants and by optimizing distribution. Also, an adequate number of implants should be positioned to facilitate splinting and protection from the possible effects of micromotion.
5. Clinical stability of dental implants should be achieved. This is made possible by selecting patients who exhibit adequate bone quality and quantity, by selecting an implant with a rough surface and adequate dimension, and by using good clinical technique to maintain contact between the implants and bone.

The following are restorative considerations:

1. Where possible, a clear advantage for the patient should be established prior to treatment.
2. Where possible, the biomechanical effects of the provisional restoration should be controlled by (a) limiting and distributing occlusal contact in centric occlusion or maximum intercuspation, (b) removing all excursive contacts from the provisional restorations, (c) limiting the effects of cantilevers and off-axis loading, and (d) splinting implants together where possible.
3. Traditional prosthodontic procedures associated with accuracy of fit and passivity, evaluation of occlusal scheme, and assessment of patient satisfaction should be encouraged.
4. Where possible, provisional restorations should remain in place throughout the healing process, allowing adequate healing of the hard and soft tissues in contact with the implants and the prosthesis.
5. Clear parameters are required to evaluate the outcome of the restorative treatment.

Another consensus (Ganeles and Willsmijer 2004) stated that most publications that address immediate and early loading indicated that implant survival with immediate restoration was comparable to the results with conventional and early loading protocols. However, they stated that these conclusions may be misleading statistical phenomena of the authors, because most publications were written by exceptionally experienced, highly skilled practitioners working under tightly controlled clinical conditions on a relatively small, statistically inconclusive number of implants and patients. Limited data suggest that immediate restoration of implants in the esthetic zone might facilitate and stabilize gingival architecture more than a staged approach. They also stated that there is no evidence that suggests that deleterious gingival complications can be directly attributed to immediate restoration or loading protocols.

Others (Chiapasco 2004) stated that limited histological data supporting the reliability of immediate loading under various clinical conditions further reduce the current possibility of widespread use of immediate or early loading of implants in all clinical situations. Only sparse data are available, and the use of immediate or early loading of fixed implant-supported prostheses in the maxilla is not supported by sufficient data to consider this treatment modality as routine, although preliminary results seem to be encouraging.

A study (Neugebauer et al. 2006) confirmed that only when torque applied to the implant insertion was more than 35 Ncm in immediately loaded implants did a higher degree of bone formation and remodeling show in comparison to unloaded implants. Immediately loaded implants also demonstrated a prevalence of transversely oriented collagen fibers in the peri-implant bone. The study used four to six immediately loaded and unloaded dental implants with a microstructured surface that were placed in the mandible and the maxilla in seven minipigs. A total of 85 implants were placed. All of the implants were retrieved after a four-month healing period and histomorphometry was performed. The study aimed to prove a relationship between the insertion torque of dental implants (more than 35 Ncm) in relation to the formation of secondary osteons. The study confirmed the presence of secondary osteons formation and a higher quantity of collagen fibers with a more parallel orientation. This was a logical explanation for the benefits of immediate loading concept on the bone remodeling and formation rate.

References

al-Ansari, B.H., and R.R. Morris. 1998. Placement of dental implants without flap surgery: A clinical report. *Int J Oral Maxillofac Implants*, (13), pp. 861–865.

Aparicio, C., B. Rangert, and L. Sennerby. 2003. Immediate/early loading of dental implants: A report from the Sociedad Espanola de Implantes World Congress Consensus Meeting in Barcelona, Spain, 2002. *Clin Implant Dent Relat Res*, 5, pp. 57–60.

Araujo, M., F. Sukekava, I. Wennstrom, et al. 2005. Ridge alterations following implant placement in fresh extraction sockets: an experimental study in the dog. *J Clin Periodontol*, 32, pp. 645–652.

Artzi, Z., and C. Nemcovsky. 1997. Bone regeneration in extraction sites. Part 1: The simultaneous approach, *Implant Dent*, (6), pp. 175–181.

Auty, C., and A. Siddiqui. 1999. Punch technique for preservation of interdental papillae at nonsubmerged implant placement. *Implant Dent*, (8), pp. 160–166.

Balshi, T.J., and G.J. Wolfinger. 1997. Immediate loading of Branemark implants in edentulous mandibles: A preliminary report. *Implant Dent*, 6, pp. 83–88.

Becker, W., B. Becker, L. Berg, J. Prichard, R. Caffesse, and E. Rosenberg. 1988. New attachment after treatment with root isolation procedures: Report for treated Class III and Class II furcation and vertical osseous defects. *Int J Periodontics. Restorative Dent*, (8), pp. 8–23.

Becker, W., and B.E. Becker. 1990. Guided tissue regeneration for implants placed into extraction sockets and for implant dehiscences: Surgical techniques and case report. Int *J Periodontics Restorative Dent*, 10, pp. 377–391.

Becker, W., C. Dahlin, B.E. Becker, et al. 1994. The use of e-PTFE barrier membranes for bone promotion around titanium implants placed into extraction sockets: A prospective multi-center study. *Int J Oral Maxillofac Implants*, 9, pp. 31–40.

Becker, B.E., W. Becker, A. Ricci, and N. Geurs. 1998. A prospective clinical trial of endosseous screw-shaped implants placed at the time of tooth extraction without augmentation, *J Periodontol*, (69), pp. 920–926.

Becker, W., C. Ochsenbein, L. Tibbetts, et al. 1997. Alveolar bone anatomic profiles as measured from dey skulls. Clinical ramifications. *J Clin Periodontol*, (24), pp. 727–731.

Becker, W. 2005. Immediate implant placement: diagnosis, treatment planning and treatment steps/or successful outcomes. *J Calif Dent Assoc.*, Apr, 33, (4), pp. 303–10.

Bengazi, F., J.L. Wennstrom, and U. Lekholm. 1996. Recession of the soft tissue margin at oral implants. *Clin Oral Implant Res*, (7), pp. 303–310.

Block, M.S., and J.N. Kent. 1991. Placement of endosseous implants into tooth extraction sites. *J Oral Maxillofac Surg*, 49, pp. 1269–1276.

Botticelli, D., T. Berglundh, and J. Lindhe. 2004. Hard tissue alterations following immediate implant placement in extraction sites. *Journal of Clinical Periodontology*, 31, pp. 820–828.

Branemark, P.I., B.O. Hansson, R. Adell, et al. 1977. Osseointegrated implants in the treatment of the edentulous jaw: Experience from a 10-year period. *Scand J Plast Reconstr Surg Suppl.*, 16, pp. 1–132.

Branemark, P.I., P. Engstrand, H. Ohrnell, et al. 1999. Branemark Novum: A new treatment concept for rehabilitation of the edentulous mandible. Preliminary results from a prospective clinical follow-up study. *Clin Implant Dent and Related Research*, 1, pp. 2–16.

Bunyaratavay, P., and H.L. Wang. 2001. Collagen membranes: A review. *J Periodontol*, (2), pp. 215–229.

Campelo, L., and J. Camara. 2002. Flapless implant surgery: A 10-year retrospective analysis. *Int J Oral Maxillofac Implants*, 17, pp. 271–267.

Chiapasco, M. 2004. Early and Immediate Restoration and Loading of Implants in Completely Edentulous Patients. *Int J Oral Maxillofac Implants*, 19, (SUPPL), pp. 76–91.

Cochran, D.L., J.S. Hermann, R.K. Schenk, et al. 1997. Biologic width around titanium implant: A histometric analysis of the implant gingival junction around unloaded and Loaded non submerged implants in the canine mandible. *J Periodontol*, (68), pp. 186–198.

Cochran, D.L., R. Schenk, J.M. Wozney, and A.A. Jones. 1999. Recombinant human BMP protein-2 stimulation of bone formation around endosseous dental implants. *J Periodontol*, 70, pp. 139–150.

Cornelini, R., A. Scarano, U. Covani, G. Petrone, and A. Piattelli. 2000. Immediate one-stage post extraction implant: A human clinical and histologic case report. *Int J Oral Maxillofac Implants*, 15:432–437.

Covani, U., C. Bortolaia, A. Barone, et al. 2004a. Bucco-Lingual Crestal Bone Changes After Immediate and Delayed Implant Placement. *J Periodontol*, 75, pp. 1605–1612.

Covani, U., A. Barone, R. Roberto Cornelini, et al. 2004b. Soft Tissue Healing Around Implants Placed Immediately After Tooth Extraction Without Incision: A Clinical Report. *Int J Oral Maxillofac Implants*, 19, pp. 549–553.

Degidi, M., and A. Piattelli. 2003. Immediate functional and non-functional loading of dental implants: A 2- to 60-month follow-up study of 646 titanium implants. *J Periodonto1*, 74, pp. 225–241.

Drago, C., and R. Lazzara. 2004. Immediate Provisional Restoration of Osseotite Implants: A Clinical Report of 18-month Results. *J Oral Maxillofac Implants*, 19, pp. 534–541.

Dreesman, H. 1892. Uber Knochenplombierung. *Bietr Klin Chir*, (9), p. 804.

Edel, A. 1995. The use of a connective tissue graft for closure over immediate implants covered with an occlusive membrane. *Clin Oral Implant Res*, (6), pp. 60–65.

El Askary, A.S. 2001. Multifaceted aspects of implant esthetics: the anterior maxilla. *Implant Dent*, 10, pp. 182–191.

Evian, C.I., and S. Cutler. 1994. Autogenous gingival grafts as epithelial barriers for immediate implants: Case reports. *J Periodontol*, (65), pp. 201–210.

Ganeles, J., M.M. Rosenberg, R.L. Holt, and L.H. Reichman. 2001. Immediate loading of implants with fixed restorations in the completely edentulous mandible: Report of 27 patients from a private practice. *Int J Oral Maxoillofac Implants*, 16 pp. 418–426.

Ganeles, J., and D. Willsmijer. 2004. Early and Immediately Restored and Loaded Dental Implants for Single Tooth and Partial-Arch Applications. *Int J Oral Maxillofac Implants*, 19 (SUPPL), pp. 92–102.

Gelb, D.A. 1993. Immediate implant surgery: Three-year retrospective evaluation of 50 consecutive cases. *Int J Oral Maxillofac Implants*, 8, pp. 388–399.

Gher, M.E., G. Quintero, D. Assad, et al. 1994a. Bone grafting and guided bone regeneration for immediate implants in humans. *J Periodontol*, (65), pp. 881–891.

Gher, M.E., G. Quintero, J.B. Sandifer, et al. 1994b. Combined dental implant and guided tissue regeneration therapy in humans. *Int J Periodontics Restorative Dent*, (14), pp. 332–347.

Gotfredsen, K., L. Nimb, D. Buser, et al. 1993. Evaluation of guided bone regeneration around implants placed into fresh extraction sockets: An experimental study in dogs. *J Oral Maxillofac Surg*, (51), pp. 879–884.

Gottlow, J., D. New, J. Lindhe, T. Karring, and J. Wennstrom. 1986. New attachment formation in the human periodontium by guided tissue regeneration. Case reports. *J Clin Periodontol*, (13), pp. 604–616.

Hammerle, C.H., S.T. Chen, T.G. Wilson Jr., et al. 2004. Consensus statements and recommended clinical procedures regarding the placement of implants in extraction sockets. *Int J Oral Maxillofac Implants*, 19 Suppl, pp. 26–8.

Jovanovic, S.A., H. Spickerman, and E.J. Richrer. 1992. Bone regeneration around titanium dental implants in dehisced sites: A clinical study. *Int J Oral Maxillofac Implants*, (13), pp. 29–45.

Kan, J.Y., and K. Rungcharassaeng. 2000. Immediate placement and provisionalization of maxillary anterior single implants: A surgical and prosthodontic rationale. *Pract Periodont Aesthet Dent*, 12, pp. 817–824.

Kan, J., K. Rungcharassaeng, and J. Lozada. 2003. Immediate Placement and Provisionalization of Maxillary Anterior Single Implants: 1-Year Prospective Study. *Int J Oral Maxillofac Implants*, 18, pp. 331–339.

Kay, L.W. 1970. The dental implications of the maxillary antrum. *J Ir Dent Assoc*, (16), pp. 10–19.

Landsberg, C.J., and N. Bichacho. 1998. Implant placement without flaps: A single-stage surgical protocol—Part 1. *Pract Periodont Aesthet Dent*, (10), pp. 1033–1039.

Landsberg, C.J., and N. Bichacho. 1999. Implant placement without flaps: A single-stage protocol—Part 2. Utilizing a two-stage surgical protocol. *Pract Periodont Asthet Dent*, (11), pp. 169–176.

Lang, N.P., C.H. Hammede, U. Bragger, B. Lehman, and S.R. Nyman. 1994. Guided tissue regeneration in jawbone defects prior to implant placement. *Clin Oral Implant Res*, (5), pp. 92–97.

Lazarra, R.J. 1989. Immediate implant placement into extraction sites: Surgical and restorative advantages. *Int J Periodont Rest Dent*, 9, pp. 332–343.

Lekholm, U., W. Becker, C. Dahlin, et al. 1993. The role of early versus late removal of GTAM membranes on bone formation at oral implants placed into immediate extraction sockets: An experimental study in dogs. *Clin Oral Implant Res*, (4), pp. 121–129.

Lekovic, V., P.M. Camargo, P.R. Klokkevold, et al. 1998. Preservation of alveolar bone in extraction sockets using bioabsorbable membranes. *Periodontol*, 69, pp. 1044–9.

Mellonig, J.T., and M. Nevins. 1995. Guided bone regeneration of bone defects associated with implants: An evidence based outcome assessment. *Int J Periodontics Restorative Dent*, (15), pp. 168–185.

Meredith, N., D. Alleyne, and P. Cawley. 1996. Quantitative determination of the stability of the implant-tissue interface using resonance frequency analysis. *Clin Oral Implants Res*, 7, pp. 261–7.

Minabe, M. 1991. Critical review of the biologic rationale for guided tissue regeneration. *J Periodontol*, (62), pp. 171–179.

Morton, D., R. Jaffin, and H. Weber. 2004. Immediate Restoration and Loading of Dental Implants: Clinical Considerations and Protocols. *Int J Oral Maxillofac Implants*, 1, 9 (SUPPL), pp. 103–108.

Nemkovesky, C.E., A. Artzi, and O. Moses. 2000. Rotated palatal flap in immediate implant procedures. *Clin Oral Implant Res*, (11), p. 83.

Neugebauer, J., T. Traini, U. Thams, et al. 2006. Peri-Implant Bone Organization Under Immediate Loading State. Circularly Polarized Light Analyses: A Minipig Study. *J Periodontol*, 77, pp. 152–160.

Novaes Jr., A.B., and A.B. Novaes. 1997. Soft tissue management for primary closure in guided bone regeneration: Surgical technique and case report. *Int J Oral Maxillofac Implants*, (12), pp. 84–87.

Paolantonio, M., M. Dolci, A. Scarano, et al. 2001. Immediate implantation in fresh extraction sockets. A controlled clinical and histological study in man. *Journal of Periodontology*, 72, pp. 1560–1571.

Pow, E., and A. McMillan. 2004. A Modified Implant Healing Abutment to Optimize Soft Tissue Contours: A Case Report. *Implant Dent*, 13, 297–300.

Rosenquist, B., and B. Grenthe. 1996. Immediate placement of implants into extraction sockets: Implant survival. *Int J Oral Maxillofac Implants*, (11), pp. 205–209.

Rosenquist, B. 1997. A comparison of various methods of soft tissue management following the immediate placement of implants into extraction sockets. *Int J Oral Maxillofac Implants*, (12), pp. 43–51.

Rosenquist, B.O., and M. Ahmad. 2000. The immediate replacement of teeth by dental implants using homologous bone membranes to seal the sockets: Clinical and radiographic finding. *Clin Oral Implant Res*, 110, pp. 572–582.

Schwartz, D.A., and G. Chaushu. 1998. Immediate implant placement: A procedure without incisions. *J Periodontol*, (69), pp. 743–750.

Schwartz-Arad, D., and G. Chaushu. 1997. Placement of implant into fresh extraction sites: to 7 year's retrospective evaluation of 95 immediate implants. *J Periodontol*, 68, pp. 111–116.

Simion, M., M. Baldoni, P. Rossi, and D. Zaffe. 1994. A comparative study of the effectiveness of e-PTFE membranes with and without early exposure during the healing period. *Int J Periodontics Restorative Dent*, (14), pp. 167–180.

Tarnow, D.P., S. Emtiaz, and A. Classi. 1997. Immediate loading of threaded implants at stage 1 surgery in edentulous arches: Ten consecutive case reports with 1- to 5-year data. *Int J Oral Maxillofac Implants*, 12, pp. 319–324.

Tsirlis, A. 2005. Clinical Evaluation of Immediate Loaded Upper Anterior Single Implants. *Implant Dent*, 14, p. 94103.

Von Rehrman, A. 1936. Eine Methode zur Schliessung von Keiferhohlen Perforationen. *Dtsch Zahnaerzth Wochen-Schr*, (39), p. 1137.

Wang, H.L., and W.J. Carroll. 2000. Using absorbable collagen membranes for guided tissue regeneration, guided bone regeneration and to treat gingival recession.

Compendium, (21), pp. 399–410.

Wilson, T.G., R. Schenk, D. Buser, and D. Cochran. 1998. Implants placed in immediate extraction sites: A report of histologic and histometric analyses of human biopsies. *Int J Oral Maxillofac Implants*, 13, pp. 333–341.

Wilson Jr, T.G., J. Carnio, R. Schenk, et al. 2003. Immediate implants covered with connective tissue membranes: human biopsies. *J Periodontol*, 74, (3), pp. 402–9.

Zarb, G.A., and A. Schmitt. 1994. Osseointegration and the edentulous predicament: The 10-year Toronto Study. *Br Dent J*, 170, pp. 439–444.

Chapter 7

Socket Augmentation: Rationale and Technique

Hom-Lay Wang and Rodrigo F. Neiva

Introduction

Tooth extraction, either traumatic or atraumatic, results in alveolar bone loss, both in width and height (Bays 1986, Mecall and Rosenfeld 1996, Mecall and Rosenfeld 1992, Mecall and Rosenfeld 1991). An average of 40% to 60% of original height and width is expected to be lost after tooth extraction, with the greatest loss happening within the first year (Sevor and Meffert 1992, Polizzi et al. 2000, Grunder et al. 1999, Werbitt and Goldberg 1992, Werbitt and Goldberg 1991). This can negatively influence bone volume that is needed for future dental implant placement as well as proper ideal esthetic restoration. Research has demonstrated that the alveolar ridge at the maxillary anterior area can be reduced by 23% in the first six months after tooth extraction, and an additional 11% in the following five years (Artzi et al. 2000). In the posterior mandible, resorption happens primarily in the buccal/labial direction, resulting in a lingual displacement of alveolar crest (Artzi et al. 2000).

The rate of reduction of residual alveolar ridges has shown to be greater in mandibular (0.4 mm/year) than in maxillary arches (0.1 mm/year) (Nemcovsky and Serfaty 1996). This often resulted in 1 mm vertical bone resorption (corresponding to 2 mm soft tissue recession) (Wang et al. 2004a, Iasella et al. 2003) and 2–2.5 mm of horizontal bone resorption. This is more evident in the buccal plate due to a greater amount of bundle bone (Araujo and Lindhe 2005). Recent evidence has shown that even with an immediate implant placement, a buccal bone resorption cannot be avoided (Botticelli et al. 2005, Araujo et al. 2005). As a consequence, the resorption may prevent ideal implant placement, thus compromising the optimal esthetic and functional outcomes (Howell et al. 1997). Socket augmentation allows clinicians to preserve alveolar bone height, potentially regenerating new bone, and thus may maintain the soft tissue height. This, in turn, could facilitate ideal implant placement with optimal esthetics.

Augmentation of the extraction socket at the time of tooth extraction using a variety of bone grafts (also known as *socket augmentation, socket preservation*, and *ridge preservation*) has been attempted and assessed in many studies (Ashman and Lopinto 2000, Froum and Orlowski 2000, Froum et al. 2002). Several techniques have also been developed in an attempt to minimize alveolar ridge resorption while promoting new bone formation (Bartee 2001a, Becker et al. 2002, Fowler et al. 2000). Immediate implant placement and bone augmentation in extraction sockets have been suggested to minimize or prevent this clinical dilemma (Ashman and Lopinto 2000, Froum and Orlowski 2000, Froum et al. 2002). Generally, these procedures are primarily aimed at preserving the current bone level and, hopefully, regenerating new bone.

This chapter describes the rationale behind socket augmentation and proposes a decision tree to guide clinicians in selecting a certain socket augmentation procedure to not only minimize alveolar bone loss, but also to promote bone formation.

Rationale

The rationale for alveolar ridge preservation relies on the knowledge that alveolar ridge resorption is an unavoidable sequelae of tooth loss (Bays 1986). Attempts to overcome the detrimental effects of alveolar ridge deficiency have included retention of residual root tips, mucogingival surgeries to deepen the vestibule or to improve esthetics of fixed bridges, immediate implant placement, and, more recently, bone augmentation in extraction sockets. The more recent approach was developed not only to maintain a more esthetic gingival profile but also to preserve adequate dimensions for dental implant placement. Reports in the literature have demonstrated the importance of this approach in implant dentistry. A study (Lekovic et al. 1997) compared the outcome of alveolar ridge preservation with or without absorbable barrier membranes. At six months, significantly less crestal bone loss (–0.38 mm versus –1.50 mm), more internal socket fill (–5.81 mm versus –3.94 mm), and less horizontal ridge resorption (–1.31 mm versus –4.56 mm) were found in the membrane group than in the control. As this study suggested, successful early alveolar ridge augmentation (preservation) procedures may reduce or eliminate the need for future ridge augmentation.

A randomized, controlled, masked clinical trial was performed with 24 patients. Subjects received either extraction alone or socket augmentation using tetracycline hydrated freeze-dried bone allograft (FDBA) and a collagen membrane. Histological analysis demonstrated greater bone formation in augmented sites after a six-month healing period. The most predictable maintenance of ridge width, height, and position was achieved when a socket augmentation procedure was employed. The control group experienced on average 1 mm of crestal bone loss, while augmented sites gained on average 1.3 mm of ridge height (Iasella et al. 2003). As both studies suggested, successful early alveolar ridge augmentation (preservation) procedures may reduce or eliminate the need for future ridge augmentation.

Immediately after tooth extraction, bleeding occurred and blood clots formed. Within 48 to 72 hours, inflammatory cells including neutrophil granulocytes, monocytes, and fibroblasts migrated into the wound site along the fibrin network. This resulted in wound cleansing. Then the blood clot was slowly replaced by granulation tissue. Granulation tissue formed from the apical end to the coronal aspect. At 96 hours, the blood clot started contraction and began proliferation of the oral epithelium. At this time, osteoclasts were visible at the margins of the alveolus. At around seven days, young connective tissue and primary osteoid and epithelial proliferation were occurring. At 21 days, formation of connective tissue, mineralization of osteoid, and re-epithelialization were noted. At six weeks, soft tissue wound closure with woven bone (e.g., primary bone, immature bone) formation was identified. Bone continues to model and remodel to form lamellar bone (secondary bone or mature bone) and bone marrow (Amler 1969). This process can take up to six months.

Alveolar ridge atrophy is a common sequel of tooth loss following the above healing events. Various bone-grafting materials and techniques have been used and attempted and have shown positive results in many clinical scenarios (Amler 1969, Cranin et al. 1995, Ashman 1995, Bartee 1995). Osteogenic graft materials supply viable osteoblasts that form new bone, whereas osteoinductive grafts stimulate pluripotential mesenchymal cells to differentiate into osteoblasts that can form new bone. Osteoconductive graft materials, however, merely act as a lattice for cell growth, permitting osteoblasts from the wound margins to infiltrate the defect and migrate across the graft (Feinberg and Fonseca 1986). These grafting materials have shown to not only aid in osteoconduction of osteogenic cells by preserving the space and excluding unwanted cells from the wound, but also to promote formation of new bone (Iasella et al. 2003, Becker et al. 1996, Pinholt et al. 1992, Pinholt et al. 1990).

Autologous grafts are considered to be the ideal material for bone-grafting procedures since they possess osteogenic, osteoinductive, and osteoconductive properties (Schallhorn 1968). Transplantation of living cells increases the possibility of retained cell viability and graft revascularization (Maatz et al. 1952a, 1952b, 1953, 1954). In addition, autologous grafts do not present a risk of disease transmission since the donor and recipient are the same individual (Goldberg and Stevenson 1987). However, they do increase the risk of additional pain, infection, and donor site morbidity since an additional surgical procedure is necessary for harvesting (Feinberg and Fonseca 1986). Hence, bone substitutes have gained increasing acceptance as alternatives to autologous bone for patients requiring bone augmentation in an effort to decrease the morbidity associated with autologous graft harvesting (Russell 2000).

Allografts, xenografts, and alloplasts come in many forms, and data support their safety, clinical applicability, and low antigenicity (Buck and Malinin 1994). Bone graft materials have been used to augment bony defects adjacent to dental implants and to repair chronic extraction socket defects, with and without the use of barrier membranes (Brugnami et al. 1999, Kassolis et al. 2000, Simion et al. 1996). When combined with barrier membranes, bone graft materials have also been shown to prevent collapse of the barrier membrane (Nevins and Mellonig 1992, 1994; Mellonig and Nevins 1995; Mellonig et al. 1998). Xenografts and alloplasts have also been applied to correct bony defects adjacent to dental implants and preserve the alveolar ridge prior to implant placement, showing promising results (Smiler 2001). Despite lack of osteoinductivity, these materials have shown results comparable with those achieved with allografts (Froum and Orlowski 2000).

Because these materials are mineralized, their osteoconductive property is enhanced due to formation of a more rigid scaffold for new bone formation (Camargo et al. 2000, Aichelmann-Reidy and Yukna 1998, Yukna et al. 2001). However, some reports have shown negative results when an alveolar ridge preservation was attempted, possibly due to use of inadequate techniques and/or materials (Cohen 1995, Tal 1999, Zitzmann et al. 1999, Zubillaga et al. 2003). For example, negative results have occurred when a combination of demineralized freeze-dried bone allograft (DFDBA) (Regenafill,

Regeneration Technologies, Inc., Alachua, FL, USA) and a bioabsorbable membrane (Resolut XT, W.L. Gore and Associates, Inc., Flagstaff, AZ, USA) were evaluated for socket augmentation. The negative results were attributed to the slow resorption of the gelatin carrier of the graft material (Zubillaga et al. 2003).

The utility of barrier membranes in socket augmentation procedures has also been evaluated. Research has demonstrated the utility of absorbable and nonabsorbable barrier membranes in preserving alveolar ridges following tooth extraction (Wang and Carroll 2001, Bartee 2001b). When combined with barrier membranes, bone graft materials have also been shown to prevent collapse of the barrier membrane (Nevins and Mellonig 1992, Wang et al. 2005, Mellonig and Nevins 1995). Collagen membranes are preferable due to their absorbable property that eliminates the second membrane retrieval procedure and are highly biocompatible with the surrounding oral tissues (Wang et al. 2004a, Sableman 1985, Postlethwaite et al. 1978).

The integrity and thickness of the buccal plate and the presence of periapical lesions are among the factors that have been associated with compromised healing capacity of extraction sockets. The presence of a thick buccal plate (>1 mm) is important since ridge collapse is initiated by a lingual depression of this socket wall (Korsnes 2002). In addition, data from our unpublished study also indicated that when buccal plates are thicker than 1 mm at 2–3 mm below the alveolar crest, no grafting material is needed since these sites heal similarly to traditional exodontia (Covani et al. 2003). Thick buccal plates are less susceptible to resorption due to the increased vascularity and mineral component (Goldschlag et al. 1994, O'Brien 1994, Barboza 1999). Hence, absence or thinning of the socket wall may predispose the site to ridge deficiency if the socket is not adequately managed.

Ridge deficiency after traditional exodontia has also been associated with sites presenting periapical pathologies (Block et al. 2002). Hence, these sites require more careful intervention, and bone grafting is sometimes encouraged only if the infection can be completely eliminated. Immediate implant placement is also indicated to reduce the amount of bone loss and to assist in space maintenance during the healing process. However, this approach is technique-sensitive and requires a higher level of experience since preparation of implant osteotomy in extraction sockets can be challenging (Paolantonio et al. 2001). This technique is often limited to single-rooted teeth since sockets of multirooted teeth rarely provide ideal location for implant placement due to the inability to achieve primary stability. The immediate implant placement is also contraindicated in sites presenting with active infections.

Techniques

Local anesthetic can be administered after a complete medical history has been reviewed and no contraindications for a surgical procedure have been found. Radiographic analysis of the surgical site should be considered for root anatomy, which aids in determining the ideal pathway for exodontia. The extraction initiates with sulcular incisions performed with a 15-C scalpel to rupture the supracrestal attachment apparatus, which is primarily composed of epithelial and connective tissue attachments to the tooth surface.

Periotomes are then applied to luxate the periodontal ligament (PDL) space. Straight periotomes are indicated for use on single-rooted teeth, while angled periotomes allow access to posterior multirooted teeth. These instruments are used in a similar manner for extraction of intact teeth or removal of retained root fragments. The instrument is used first to completely rupture the gingival fibers at the cervical area of the tooth, as shown in Figures 7.1A–F. During this procedure, the long axis of the blade should be angled converging at approximately 20 degrees from the tooth long axis. This maneuver ensures that the tip of the periotome blade is located

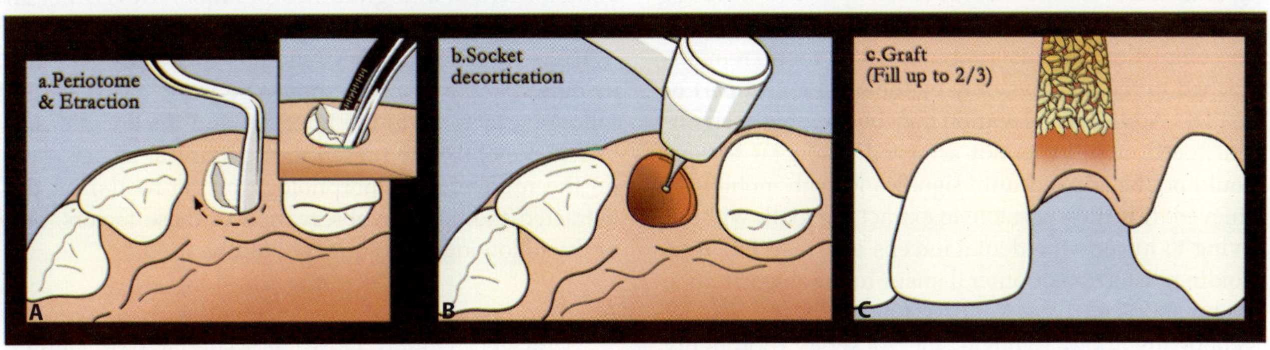

Figure 7.1. **A.** Atraumatic tooth extraction. **B.** Bleeding is stimulated with curettes or rotary instruments. **C.** Bone graft fills two-thirds of the socket depth. Reproduced from Wang H-L, Kiyonobu K, Neiva RF. Socket Augmentation: Rational & technique. *Implant Dentistry*, 2004; 13(4): 286–296.

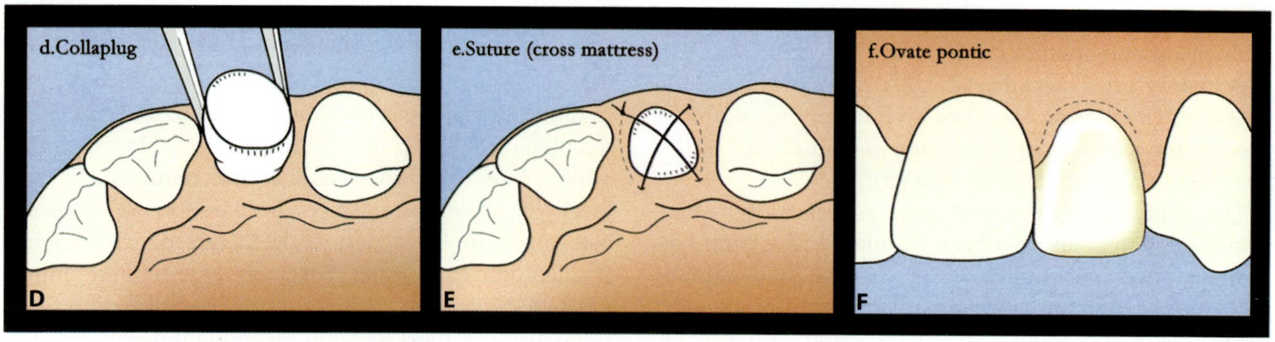

Figure 7.1. **D.** Wound dressing material fills the remaining one-third of the socket. **E.** A cross-mattress suture is applied. **F.** Ovate pontics are used for soft tissue development. Reproduced from Wang H-L, Kiyonobu K, Neiva RF. Socket Augmentation: Rational & technique. *Implant Dentistry*, 2004; 13(4): 286–296.

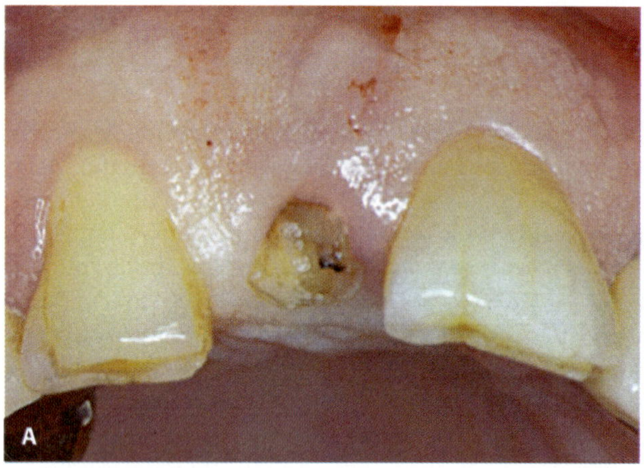

Figure 7.2A. Preoperative view.

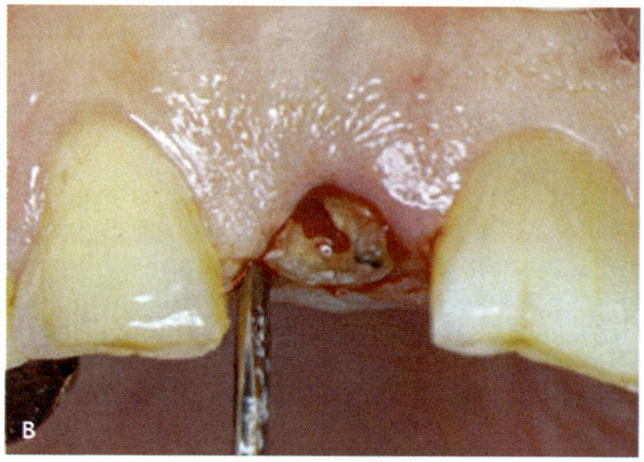

Figure 7.2B. Periotomes facilitate rupture of the supracrestal attachment apparatus.

within the crest of the alveolar bone only, thus preventing the blade from sliding out of the ridge and lacerating the gingiva. It is necessary to repeat this procedure to ensure that all gingival fibers are ruptured.

The instrument is then inserted into the PDL and moved repeatedly in a mesiodistal direction, on the whole circumference of the root, resulting in the widening of the PDL. It is possible to reach up to two-thirds of the root length by repeatedly using this maneuver. With the completion of this procedure, the tooth remains attached to the alveolus only by the most apical part of the PDL. Additional elevation may be required if significant tooth mobility is not achieved. A dental forceps should not be applied until significant tooth mobility is achieved. It is then possible to extract the tooth without having to intrude the dental forceps into the PDL, thus avoiding distortion or other damage to the alveolar bone (Quinn and Kent 1984, Kentros et al. 1985).

Following tooth removal, the socket is thoroughly curetted of all soft tissue debris. Bleeding should be stimulated from the osseous base if absent. The key for maximum bone fill is adequate bleeding from the bone, since blood contains fundamental proteins and growth factors for bone healing (Becker et al. 1996). Profuse bleeding can be easily achieved by scraping the walls of the socket with either curettes or rotary instruments. This procedure also triggers the regional acceleratory phenomena (RAP), which is known to stimulate new bone formation and graft incorporation (Trevisan et al. 2002, Melsen 1999).

The extraction socket should then be carefully inspected and a decision should be made based on the following factors: (a) the integrity and thickness of the buccal plate; (b) the presence of periapical lesions; and (c) the number and morphology of the root(s) on the extracted tooth. After observation of these factors, one of the following techniques should be used:

A. Traditional Socket Management with or without Collagen Wound Dressing Material (see Figures 7.2A–H, which illustrate socket management when buccal plate is ≥1 mm thickness):

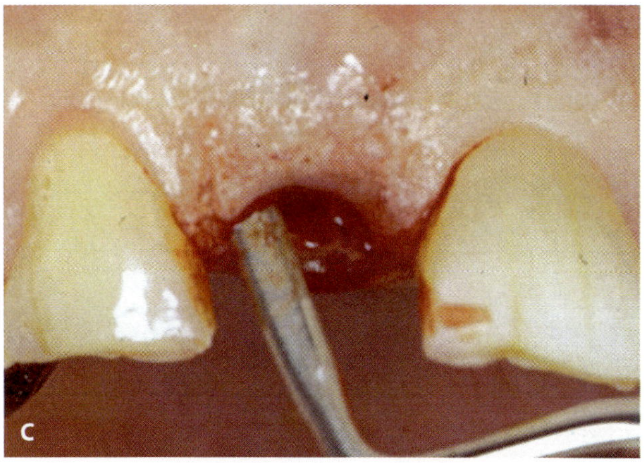

Figure 7.2C. Use of periotomes to luxate surrounding periodontal ligament space.

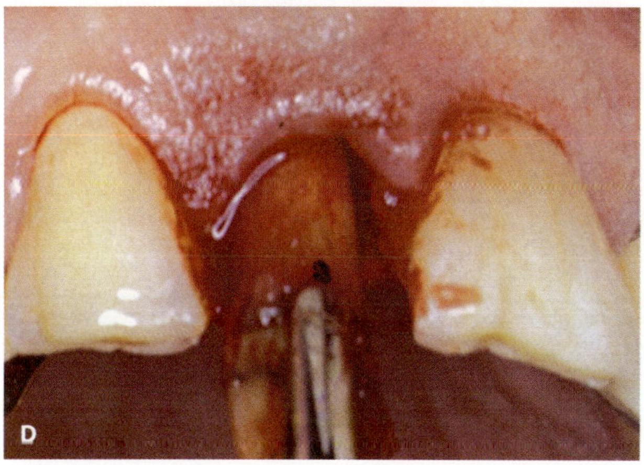

Figure 7.2D. Tooth extraction occurs with minimal trauma to the surrounding tissue.

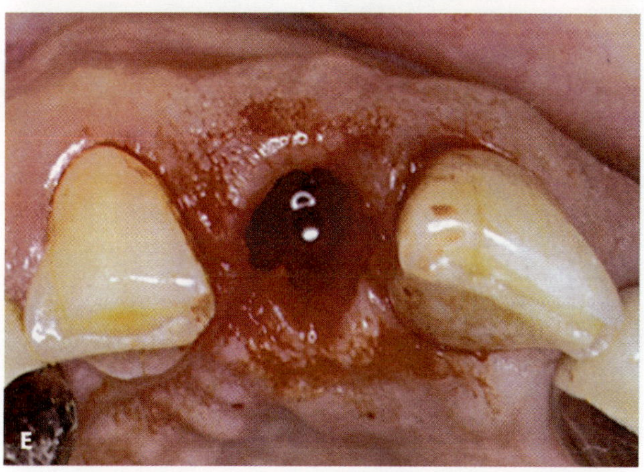

Figure 7.2E. The socket is free of infection and presents profuse bleeding.

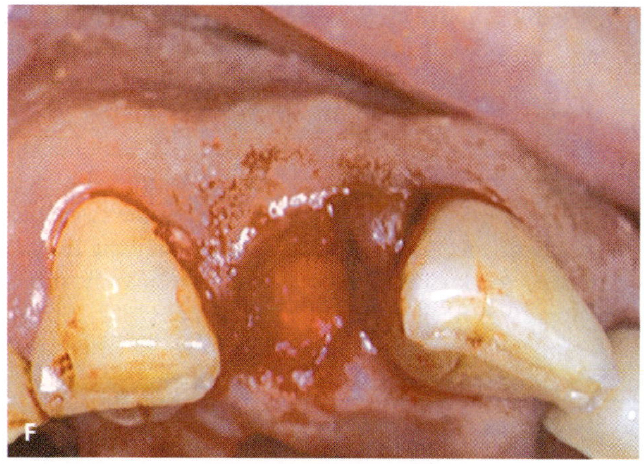

Figure 7.2F. A wound dressing material (CollaPlug®, Zimmer Dental, Carlsbad, CA, USA) covers the augmented extraction socket.

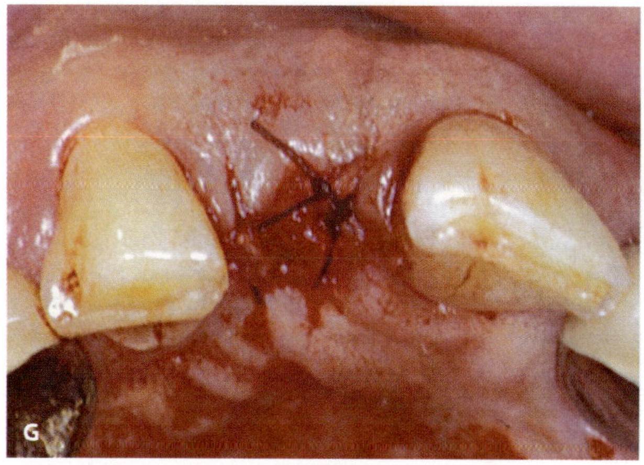

Figure 7.2G. A cross-mattress suture is placed to stabilize the wound.

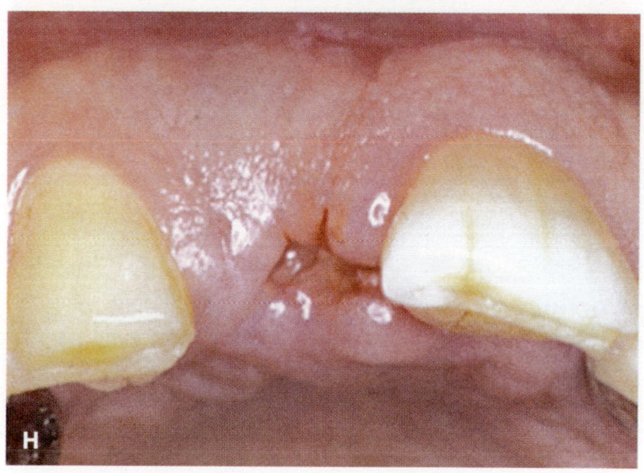

Figure 7.2H. Postoperative view 14 days after socket augmentation.

The buccal socket wall should be measured for its thickness with the aid of a boley gauge caliper at approximately 2–3 mm below the alveolar crest. The tip of the caliper should pass through the soft tissue for a more accurate measurement. If a thick buccal plate is found (>1 mm), no bone grafting is needed because thick buccal plates are less prone to future bone resorption. Research has shown that buccal plates thicker than 1 mm have significantly more favorable healing capacity (Korsnes 2002, Spray et al. 2000). Hence, bone grafting is often not required. However, if dehiscence or fenestration is noted then the socket should be treated with the layers technique (see "B. Layers Technique" below).

An absorbable collagen dressing material (CollaPlug, Zimmer Dental, Inc., Carlsbad, CA, USA) could be used to promote clot stabilization. Collagen is a hemostatic agent and possesses the ability to stimulate platelet aggregation and enhance fibrin linkage, which may lead to initial clot formation, stability, and maturation (Sableman 1985). Furthermore, collagen has been demonstrated to be chemotatic for fibroblasts in vitro (Postlethwaite et al. 1978). This property could enhance cell migration and promote primary wound coverage that is fundamental for bone growth. A cross-mattress suture is then used to secure the collagen dressing material in the socket for the initial 14 days of the healing process.

B. Layers Technique (see Figures 7.3A–J, which illustrate socket management when buccal plate is ≤1 mm thickness):

The layers technique was developed to maximize bone healing in sockets with compromised healing potential. A combination of a bone replacement graft and a collagen wound dressing material should be used when the buccal socket wall is

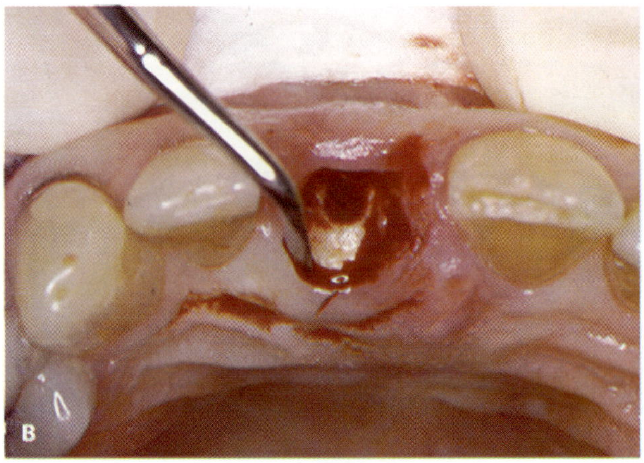

Figure 7.3B. Periotomes facilitate rupture of the supracrestal attachment apparatus. Reproduced from Wang H-L, Kiyonobu K, Neiva RF. Socket Augmentation: Rational & technique. *Implant Dentistry*, 2004; 13(4): 286–296.

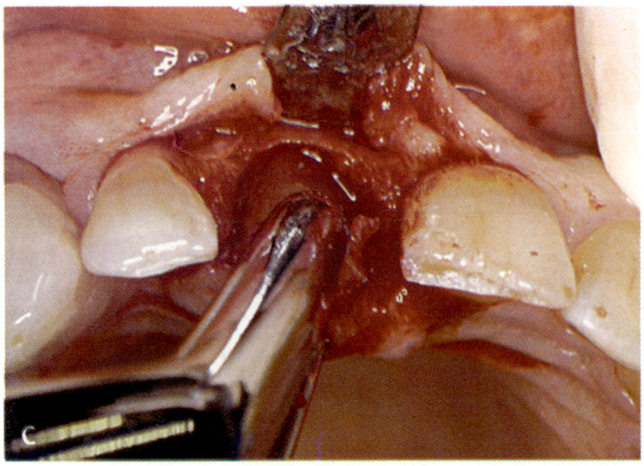

Figure 7.3C. Tooth extraction occurs with minimal trauma to the surrounding tissue. Reproduced from Wang H-L, Kiyonobu K, Neiva RF. Socket Augmentation: Rational & technique. *Implant Dentistry*, 2004; 13(4): 286–296.

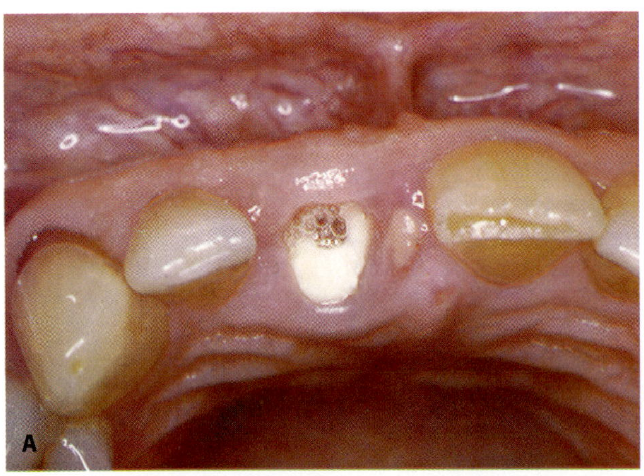

Figure 7.3A. Preoperative view. Reproduced from Wang H-L, Kiyonobu K, Neiva RF. Socket Augmentation: Rational & technique. *Implant Dentistry*, 2004; 13(4): 286–296.

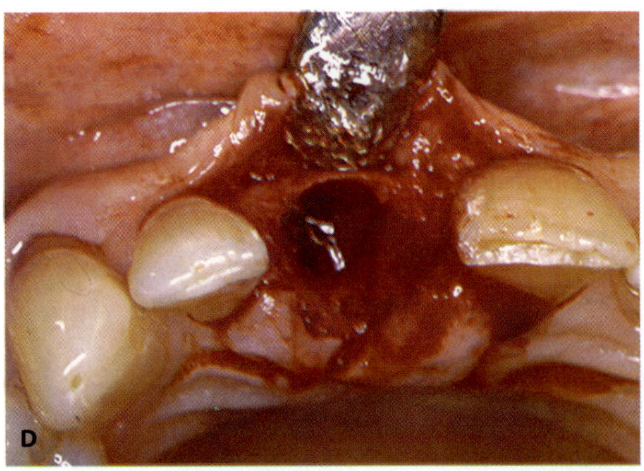

Figure 7.3D. The socket is free of infection and presents profuse bleeding. Reproduced from Wang H-L, Kiyonobu K, Neiva RF. Socket Augmentation: Rational & technique. *Implant Dentistry*, 2004; 13(4): 286–296.

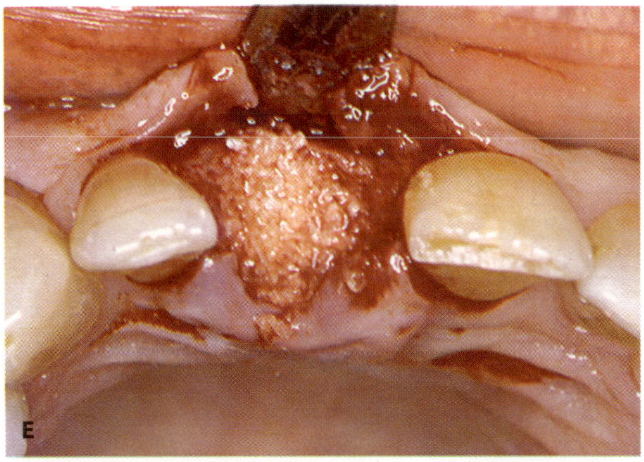

Figure 7.3E. The bone-graft material is inserted into the extraction socket (Puros®, Zimmer Dental, Carlsbad, CA, USA). Reproduced from Wang H-L, Kiyonobu K, Neiva RF. Socket Augmentation: Rational & technique. *Implant Dentistry*, 2004; 13(4): 286–296.

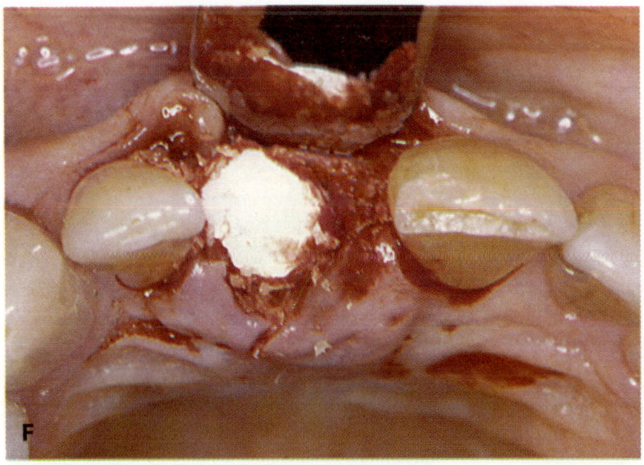

Figure 7.3F. A wound dressing material (CollaPlug®, Zimmer Dental, Carlsbad, CA, USA) covers the augmented extraction socket. Reproduced from Wang H-L, Kiyonobu K, Neiva RF. Socket Augmentation: Rational & technique. *Implant Dentistry*, 2004; 13(4): 286–296.

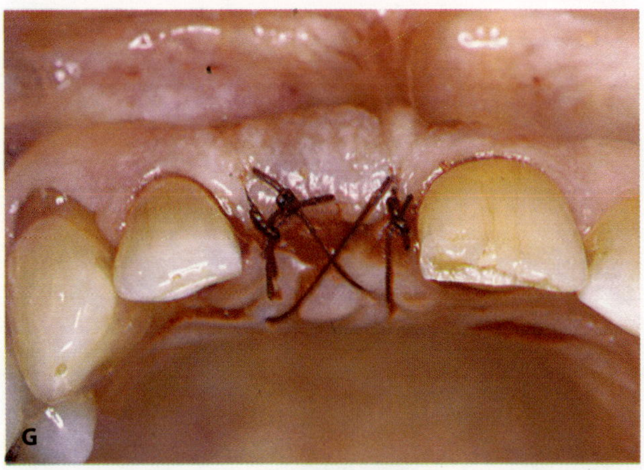

Figure 7.3G. A cross-mattress suture is placed to stabilize the wound. Reproduced from Wang H-L, Kiyonobu K, Neiva RF. Socket Augmentation: Rational & technique. *Implant Dentistry*, 2004; 13(4): 286–296.

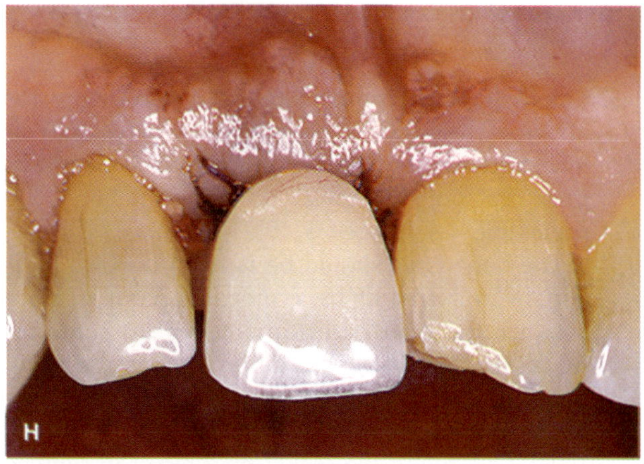

Figure 7.3H. An ovate pontic is used for soft tissue development. Reproduced from Wang H-L, Kiyonobu K, Neiva RF. Socket Augmentation: Rational & technique. *Implant Dentistry*, 2004; 13(4): 286–296.

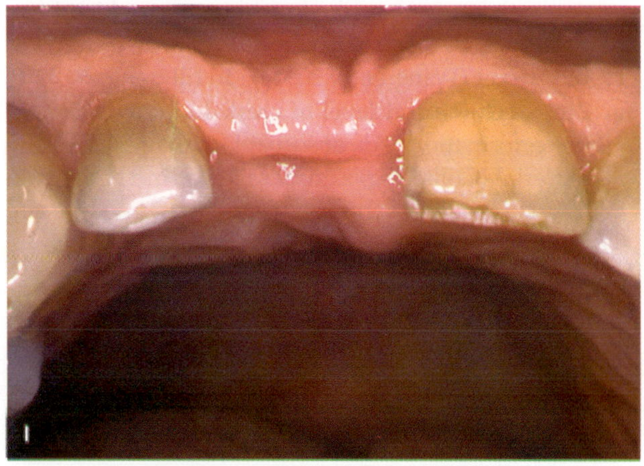

Figure 7.3I. Postoperative view 14 days after socket augmentation. Reproduced from Wang H-L, Kiyonobu K, Neiva RF. Socket Augmentation: Rational & technique. *Implant Dentistry*, 2004; 13(4): 286–296.

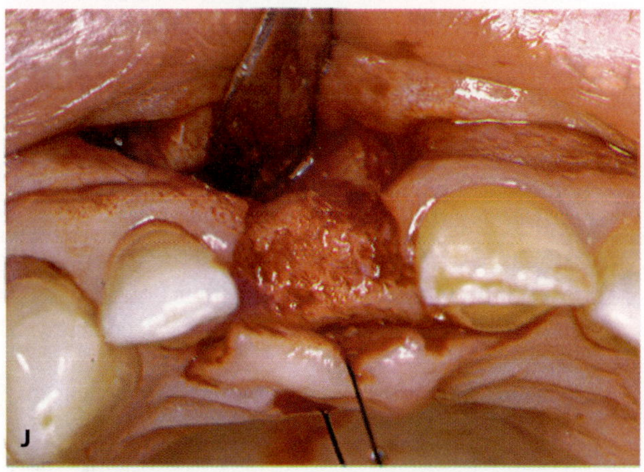

Figure 7.3J. Reentry 120 days later showing complete bone fill. Reproduced from Wang H-L, Kiyonobu K, Neiva RF. Socket Augmentation: Rational & technique. *Implant Dentistry*, 2004; 13(4): 286–296.

≤1 mm thick at approximately 2–3 mm below the alveolar crest and/or occurrence of dehiscence or fenestrations are found. Mineralized bone grafts that are quickly replaced by host bone are preferable.

The bone graft should be tamped down lightly, and overfill should be avoided. Adequate space between the graft particles is critical to allow for revascularization to spread throughout the graft, bringing the proteins and growth factors necessary for new bone growth (Becker et al. 1992, Mellonig 1996). Overfilling the socket may result in sequestration of the graft particles, which may lead to infectious processes that may negatively influence bone formation (Sclar 1999). Hence, bone grafts should be placed only up to or 2 mm below the level of the alveolar crest. This is slightly different from our previously described technique in which bone graft materials were used to fill up to two-thirds of the socket (Wang et al. 2004a). To fill bone grafts to 2 mm below or at level of crest do allow for more bone formation. An absorbable collagen dressing material (CollaPlug, Zimmer Dental Inc., Carlsbad, CA, USA) should then be trimmed and adapted to seal the coronal portion of the socket. This material not only provides wound stabilization but also facilitates soft tissue healing over the grafted area. A cross-mattress suture is then used to secure the collagen dressing material in the socket for the initial 14 days of the healing process.

Recently, a Puros-plug layers technique was developed by Korsnes at the University of Michigan School of Dentistry (unpublished data by Korsnes 2002) to promote socket bone formation. This technique uses solvent-preserved mineralized cancellous allografts (Puros®, Zimmer Dental Inc., Carlsbad, CA, USA) that are then covered with an absorbable collagen dressing material as previously described. The histologic data obtained from our unpublished data indicated 68% of vital bone, 5% of residual particle, and 27% of connective tissue. This is similar to the human host bone component. Sites that may also benefit from using this technique include those with thin bone ≤1 mm, periapical pathologies, and sockets of multirooted teeth associated with loss of the interradicular bone.

C. Guided Bone Regeneration (GBR) (see Figures 7.4A–F):
Cases in which the buccal plate is absent or was lost during exodontia require a different approach. GBR techniques associated with or without immediate implant placement are required to treat these ridge defects. A delayed implant placement approach is indicated when primary stability of the implant

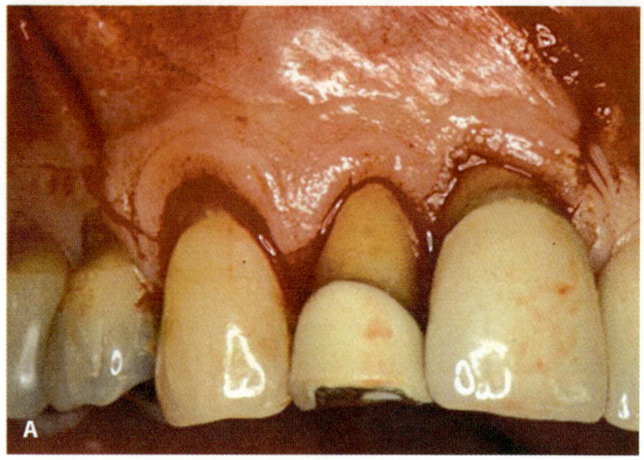

Figure 7.4A. Preoperative view of tooth No. 7.

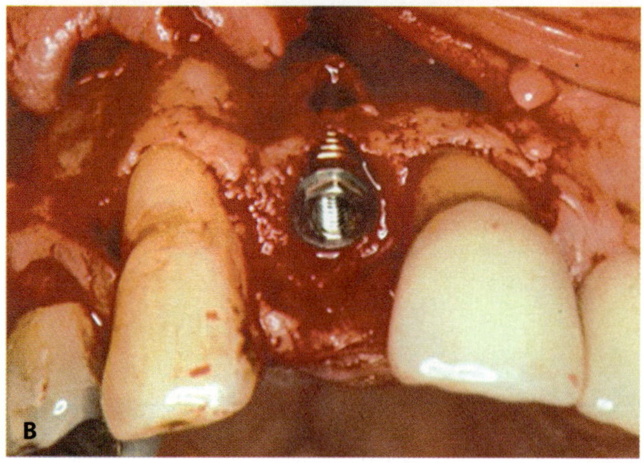

Figure 7.4B. Implant is placed immediately after extraction. Note significant dehiscence/fenestration defect.

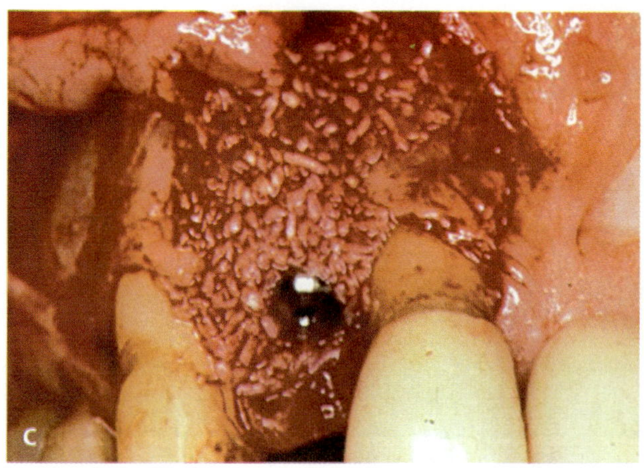

Figure 7.4C. Layers of bone-grafting material are applied (sandwich bone augmentation).

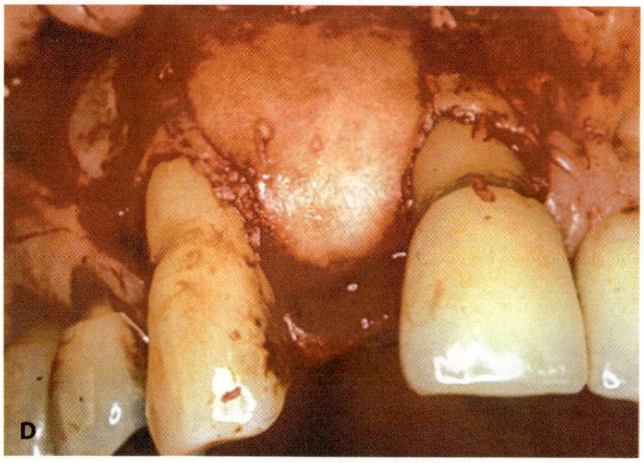

Figure 7.4D. Absorbable collagen membrane is trimmed and adapted.

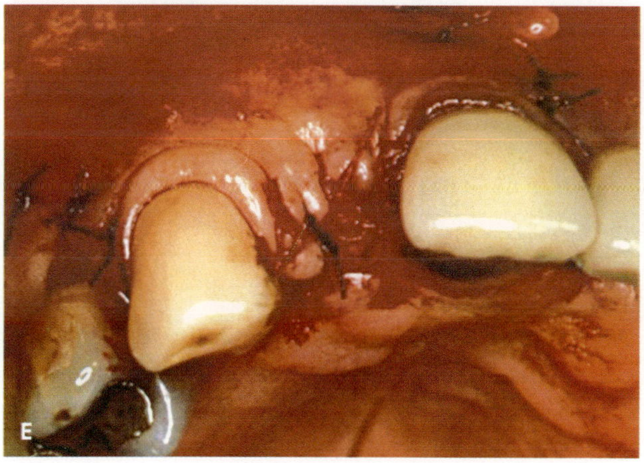

Figure 7.4E. Primary wound closure is achieved with coronal flap advancement.

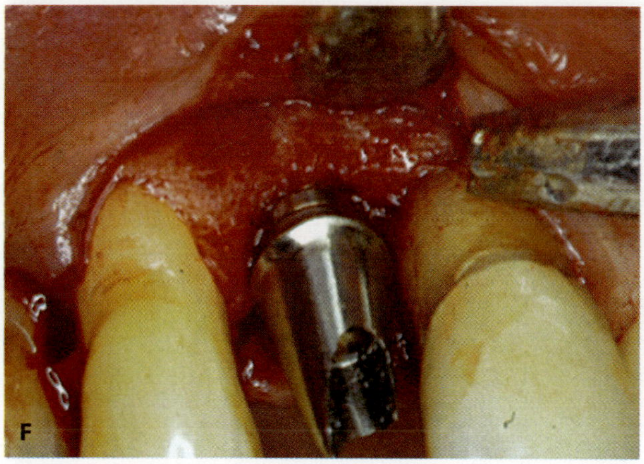

Figure 7.4F. Complete defect fill is observed 6 months later.

cannot be predictably achieved, particularly in sockets of bi- or multirooted teeth. In these cases GBR techniques, such as the "sandwich bone augmentation," are indicated (Wang et al. 2004b).

In this technique, layers of different bone-grafting materials are used to maximize new bone formation. The inner layer of bone graft is composed of a combination of osseous coagulum (autogenous bone collected during implant osteotomy preparation) and fast-absorbing allograft materials. Fast-absorbing graft materials (e.g., FDBA) allow quick bone turnover via creeping substitution and therefore promote bone formation and possible achievement of greater bone-to-implant contact (Goldberg and Stevenson 1987, Lyford et al. 2003). Osseous coagulum provides living cells in close contact with the recipient area. Allografts may possess osteoinductive properties by release of bone morphogenic proteins (BMP) in addition to osteoconductivity by serving as an ideal scaffold for osteoblast migration and proliferation. The outer layer of bone graft material is comprised of a slow-absorbing grafting material, such as human cortical bone or bovine hydroxyapatite (HA). Human cortical bone (e.g., Puros cortical bone, Zimmer Dental Inc., Carlsbad, CA, USA) or bovine HA acts as a scaffold/space occupier by preserving and/or maintaining the space that is essential for bone augmentation procedures. Human cortical bone undergoes a slower absorption process, called *reversed creeping substitution*, allowing time for the inner bone to mature (Goldberg and Stevenson 1987, Lyford et al. 2003).

A collagen membrane should then be applied to cover the grafted site to facilitate wound stability and exclude unwanted cells. The mucoperiosteal flap is then coronally repositioned for complete wound coverage with passive tension. Bone regeneration, once activated, progresses in a programmed sequence through a series of maturation steps, which closely resemble the pattern of bone development and growth (Fugazzotto 2002). Implant placement should not be performed before a five- to six-month healing period.

D. Immediate Implant Placement Together with GBR (see Figures 7.5A–I):

It is true that immediate implant placement with GBR could achieve a success rate similar to those of the staged approach (first socket augmentation then implant surgery) (Araujo et al. 2005, Schenk et al. 1994). When the socket is free from infection, such as residual endodontic or periodontal infection, the clinician is confident in the procedure he is performing–especially in the case of a GBR grafting procedure–and primary implant stability has been

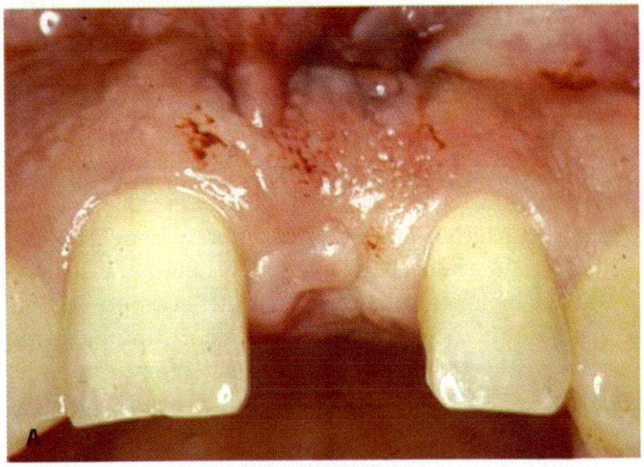

Figure 7.5A. Preoperative view showing inadequate ridge width. Augmentation of horizontal ridge defect in conjunction with implant placement using sandwich bone augmentation technique is to be performed. Reproduced from Wang H-L, Boyapari L. "PASS" principles for predictable bone regeneration. *Implant Dentistry*, 2006; 15(1): 10–17.

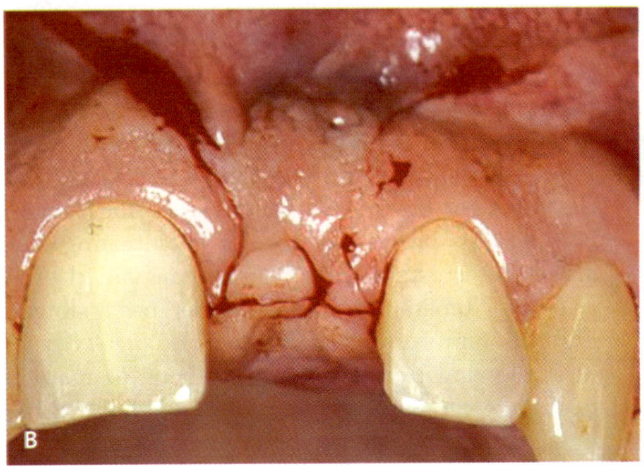

Figure 7.5B. Initial incisions show two divergent vertical releasing incisions. Reproduced from Wang H-L, Boyapari L. "PASS" principles for predictable bone regeneration. *Implant Dentistry*, 2006; 15(1): 10–17.

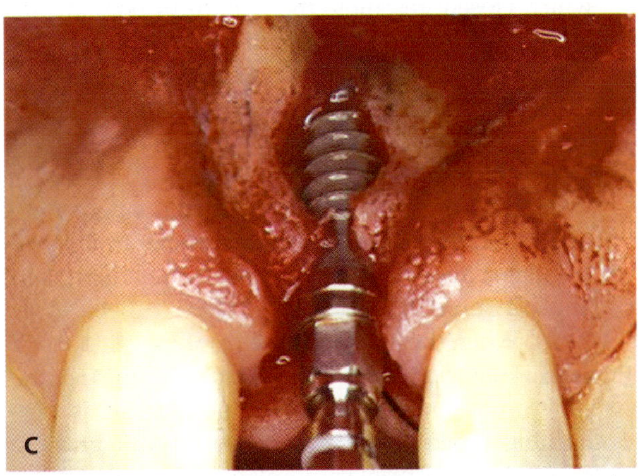

Figure 7.5C. Implant placement with horizontal ridge deficiency. Reproduced from Wang H-L, Boyapari L. "PASS" principles for predictable bone regeneration. *Implant Dentistry*, 2006; 15(1): 10–17.

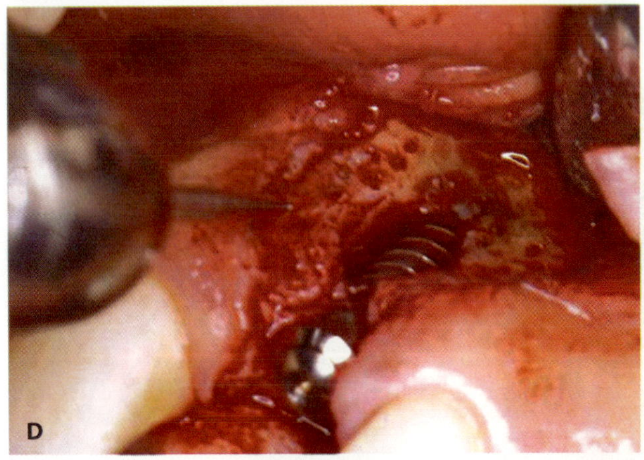

Figure 7.5D. Intrabone bone marrow penetration to stimulate regional acceleratory phenomenon (RAP) using one-half round bur. Reproduced from Wang H-L, Boyapari L. "PASS" principles for predictable bone regeneration. *Implant Dentistry*, 2006; 15(1): 10–17.

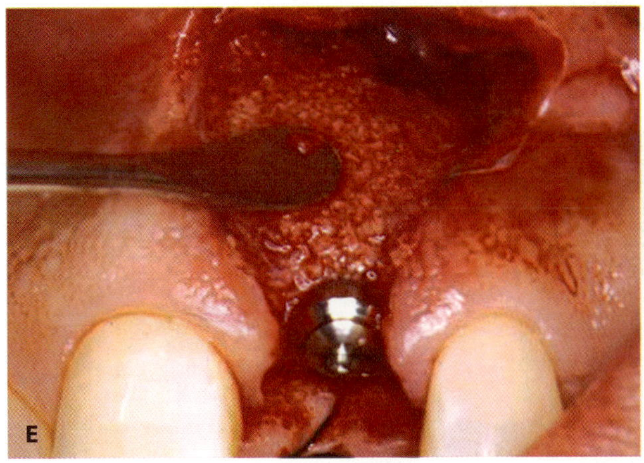

Figure 7.5E. Sandwich bone augmentation. Inner layer of bone graft. Human mineralized cancellous bone (Puros®, Zimmer Dental, Inc., Carlsbad, CA, USA) was placed to the adjacent bone level. Reproduced from Wang H-L, Boyapari L. "PASS" principles for predictable bone regeneration. *Implant Dentistry*, 2006; 15(1): 10–17.

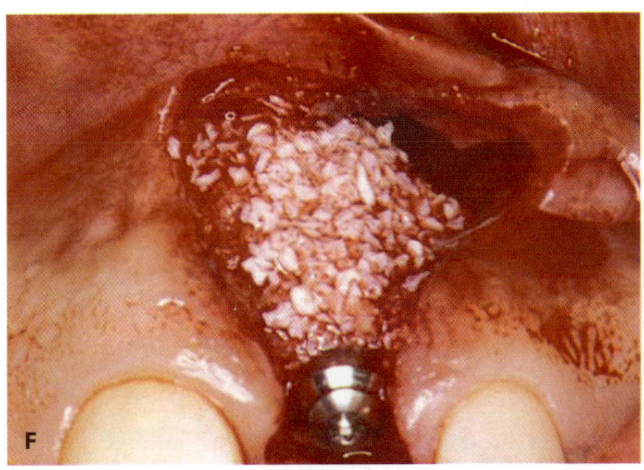

Figure 7.5F. Sandwich bone augmentation. Outer layer of bone graft. Human mineralized cortical bone (Puros®, Zimmer Dental, Inc., Carlsbad, CA, USA) was placed against the inner layer at least 2–3 mm beyond the inner layer should be achieved. Reproduced from Wang H-L, Boyapari L. "PASS" principles for predictable bone regeneration. *Implant Dentistry*, 2006; 15(1): 10–17.

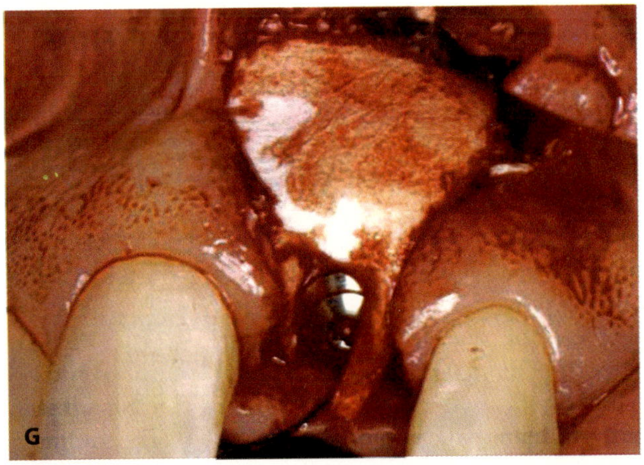

Figure 7.5G. Sandwich bone augmentation. Absorbable collagen (Bio-Mend™, Zimmer Dental, Inc., Carlsbad, CA, USA) was used to cover the bone grafts to promote primary wound coverage as well as to protect the underneath bone grafts. Reproduced from Wang H-L, Boyapari L. "PASS" principles for predictable bone regeneration. *Implant Dentistry*, 2006; 15(1): 10–17.

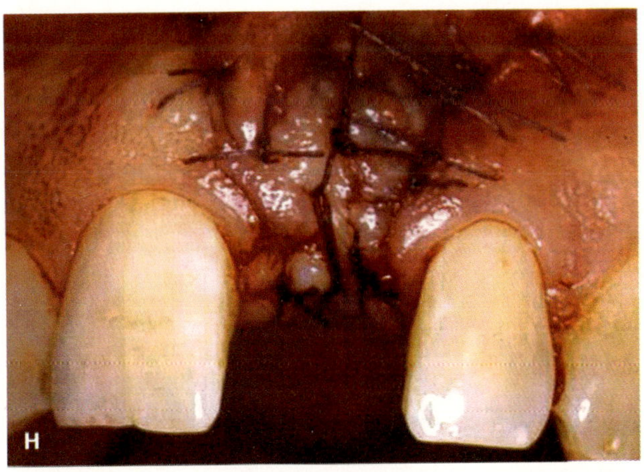

Figure 7.5H. Suture with 4-0 and 5-0 Vicryl suture (primary coverage with passive flap tension). Reproduced from Wang H-L, Boyapari L. "PASS" principles for predictable bone regeneration. *Implant Dentistry*, 2006; 15(1): 10–17.

achieved, an immediate implant placement can be performed. If any of these criteria cannot be fulfilled, a staged socket augmentation is recommended.

The sandwich bone augmentation GBR technique is often the primary choice of authors. As reported in the literature, an average of 80% of bone height gain as well as ≥1.7 mm bone thickness gain was achieved when this technique was employed (Park and Wang 2005a, Park 2006). Sutures are generally removed 10 to 14 days after surgery. Implant uncovering and subsequent restorative treatment should not be performed before a five- to six-month healing period. (See Figure 7.6.)

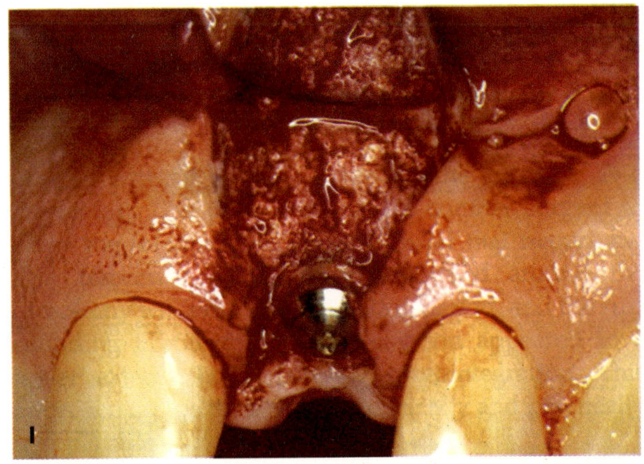

Figure 7.5I. Reentry at 6 months showing new bone formation. Reproduced from Wang H-L, Boyapari L. "PASS" principles for predictable bone regeneration. *Implant Dentistry*, 2006; 15(1): 10–17.

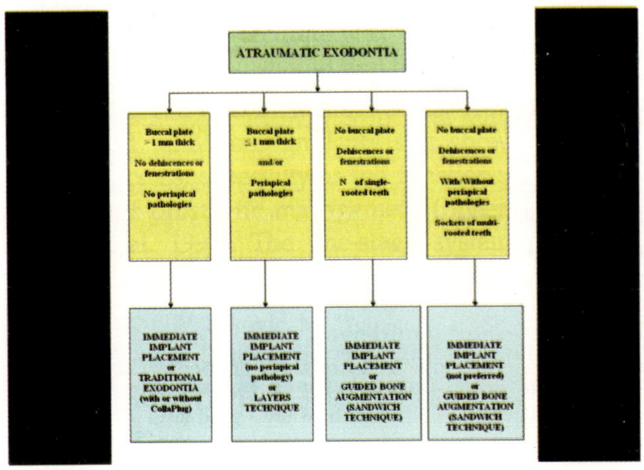

Figure 7.6. Decision making on socket augmentation procedure.

Postoperative Instruction

Postoperative care includes rinsing twice daily with warm salt water for the first two weeks before switching to twice daily rinsing with 0.12% chlorhexidine gluconate for the next two weeks. Systemic antibiotic prophylaxis is not recommended unless signs of active infection are found. If indicated, antibiotics such as 500 mg amoxicillin three times/day (t.i.d.) for 10 days, or in cases of allergy to penicillin and derivatives, azithromycin 500 mg/day for three days, should be prescribed. Pain medications such as ibuprofen are often prescribed to help relieve discomfort associated with the procedure.

The healing process should be monitored radiographically, and implant placement or stage-two surgery can usually be performed four months after treatment. Radiolucencies persisting for more than four months are indicative of inadequate graft incorporation, frequently requiring an additional procedure for debridement of the graft particles and possibly a new grafting procedure.

Discussion

Before implant therapy was introduced, little attention was paid to the faith of alveolar ridges following tooth extraction. Nowadays atrophic ridges can negatively influence or prohibit implant placement and/or result in poor esthetic outcomes and inadequate implant placement. Hence, ridge resorption caused by tooth extraction should be prevented. The techniques presented in this chapter should facilitate decision making on socket augmentation procedures. Positive outcomes have been constantly observed, with minimal ridge morphologic changes. Augmented sockets have shown not only adequate morphology, but also density, noticeable during implant osteotomy preparation. As a consequence, soft tissue profile has often been preserved, maximizing the esthetic outcome. Implants placed in fresh extraction sockets combined with the sandwich bone augmentation technique have shown successful osseointegration and coverage of the threads exposed during placement (Wang et al. 2004b, Park and Wang 2005a, Park 2006). The techniques presented here have been extensively used by authors with positive outcomes. Augmented sockets have shown not only adequate morphology, but also density, noticeable during implant osteotomy preparation. As a consequence, soft tissue profile has been constantly preserved, maximizing the esthetic outcome.

Many bone-grafting materials have been suggested for socket augmentation (Sclar 1999, Park 2006, Serino et al. 2003, Vasilic et al. 2003). These include autogenous bone, DFDBA (Becker et al. 1994), mineralized FDBA (Feuille et al. 2003), bovine HA (Artzi et al. 2000, Sclar 1999), and alloplasts (Froum and Orlowski 2000). When the bone-forming capacity of DFDBA in extraction sockets was histologically evaluated (Becker et al. 1994), the biopsies showed that DFDBA-grafted sites had no evidence of new bone formation and that there was no evidence of osteoclastic resorption of the graft particles, while the autograft-treated sites revealed vascular channels with woven and lamellar bone. The evidence suggests that DFDBA may not be a good material for socket augmentation (Becker et al. 1994).

A potential delay in osteogenic cell ingrowth has also been observed when a demineralized bone matrix immersed in a glycerol carrier (Zubillaga et al. 2003, Korsnes 2002). However, DFDBA combined with barrier membranes has been shown to overcome these possible deficiencies (Brugnami et al. 1999). Recently, a human bone mineralized graft (Puros®, Zimmer Dental Inc., Carlsbad, CA, USA) was introduced. It constitutes a mineralized bone allograft material processed through unique solvent-preserved processes for tissue preservation and viral inactivation, which differ from the standard cryo-preserved process. Data have demonstrated that after standard tissue bank processing and limited gamma radiation, the bone appears to remain intact, providing excellent bone matrix and load-bearing capabilities (Günther et al. 1996).

Research has demonstrated lamellar bone formation as quickly as 15 days after implantation of this material in the tibia of rabbits and almost complete disappearance in 60 days (Günther et al. 1996, Dalkyz et al. 2000). These findings suggest that this material may be a good alternative for socket augmentation procedures. Our group uses either FDBA or human mineralized bone as the primary bone graft for this type of procedure. These materials have optimal osteoconductive properties, and may also be osteoinductive by releasing BMPs, which could induce osteogenesis from surrounding bone (Park and Wang 2005a, Tsao et al. 2006, Urist 1965, Urist and Iwata 1973). In addition, most of these materials have shown to be resorbed and consequently replaced with host bone within 2–4 months, which facilitates future implant placement (Gapski et al. 2006, unpublished data by Korsnes 2002). The Puros-plug layers technique is slightly different from the previously described Bio-Col technique (Sclar 1999). The Bio-Col technique uses bovine HA bone graft on the bottom two-thirds and then is covered with an absorbable collagen dressing. CollaPlug is used for the top one-third, and then it is sealed with tissue glue (Isodent, Ellman International, Hewlett, NY, USA). The author claims that this technique prevents loss of both hard and soft tissues, reduces the number of surgical interventions, and provides optimum esthetics with greater predictability, even though some studies have shown the remaining bovine HA particle even after four months healing (Artzi et al. 2000). Future investigations to compare these two techniques are desired.

The utility of barrier membranes in socket augmentation procedures has also been evaluated. Data have suggested that membrane-covered sites presented with significantly less ridge atrophy than control sites (Lekovic et al. 1997). This implies that the use of membranes during socket augmentation is beneficial. Difficulties associated with barrier membrane use during socket augmentation include (a) the potential reduction of keratinized gingiva, (b) alterations of gingival contours, and (c) migration of the mucogingival junction, as a result of coronal displacement of the flap to achieve soft tissue closure over the membrane. Even with these drawbacks, some studies have demonstrated success in the use of a variety of membranes for socket augmentation, including nonabsorbable, absorbable, and acellular dermal allografts (Wang et al. 2004a, Zitzmann 1999). Recently, an acellular dermal matrix (AlloDerm, Lifecore Biomedical, Oral Restorative Division, Chaska, MN,

USA) has been used as a barrier membrane with a DFDBA for ridge preservation (Fowler et al. 2000, Park and Wang 2005b). A series of cases demonstrated an acceptable esthetic result with no apparent loss of ridge height or width. However, future studies in this area are certainly needed to further confirm this observation.

Reports in the literature have suggested the use of other materials, such as xenografts and alloplasts (Yang et al. 2000, Ashman 2000, Wiesen and Kitzis 1998). However, these reports were primarily case study series. Future controlled clinical trials are encouraged to validate the findings of the various case reports found in the literature, including the technique presented in this chapter, to provide needed scientific evidence.

References

Aichelmann-Reidy, M.E., and R.A. Yukna. 1998. Bone replacement grafts. The bone substitutes. *Dent Clin North Am*, 42, pp. 491–503.

Amler, M.H. 1969. The time sequence of tissue regeneration in human extraction wounds. *Oral Surgery*, 27, pp. 309–318.

Artzi, Z., H. Tal, and D. Dayan. 2000. Porous bovine bone mineral in healing of human extraction sockets. Part 1: histomorphometric evaluations at 9 months. *J Periodontol*, 71, pp. 1015–1023.

Araujo, M.G., and J. Lindhe. 2005. Dimensional ridge alterations following tooth extraction. An experimental study in the dog. *J Clin Periodontol*, 32, pp. 212–218.

Araujo, M.G., F. Sukekava, J.L. Wennstrom, and J. Lindhe. 2005. Ridge alterations following implant placement in fresh extraction sockets: An experimental study in the dog. *J Clin Periodontol*, 32, pp. 645–652.

Ashman, A. 1995. Ridge preservation: the new buzzword in dentistry. *Implant Soc*, 6, pp. 1–7.

Ashman, A. 2000. Postextraction ridge preservation using a synthetic alloplast. *Implant Dent*, 9, pp. 168–176.

Ashman, A., and J. Lopinto. 2000. Placement of implants into ridges grafted with bioplant HTR synthetic bone: histological long-term case history reports. *J Oral Implantol*, 26, pp. 276–290.

Barboza, E.P. 1999. Localized ridge maintenance using bone membrane. *Implant Dent*, 8, (2), pp. 167–172.

Bartee, B.K. 1995. A simplified technique for ridge preservation after tooth extraction. *Dent Today*, 14, pp. 62–67.

Bartee, B.K. 2001a. Extraction site reconstruction for alveolar ridge preservation. Part 1: rationale and materials selection. *J Oral Implantol*, 27, pp. 187–193.

Bartee, B.K. 2001b. Extraction site reconstruction for alveolar ridge preservation. Part 2: membrane-assisted surgical technique. *J Oral Implantol*, 27, (4), pp. 194–197.

Bays, R. 1986. The pathophysiology and anatomy of edentulous bone loss. *Reconstructive Preprosthetic Oral and Maxillofacial Surgery*, 1st ed, pp. 1–17.

Becker, W., S.E. Lynch, U. Lekholm, B.E. Becker, R. Caffesse, K. Donath, et al. 1992. A comparison of ePTFE membranes alone or in combination with platelet-derived growth factors and insulin-like growth factor-I or demineralized freeze-dried bone in promoting bone formation around immediate extraction socket implants. *J Periodontol*, 63, (11), pp. 929–940.

Becker, W., B.E. Becker, and R. Caffesse. 1994. A comparison of demineralized freeze-dried bone and autologous bone to induce bone formation in human extraction sockets. *J Periodontol*, 65, pp. 1128–1133.

Becker, W., M. Urist, B.E. Becker, W. Jackson, D.A. Parry, M. Bartold, et al. 1996. Clinical and histologic observations of sites implanted with intraoral autologous bone grafts or allografts. 15 human case reports. *J Periodontol*, 67, pp. 1025–1033.

Becker, W., P. Hujoel, and B.E. Becker. 2002. Effect of barrier membranes and autologous bone grafts on ridge width preservation around implants. *Clin Implant Dent Relat Res*, 4, pp. 143–149.

Block, M.S., I. Finger, and R. Lytle. 2002. Human mineralized bone in extraction sites before implant placement: preliminary results. *J Am Dent Assoc*, 133, (12), pp. 1631–1638.

Botticelli, D., T. Berglundhl, and J. Lindhe. 2005. Hard tissue alterations following implant placement in extraction sites. *J Clin Periodontol*, 31, pp. 820–828.

Brugnami, F., P.R. Then, H. Moroi, S. Kabani, and C.W. Leone. 1999. GBR in human extraction sockets and ridge defects prior to implant placement: clinical results and histologic evidence of osteoblastic and osteoclastic activities in DFDBA. *Int J Periodontics Restorative Dent*, 19, pp. 259–267.

Buck, B.E., and T.I. Malinin. 1994. Human bone and tissue allografts. Preparation and safety. *Clin Orthop*, pp. 8–17.

Camargo, P.M., V. Lekovic, M. Weinlaender, P.R. Klokkevold, E.B. Kenney, B. Dimitrijevic, et al. 2000. Influence of bioactive glass on changes in alveolar process dimensions after exodontia. *Oral Surg Oral Med Oral Pathol Oral Radiol Endod*, 90, pp. 581–586.

Cohen, E.S. 1995. Ridge enhancement and socket preservation utilizing the subepithelial connective tissue graft: a case report. *Pract Periodontics Aesthet Dent*, 7, pp. 53–58, quiz 60.

Covani, U., R. Cornelini, and A. Barone. 2003. Bucco-lingual bone remodeling around implants placed into immediate extraction sockets: a case series. *J Periodontol*, 74, (2), pp. 268–273.

Cranin, A.N., A. Simons, M. Klein, A. Sirakian, A. Ashman, B.H. Colmery III. 1995. The use of a particulate, microporous, calcified copolymer as a ridge maintenance device in dogs. *J Vet Dent*, 12, pp.53–58.

Dalkyz, M., A. Ozcan, M. Yapar, N. Gokay, and M. Yuncu. 2000. Evaluation of the effects of different biomaterials on bone defects. *Implant Dent*, 9, pp. 226–235.

Feinberg, S.E., and R.J. Fonseca. 1986. Biologic aspects of transplantation of grafts. In: Davis, W.H., editor. *Reconstructive Preprosthetic Oral and Maxillofacial Surgery*. 1st ed. Philadelphia: WB Saunders.

Feuille, F., C.I. Knapp, M.A. Brunsvold, and J.T. Mellonig. 2003. Clinical and histologic evaluation of bone-replacement grafts in the treatment of localized alveolar ridge defects. Part 1: Mineralized freeze-dried bone allograft. *Int J Periodontics Restorative Dent*, 23, pp. 29–35.

Fowler, E.B., L.G. Breault, and G. Rebitski. 2000. Ridge preservation utilizing an acellular dermal allograft and demineralized freeze-dried bone allograft: Part I. A report of 2 cases. *J Periodontol*, 71, pp. 1353–1359.

Froum, S., and W. Orlowski. 2000. Ridge preservation utilizing an alloplast prior to implant placement—clinical and histological case reports. *Pract Periodontics Aesthet Dent*, 12, pp. 393–402, quiz 404.

Froum, S., S.C. Cho, E. Rosenberg, M. Rohrer, and D. Tarnow. 2002. Histological comparison of healing extraction sockets implanted with bioactive glass or demineralized freeze-dried bone allograft: a pilot study. *J Periodontol*, 73, pp. 94–102.

Fugazzotto, P.A. 2002. Implant placement in maxillary first premolar fresh extraction sockets: description of technique and report of preliminary results. *J Periodontol*, 73, (6), pp. 669–674.

Gapski, R., R. Neiva, T. Oh, and H. Wang. 2006. Histological analyses of human hydroxyapatite grafting material in sinus elevation procedures: a case series. *Int J Periodontics Restorative Dent*, 26, pp. 59–69.

Goldberg, V.M., and S. Stevenson. 1987. Natural history of autografts and allografts. *Clin Orthop Related Res*, 225, pp. 7–15.

Goldschlag, D., M. Haghpassand, and P.N. Baer. 1994. An alternative method for treating buccal osseous defects. *Periodontal Clin Investig*, 16, (2), pp. 10–12.

Grunder, U., G. Polizzi, R. Goene, N. Hatano, P. Henry, W.J. Jackson, et al. 1999. A 3-year prospective multicenter follow-up report on the immediate and delayed-immediate placement of implants. *Int J Oral Maxillofac Implants*, 14, pp. 210–216.

Günther, K.P., H.-P. Scharf, H.-J. Pesch, and W. Puhl. 1996. Osteointegration of solvent-preserved bone transplants in an animal model. *Osteologie*, 5, pp. 4–12.

Howell, T.H., J. Fiorellini, A. Jones, M. Alder, P. Nummikoski, M. Lazaro, et al. 1997. A feasibility study evaluating rhBMP-2/absorbable collagen sponge device for local alveolar ridge preservation or augmentation. *Int J Periodontics Restorative Dent*, 17, pp. 124–139.

Iasella, J.M., H. Greenwell, R.L. Miller, M. Hill, C. Drisko, A.A. Bohra, et al. 2003. Ridge preservation with freeze-dried bone allograft and a collagen membrane compared to extraction alone for implant site development: a clinical and histologic study in humans. *J Periodontol*, 74, pp. 990–999.

Iasella, J.M., H. Greenwell, R.L. Miller, M. Hill, C. Drisko, A.A. Bohra, et al. 2003. Ridge preservation with freeze-dried bone allograft and a collagen membrane compared to extraction alone for implant site development: a clinical and histologic study in humans. *J Periodontol*, 74, pp. 990–999.

Kassolis, J.D., P.S. Rosen, and M.A. Reynolds. 2000. Alveolar ridge and sinus augmentation utilizing platelet-rich plasma in combination with freeze-dried bone allograft: case series. *J Periodontol*, 71, pp. 1654–1661.

Kentros, G.A., S.J. Filler, and S.S. Rothstein. 1985. Six month evaluation of particulate Durapatite in extraction sockets for the preservation of the alveolar ridge. *Implantologist*, 3, pp. 53–62.

Korsnes, J. 2002. The effects of a demineralized bone matrix on healing of extraction sockets. Master Thesis, University of Michigan, School of Dentistry, Unpublished data.

Lekovic, V., E.B. Kenney, M. Weinlaender, T. Han, P. Klokkevold, M. Nedic, et al. 1997. A bone regenerative approach to alveolar ridge maintenance following tooth extraction. Report of 10 cases. *J Periodontol*, 68, pp. 563–570.

Lyford, R.H., M.P. Mills, C.I. Knapp, E.T. Scheyer, and J.T. Mellonig. 2003. Clinical evaluation of freeze-dried block allografts for alveolar ridge augmentation: a case series. *Int J Periodontics Restorative Dent*, 23, pp. 417–425.

Maatz, R., W. Lentz, and R. Graf. 1952a. Experimental principles in transplantation of preserved bones. *Langenbecks Arch Klin Chir Ver Dtsch Z Chir*, 273, pp. 850–855.

Maatz, R., W. Lentz, and R. Graf. 1952b. Bone tissue formation by preserved particles; bone banks. *Zentralbl Chir*, 77, pp. 1376–1382.

Maatz, R. 1953. Biological principles of healing of bone wounds. *Dtsch Med J*, 4, pp. 255–260.

Maatz, R., W. Lentz, and R. Graf. 1954. Spongiosa test of bone grafts for transplantation. *J Bone Joint Surg Am*, 36-A, pp. 721–731.

Mecall, R.A., and A.L. Rosenfeld. 1991. Influence of residual ridge resorption patterns on implant fixture placement and tooth position. 1. *Int J Periodontics Restorative Dent*, 11, pp. 8–23.

Mecall, R.A., and A.L. Rosenfeld. 1992. The influence of residual ridge resorption patterns on implant fixture placement and tooth position. 2. Presurgical determination of prosthesis type and design. *Int J Periodontics Restorative Dent*, 12, pp. 32–51.

Mecall, R.A., and A.L. Rosenfeld. 1996. Influence of residual ridge resorption patterns on fixture placement and tooth position, Part III: Presurgical assessment of ridge augmentation requirements. *Int J Periodontics Restorative Dent*, 16, pp. 322–337.

Mellonig, J.T., and M. Nevins. 1995. Guided bone regeneration of bone defects associated with implants: an evidence-based outcome assessment. *Int J Periodontics Restorative Dent*, 15, pp. 168–185.

Mellonig, J.T., and M. Nevins. 1995. Guided bone regeneration of bone defects associated with implants: an evidence-based outcome assessment. *Int J Periodontics Restorative Dent*, 15, (2), pp. 168–185.

Mellonig, J.T. 1996. Bone allografts in periodontal therapy. *Clin Orthop*, (324), pp. 116–125.

Mellonig, J.T., M. Nevins, and R. Sanchez. 1998. Evaluation of a bioabsorbable physical barrier for guided bone regeneration. Part I. Material alone. *Int J Periodontics Restorative Dent*, 18, pp. 139–149.

Melsen, B. 1999. Biological reaction of alveolar bone to orthodontic tooth movement. *Angle Orthod*, 69, pp. 151–158.

Nemcovsky, C.E., and V. Serfaty. 1996. Alveolar ridge preservation following extraction of maxillary anterior teeth. Report on 23 consecutive cases. *J Periodontol*, 67, pp. 390–395.

Nevins, M., and J.T. Mellonig. 1992. Enhancement of the damaged edentulous ridge to receive dental implants: a combination of allograft and the GORE-TEX membrane. *Int J Periodontics Restorative Dent*, 12, pp. 96–111.

Nevins, M., and J.T. Mellonig. 1994. The advantages of localized ridge augmentation prior to implant placement: a staged event. *Int J Periodontics Restorative Dent*, 14, pp. 96–111.

O'Brien T.P., J.E. Hinrichs, and E.M. Schaffer. 1994. The prevention of localized ridge deformities using guided tissue regeneration. *J Periodontol*, 65, (1), pp. 17–24.

Paolantonio, M., M. Dolci, A. Scarano, D. d'Archivio, G. di Placido, V. Tumini, et al. 2001. Immediate implantation in fresh extraction sockets. A controlled clinical and histological study in man. *J Periodontol*, 72, (11), pp. 1560–71.70.

Park, S.-H., and H.-L. Wang. 2005a. Mucogingival pouch flap (MPF) for sandwich bone augmentation. *Implant Dentistry*, 14, (4), pp. 349–356.

Park, S.-H., and H.-L. Wang. 2005b. Management of localized buccal dehiscence defect with allografts and acellular dermal matrix. Submitted for publication in *Int J Perio Rest Dent*, October.

Park, S.-H. 2006. Comparison of two absorbable membranes in guided bone regeneration on implant dehiscence defects in humans. University of Michigan, Thesis 2006 (Submitted for publication).

Pinholt, E.M., G. Bang, and H.R. Haanaes. 1990. Alveolar ridge augmentation by osteoinduction in rats. *Scand J Dent Res*, 98, pp. 434–441.

Pinholt, E.M., H.R. Haanaes, M. Roervik, K. Donath, and G. Bang. 1992. Alveolar ridge augmentation by osteoinductive materials in goats. *Scand J Dent Res*, 100, pp. 361–365.

Polizzi, G., U. Grunder, R. Goene, N. Hatano, P. Henry, W.J. Jackson, et al. 2000. Immediate and delayed implant placement into extraction sockets: a 5-year report. *Clin Implant Dent Relat Res*, 2, pp. 93–99.

Postlethwaite, A.E., J.M. Seyer, and A.H. Kang. 1978. Chemotactic attraction of human fibroblasts to type I, II, and III collagens and collagen-derived peptides. *Proc Natl Acad Sci USA*, 75, (2), pp. 871–875.

Quinn, J.H., and J.N. Kent. 1984. Alveolar ridge maintenance with solid nonporous hydroxylapatite root implants. *Oral Surg Oral Med Oral Pathol*, 58, pp. 511–521.

Russell, J.L. 2000. Grafton demineralized bone matrix: Performance consistency, utility, and value. *Tissue Engineering*, 6, pp. 435–440.

Sableman, E. 1985. Biology, Biotechnology, and Biocompatibility of Collagen. *Biocompatibility of Tissue Analogs*. CRC Press, First edition, Boca Raton, FL, 27.

Schallhorn, R.G. 1968. The use of autogenous hip marrow biopsy implants for bony crater defects. *J Periodontol*, 39, pp. 145–147.

Schenk, R.K., D. Buser, W.R. Hardwick, and C. Dahlin. 1994. Healing pattern of bone regeneration in membrane-protected defects: a histologic study in the canine mandible. *Int J Oral Maxillofac Implants*, 9, (1), pp. 13–29.

Sclar, A.G. 1999. Preserving alveolar ridge anatomy following tooth removal in conjunction with immediate implant placement. The Bio-Col Technique. *Atlas Oral Maxillofac Surg Clin North Am*, 7, pp. 39–59.

Serino, G., S. Biancu, G. Iezzi, and A. Piattelli. 2003. Ridge preservation following tooth extraction using a polylactide and polyglycolide sponge as space filler: a clinical and histological study in humans. *Clin Oral Implants Res*, 14, pp. 651–658.

Sevor, J.J., and R. Meffert. 1992. Placement of implants into fresh extraction sites using a resorbable collagen membrane: case reports. *Pract Periodontics Aesthet Dent*, 4, pp. 35–41.

Simion, M., P. Trisi, and A. Piattelli. 1996. GBR with an e-PTFE membrane associated with DFDBA: histologic and histochemical analysis in a human implant retrieved after 4 years of loading. *Int J Periodontics Restorative Dent*, 16, pp. 338–347.

Smiler, D.G. 2001. Comparison of anorganic bovine mineral with and without synthetic peptide in a sinus elevation: a case study. *Implant Dent*, 10, pp. 139–142.

Spray, J.R., C.G. Black, H.F. Morris, and S. Ochi. 2000. The influence of bone thickness on facial marginal bone response: stage 1 placement through stage 2 uncovering. *Ann Periodontol*, 5, (1), pp. 119–128.

Tal, H. 1999. Autogenous masticatory mucosal grafts in extraction socket seal procedures: a comparison between sockets grafted with demineralized freeze-dried bone and deproteinized bovine bone mineral. *Clin Oral Implants Res*, 10, pp. 289–296.

Trevisan, C., S. Ortolani, M. Monteleone, and E.C. Marinoni. 2002. Regional migratory osteoporosis: a pathogenetic hypothesis based on three cases and a review of the literature. *Clin Rheumatol*, 21, pp. 418–425.

Tsao, Y.-P., R. Neiva, K. Al-Shammari, T.-J. Oh, and H.-L. Wang. 2006. Effects of a mineralized human cancellous bone allograft in regeneration of mandibular class II furcation defects. *J Periodontol*, 77, pp. 416–425.

Urist, M.R. 1965. Bone: formation by autoinduction. *Science*, 150, pp. 893–899.

Urist, M.R., and H. Iwata. 1973. Preservation and biodegradation of the morphogenetic property of bone matrix. *J Theor Biol*, 38, pp. 155–167.

Vasilic, N., R. Henderson, T. Jorgenson, E. Sutherland, and R. Carson. 2003. The use of bovine porous bone mineral in combination with collagen membrane or autologous fibrinogen/fibronectin system for ridge preservation following tooth extraction. *J Okla Dent Assoc*, 93, pp. 33–38.

Wang, H.L., and M.J. Carroll. 2001. Guided bone regeneration using bone grafts and collagen membranes. Quintessence Int, 32, (7), pp. 504–515.

Wang, H.-L., K. Kiyonobu, and R.F. Neiva. 2004a. Socket augmentation: rationale and technique. *Implant Dent*, 13, pp. 286–296.

Wang, HL, C Misch, and RF Neiva. 2004b. "Sandwich" bone augmentation technique: rationale and report of pilot cases. *Int J Periodontics Restorative Dent*, 24, (3), pp. 232–245.

Wang, H.-L., T. Itose, R.F. Neiva, and J.L. Shotwell. 2005. Multidisciplinary treatment approach for enhancement of implant esthetics. *Implant Dentistry*, 14, (1), pp. 21–29.

Werbitt, M.J., and P.V. Goldberg. 1991. Immediate implantation. Preservation of bone volume and osseous regeneration. *J Parodontol*, 10, pp. 157–166.

Werbitt, M.J., and P.V. Goldberg. 1992. The immediate implant: bone preservation and bone regeneration. *Int J Periodontics Restorative Dent*, 12, pp. 206–217.

Wiesen, M., and R. Kitzis. 1998. Preservation of the alveolar ridge at implant sites. *Periodontal Clin Investig*, 20, pp. 17–20.

Yang, J., H.M. Lee, and A. Vernino. 2000. Ridge preservation of dentition with severe periodontitis. *Compend Contin Educ Dent*, 21, pp. 579–583, quiz 584.

Yukna, R.A., G.H. Evans, M.B. Aichelmann-Reidy, and E.T. Mayer. 2001. Clinical comparison of bioactive glass bone replacement graft material and expanded polytetrafluoroethylene barrier membrane in treating human mandibular molar class II furcations. *J Periodontol*, 72, pp. 125–133.

Yukna, R.A., P. Castellon, A.M. Saenz-Nasr, K. Owens, J. Simmons, T.H. Thunthy, et al. 2003. Evaluation of hard tissue replacement composite graft material as a ridge preservation/augmentation material in conjunction with immediate hydroxyapatite-coated dental implants. *J Periodontol*, 74, pp. 679–686.

Zitzmann, N.U., P. Scharer, and C.P. Marinello. 1999. Factors influencing the success of GBR. Smoking, timing of implant placement, implant location, bone quality and provisional restoration. *J Clin Periodontol*, 26, pp. 673–682.

Zubillaga, G., S. Von Hagen, B.I. Simon, and M.J. Deasy. 2003. Changes in alveolar bone height and width following post-extraction ridge augmentation using a fixed bioabsorbable membrane and demineralized freeze-dried bone osteoinductive graft. *J Periodontol*, 74, pp. 965–975.

Chapter 8

The Interimplant Papilla

Abd El Salam El Askary

Biological Facts

Optimal esthetics for implant-supported restorations in the anterior maxilla may be more difficult to obtain than implant osseointegration. The ability to predictably preserve or reproduce interimplant papillae is extremely important in the replacement of maxillary anterior teeth. The interproximal papilla that is related to an implant site has been an important topic of clinical research recently, probably due to the increased demand for esthetic restoration by patients. This in turn challenges clinicians to create harmonious gingival contours around dental implant-supported restorations, which depend to a great extent on the presence of healthy natural-looking peri-implant soft issue architecture (El Askary 2000a).

The presence of the interproximal papillae around implant-supported restorations allows symmetrical soft tissue margins and a state of harmony between natural teeth and dental implant components (Tarnow et al. 1996). This harmony and tissue symmetry leads to a natural-looking restoration that does not obscure vision. On the other hand, the slightest change in the level of the interproximal papillae around dental implants due to pathologic reasons or poor soft tissue handling during implant treatment can lead to major esthetic and phonetic complications that are often difficult to correct. That is what makes the peri-implant–supported tissues a delicate clinical issue to handle.

The sequence of losing the interproximal papilla starts immediately after tooth extraction. The thin adjacent alveolar bone (interradicular bone) starts to undergo a rapid process of resorption, probably due to the following reasons: (1) the thin nature of the alveolar bone (which allows faster resorption), (2) reduced blood supply to the crest of the interradicular bone at this particular area, (3) the possible direct contamination of the interradicular bone by oral bacteria as a result of tooth extraction, and (4) most importantly, the absence of the Sharpey's fibers that stimulate continuous bone remodeling and thus maintain healthy marginal levels. (See Figures 8.1A–B.) Sharpey's fibers are totally responsible for maintaining the shape of the interdental papilla without any other proximal support, unlike the case in which the papilla is located between two implants. The collar of the implant prosthetic components interface is not attached to the surrounding gingival tissues by any fibers because there is no cementum and because the nature of the circular orientation of the fibrous tissues around dental implants. Therefore, the final outcome of papilla presence between dental implants is unlikely to occur. (See Figure 8.2A–B.) The importance of presurgical planning and predicting the prognosis of the presence of the papilla between dental implants reaches an important level when replicating natural appearance (El Askary 2002). (See Figures 8.3A–B.)

As a consequence of tooth extraction, the interdental papilla remodels in a sloping fashion from the palatal to the more apical facial osseous plate, and becomes depressed in comparison with the healthy adjacent marginal tissue (Engquist et al. 1995). Unfortunately, the lost interdental papilla usually cannot regenerate to regain its original dimensions (Holmes 1965). The nature of the interimplant (scar-like) soft tissues also complicates the overall clinical prognosis and mandates special reconstructive procedures. The greatest challenge today in implant and periodontal plastic surgery is the reconstruction of lost or incomplete interproximal papillae.

Many clinical efforts have attempted to reconstruct the missing interproximal papillae by using guided tissue regenerative (GTR) procedures (Tinti et al. 1987), augmenting procedures (Salama et al. 1995), free gingival grafts (Miller 1982), coronally positioned flaps (Harvey 1965), pedicle grafts (Nelson 1987), and pontic development techniques (El Askary 2000a). Unfortunately, no single surgical technique for papilla regeneration seems to offer complete predictable long-term clinical success. This chapter highlights the current and future methods for regenerating the papilla and their clinical predictability.

To assess and classify the different clinical conditions of the interdental papillae, Nordland and Tarnow (1998) have reported the deferent clinical conditions of the interdental papillae according to their marginal level. They subdivided the interdental papillae into three classes (see Figures 8.4A–D):

- Class I: Tip of the interdental papilla lies between the interdental contact point and the most coronal extent of the interproximal cementoenamel junction (CEJ) (space is present, but interproximal CEJ is not visible).
- Class II: Tip of the interdental papilla lies at or apical to the interproximal CEJ (interproximal CEJ is visible).
- Class III: Tip of the interdental papilla lies level with or apical to the facial CEJ.

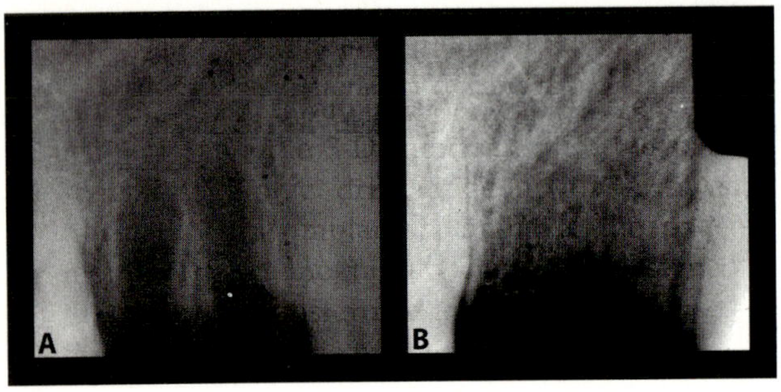

Figure 8.1. A. The papilla bone support at the time of tooth extraction. B. The bone support of the papilla is totally lost due to bone resorption 6 weeks' postextraction.

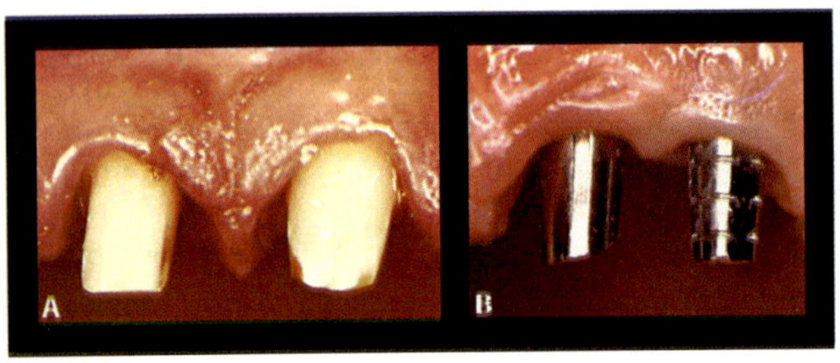

Figure 8.2. A. The Sharpey's fibers are responsible for maintaining the shape of the interdental papilla between natural teeth. B. Absences of interimplant papilla between dental implants due to the absence of Sharpey's fibers.

Tarnow and others (1992) developed a useful classification for clinically identifying the predictability of the presence of interdental papillae. They concluded that when the measurement from the contact point of the natural tooth to the crest of the bone was 5 mm or less, the papilla was present almost 100% of the time; when the

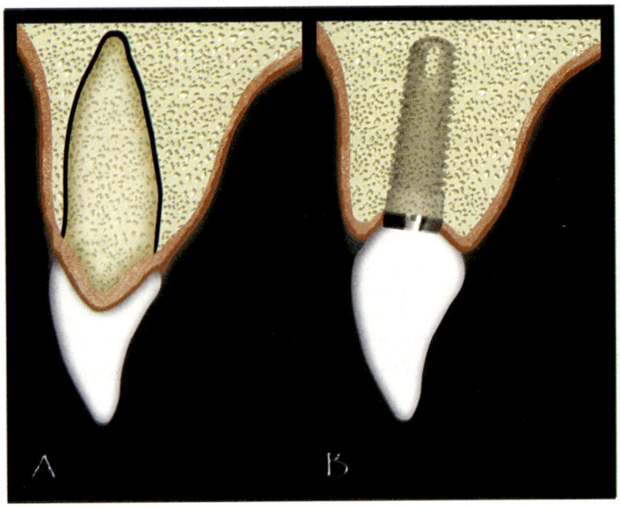

Figure 8.3A, B. An illustration showing the difference between implants and natural teeth in terms of papilla predictability.

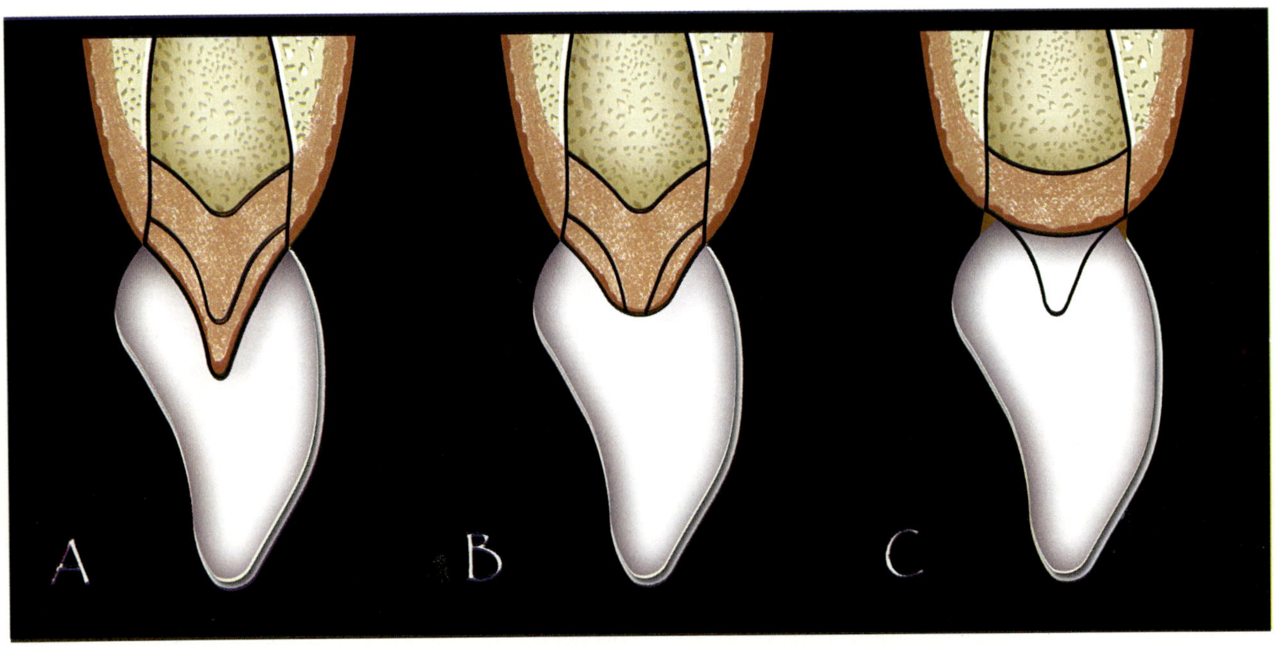

Figure 8.4. A. Class I Nordland classification. B. Class II Nordland classification. C. Class III Nordland classification.

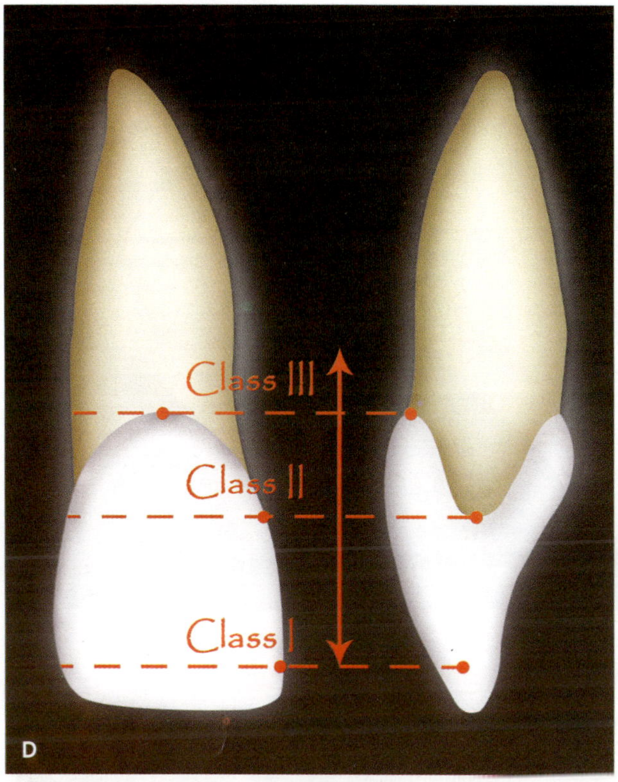

Figure 8.4D. Nordland classification legend.

distance was 6 mm, the papilla was present 56% of the time; and when the distance was 7 mm or more, the papilla was present only 27% of the time or less. (See Figure 8.5A–C.) This classification is considered to be the ultimate clinical parameter for predicting the presence of the papilla around dental implants in single-tooth situations and not in-between two adjacent implants situations.

Salama and others (1998) proposed another interesting classification that furnished a prognostic classification system for the peri-implant papillae. Their three classes are based on the available interproximal height of bone (IHB) in relation to the prognosis of the peri-implant papillae. In Class 1, IHB is 4–5 mm (measured from the apical extent of the future contact point of the restoration to the crest of bone), suggesting an optimal prognosis; in Class 2, an IHB of 6–7 mm shows a guarded prognosis; and in Class 3, the IHB is greater than 7 mm, indicating a poor prognosis, as shown in Figures 8.6A–D.

Another similar classification that offered clinical differentiation and prediction of the interimplant papilla was developed recently by Gastaldo and others (2004). They evaluated 48 patients with 96 interproximal sites in Group 1 and 80 in Group 2. The distance from the base of the contact point to the bone crest was called D1, the distance between tooth and implant or between two

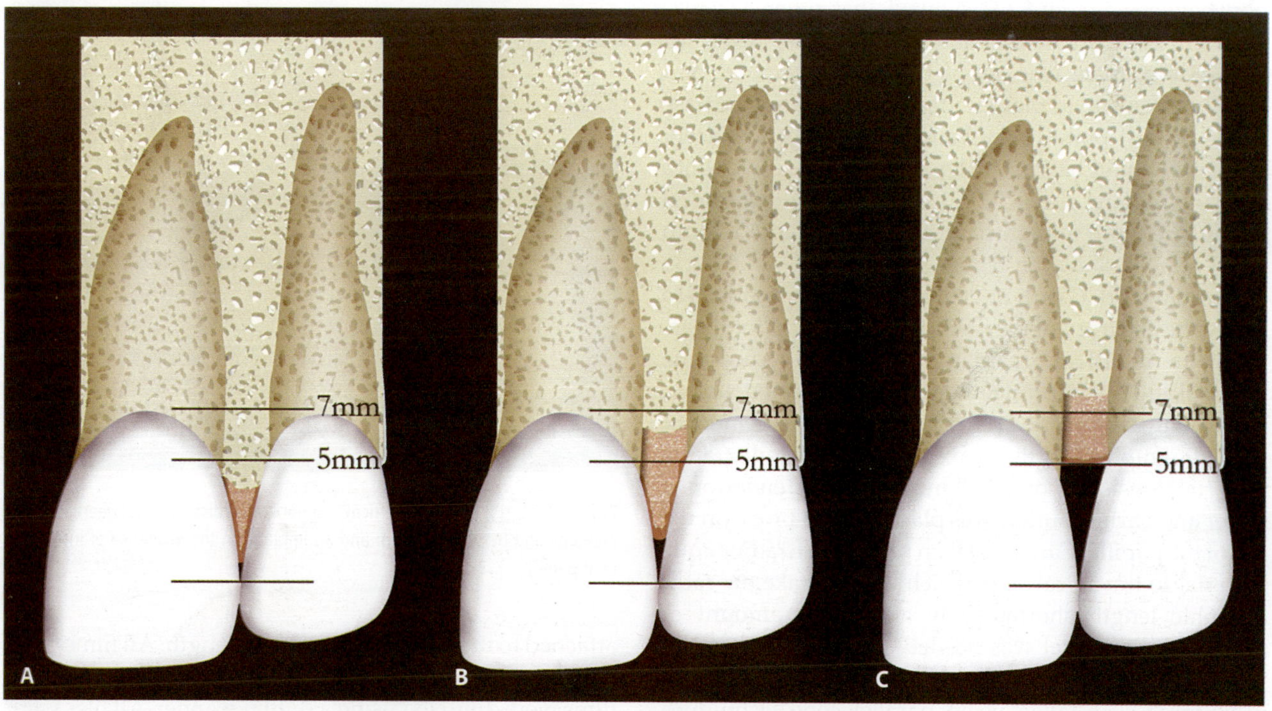

Figure 8.5A, B, C. Tarnow and others classification to assess predictability of interdental papillae.

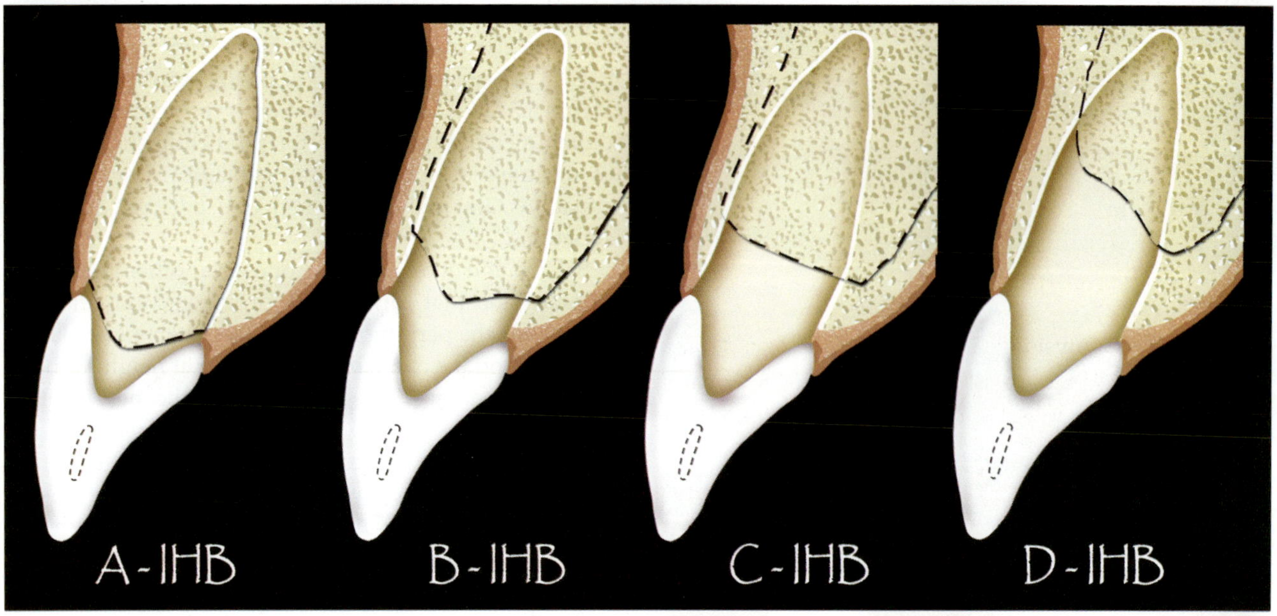

Figure 8.6A, B, C, D. Salama and others classification of the interproximal height of bone.

implants was called D2, and the distance from the base of the contact point to the tip of the papillae was called D3. In both groups, when D2 was 3, 3.5, or 4 mm, the papilla was present most of the time ($P < 0.05$), and when D2 was 2 or 2.5 mm, the papilla was absent 100% of the time ($P < 0.05$). Further, in Group 2 when D1 was between 3 and 5 mm, the papilla was present most of the time ($P < 0.05$). For both groups, analysis of the interaction between D1 and D2 showed that when D2 was ≤2.5 mm, the papilla was absent; otherwise, when D2 was ≥3 mm, there was an interaction between D1 and D2. They concluded that the ideal distance from the base of the contact point to the bone crest between adjacent implants should be 3 mm. The distance between a tooth and an implant should be 3–5 mm. The ideal lateral spacing between implants and an adjacent natural tooth is 3–4 mm, as shown in Figure 8.7.

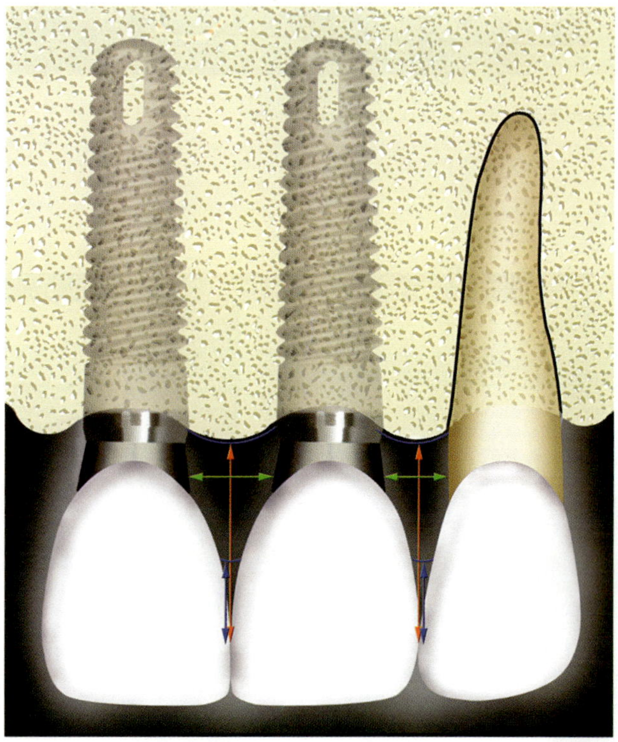

Figure 8.7. Effect of the vertical and horizontal distances between adjacent implants and between a tooth and an implant on the incidence of interproximal papilla.

A recent work (Lee et al. 2005a) has been introduced to verify the accuracy of the noninvasive method for measuring the interdental papilla height using radiopaque material and a periapical radiograph. The method did not include any clinical intervention. For the measurement of the radiographic length (RL) of the papilla, a radiopaque material consisting of a 2:1 mixture of an endodontic sealer and barium sulfate was placed with a probe on the top of the papilla. Care was taken not to place radiopaque material to the apical side, which would make the radiographic length shorter. Only a minimal amount of radiopaque material was needed since the radiopacity was greatly enhanced by the contrast media. A periapical radiograph was taken using parallel cone techniques with an XCP device, along with a 5-mm metal ball bearing attached to the teeth to calibrate the length. All films were developed using the same automatic processor and the films were digitized using a digital scanner. All files were then transferred to a personal computer and examined to calculate the length between the crestal bone and the top of papilla. The length between the most coronal portions of the crestal bone to the radiopaque material was measured with the computer-aided device. The study involved 142 interproximal papillae in 40 patients with chronic periodontitis. The distance between the radiopaque material and most coronal portion of the crestal bone (RL of the papilla) was measured.

Bone probing length (BPL) at the interdental papilla was performed after local anesthesia. After flap elevation, the actual length (AL) of the papilla was measured. A correlation analysis was performed between AL-RL and AL-BPL using Pearson's correlation coefficients. Results suggested that the method using a radiopaque material and periapical radiograph could be used to measure the length of the interdental papilla predictably instead of the other invasive methods that could lead to papillary recession. All of these previous methods mentioned were based on measuring the distance from the contact point or the crown to the osseous crest. However, the distance from the osseous crest to the contact point is not a constant reference, because the contact point can vary in position according to the laboratory fabrication that makes those measurements only valid for natural dentition. As a result, the measurements are variable. (See Figure 8.8A–B.) Subsequently, a promising protocol of a study has been introduced by Tarnow and others (2003) that aims to measure the height of the soft tissue above the osseous crest. It would offer more stable readings and better measurement prediction. A total of 136 interimplant papillary heights were examined in 33 patients. A standardized periodontal probe was placed vertically from the height of the papilla to the crest of bone. The measurements were approximated to the nearest millimeter. The mean height of papillary tissue between two adjacent implants was 3.4 mm, with a range of 1–7 mm. They recommended that only 2, 3, or 4 mm of soft tissue height (average 3.4 mm) can be expected to form over the interimplant crest of bone, which represents a deficiency of 1 to 2 mm of what is needed to duplicate the interproximal papillae of the adjacent teeth. (See Figure 8.9.)

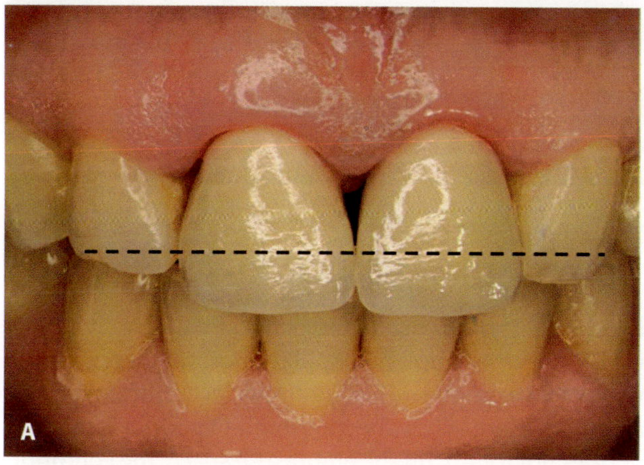

Figure 8.8A. The level of the contact point of any given implant supported restoration can be modified according to the laboratory technician's preference. Note the black lines indicate a further incisal position of the contact point.

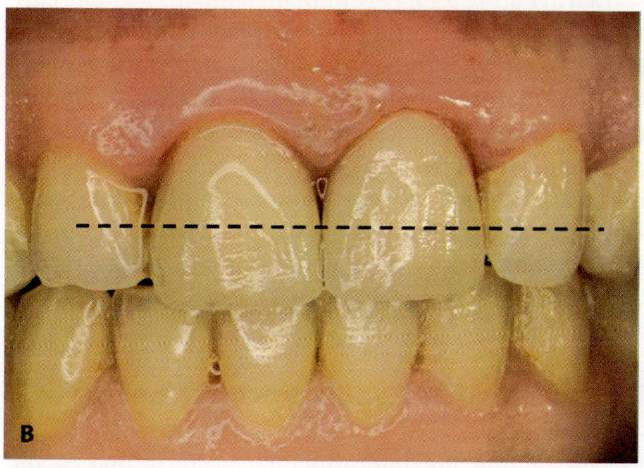

Figure 8.8B. The black lines indicate that the contact point is moved to an apical position in the same patient, which means that the contact point is not a stable reference for any research measurements.

Morphology and Nomenclature of the Interproximal Papillae

The morphological configurations of the interdental papilla depend on several factors, such as the volume of the underlying osseous support, the proximal surface topography of the adjacent teeth, and the assistance of the Sharpey's fibers. The osseous structure of the interdental papilla is composed of two crests or peaks that run from the labial and lingual sides. The labial crest is slightly higher than the lingual one, with an intervening distance averaging from 2–6 mm. The two crests are connected by the so-called *gingival col*, as shown in Figures 8.10A–B, which may be convex or concave in shape, or have a sawlike appearance (Holmes 1965, Cohen 1959). (See Figure 8.11.) Histologically, the interdental papilla is composed of stratified squamous epithelium covering its crest (Holmes 1965) with abundant bundles of collagenous fibers running through the lamina propria. The collagenous fibers, which run in a buccolingual direction through the lamina propria (Stahl 1963, Melcher 1962, Arnim and Hagerman 1953), may have a significant role in keeping the marginal gingival closely adhered to the neck of the tooth; thus, these fibers are responsible for maintaining both the shape and the position of the papilla. The connective tissue contains lymphocytes and plasma cells.

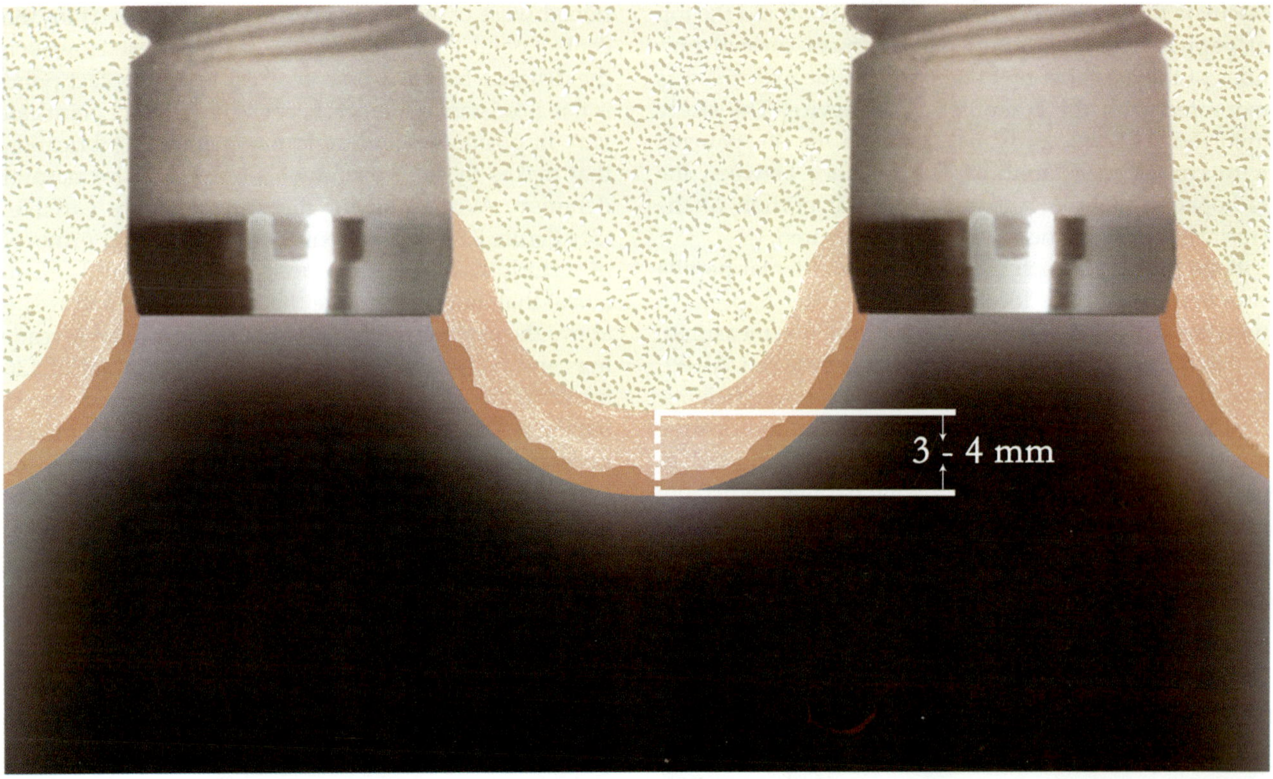

Figure 8.9. Vertical distance from the crest of bone to the height of the interproximal papilla between adjacent implants.

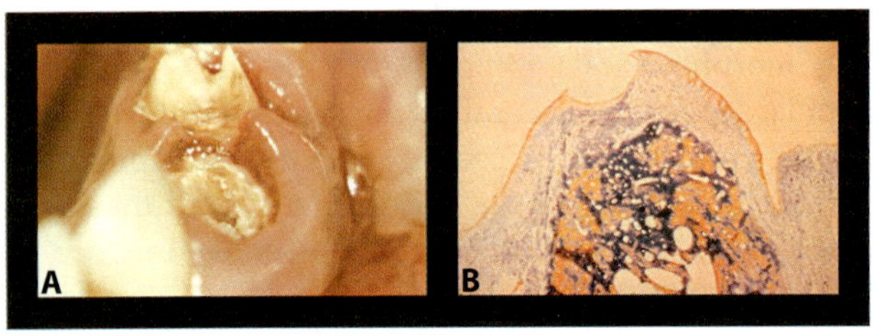

Figure 8.10. **A.** Gingival col clinically. **B.** Gingival col histologically.

Different terms have been coined to identify or distinguish between the interproximal papillae located at different clinical sites. Any given nomenclature for each condition will assist in accurate notification of any given clinical condition. The papilla that exists between natural dentition is called *interdental papilla* and the papilla located between an implant and a natural tooth is called *peri-implant papilla*, as shown in Figure 8.12. If papilla exists between two adjacent implants, it is called *interimplant papilla*. When papilla is used as a generalized term (unspecified), it can be called *interproximal papilla*. The soft tissue histological characteristics of interimplant papillae and interdental papillae are not similar at all.

The interimplant papillae have a parallel connective tissue fibers orientation (Berglundh et al. 1991). They contain a high percentage of collagen fibers with fewer fibroblasts, and have a less adequate blood supply because of the absence of the periodontal ligament. This makes the interimplant papillae more like scar tissue, which may complicate any attempts for surgical repair or reconstruction. When the interimplant papilla is missing or does not totally fill the embrasure space, the condition looks like and is called a *black triangle*. This triangle becomes an esthetic defect that disturbs the overall treatment outcome, especially in high smile line patients, as shown in Figure 8.13. Peri-implant papillae are more clinically achievable than the interimplant papillae because the topography of the CEJ at the proximal surface of the adjacent natural tooth follows a reverse scalloping toward the incisal edge. Sharpey's fibers keep the interproximal bone at the same height (Misch 1999), but this is not the case for adjacent multiple implants. In cases single-tooth implants and when the distance from the contact point to the osseous crest is optimized, the results become highly predictable. (See Figure 8.14A–B.)

Procedures for Papilla Reconstruction

Reconstructing the interimplant papilla is one of the most technique-sensitive procedures in dental implantology. It requires greater surgical skills and optimal scientific background. The nature of the interimplant papilla (scar tissues) also might compromise an optimal

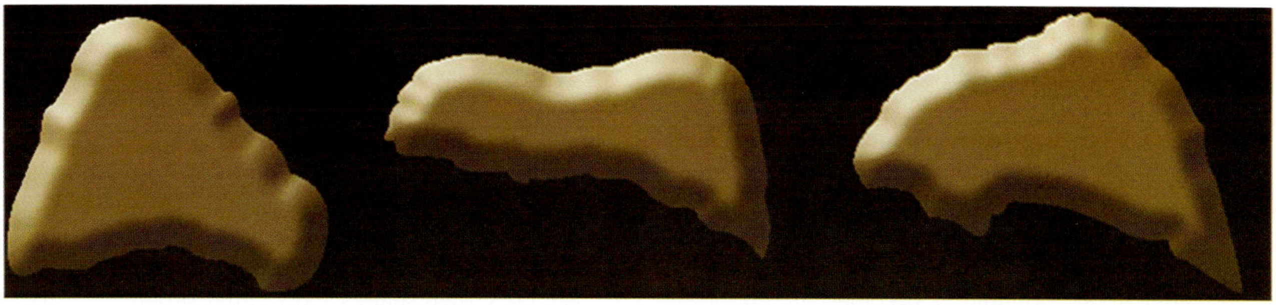

Figure 8.11. The different morphological variations of the papilla osseous structure.

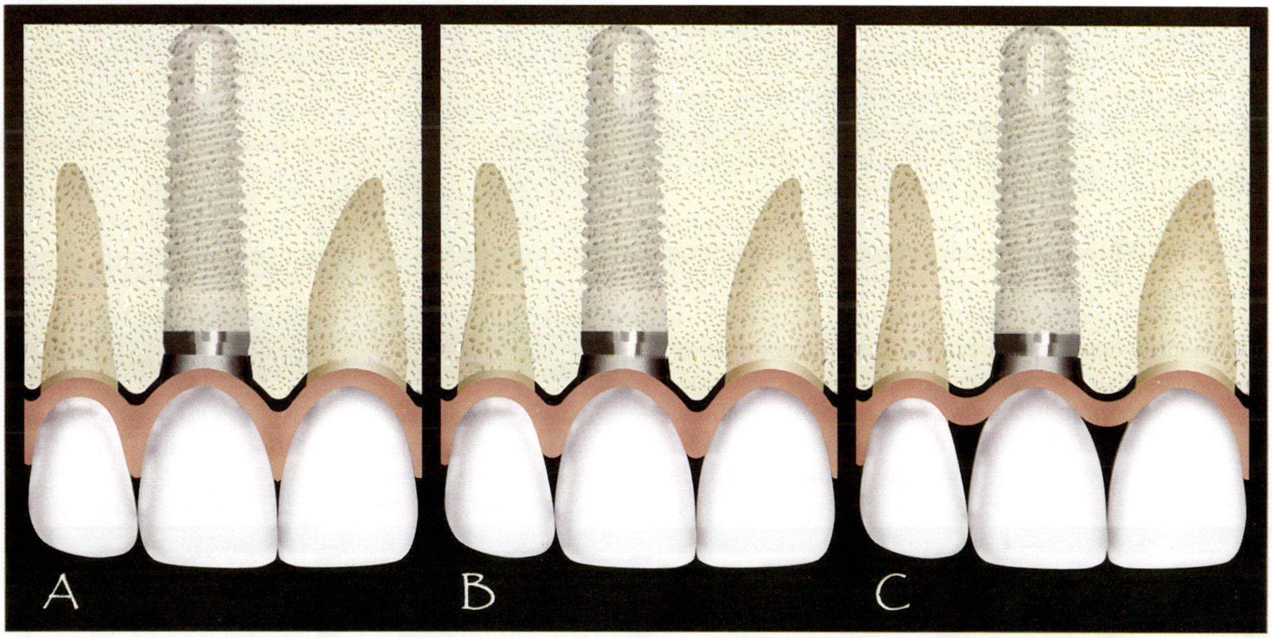

Figure 8.12. Different clinical levels of the peri-implant papilla.

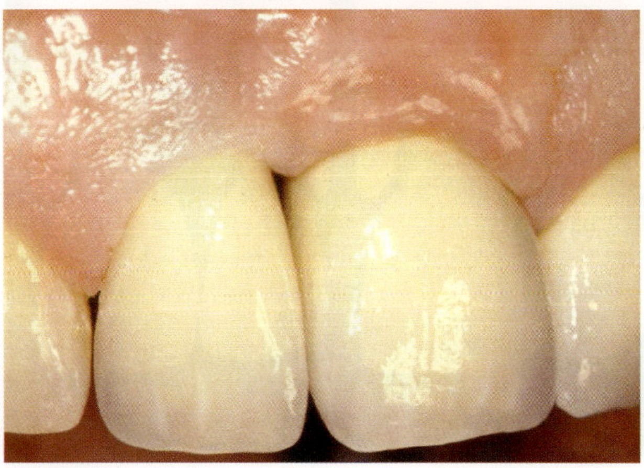

Figure 8.13. The black triangle located between two implant-supported prostheses.

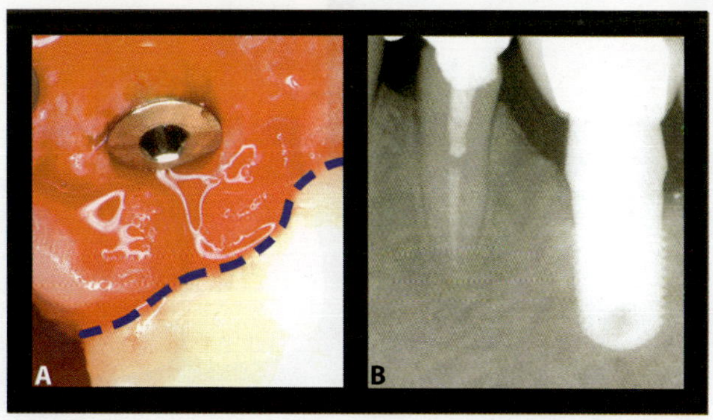

Figure 8.14A, B. The scalloping of the papilla morphology according to the fiber orientation path. And also note the bone level difference around natural teeth and around dental implants that shows the value of the gingival fibers in maintaining bone levels.

surgical reconstructive procedure; however, there are general factors that influence the treatment outcome when one is to reconstruct the inter-implant papilla:

1. Blood supply is the key factor in predicting the treatment outcome. A sufficient blood supply should be maintained in any flap design, especially in complex grafting procedures that involve both soft and hard tissues.
2. Relative tooth orientation becomes an important factor in predicting the peri-implant papilla, because restoring two missing central incisors is unlike restoring unidentical anterior teeth, such as a central and adjacent lateral incisor.
3. Optimal implant position becomes an important factor in determining the future crown contours. The three-dimensional (3-D) implant positioning in the alveolar ridge becomes an influential factor, especially the axial position that influences the distance from the contact point to the osseous crest.
4. Tissue biotypes should be carefully evaluated and recorded before the treatment begins. For example, in the thin scalloped tissue biotypes, the soft tissue volume is usually insufficient and more liable to slough when surgical procedures are being undertaken. Also, the postoperative response to trauma (recession) might complicate the overall treatment fate. In thick flat tissue biotypes, reconstruction procedures seem to be more predictable due to the sturdy nature of the soft tissue and the underlying osseous structure. Therefore, when treating a patient with a thin scalloped tissue biotype, minimally invasive methods should be undertaken with very minimal soft tissue displacement.
5. In tooth morphology, the triangular crown shape seems to negatively influence the volume and height of the gingival embrasure, thus affecting the overall size of the interimplant papilla. On the other hand, square crown shapes show better prognosis. Attenuated tapered roots seem to allow more interradic-

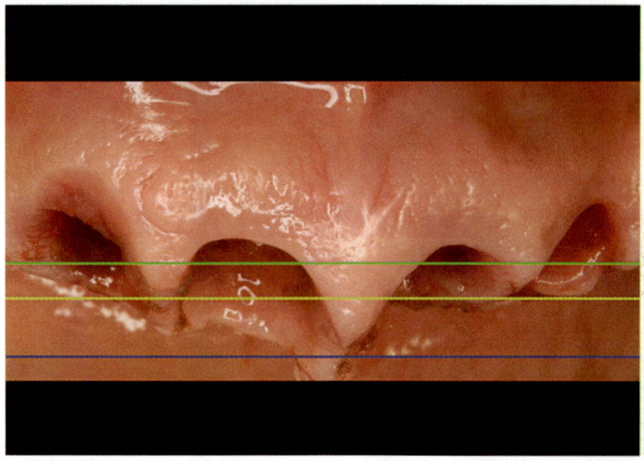

Figure 8.15. Note that the levels of the papilla between the two central incisors exhibit different heights than in between a central and a lateral incisor and also a lateral incisor and a canine.

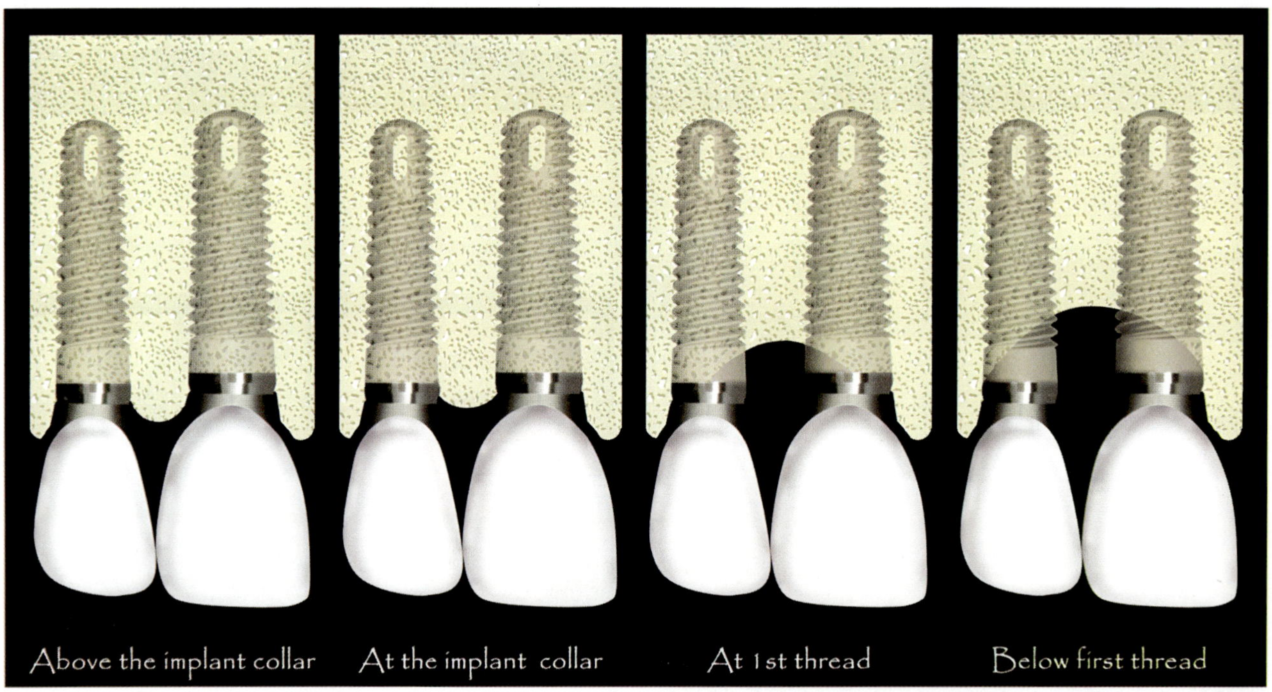

Figure 8.16. Osseous marginal condition between two adjacent implants regarding bone level above the collar of the implant, at the collar, at the first thread, and bone level below the first thread.

ular bone than wider roots, which influences the diameter of the future implant to be used, as shown in Figure 8.15.

6. When reviewing the status of the osseous crestal level, the height of the osseous crest determines the predictability of the interimplant papilla. In cases of severe osseous resorption, the papillary morphology as well as the soft tissues will be compromised; therefore a staged approach should be undertaken. The current thought is to improve the osseous topography until a stable level is reached, and then proceed with implant installation procedures. (See Figure 8.16.)
7. The clinician needs to consider the platform size of the implant. Recently platform switching has been introduced to many esthetic implantology procedures. Switching the platform of the implant diameter to a smaller diameter at the interface level favors the biological width development in the horizontal direction to compensate for the vertical one, thereby minimizing postoperative bone resorption and helping to maintain stable soft tissue margins (D. Tarnow, personal communications, December 2004, NYU, NY, USA). Platform switching seems to make sense because with experience, osseous levels were found to be more stable with the use of narrow platforms. This current thought has led to many new implant designs. (See Figure 8.17A.) Also, shaping the subgingival prosthetic components to be narrower and constricted subgingivally has led to better soft tissue marginal results. (See Figures 8.17B–G.)
8. Keeping an optimal distance between adjacent implants and between natural teeth and adjacent implants is vital in restoring natural soft tissue margins and prosthetic contours. There is no definite guideline that dictates a certain distance to be kept between dental implants, and nor should there be because the variations in teeth shape as well as the implant diameters are countless. When possible, a logical spacing should be maintained that will not jeopardize or infringe on any biological areas.
9. Recently several attempts have been made to introduce new implant designs with scalloped features. While clinicians worldwide do not yet find this to yield predictable results, it is the author's opinion that the designs will show promising results in the future. Scalloped designs can be helpful in

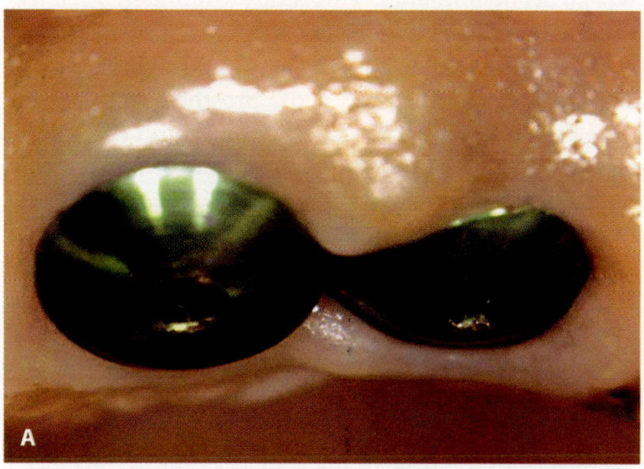

Figure 8.17A. The use of wide implant diameters seemed to induce more tissue loss.

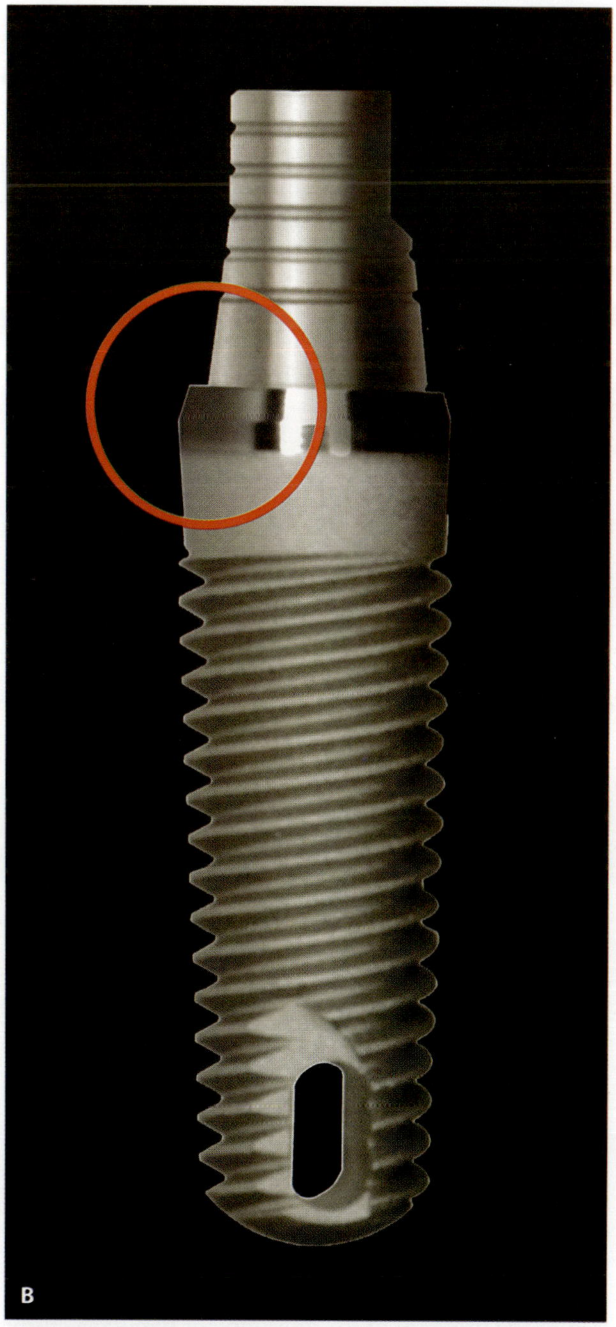

Figure 8.17B. Platform switching.

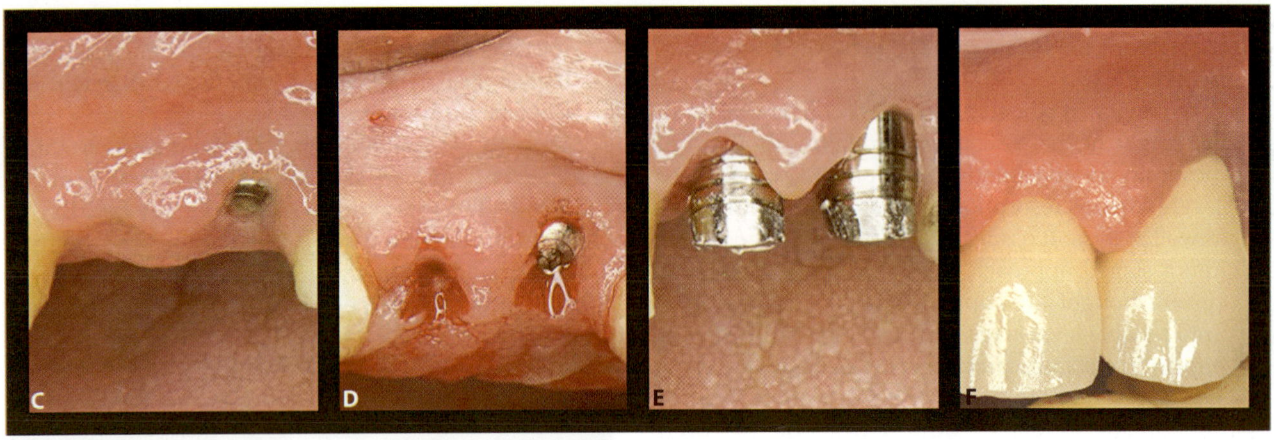

Figure 8.17. **C.** A two adjacent implants at the time of the second-stage surgery. Note the use of very small diameter healing abutments. **D.** Soft tissue punch to uncover the implants. **E.** Abutments connected. Note the development of the papilla between implants due to platform switching. **F.** The case restored finally.

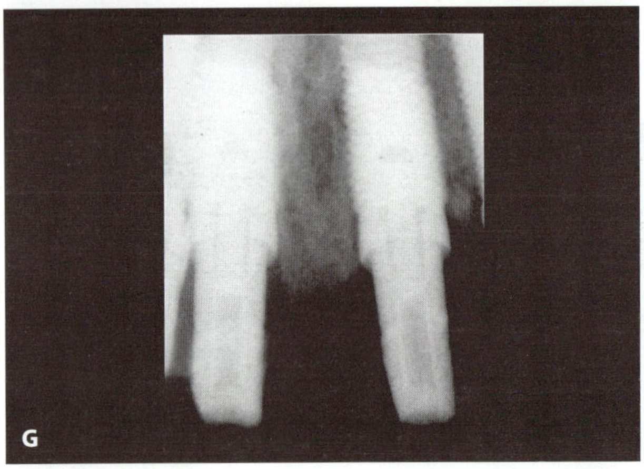

Figure 8.17G. Radiographic view showing the bone levels maintained between implants when platform switching is used.

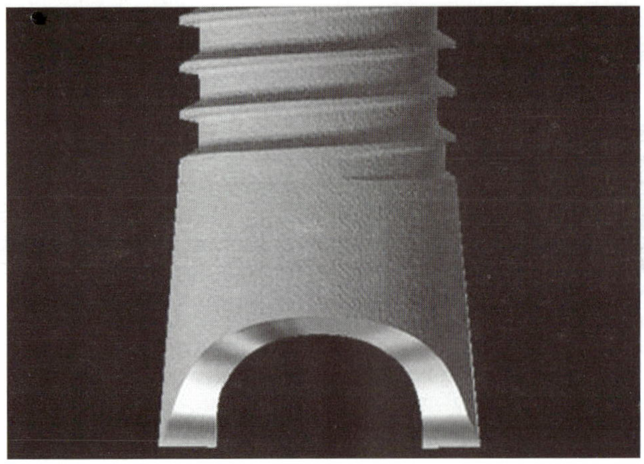

Figure 8.18. A scalloped implant design.

maintaining proximal osseous contours at stable levels in immediate implant placement; however, in delayed implant placement therapy, it is necessary for the bone-grafting procedure to regenerate bone on the scalloped margins. (See Figure 8.18.)

Soft Tissue Procedures for Reconstruction of the Interimplant Papillae

Because of the fragile nature of the peri-implant soft tissue, reduced blood supply at the soft tissue ends, and the postoperative soft tissue remodeling factor, most of the soft tissue methods have attained neither great success nor predictable long-term clinical results. This explains the poor prognosis of any surgical reconstruction attempt to reconstruct the interimplant papilla.

To quantify the value of the keratinized tissues in relation to the presence of the interimplant papilla, a study (Lee et al. 2005b) evaluated the effect of the width of the keratinized mucosa as well as the distance from the base of the contact point to the crestal bone. The study also examined the effect of the horizontal distance between two adjacent implants. This study examined 72 interproximal papillae between two adjacent implants (interimplant papilla) in 52 patients who had implants placed adjacent to each other and had a prosthesis in place for more than one year. The radiographic length (RL) of the papilla, the width of the keratinized mucosa (WK) from the tip of the papilla, and the vertical distance between the base of the contact point and interimplant crestal bone level (CC) were measured. The horizontal distance (HD) between the two implants at the fixture-abutment interface level was also measured.

The study stated that a wider WK indicates that mucosa around the implants was more voluminous and had a thicker peri-implant biotype, leading to the thicker RL. The distance from the base of the contact point to the crestal bone did not influence the length of the interproximal papilla between two implants. The papilla fill was closely related with the HD between two implants. When the distance was less than 2.5 mm, there was an absence of papilla fill. However, in this study, the radiographic dimension of the papilla, not the papilla fill, was measured, and the implant system was arbitrarily selected so that the influence of HD on a specific design was eliminated.

Several soft tissue surgical procedures have been introduced in an attempt to reconstruct the missing papillary tissues. These include coronally positioned flaps in combination with connective tissue grafts (Han and Takei 1996), coronally positioned palatal sliding flaps (Tinti and Parma-Benfenati 1995), and Beagle's technique (Beagle 1992). Beagle's technique entails performing a palatal pedicle flap that is folded and tied on itself on the facial side to increase the height of the interimplant papilla. Regrettably, this method did not attain a high success rate because of the compromised blood supply of the small-sized pedicle, as shown in Figures 8.19A–C. Alternatively, Han and Takei (1996) described a technique that uses a pedicle graft with a semilunar incision and total coronal displacement of the gingival unit.

Others have disclosed several methods for minimizing gingival recession around dental implants to improve the interimplant papilla contours (Israelson and Plemons 1993). Azzi and others (1998) employed a connective tissue graft to be placed on the defective area and then tucked under buccal and palatal flaps, thus providing the graft with an adequate blood supply. The method requires two buccal and lingual marginal partial-thickness incisions at the compromised site. A wedge-shaped graft is harvested from the tuberosity and then shaped and trimmed to obtain two connective tissue extensions with an epithelial crest on the center. When both flaps cover the connective tissue ends of the graft, the epithelial crest stays exposed to increase the height of the interimplant papilla, as shown in Figures 8.20A–C.

The author has introduced a modified lateral sliding flap. The procedure entails moving a tongue-like process from an intact papilla location to a deficient papilla location. This method did not attain any promising clinical success. (See Figures 8.21A–D.)

Nonpedicled connective tissue grafts were used to add bulk to the interimplant papilla. The method entails harvesting a thick piece of connective tissue from the palate and introducing it to the defective site, then pushing it in an incisal direction to reshape the papilla. A free gingival graft then is placed and sutured to prevent the apical migration of the flap. The graft should be slightly thicker than the mucosa in the interimplant region. Care must be taken to adapt this inlay graft on the buccal and lingual to the existing mucosa, to help reestablish collateral circulation so that the grafts will heal with almost no shrinkage. The resulting volume of soft tissue is sufficient for the creation of papillae. The soft tissue must be allowed four to six weeks to heal.

The use of nonpedicled connective tissue grafts to treat defective interimplant papilla has led to questions regarding how long this tissue will support the papilla

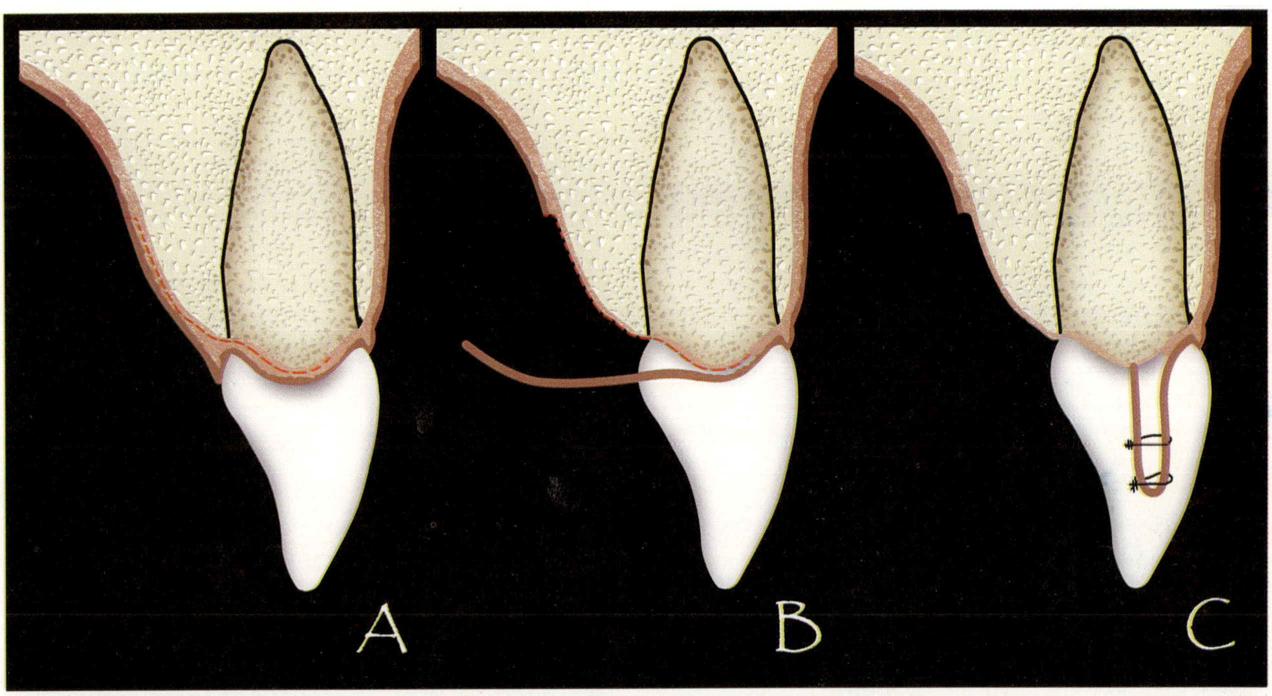

Figure 8.19A, B, C. Beagle's technique.

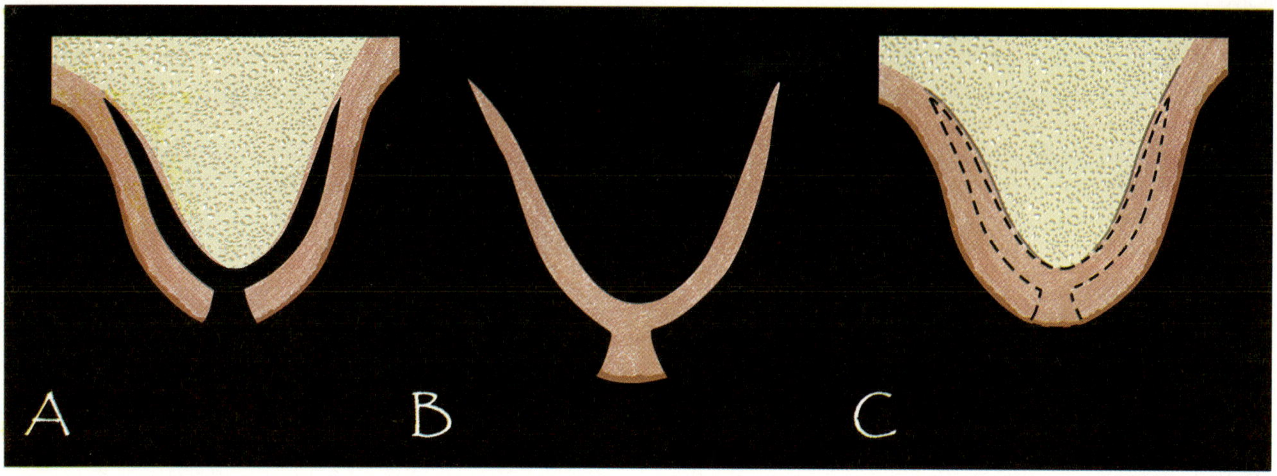

Figure 8.20. **A.** Illustration showing Azzi and others' technique for regenerating the interdental papilla with a connective tissue graft showing the crestal incision with the labial and lingual partial thickness flaps reflected. **B.** Illustration showing the preparation of the composite connective tissue graft. **C.** The graft secured in place.

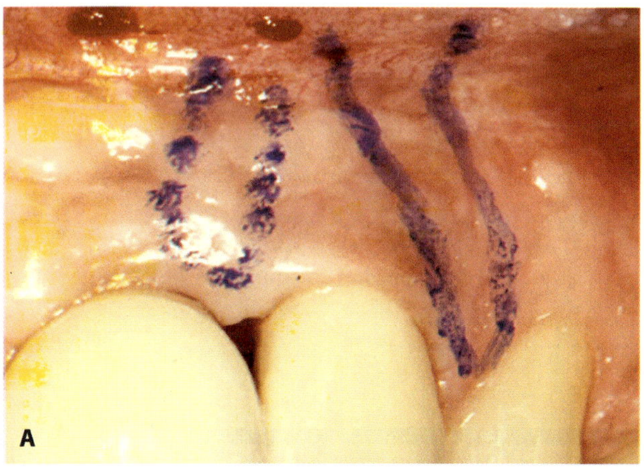

Figure 8.21A. The blue lines show a modified lateral sliding pedicle flap design that is thought to improve the position of the inter-implant papilla.

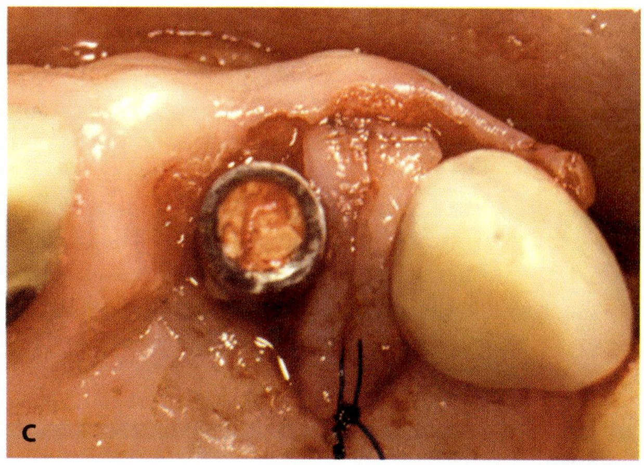

Figure 8.21C. The pedicle flap is sutured.

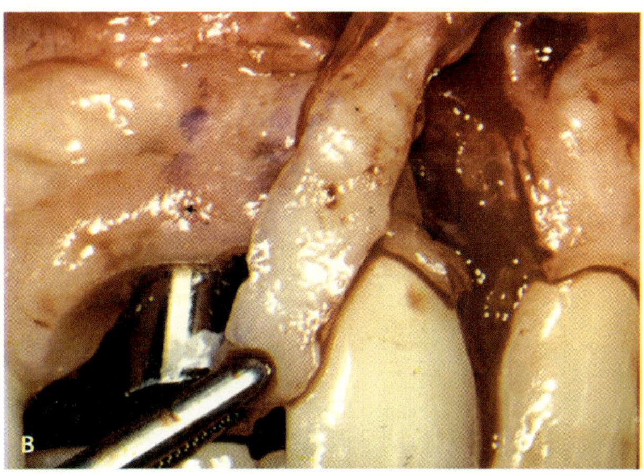

Figure 8.21B. A partial thickness pedicle flap is being displaced laterally to fill the papillary space.

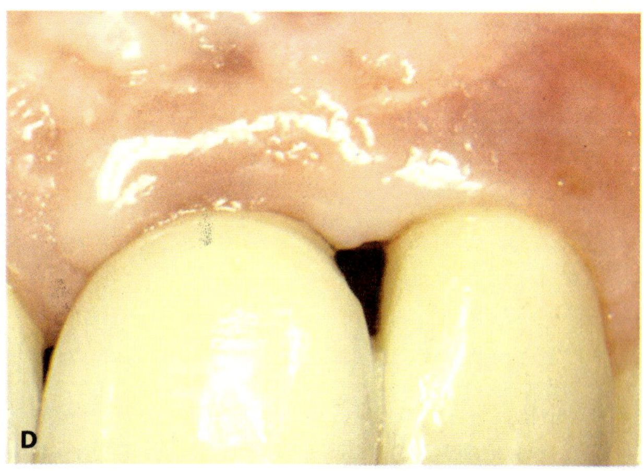

Figure 8.21D. The procedure did not provide any clinical success.

before it starts a remodeling path. (See Figures 8.22A–D.) The use of a minimally invasive second-stage surgery has revealed successful postoperative results. For instance, using narrower platform implants with the healing abutments connected to it at the time of implant installation and attempting a complete soft tissue closure on top of it has revealed clinical success due to the relationship between platform switching and the formation of biological width. It is only in cases of peri-implant papilla conditions that limited incision lines to the keratinized bands at the time of the second-stage surgery have led to enhanced postoperative results.

Misch and others (2004) introduced the split finger technique to bulk the soft tissue around a peri-implant papilla. The method has shown high predictability and clinical efficiency. It entails reflecting a palatal flap at the time of the second-stage surgery and splitting it into two halves, then suturing each half to the labial closest flap.

Adriaenssens and others (1999) described a similar approach to enhance the papilla formation around dental implants in the second-stage surgery in both single- or multiple-teeth situations. The method is called the Palatal Sliding Strip Flap and it helps form the papillae between implants and between natural teeth in the anterior area of the maxilla. The flap is designed and managed so that the palatal attached mucosa slides in a labial direction to create papillae and at the same time augment the labial ridge. The procedure entails an incision that allows the dissection of the masticatory mucosa from the underlying bone with a full-thickness sulcular approach in a labiopalatal direction perpendicular to the ridge crest, both on the mesial and distal aspects of the implant. A full-thickness horizontal incision is extended from the distal to the mesial on the palatal side comprising approximately two-thirds of the distance between the two teeth. Two incisions are then made parallel to each

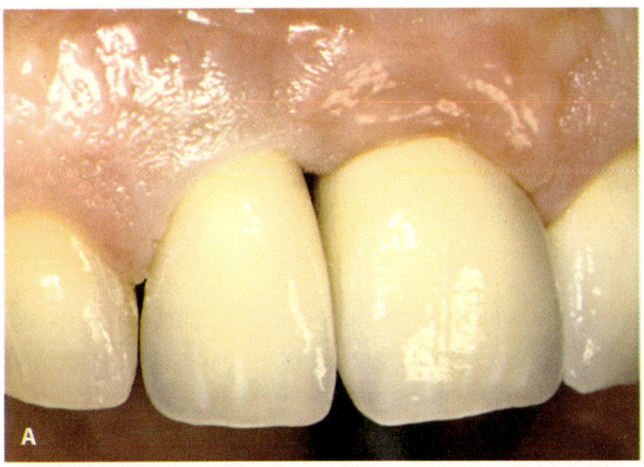

Figure 8.22A. Preoperative view of a black triangle between two implant-supported restorations.

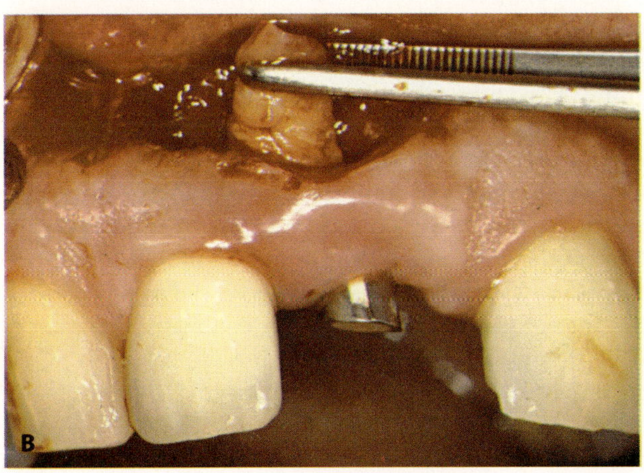

Figure 8.22B. The connective tissue graft is interceded and secured to the site.

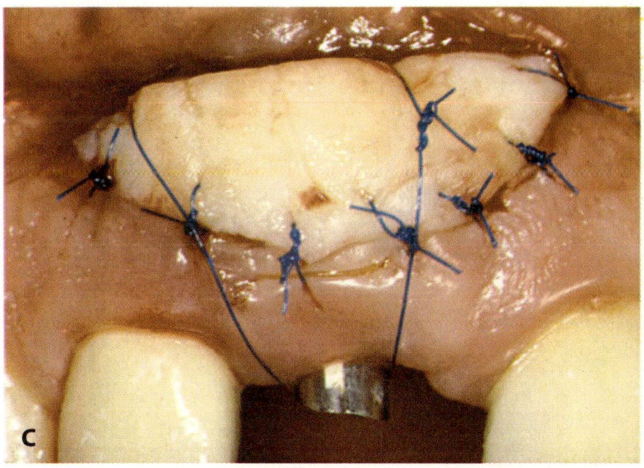

Figure 8.22C. Free gingival graft is placed to prevent tissue creeping.

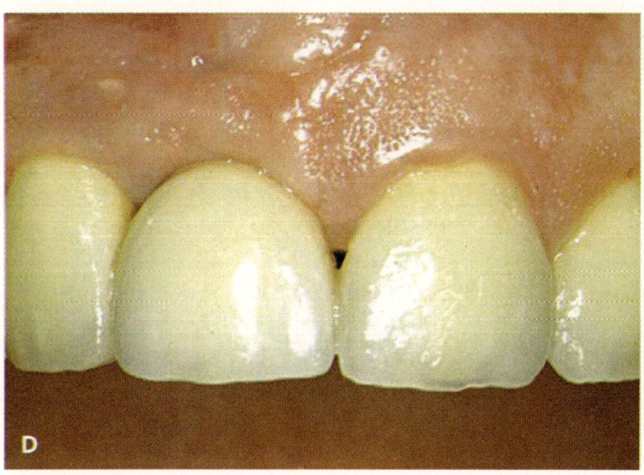

Figure 8.22D. Final case resorted with moderate improvement in the papillary levels.

other in a labiopalatal direction to create a partial thickness flap extending in the palate, leaving the periosteum intact. This extension portion is designed into a strip to be located at the mesial aspect of the implant. A partial-thickness horizontal dissection is made to connect the two parallel incisions to form the sliding palatal strip. A final incision dissects the masticatory mucosa from the bone and incorporates the partial-thickness incision into a full-thickness incision in a labial direction.

Once the incisions are made, the partial- and full-thickness flaps are prepared for flap elevation. The partial-thickness flap with a strip is raised to uncover the implant. The healing abutment is connected, and a semilunar incision is made to the distal, away from the side of the strip. Care must be taken so that the semilunar incision is coronal to the CEJ or the gingival line of the adjacent teeth, otherwise the healing abutment will displace the flap apically and the final gingival margin will heal apical to the gingival line of the adjacent teeth. The semilunar incision provides a second strip, which gives two pedicles. The distal pedicle created by the semilunar bevel incision is rotated 90 degrees in the palatal direction around the healing abutment. The mesial pedicle with the partial-thickness component from the palate fills the interproximal space. This flap manipulation between the teeth and the healing abutment allows the reconstruction of two papillae at one time. The buccal soft tissue augmentation is related to the support by the healing abutment and the buccal repositioning of the flap. Simple sutures are used around each newly formed papilla to maintain the flap in position.

In the case of two adjacent implants, the flap design for multiple restorations in the anterior maxilla follows the general principle of a palatal strip of split-thickness tail harvested from the palate, combined with a full-thickness flap displaced in the midpalate toward the sulcus of adjacent tooth. The difference is in the location of the palatal strip and the semilunar incisions. The palatal strip of split-thickness connective tissue tail harvested from the palate must be made between the implants. A full-thickness incision displaced in the midpalatal area dissects the masticatory mucosa toward each adjacent tooth. A final incision dissects the masticatory mucosa from the bone over the ridge crest, creating a full-thickness sulcular incision. Once the incisions are made, the partial- and full-thickness flaps are prepared for elevation. The partial-thickness flap with a strip adjacent to the distal tooth is raised to uncover the implants and their cover screws. The healing abutments are connected, allowing the flap to be sustained on the buccal side. Two semilunar incisions are made toward the contralateral side of the strip. Care must be taken that the semilunar incision is coronal to the CEJ, otherwise the healing abutment will displace the flap apically. The two semilunar incisions provide two small pedicles. They are rotated in the palatal direction, each one creating a tissue augmentation in the interproximal space between the tooth and the implant. The palatal strip of partial thickness is foiled to fill the interproximal space between the adjacent implants.

All soft tissue solutions to restore the interimplant papilla offer less predictable long-term results because of the fragile nature of the oral soft tissues and reduced blood supply at its marginal ends. Oral bacteria and smoking complicate healing to a great extent. Soft tissue procedures can be used only in single fairly small papillary defects.

Osseous Regenerative Methods for Reconstructing the Inter-implant Papilla

The natural appearance of the peri-implant soft tissue contours reflects the condition of the underlying osseous structure. Two anatomic structures are important for the final appearance of the interimplant papilla: the interproximal bone height and the height and thickness of the facial bone wall. The interproximal crest height plays a role in the presence or absence of peri-implant papillae, as shown in Figure 8.23A. It has been shown that the height of peri-implant papillae in single-tooth conditions depends on the interproximal bone height of the adjacent teeth (Tarnow et al. 1992, Choquet et al. 2001, Kan et al. 2003). (See Figures 8.23B–J.) Clinical situations with reduced vertical bone height on adjacent teeth are challenging, because it is almost clinically impossible to regain this lost vertical height. The height and thickness of the labial bone is important for long-term soft tissue marginal stability around implants and adjacent teeth (Buser and von Arx 2000, Buser et al. 2004).

Based on Holmes' findings (1965), a major consensus valued the importance of regenerating the underlying osseous support. The aim is to regain the overall lost tissue height between adjacent implants (El Askary 2000a). Salama and others (1998) stated that "successful and predictable esthetic results can be accomplished only when underlying labial and inter-proximal osseous support has been therapeutically provided." This statement was a turning point for many clinicians to regenerate the osseous support (the foundation) of the interimplant papilla, which might be more predictable than soft tissue procedures. An early trial to reconstruct the interimplant papilla through osseous regeneration was presented through reports on cases in which mini-cortical screws were applied to tent a guided bone regeneration (GBR) membrane to create a space for osseous regeneration (Salama et al. 1995).

Few methods that focused mainly on the osseous support of the inter implant papilla have been recorded

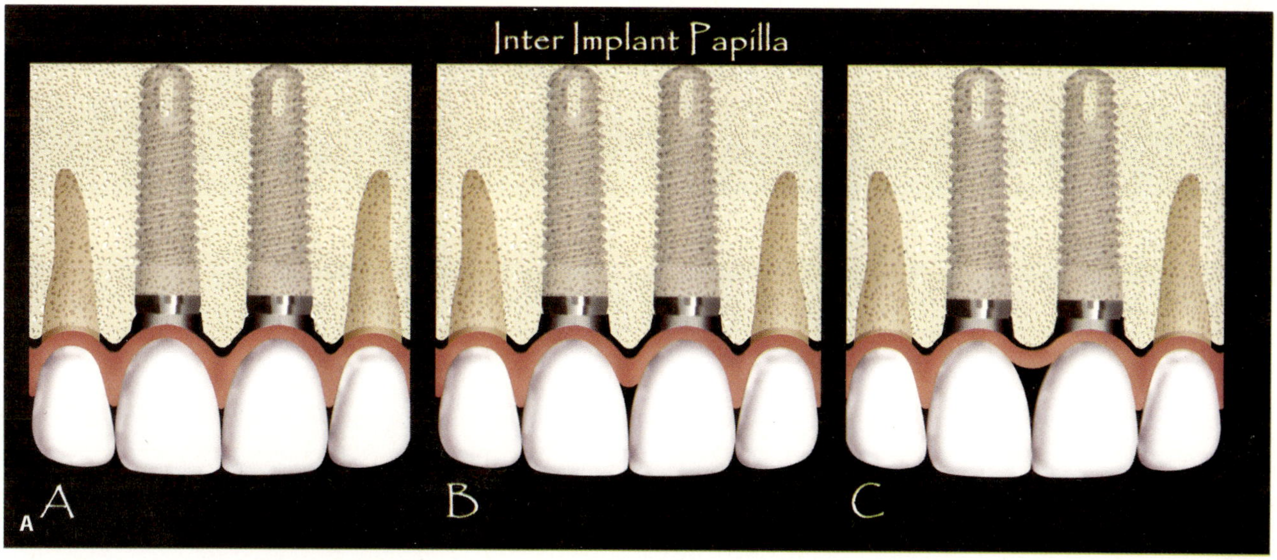

Figure 8.23A. The different clincal inter papilla levels.

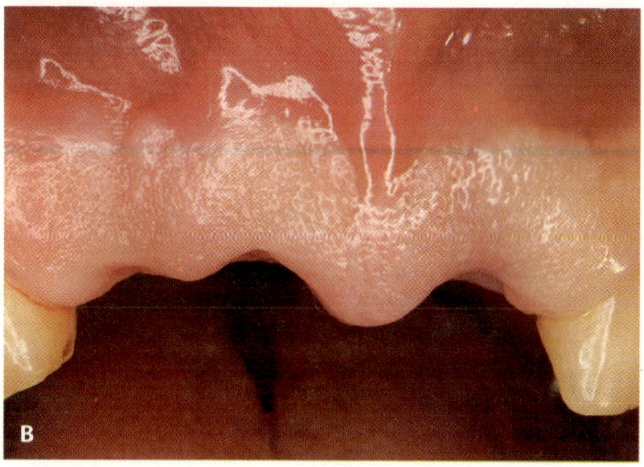

Figure 8.23B. Preoperative view showing asymmetrical papillary levels due to deficient osseous support.

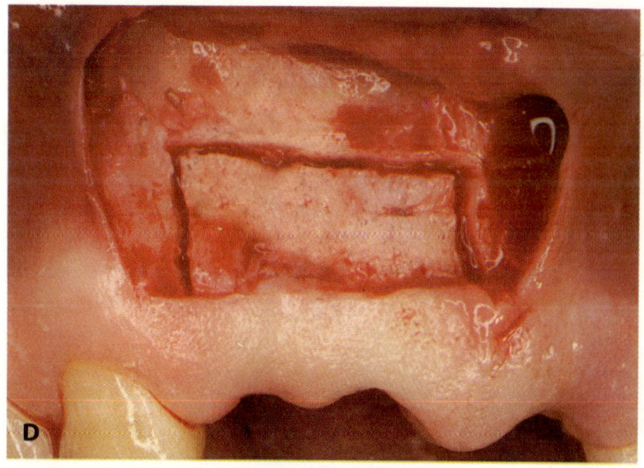

Figure 8.23D. Mucoperiosteal flap is being reflected and complete osteotomy is made at the place of the defect.

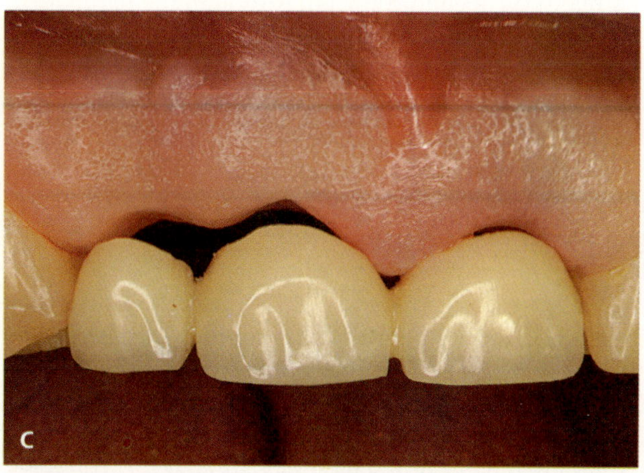

Figure 8.23C. The surgical template in place showing the amount of tissue deficiency.

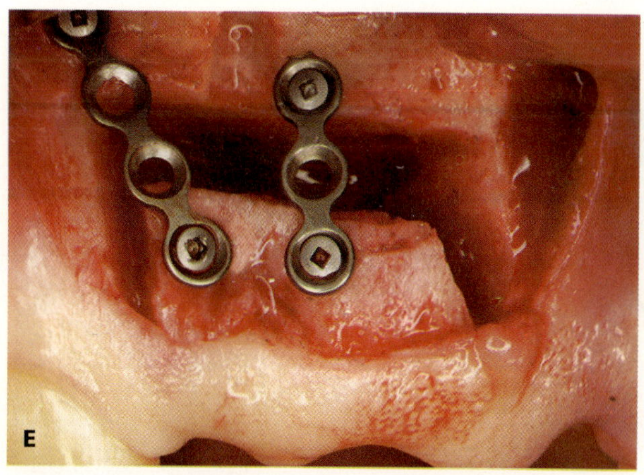

Figure 8.23E. The bone block is moved to an incisal direction in order to move the bone support of the papillae to its original position. The bone block is being stabilized at its new position via two titanium microplates.

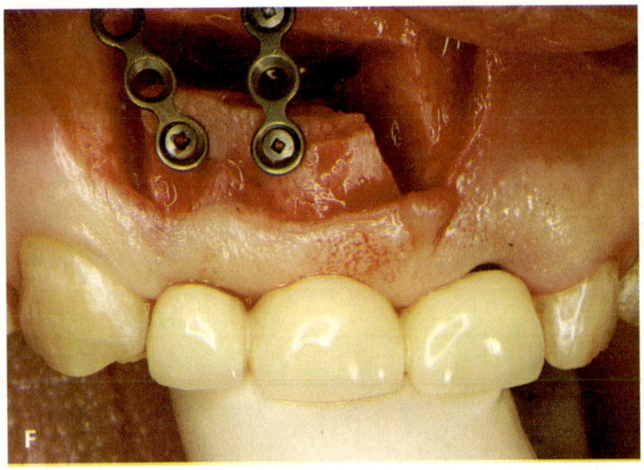

Figure 8.23F. The surgical template is placed to check the amount of bone displaced incisally.

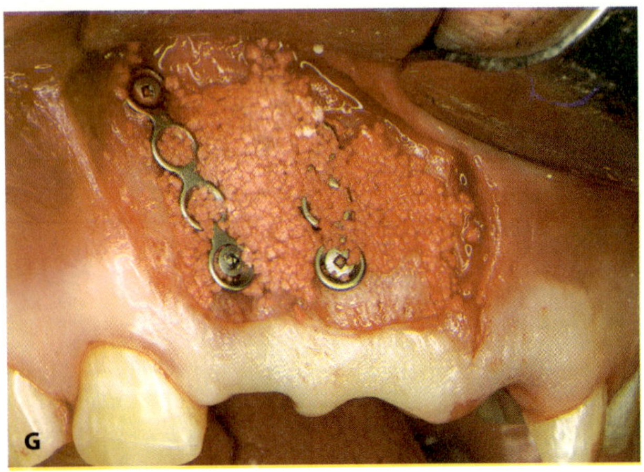

Figure 8.23G. The resultant space is filled with bone-grafting particulated graft.

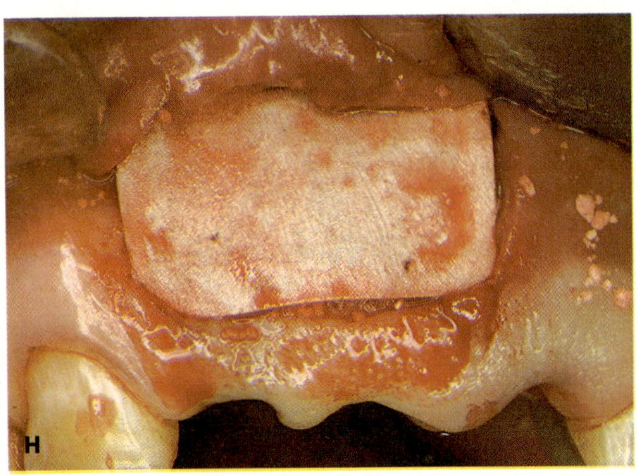

Figure 8.23H. BioMend collagen membrane is being placed to cover the bone graft.

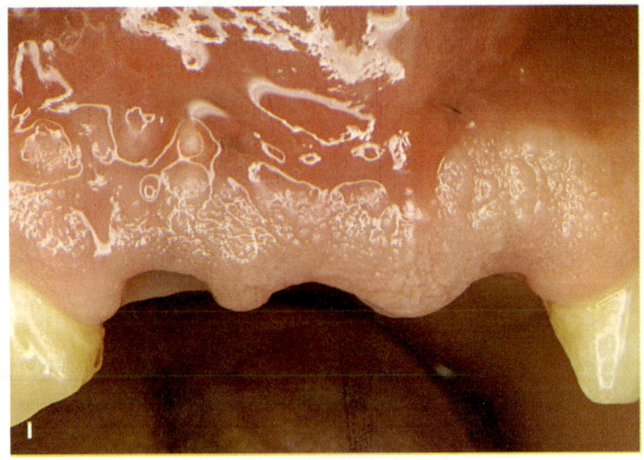

Figure 8.23I. Five weeks' posthealing showing the improvement of the papillary contours.

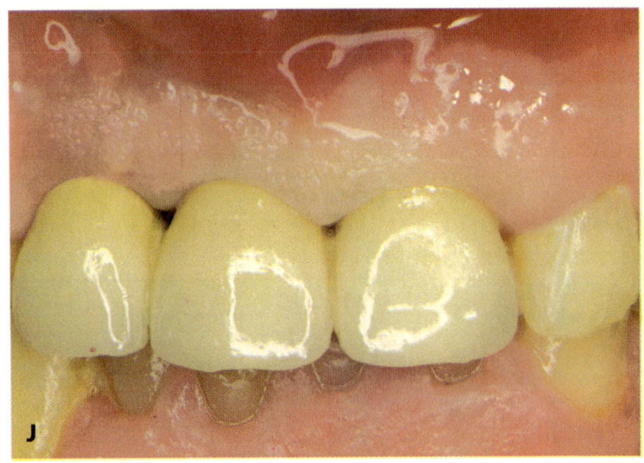

Figure 8.23J. The case is finally restored.

in the literature. An interimplant papilla regenerative template has been introduced. Although the template is still in its preliminary experimental stages, it showed acceptable clinical success (El Askary 2000a).

Interimplant Papilla Regenerative Template

The author introduced this technique in 1999. The interimplant papilla regenerative template (El Askary 2000a) is a carrier fabricated from pure titanium. It acts as a housing for any bone-grafting material that is to be placed on the alveolar ridge to regenerate an osseous foundation for the interimplant papilla. The template is shown in Figure 8.24. The template is to be placed at the time of implant insertion, thereby eliminating the need for any additional surgical procedure. (See Figure 8.25.) Other advantages of the template are that it carries and protects the bone-graft material and separates the bone-grafting mix from the undesired fibroblast and epithelial cells, which favors graft predictability. The use of the template requires a space of not less than 3 mm between two adjacent implants.

After the implants are inserted, the interimplant bone is decorticated to allow for a pool of cellular activity to the graft. The preferred grafting mix used with the template is 50% autogenous bone chips harvested from the drilling procedure and 50% allograft bone chips (Porous, Zimmer Dental, Carlsbad, CA, USA). The use of 100% autogenous chips can provide a more predictable clinical outcome but is liable for greater postoperative remodeling and resorption.

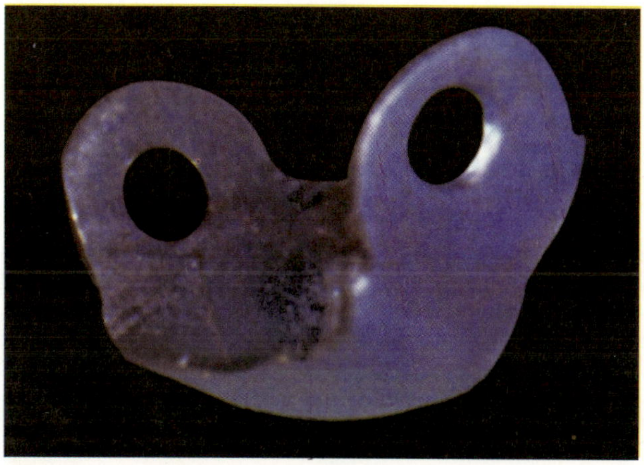

Figure 8.24. Interimplant papilla regenerative template.

The template is then placed on the alveolar ridge with its two perforated ends facing the sides of the alveolar ridge. Two GBR fixation pins (Autotac System, Biohorizons, AL, USA) are fitted into the perforated ends of the template to stabilize and secure it. Soft tissue requires some manipulation to achieve complete tension-free closure, which is extremely valuable to the template survival. At the time of the second-stage surgery, the template is removed, revealing the regenerated bone, and the flap is then sutured and left to heal. After soft tissue healing is complete, the provisional prosthesis might be used to develop a natural emergence profile. Care must be exercised so that the provisional prosthesis margins exert no pressure on the newly formed bone. (See Figures 8.26A–C and 8.27A–H.)

While the use of templates has revealed exciting clinical results, in some cases they showed exposure through the mucosa. This was considered one of the major complications in the use of templates with thin scalloped tissue biotype patients. The long-term use of the template has raised the concern for postoperative bone resorption due to loading because of the tendency

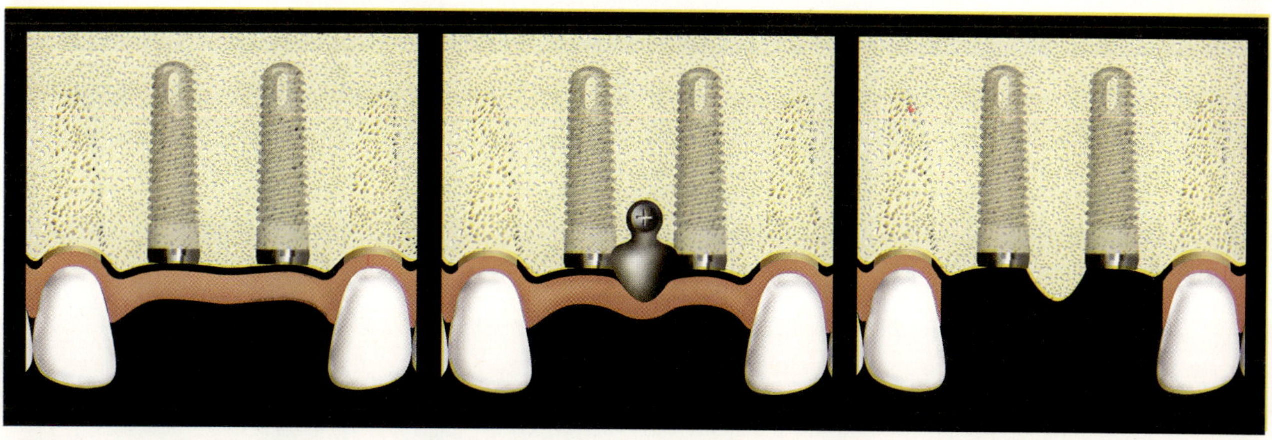

Figure 8.25. An illustration showing the clinical use of the template.

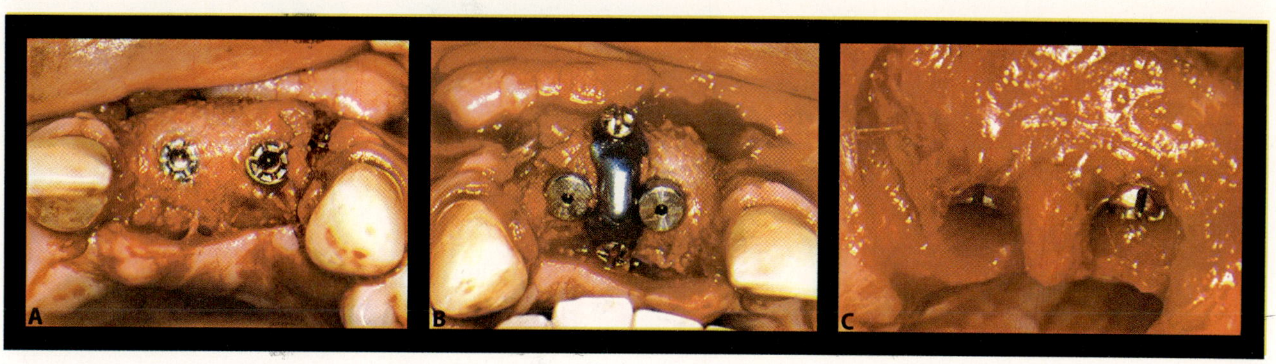

Figure 8.26. **A.** Two adjacent implants placed. **B.** The template secured in place with two fixation screws. **C.** The bone regenerated between the two implants after template removal in second-stage surgery.

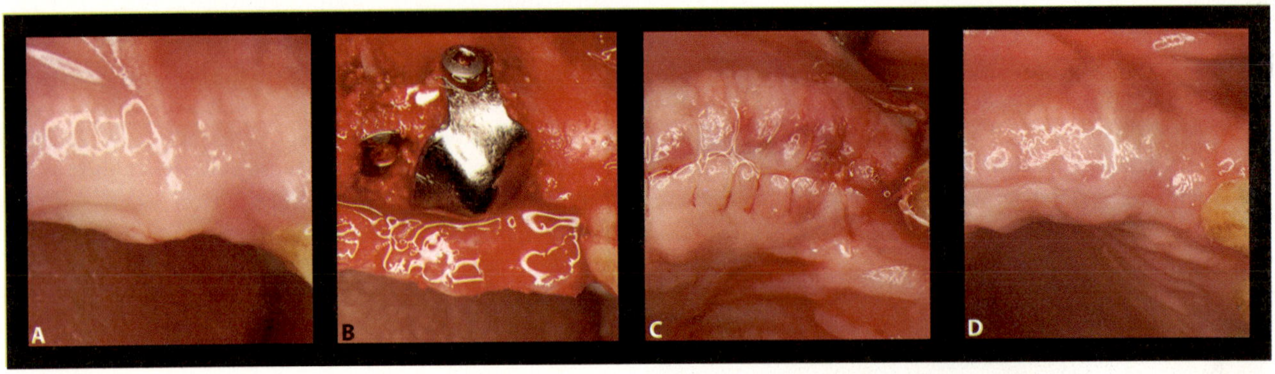

Figure 8.27. **A.** Edentulous maxillary alveolar ridge. **B.** The regenerative template placed between two implants. **C.** The flap sutured. **D.** The postoperative healing clinical condition.

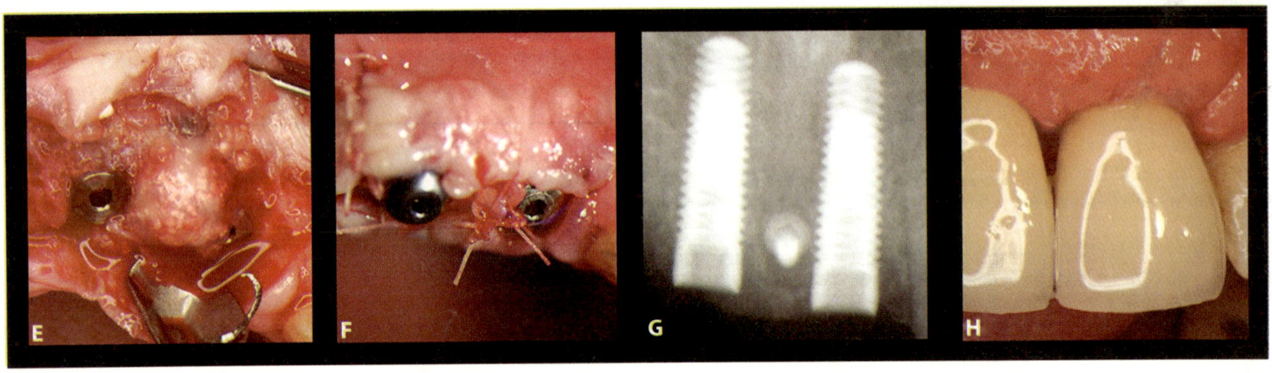

Figure 8.27. **E.** The second-stage surgery revealing the bone regenerated between implants. **F.** Healing abutments connected with connective tissue graft being placed on top of the grafted bone for protection. **G.** Radiographic view showing the grafted bone between the implants. **H.** The case restored with moderate papilla fill.

to form a biological width and because of the bacterial population at the implant interface at the implant abutment connection. (See Figure 8.28.)

These complications might be overcome by using slowly resorbable bone-grafting materials. In the future, using resorbable materials made from polyacrylic acid products and using self-retained templates instead of using the membrane taks currently are being considered. With the introduction of the scalloped implants, this template becomes more valuable because now it can regenerate bone between the two scalloped peaks of two adjacent implants with no fear of postoperative bone resorption because the regenerated bone will be far from the implant abutment connection.

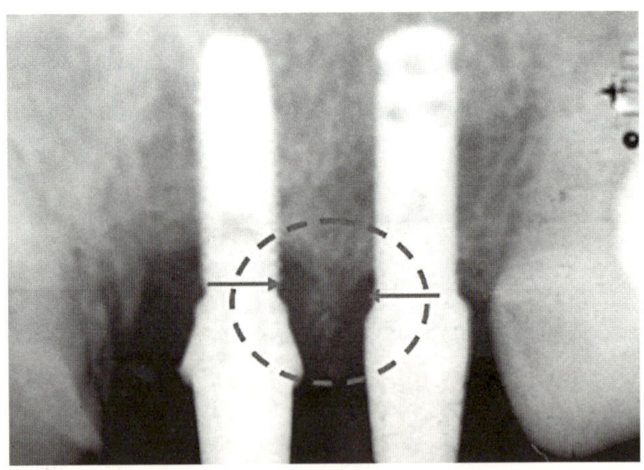

Figure 8.28. Postloading bone resorption between implants.

The Use of Miniautogenous Blocks

Miniautogenous bone blocks have been tested as a method of creating a basal foundation of an interimplant papilla. The method entails harvesting a small graft from an intraoral site and stabilizing it to the recipient site with a microtitanium screw, as shown in Figure 8.29. Harvesting a corticocancellous has been suggested as a way to minimize the surgical trauma and morbidity. The core graft is then returned to its place in an upright position, leaving a bone peak extruding in a higher position to support the papilla, as shown in Figures 8.30A–E. The graft is fastened with microtitanium screws to the underlying site. (See Figures 8.31A–H.) However, this method did not reveal a higher success rate due to the smaller size of the core graft.

The Use of Distraction Osteogenesis

Alveolar distraction osteogenesis is widely documented in the literature (Block et al. 1996, Lazar et al. 2000, Beitan 1967). It is a biologic process by which new alveolar bone is formed following a gradual separation of a block of bone from the ridge. This process is used mainly to correct alveolar deformities in ridge height. In 1996, distraction osteogenesis was introduced as a promising method for restoring a deficient alveolar ridge to its original size. The technique was taken from orthopedic surgery, has been used in the elongation of tubular bone in children, and now is predictably used in restoring severe atrophy of the alveolar ridge (Lazar et al. 2000). It eliminates the need for donor site surgery and reduces the risk of morbidity in comparison with the autogenous grafting procedures (Beitan 1967).

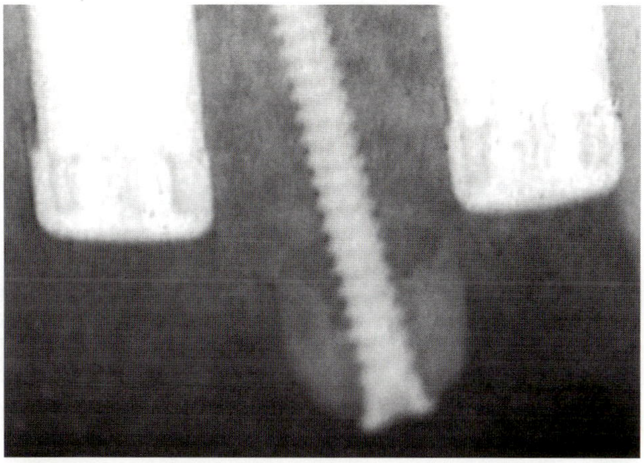

Figure 8.29. Miniautogenous block is used to support the interimplant papilla.

Alveolar distraction osteogenesis entails exposure of the ridge by a mucoperiosteal flap, sectioning (osteotomy) and mobilization of the alveolar bone, and attachment of the distraction device. Following an initial rest period, the distraction device is activated, typically moving at a rate of 1 mm per day. The device must be activated in accordance with the required height of the alveolar ridge (up to 15 mm). Clinical and radiological evaluations are carried out to monitor the regeneration process and determine when the desired height or width has been reached. The device is then removed following another rest period, which allows consolidation of

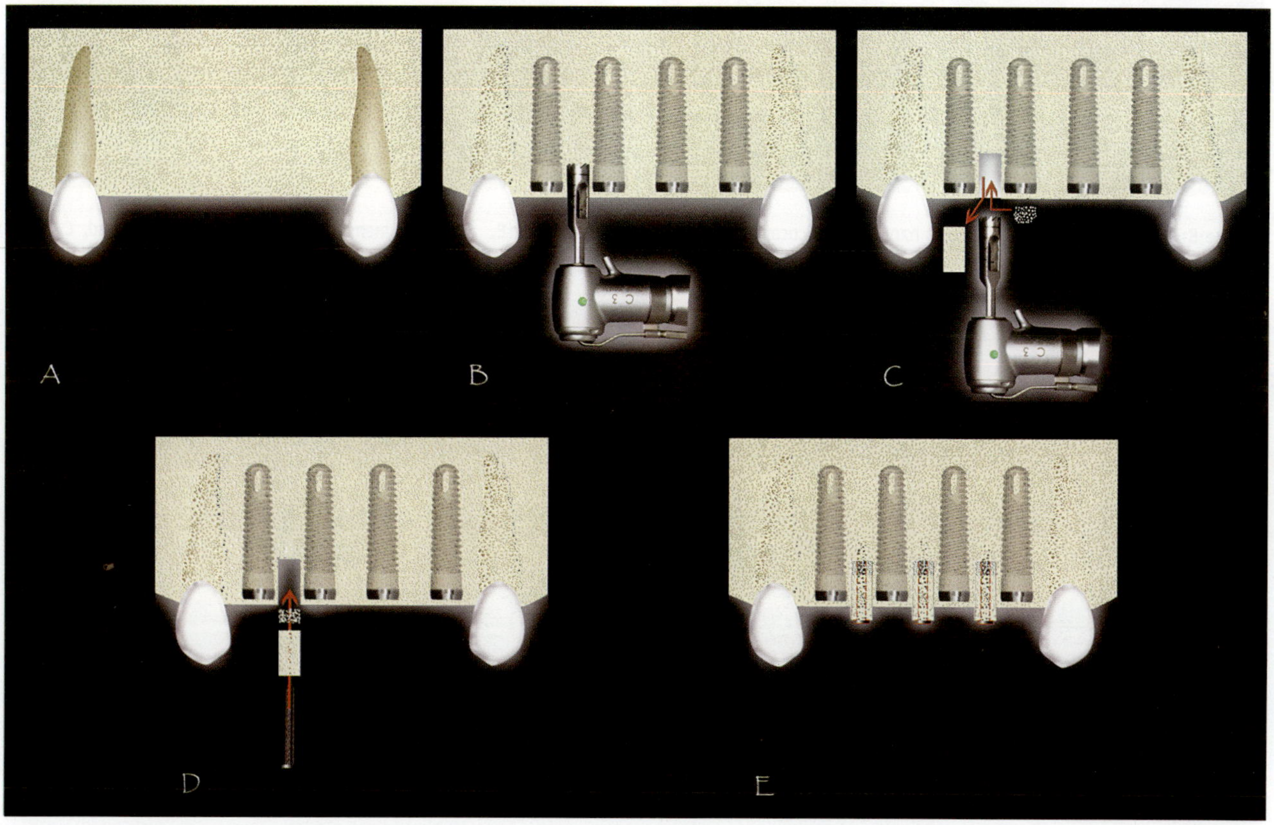

Figure 8.30A, B, C, D, E. An illustration showing the use of the trephine graft technique for papillary reconstruction.

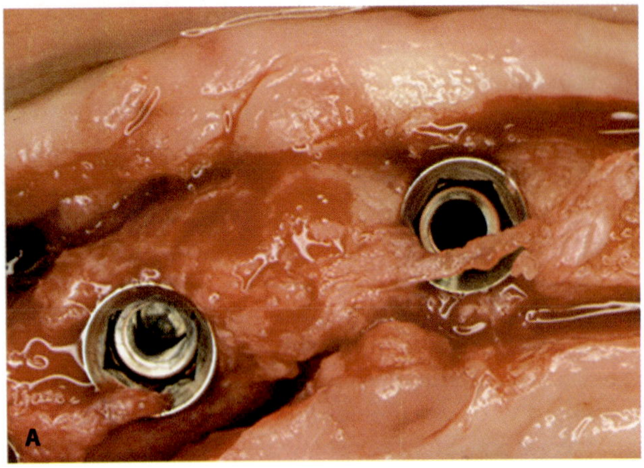

Figure 8.31A. Implants are placed in the ridge according to a 3D protocol.

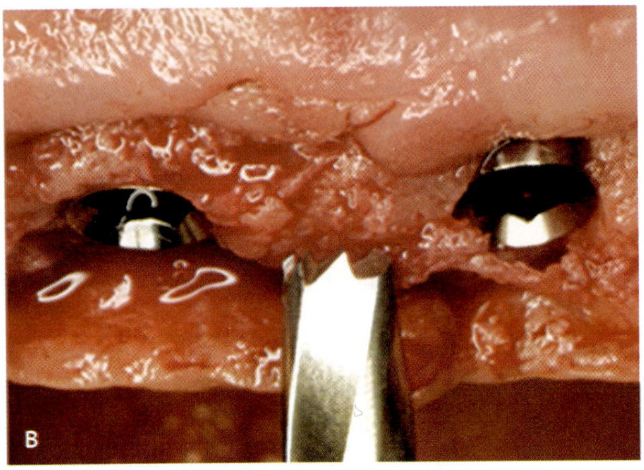

Figure 8.31B. A trephine drill is used to harvest a corticocancellous core.

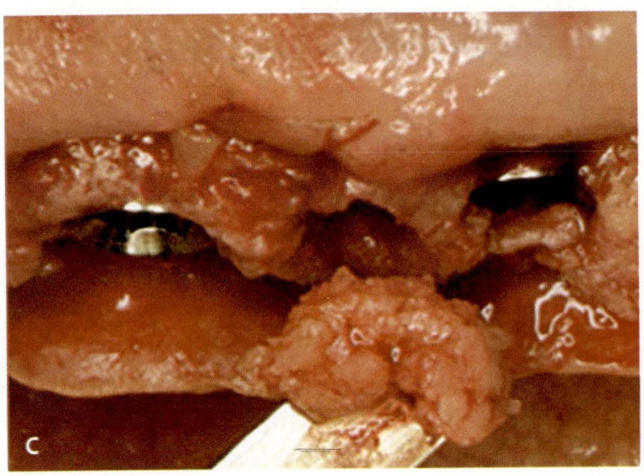

Figure 8.31C. Adding alloplast bone graft material to the osteotomy.

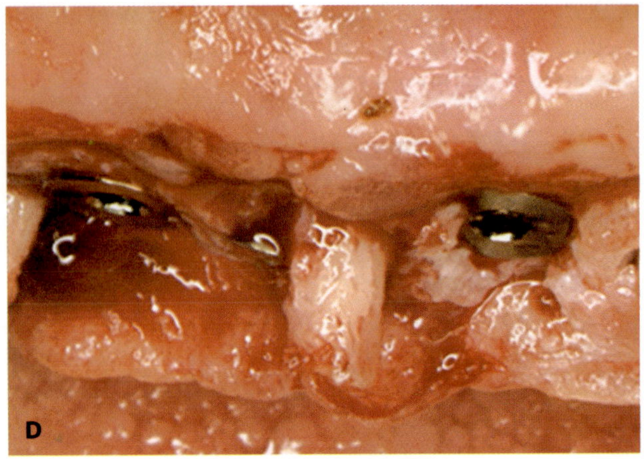

Figure 8.31D. Placing the core in place in a higher position.

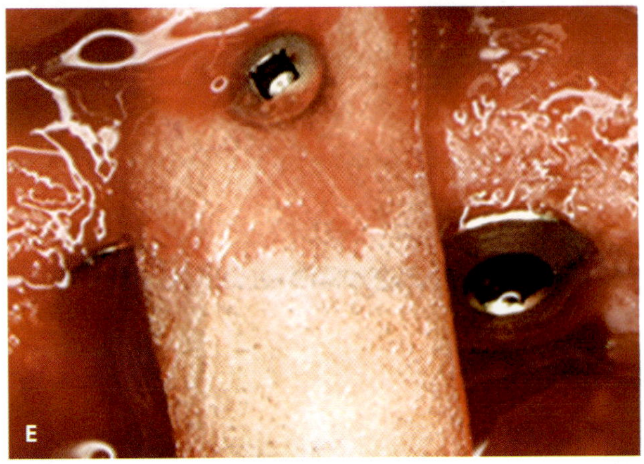

Figure 8.31E. BioMend membrane (Zimmer Dental, Carlsbad, CA, USA) placed to cover the graft.

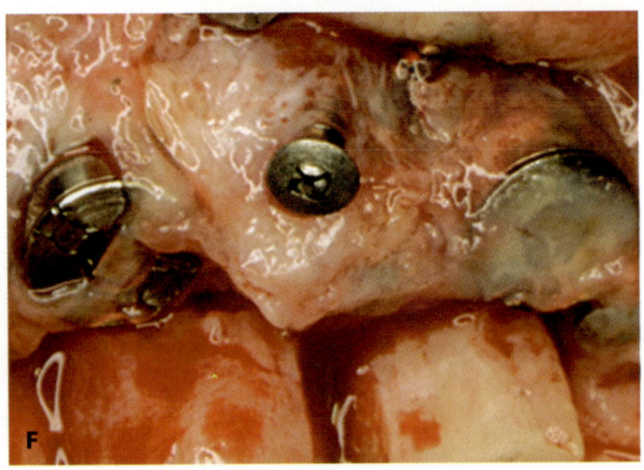

Figure 8.31F. Regenerated bone at the second-stage surgery.

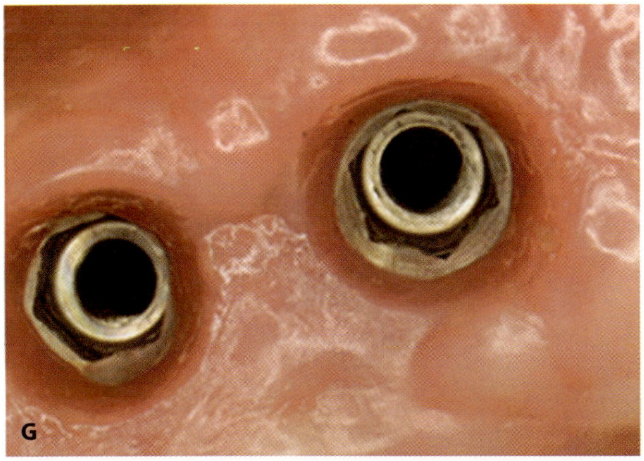

Figure 8.31G. Postsecond-stage surgery healing.

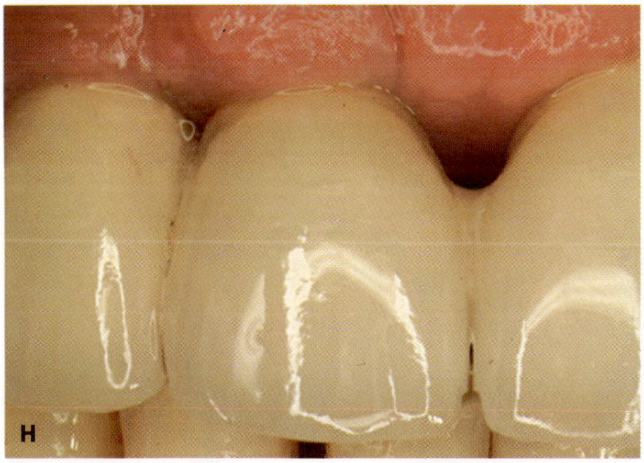

Figure 8.31H. The final restoration in place with limited papillary height is being regenerated.

newly generated bone with native bone. Implants may then be placed in the regenerated site. Distraction osteogenesis has the advantage of inducing rapid bone formation. The current thinking on reconstructing an osseous base for the inter-implant papilla is to increase the osseous height via osteodistraction beyond its normal levels, then place the implants in their optimal position, leaving the interimplant bone at a higher level to support the future interimplant papilla (Moy 2001). (See Figures 8.32A–I.) The use of distracting devices is limited to one osseous dimension as well as its complexity in clinical handling and soft tissue closure. Furthermore, it is not tolerated by many patients.

Osseous regenerative methods to restore the interimplant papilla:

1. Do not offer a highly predictable success rate
2. Require superior surgical skills

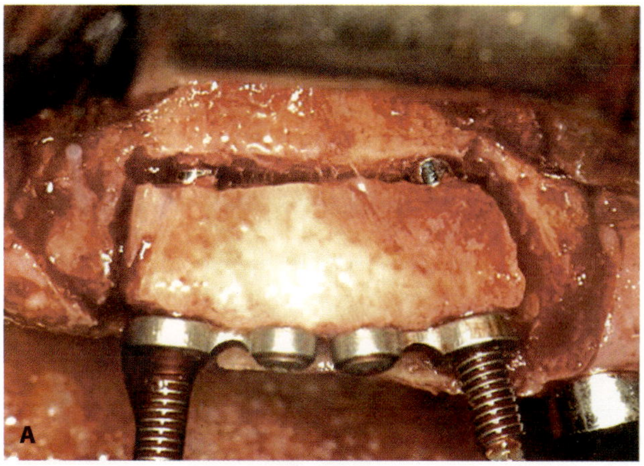

Figure 8.32A. Distractor device in place after the osteotomy is performed.

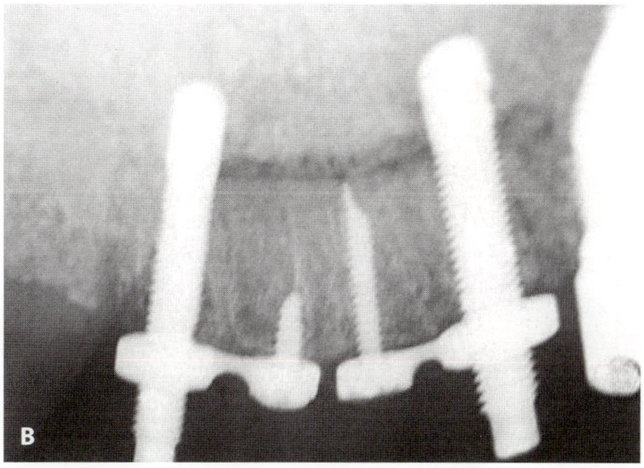

Figure 8.32B. Distractor in place radiographically.

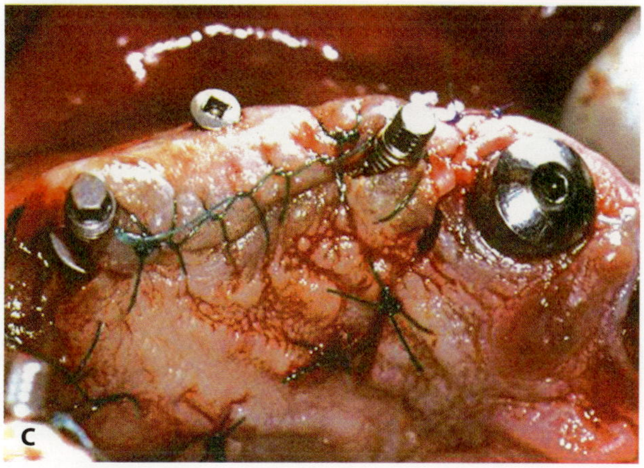

Figure 8.32C. Soft tissue closure.

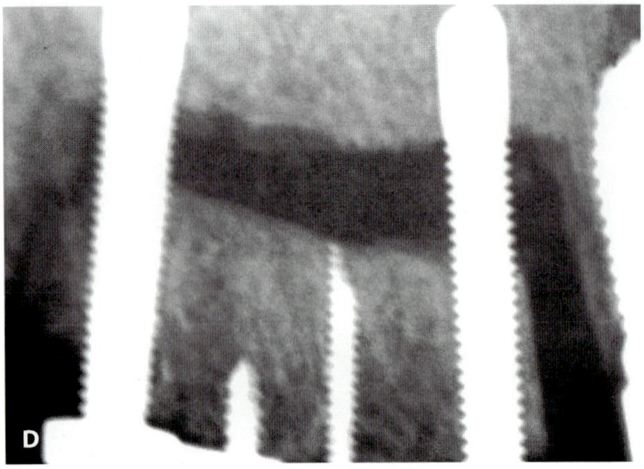

Figure 8.32D. Distracted bone radiographically.

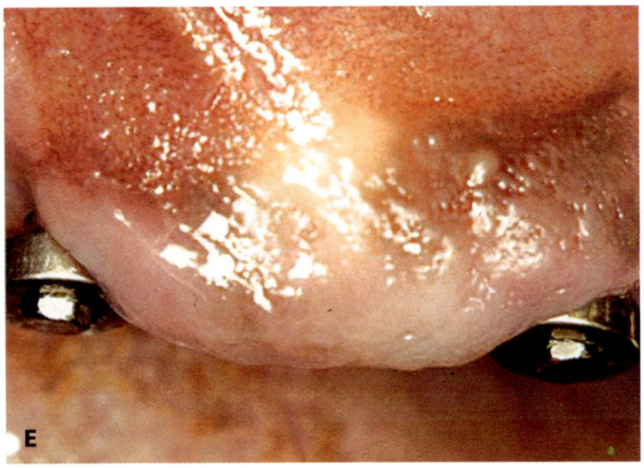

Figure 8.32E. Distracted bone after the completion of distraction procedure.

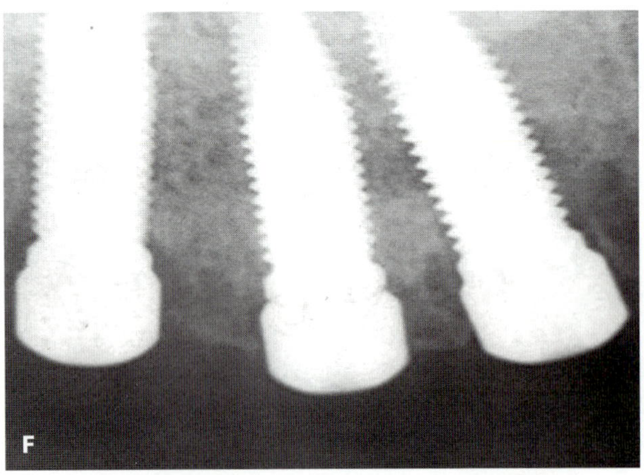

Figure 8.32F. Implant in place. Note the osseous levels around the implant collars.

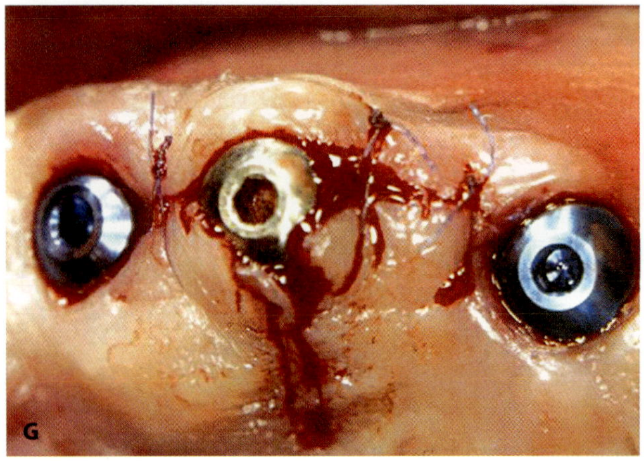

Figure 8.32G. Second-stage surgery performed.

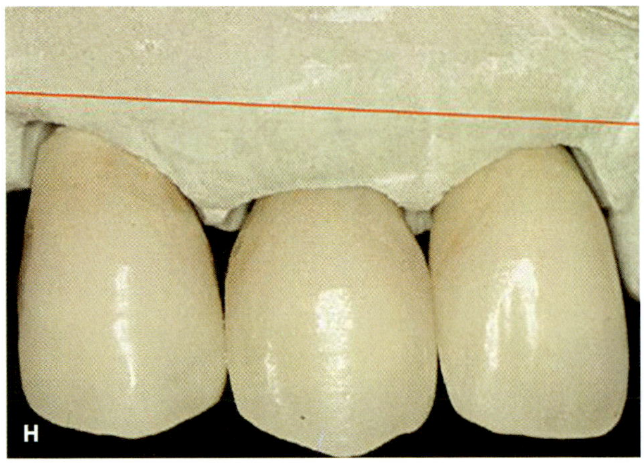

Figure 8.32H. Final prosthesis on the model. Note the amount of bone height gain.

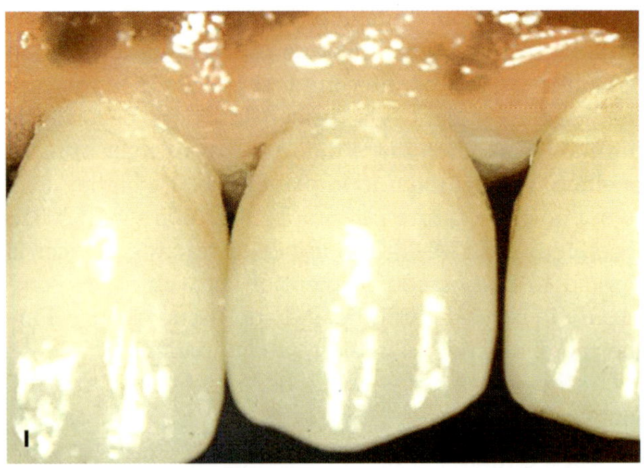

Figure 8.32I. Final prosthesis insertion. Note the improved papillary height.

3. Require a wider space between implants
4. Increase the risk of graft morbidity
5. Must modify the soft tissue margins to allow for total closure
6. Decrease. the size of the papilla via postoperative resorption and remodeling

Orthodontic Solutions

Orthodontic methods have revealed great clinical success in regenerating the interimplant papilla only when immediate implant placement is the treatment of choice. (See Figure 8.33.) Forced eruption of the unsalvageable teeth is used to move the entire attachment apparatus to an incisal direction, thus moving the papillary level in the desired direction. If the unsalvageable tooth or teeth are moved slowly in an incisal direction, new bone deposits above the root apex and an increase in the level of the attached mucosa and the proximal papillae occurs at the cervical level (Beitan 1967, Ingber 1974, Ingber 1976). Forced eruption should fulfill the following clinical requirements:

1. Extrusion should be brought about at a speed that does not exceed the rate of bone deposition (i.e., slow speed).
2. The tooth to be removed must be allowed to move only in an axial direction without tipping, which might cause penetration of the labial plate.
3. A light eruptive force of 25–30 g will result in the coronal migration of the entire attachment apparatus (Zaher 2000).

The merit of using forced eruption to regenerate the interimplant papilla is that when extruding the entire supporting structure, the attachment levels will move in further incisal levels exceeding its normal biological levels. Then, upon performing sequential tooth extractions (in the case of multiple adjacent units) and restoring them with dental implants, the biological levels acquire their natural contours, which keep the papilla in place. (See Figures 8.34A–I.) Orthodontic solutions are considered to be a highly predictable treatment modality in restoring the interimplant papilla; however, there is the potential for loss of proximal alveolar bone support. This may reduce or eliminate the fill of interproximal papillae, which is not favorable in anterior esthetic regions. Orthodontic extrusion eventually increases the treatment time and places additional costs on the patient. It is only used when immediate implant placement protocol is selected.

Prosthetic Solutions

Using the commonly known prosthetic methods to enhance the papillary shape or to hide any existing artifacts has benefited many patients and solved many clinical dilemmas. For example, soft-tissue-colored

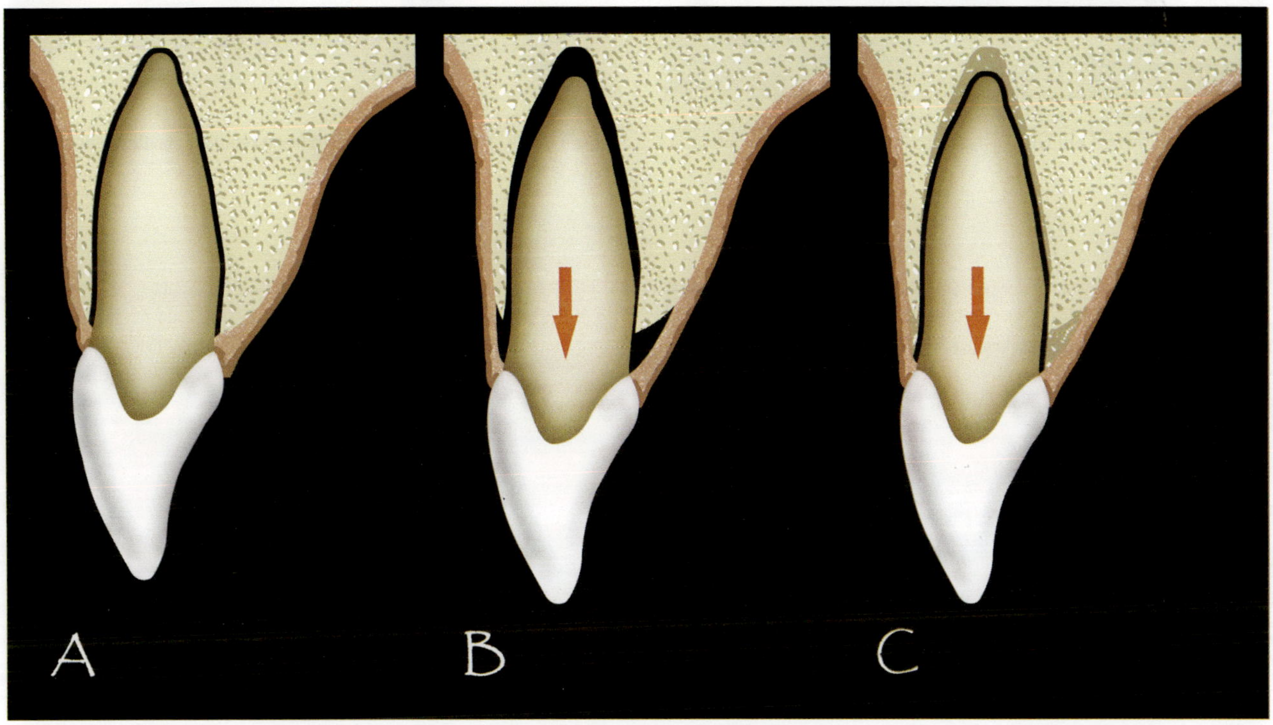

Figure 8.33. An illustration showing forced eruption.

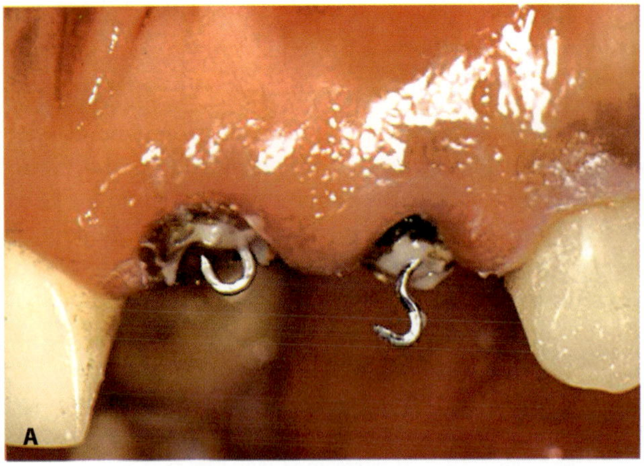

Figure 8.34A. Preoperative picture of hopeless maxillary central and lateral left incisors to be extracted.

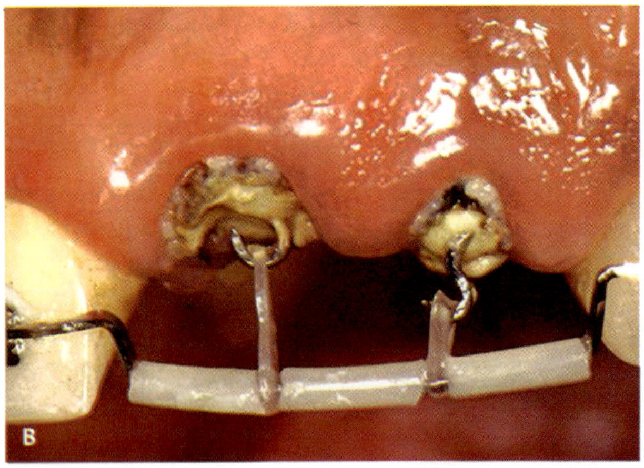

Figure 8.34B. Fixed orthodontic appliance in place for forced eruption.

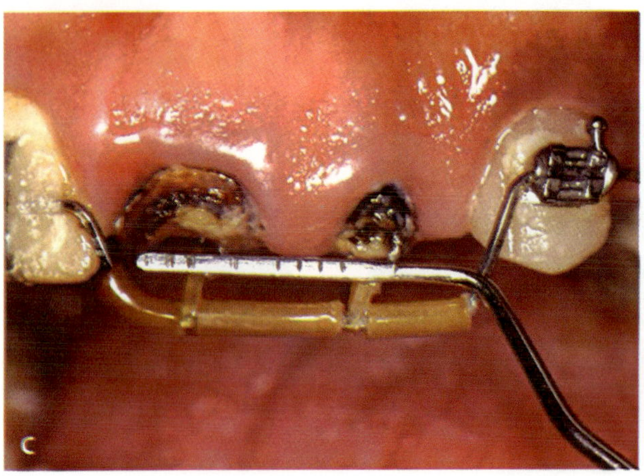

Figure 8.34C. Forced eruption occurred in incisal direction.

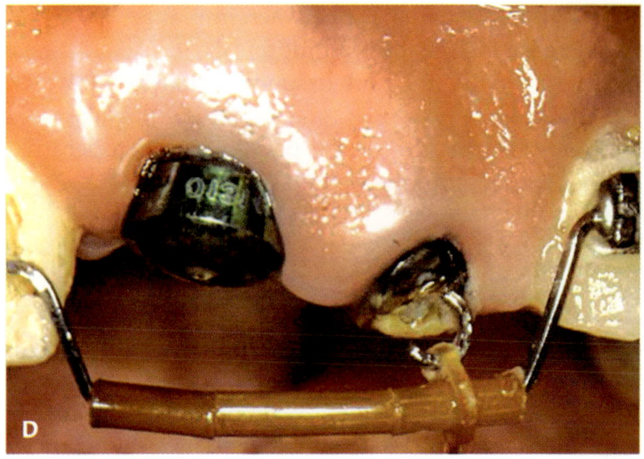

Figure 8.34D. Sequential tooth extraction and implant placement.

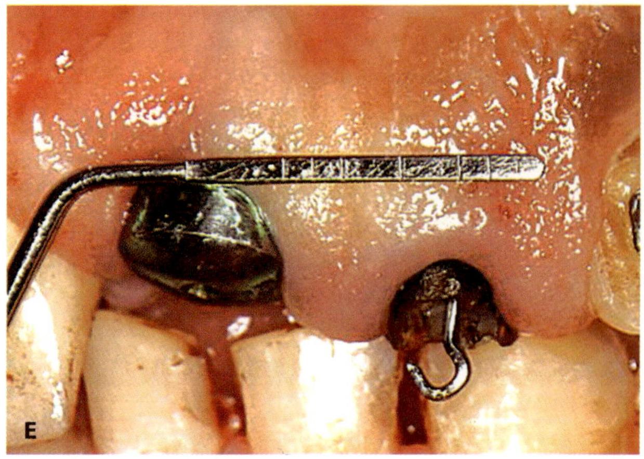

Figure 8.34E. The attachment levels being kept for 1 months' time to retain tissue levels.

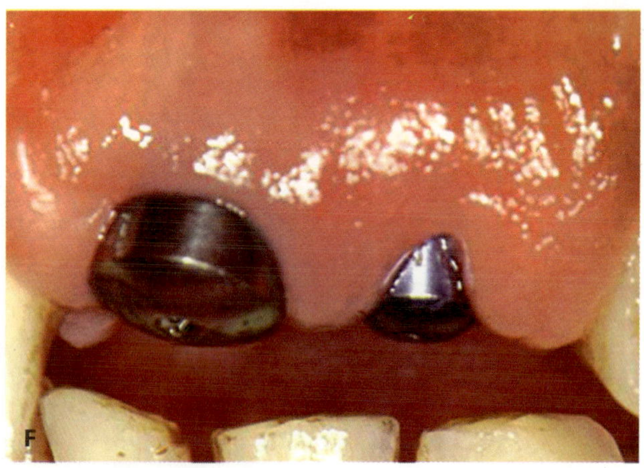

Figure 8.34F. Implant installation for the missing lateral incisor.

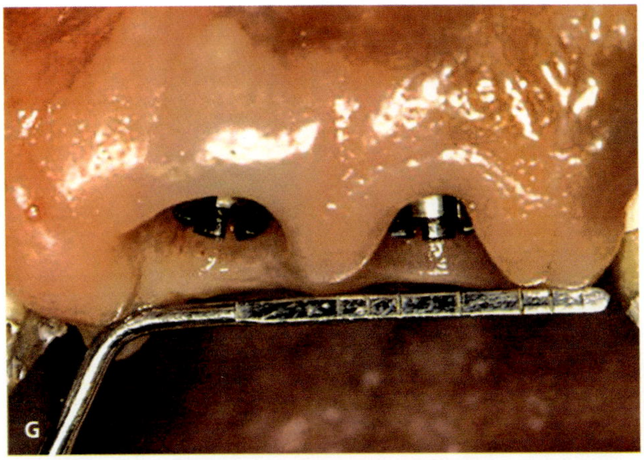

Figure 8.34G. Note the stable and improved tissue marginal levels just prior to final crowns placement.

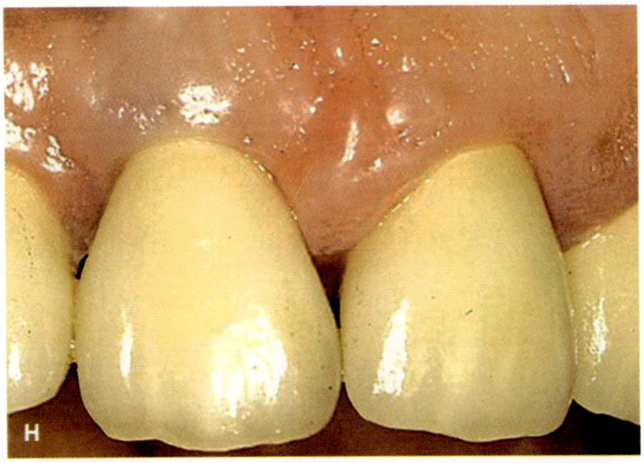

Figure 8.34H. The final case restored.

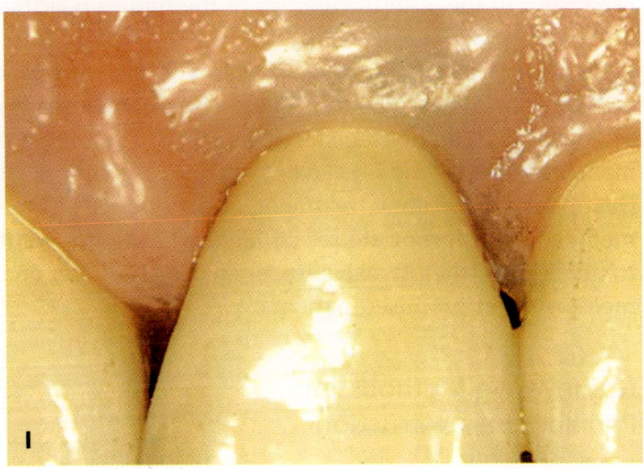

Figure 8.34I. Note the improved papillary height.

acrylic stents may be used to improve esthetic and phonetic problems associated with losing interimplant papillae that is usually accompanied by severe soft tissue loss.

Papillary illusions are yet another method used to modify the final prosthesis by moving the contact area in an apical direction, thus making the gingival embrasures smaller in size and giving the impression that the interimplant papilla fills most of the gingival embrasure space as explained earlier in this chapter. This method gives an acceptable clinical result without the need to perform any invasive surgical procedure.

An alternative method, which requires a highly experienced dental technician, is the use of pink porcelain (Cronin and Wardle 1983) to mimic the natural appearance of the papilla and the surrounding soft tissues. With this method, oral hygiene might be compromised if fabricated improperly. Furthermore, the line of demarcation between the porcelain and the soft tissues might be unpleasant, and the porcelain color usually does not match the color of the adjacent natural tissues.

A removable provisional prosthesis can influence the underlying gingival tissues at the pontic areas to create a papilla-like shape. This can be achieved by adding acrylic resin to the fitting surface of the pontic to press and conform the alveolar mucosa, forming a papilla between the two pontics, as shown in Figures 8.35A–B. Pontic development methods have been successful in restoring or duplicating the original shape of the papillary tissues. Clinical experience has shown natural-looking implant-supported prostheses when using reduced implant numbers (less than the number of the missing teeth) when compared to using the maximum implant number. The following conditions should be met when using pontic development methods: (1) long surface-treated implants must be used, (2) optimal bone quality and quantity must be used, and (3) provisional restorations for long durations to ensure soft tissue stability must be used. (See Figures 8.36A–B.)

Another prosthetic method for supporting the foundation of the interimplant papilla is the titanium papillary insert (TPI) (El Askary 2000b). TPI is composed of a pyramidal-shaped, polished titanium core 2–3 mm in height, 1 mm in width, and 3 mm in length. It was designed as foundational support for the development of interimplant papillae; it offers immediate results, and it is thought to allow for a predictable and stable esthetic outcome. The TPI is placed between adjacent implants and requires more than 3 mm of interimplant distance to ensure sufficient blood supply. A 1 mm-diameter twist drill is used to create a 5 mm-deep osteotomy, and then the insert is screwed in with cotton pliers until it is flush with the alveolar crest. Primary soft tissue closure is obtained and healing ensues. This procedure appears to have some favorable results in re-creating the

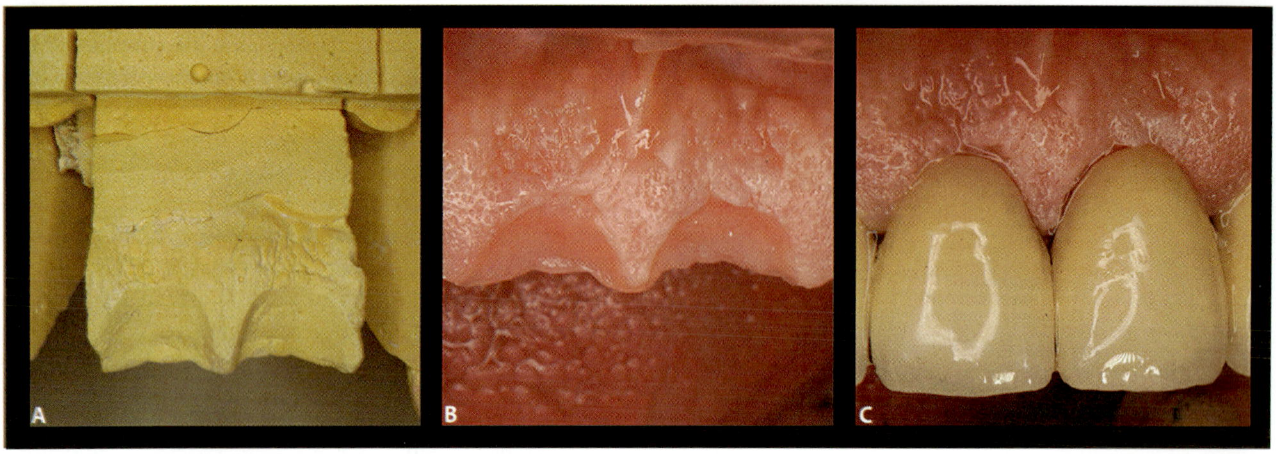

Figure 8.35. **A.** Prosthetic solution to enhance the interdental papilla by adding a resin material to the fitting surface of the removable partial denture, in order to press and reshape the pontic area. **B.** The postconfiguration effect of the alveolar ridge. **C.** The case finally restored with the interproximal papilla shaped in between the pontics.

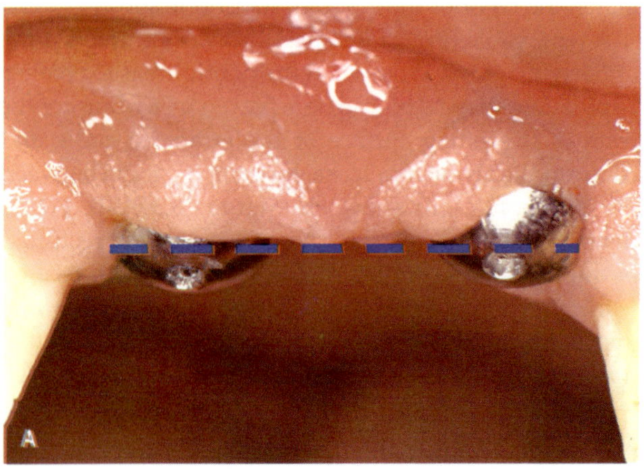

Figure 8.36A. Using maximum implants number leads to a jeopardized aesthetic result.

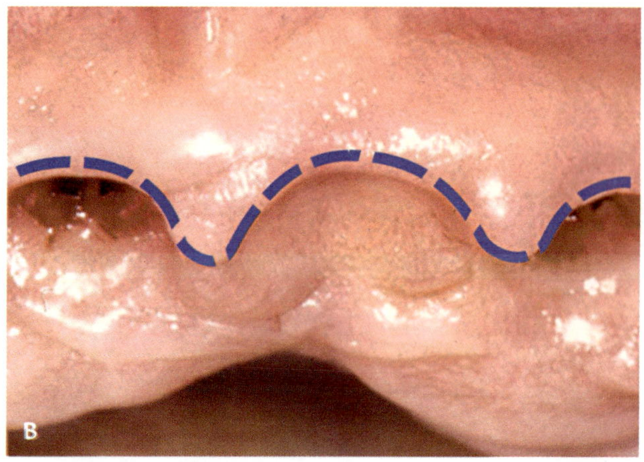

Figure 8.36B. Minimizing the number of implants leads to enhanced papillary architecture.

morphology of the interimplant papilla, despite the fact that it is not yet readily available and long-term results have not been substantiated. Currently, a modified design and a new material are being tested.

Implant-supported restorations should consider the biologic width and natural tooth scallop. The margins of restorations follow a curvilinear pattern around the circumference of the teeth, and resemble the parabolic contours of the underlying bone crest and gingival tissue contours that can be achieved using versatile implant designs. The principle behind the use of the parabolic margin, as opposed to a flat and monoplane margin, is that any bone remodeling that follows would replicate a parabolic form. Bone therefore may be maintained more coronal on the proximal surfaces than on the facial and lingual surfaces, hence preserving the bone support of the gingival papillae. The concept of a biologically derived parabolic implant design might be necessary, especially in the anterior regions of the mouth (Gadiha and Hoit 2003).

Prosthetic methods of restoring the interimplant papilla (1) are less invasive, (2) are more convenient to the patient, (3) do not regenerate a real papilla, but help mask the defects, and (4) can be used as a second line of treatment when other treatment options failed. These methods are appropriate for patients who do not want to undergo further invasive treatments, or for older and medically compromised patients.

Noninvasive Methods for Papillary Reconstruction

Interestingly, Jemt (1997) observed that the peri-implant papillae can, to some extent, regenerate without any clinical manipulation of the soft tissue one to three years after completing the implant therapy. He reasoned that plaque accumulation in the proximal areas causes gingival inflammation and hyperplasia, which subsequently leads to overgrowth of the papilla to fill the interproximal space. (See Figure 8.37A–B.) Creeping of interdental papilla onto the tooth surface (Han and Takei 1996) as well as onto porcelain crowns (Matter and Cimasoni 1976, Bell et al. 1978) has been reported in the literature. Scaling and root planning also may induce proliferation of the gingival tissues (referred to as *inflammatory hyperplasia*). This can lead to regeneration of the interdental papilla after nine months (Shapiro 1985). However, creeping of the interdental papilla around the root surface is not clinically predictable in many clinical conditions. Flapless implant placement has proven to stabilize tissue margins and lead to enhanced treatment results. Injecting collagen material in the gingival sulcus has failed due to the nature of the oral tissues as well as the bacterial medium. (See Figure 8.38.)

Recently the soft tissue ballooning concept was proven to be unsuccessful. This concept has been investigated as a technique for developing a subgingival tissue space that can be filled later with any commercially available silicon material or bone cement. The use of a micronized acellular dermal graft to provide a scaffolding of collagen and elastin has not yet proven to be a predictable treatment option. In this case, the collagen and elastin host the in-growth of fibroblast and endothelial cells, and thus revascularization occurs to the graft.

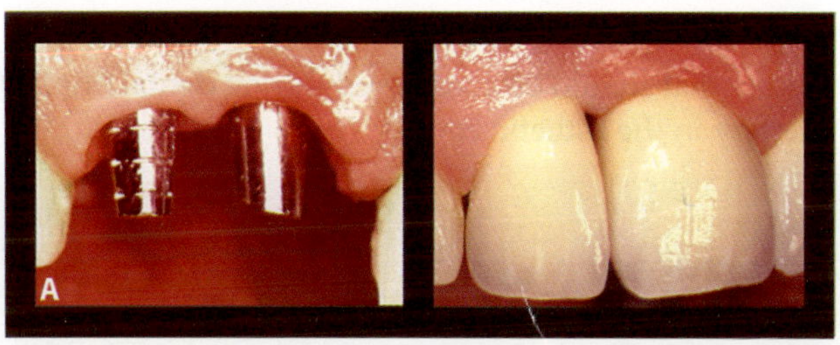

Figure 8.37A. Two adjacent implants loosing the papilla in between.

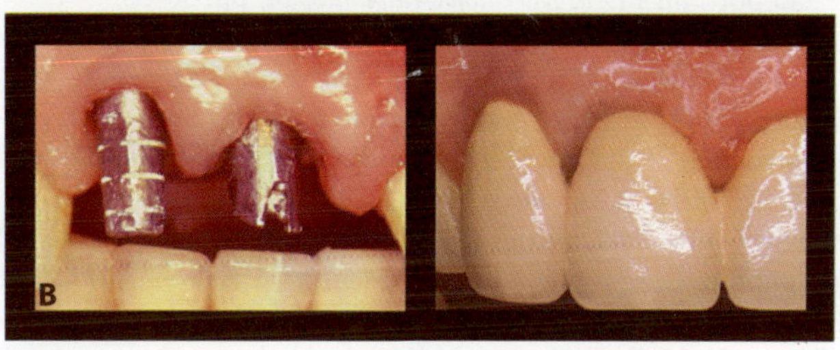

Figure 8.37B. Three years' postimplant restoration showed some improvement in the papillary levels.

Alternate immediate implant placement and provisionalization (Kan and Rungcharassaeg 2003) has been introduced to the literature to help retain the interimplant papillary levels, because simultaneous removal of adjacent teeth often results in the flattening of the interproximal osseous scallop and the subsequent collapse of the interproximal papillae due to the loss of its osseous support. One way to manage this is to approach the situation as multiple single-tooth replacements by alternating immediate implant placement and provisionalization procedures, one following the osseointegration healing period of the other. (See Figures 8.39A–C.) This way, the proximal bone on one side of the implant can always be maintained while the other side heals. At the same time, the remaining tooth form can be used as a guide for implant placement and provisionalization of the other tooth, which would not be possible if both were restored simultaneously. This technique also avoids simultaneous extraction of multiple adjacent teeth, which compromises the integrity and stability of the interproximal bone and papilla. If more than two adjacent teeth are failing, the first-stage surgery could involve two or more nonadjacent teeth to take advantage of the alternate approach without increasing the total treatment time, as shown in Figures 8.40A–B.

Conclusion

The presence of the interimplant papilla depends on the following factors: the level of the underlying bone, volume of the connective tissue, and amount of keratinized mucosa. The presence of the papilla is mainly determined by the bone attachment of the adjacent tooth, whereas the presence of a papilla between two implants depends mainly on the amount of existing bone in the interproximal area. If there is sufficient soft tissue volume, its height can be increased by applying

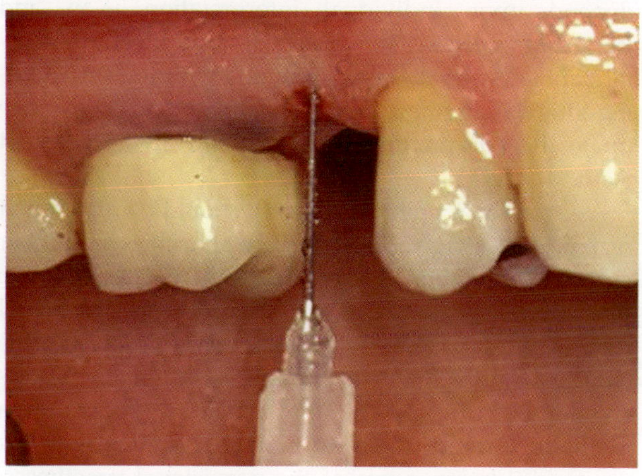

Figure 8.38. Collagen injection trial to augment the gingival tissues.

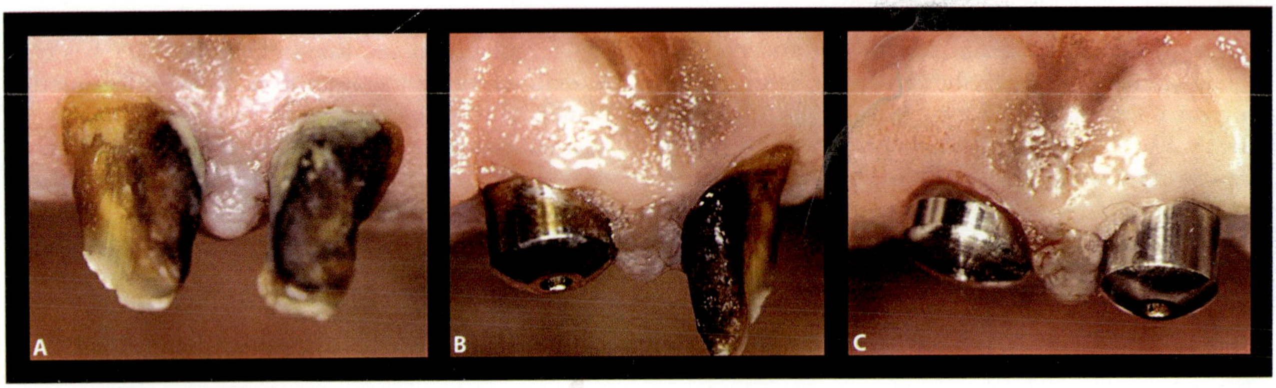

Figure 8.39A, B, C. Alternate implant placement approach in case of two adjacent implants.

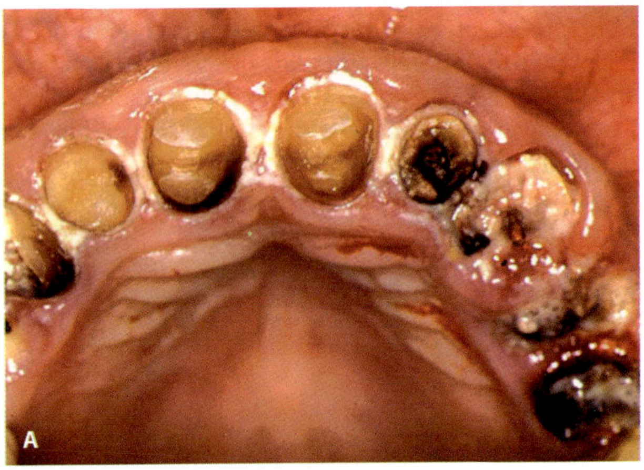

Figure 8.40A. Failed abutment teeth that planed for extraction.

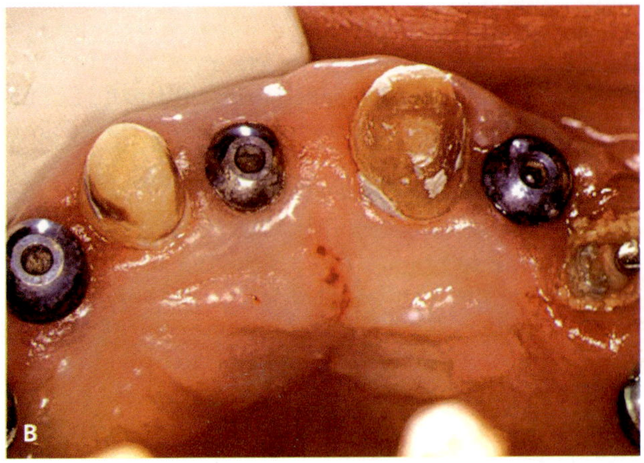

Figure 8.40B. Sequential implant placement that is thought to stabilize the papillary margins.

pressure interproximally; however, major predictable improvements are not fully expected (Grunder et al. 2005).

Interimplant papillae esthetics are subjective and depend upon individual interpretation (Kan and Rungcharassaeg 2003). Nevertheless, an ideal interdental papilla is one that is in harmony with the surrounding gingival architecture and fills the interdental space up to the interproximal contact point of the adjacent teeth.

As a personal opinion, research should be directed at regenerating gingival fibers and not to achieving higher osseous foundation. Developing and regenerating the interimplant papillae should not be based on clinical reports that lack long-term evaluations and predictable clinical results (Blatz et al. 1999). Until then, efforts should be directed to the papillary preservation methods. Careful treatment planning, optimal implant positioning, proper use of the provisional prostheses, and development of appropriate surgical skills are all factors that should be considered during dental implant therapy in the esthetic zone.

References

Adriaenssens, P., M. Hermans, A. Ingber, et al. 1999. Palatal Sliding Strip Flap: Soft Tissue Management to Restore Maxillary Anterior Esthetics at Stage 2 Surgeries: A Clinical Report. *Int J Oral Maxillofac Implants*, 14, pp. 30–36.

Arnim, A., and D. Hagerman. 1953. The connective tissue fibers of the marginal gingival. *J Am Dent Assoc*, (47), p. 271.

Azzi, R., D. Etienne, and F. Carranza. 1998. Surgical reconstruction of the interdental papilla. *Int J Periodontics Restorative Dent*, (18), pp. 467–473.

Beagle, J.R. 1992. Surgical reconstruction of the interdental papilla: Case report. *Int J Periodontics Restorative Dent*, (12), pp. 145–151.

Beitan, K. 1967. Clinical and histological observations on tooth movement during and after orthodontic treatment. *Am J Orthod*, (53), pp. 721–745.

Bell, L.A., T.A. Valluzzo, J.J. Garnick, et al. 1978. The presence of creeping attachment in human gingivae. *J Periodontol*, (49), pp. 513–517.

Berglundh, T., J. Lindhe, I. Ericsson, C.P. Marinello, B. Lijenberg, and P. Thomsen. 1991. The soft tissue barrier at implants and teeth. *Clin Oral Implant Res*, (2), pp. 81–90.

Blatz, M.B., M.B. Hurzeler, and J.R. Strub. 1999. Reconstruction of the lost interproximal papilla—Presentation of surgical and non surgical approaches. *Int J Periodontics Restorative Dent*, (19), pp. 395–406.

Block, M.S., A. Chang, and C. Crawford. 1996. Mandibular alveolar ridge augmentation in the dog using distraction osteogenesis. *J Oral Maxillofac Surg*, (54), p. 309.

Buser, D., and T. von Arx. 2000. Surgical procedures in partially edentulous patients with ITI implants. *Clin Oral Implants Res*, 11, (suppl 1), pp. 83–100.

Buser, D., W. Martin, and U. Belser. 2004. Optimizing Esthetics for Implant Restorations in the Anterior Maxilla: Anatomic and Surgical Considerations. *Int J Oral Maxillofac Implants*, 19, pp. 43–61.

Choquet, V., M. Hermans, P. Adriaenssens, et al. 2001. Clinical and radiographic evaluation of the papilla level adjacent to single-tooth dental implants. A retrospective study in the maxillary anterior region. *J Periodontol*, 2, pp. 1364–1371.

Cohen, B. 1959. Morphological factors in the pathogenesis of periodontal diseases. *Br Dent J*, (107), pp. 31–39.

Cronin, R.J., and W.L. Wardle. 1983. Loss of anterior interdental tissue: Periodontal and prosthodontic solutions. *J Prosthet Dent*, (50), pp. 505–506.

El Askary, A.S. 2000a. Inter-implant papilla reconstruction by means of a titanium guide. *Implant Dent*, (9), pp. 85–89.

El Askary, A.S. 2000b. Use of a Titanium Papillary Insert for the Construction of Interimplant Papillae. *Implant Dent*, 9, pp. 358–362.

El Askary, A.S. 2002. The use of connective tissue grafts to enhance esthetics. *J Prosthet Dent*, (87), pp. 129–132.

Engquist, B., H. Nilson, and P. Astrand. 1995. Single tooth replacement by osseointegrated Branemark implants. A retrospective study of 82 implants. *Clin Oral Implant Res*, (6), pp. 238–245.

Gadiha, M., and R. Hoit. 2003. A New Implant Design for Optimal Esthetics and Retention of Interproximal Papillae. *Implant Dent*, 12, pp. 164–169.

Gastaldo, J.F., R. Curyfi, and W.R. Sendyk. 2004. Effect of the Vertical and Horizontal Distances Between Adjacent Implants and Between a Tooth and an Implant on the Incidence of Inter-proximal Papilla. *J Periodontol*, 75, pp. 1242–1246.

Grunder, U., S. Gracis, and M. Capelli. 2005. Influence of the 3-D Bone-to-Implant Relationship on Esthetics. *Int J Periodontics Restorative Dent*, 25, pp. 113–119.

Han, T.J., and H.H. Takei. 1996. Progress in gingival papilla reconstruction. *Periodontol* 2000, (11), pp. 65–68.

Harvey, P.M. 1965. Management of advanced periodontitis. Part I. Preliminary report of method of surgical reconstruction. *N Z Dent J*, (61), pp. 180–187.

Holmes, C.H. 1965. Morphology of the interdental papillae. *J Periodontol*, (36), pp. 455–460.

Ingber, J.S. 1974. Forced eruption: Part I. A method of treating one and two wall infrabony osseous defects—Rationale and case report. *J Periodontol*, (45), pp. 199–206.

Ingber, J.S. 1976. Forced eruption: Part II. A method of treating nonrestorable teeth—Periodontal and restorative considerations. *J Periodontol*, (47), pp. 203–216.

Israelson, H., and J.M. Plemons. 1993. Dental implant, regenerative techniques and periodontal plastic surgery to restore–maxillary anterior esthetics. *Int J Oral Maxillofac Implants*, (8), pp. 555–561.

Jemt, T. 1997. Regeneration of gingival papillae after single implant treatment. *Int J Periodontics Restorative Dent*, (17), pp. 327–333.

Kan, J., and K. Rungcharassaeng. 2003. Inter-implant Papilla Preservation in the Esthetic Zone: A Report of Six Consecutive Cases. *Int J Periodontics Restorative Dent*, 23, pp. 249–259.

Kan, J.Y., K. Rungcharassaeng, K. Umezu, et al. 2003. Dimensions of peri-implant mucosa: An evaluation of maxillary anterior single implants in humans. *J Periodontol*, 4, pp. 557–562.

Lazar, F., J. Hidding, and J.E. Zöller. 2000. Preimplantologische Distrakionsosteogenese. *Impl J*, (4), pp. 18–26.

Lee, D., C. Kim, K. Park, et al. 2005a. Non-Invasive Method to Measure the Length of Soft Tissue from the Top of the Papilla the Crestal Bone. *J Periodontol*, 76, pp. 1311–1314.

Lee, D., K. Park, and S. Moon. 2005b. Dimension of keratinized mucosa and the interproximal papilla between adjacent implants. *J Periodontal*, 76, pp. 1856–1860.

Matter, J., and G. Cimasoni. 1976. Creeping attachment after free gingival grafts. *J Periodontol*, (47), pp. 574–579.

Melcher, A. 1962. The Interpapillary ligament. *Dent Practitioner Dent Rec*, (12), p. 461.

Miller, Jr., P.D. 1982. Root coverage using a free soft tissue auto graft following citric acid application. Part I. Technique. *Int J Periodontics Restorative Dent*, (2), pp. 56–70.

Misch, E.C. 1999. Single tooth implant. In: Misch, C.E, Ed. *Contemporary Implant Dentistry*. St. Louis: Mosby, pp. 397–428.

Misch, C.E., K. Al Shammari, and H.L. Wang. 2004. Creation of Interimplant Papillae through a Split-Finger Technique. *Implant Dent*, 13, pp. 20–27.

Moy, P.K. 2001. Personal communications. Barcelona, Spain.

Nelson, S. 1987. The subpedicle connective tissue graft. A bilaminar reconstructive procedure for the coverage of denuded root surfaces. *J Periodontol*, (58), pp. 95–102.

Nordland, W.P., and D.P. Tarnow. 1998. A classification system for loss of papillary height. *J Periodontol*, (69), pp. 1124–1126.

Salama, H., M. Salama, D. Garder, and P. Adar. 1995. Developing optimal peri-implant papillae within the esthetic zone: Guided soft tissue augmentation. *J Esthet Dent*, (7), pp. 125–129.

Salama, H., M.A. Salama, D. Garder, and P. Adar. 1998. The interproximal height of bone: A guidepost to predictable aesthetic strategies and soft tissue contours in anterior tooth replacement. *Pract Periodont Aesthet Dent*, (10), pp. 1131–1141.

Shapiro, A. 1985. Regeneration of interdental papilla using periodic curettage. *Int J Periodontics Restorative Dent*, (5), pp. 27–33.

Stahl, S. 1963. Morphology and healing pattern of human interdental gingivae. *J Am Dent Assoc*, (67), p. 48.

Tarnow, D.P., A.W. Magner, and P. Fletcher. 1992. The effect of the distance from the contact point to the crest of the bone on the presence or absence of the interproximal dental papilla. *J Periodontol*, (63), pp. 995–996.

Tarnow, D.P., R.N. Eskow, and J. Zamok. 1996. Aesthetics and implant dentistry. *Periodontol 2000*, (11), pp. 85–94.

Tarnow, D., N. Elian, P. Fletcher, et al. 2003. Vertical distance from the crest of bone to the height of the interproximal papilla between adjacent implants. *J Periodontol*, 74, pp. 1785–1788.

Tinti, C., G. Vincenzi, P. Cortellini, G.P. Pinti Prato, and C. Clauser. 1987. Guided tissue regeneration in the treatment of human facial recession. A 12-case report. *J Periodontol*, (58), pp. 95–102.

Tinti, C., and S. Parma-Benfenati. 1995. Coronally positioned palatal sliding flap. *Int J Periodontics Restorative Dent*, (15), pp. 298–310.

Zaher, A. 2000. Personal communications. Alexandria, Egypt.

Chapter 9

Tissue Engineering in Maxillofacial Surgery

Dritan Turhani, Elisabeth Stein, Martina Weinβenböck, and Rolf Ewers

Principles of Tissue Engineering

The term *tissue engineering* was defined in 1995 in the first issue of the magazine *Tissue Engineering* as "the use of biological and/or synthetic materials in conjunction with cells to create biologic substitutes to serve as functional tissue replacements" (*Tissue Engineering* 1995).

Tissue engineering is an interdisciplinary field that applies the principles of engineering and the life sciences toward the development of biological substitutes that restore, maintain, or improve tissue function (Langer and Vacanti 1993).

Examples of tissue engineering can be found as early as 1933 when Bisceglie (1933) encased mouse tumor cells in a polymer membrane and inserted them into the abdominal cavity of a pig. The cells lived long enough to show that they were not killed by the immune system.

Significant research activities first appeared in the 1970s. In 1975, Chick and colleagues (1975) reported their results of encapsulating pancreatic-islet cells in semipermeable membranes to aid glucose control in patients with diabetes mellitus. Replacement of the skin with cells in collagen gels, or collagen-glycosaminoglycan composites to guide regeneration, was attempted by the early 1980s and these techniques are now in clinical use (Bell et al. 1981, Burke et al. 1981). Those efforts have now expanded to include applications as diverse as skin, bone, blood vessel, kidney, and neural repair. Consistent research efforts in this field led the National Library of Medicine to introduce "Tissue Engineering" as a medical subject heading (MeSH) in 2002 (MEDLINE 1960).

Tissue engineering is at the interface of the medical implant industry and the biological revolution. This industry is in the process of being revolutionized by the continuing advances in molecular and cell biology. Recent technical advances in molecular and cell biology that result in large volumes of data, combined with bioinformatics (a new field focusing on the collection and manipulation of biological data), is producing great advances in biological knowledge and understanding. These advances will give rise to the next generation of medical implants and related therapies. Although most previous implants were mostly structural and inert, future products will be much more biologic in nature, taking advantage of and mobilizing the inherent biological power of our bodies (Ahsan and Nerem 2005).

The primary goal of all approaches in tissue engineering is the restoration of function through the delivery of living elements that become integrated into the patient. Although some techniques of guided tissue regeneration (GTR) rely on matrices alone, and other approaches rely on cells alone, most investigators in tissue engineering use cells combined with matrices to achieve new tissue formation (Vacanti and Langer 1999).

Sources of cells for implantation include autologous cells from the patient, allogeneic cells from a human donor who is not immunologically identical to the patient, and xenogeneic cells from a different species. Each category may be further delineated in terms of whether the cells are adult or embryonic stem cells (capable of both self renewal and differentiation into a variety of cell lineages) or a mixture of differentiated cells at different stages of maturation (including rare stem and progenitor cells). An autologous source of cells is most desirable because it eliminates complications associated with immune rejection of allogenic and xenogenic tissues (Griffith and Naughton 2002).

The choice of carrier material is the second important step in the development of tissue engineering strategies. The requirements for a suitable scaffold in bone tissue engineering and dental approaches will be discussed in the following paragraphs.

Tissue Engineering of Bone

Bone is a dynamic, highly vascularized tissue with a unique capacity to heal and remodel without leaving a scar (Sommerfeldt and Rubin 2001). These properties, together with its capacity to rapidly mobilize mineral stores on metabolic demand, make bone the ultimate smart material. Its main role is to provide structural support for the body. Furthermore, the skeleton also serves as a mineral reservoir, supports muscular contraction resulting in motion, withstands load bearing, and protects internal organs (Rodan 1992).

Hence, it is logical to say that major alterations in its structure due to injury or disease can dramatically alter one's body equilibrium and quality of life. Although major progress has been made in the field of bone regenerative medicine in recent years, current therapies such as autologous bone grafts still have many limitations. Moreover, and in spite of the fact that material science technology has resulted in clear improvements in the field of bone substitution medicine, no adequate bone substitute has been developed and hence large bone defects/injuries still represent a major challenge for reconstructive surgeons (Salgado et al. 2004).

Autologous bone graft, that is, bone taken from another part of the patient's own body, has been the gold standard of bone replacement for many years (Rose and Oreffo 2002, Asahina et al. 1999). Grafts of this kind are osteoconductive (they provide a scaffold on which bone cells can proliferate), osteoinductive (they induce proliferation of undifferentiated cells and their differentiation into osteoblasts), and osteogenic (they provide a reservoir of skeletal stem and progenitor cells that can form new bone), and therefore offer a variety of favorable properties. However, and although it presents relatively good percentages of success, the spectrum of cases in which it can be used is restricted because the available autologous bone supplies are limited and harvesting autologous bone is painful and entails procedures with risk of infection and donor site morbidity. Therefore, it has become necessary to develop alternative techniques to overcome these drawbacks (Yaszemski et al. 1994, Spitzer et al. 2002, Simon et al. 2002, Petite et al. 2000).

Bone tissue engineering offers a new technology that aims to overcome these limitations. The transplantation of osteogenic cells in suitable carrier systems is an encouraging new approach to further enhance the process of bone reconstitution and remodelling. Thus, such attempts must focus on synergistic interaction of these two key players. Cell sourcing is the first issue to address in the development of bioengineered bone. The characteristics of an optimal cell source include no immunorejection, no graft-versus-host disease, no tumorigenicity, immediate availability, availability in pertinent quantities, controlled cell proliferation rate, predictable and consistent osteogenic potential, as well as controlled integration into the surrounding tissues (Logeart-Avramoglou et al. 2005).

Cell-induced osteogenesis and chondrogenesis is highly dependent upon the substrate carrier that provides a permissive environment into which bone cells would migrate, proliferate, differentiate, and deposit bone matrix (i.e., osteoconduction) (Kuboki et al. 1998). Therefore, the second critical issue in the development of a transplantable bioengineering bone substitute is the quest for a suitable carrier material. Such substratum should have specific biochemical (i.e., molecules of the extracellular matrix), hysicochemical (such as surface-free energy, charge, hydrophobicity), and geometric aspects (for example, 3-D, interconnected porosity) (Jin et al. 2000, Ripamonti et al. 1992, Sampath and Reddi 1984). (See Figure 9.1.)

Tissue Engineering in Maxillofacial Surgery

Roughly 20,000 organ transplants, 500,000 joint replacements, and literally millions of dental-oral-craniofacial procedures ranging from tooth restorations to major reconstruction of facial hard and soft tissues are performed annually. According to the National Institute of Dental and Craniofacial Research, 86% of adults over 70 years have at least moderate periodontitis and more than one-quarter have lost their teeth, which has serious repercussions on health and quality of life (Albandar and Kingman 1999).

To date, artificial replacements possess significant limitations when compared with the natural original tissues in terms of function and esthetics. Bridges and dentures have been used for centuries in dentistry but require periodic maintenance or even replacement after a period of time because of usage or loss of adaptation (Taba et al. 2005).

Also in the area of maxillofacial reconstruction, the transplantation of autologous bone grafts is still the most popular way to treat extensive bone defects.

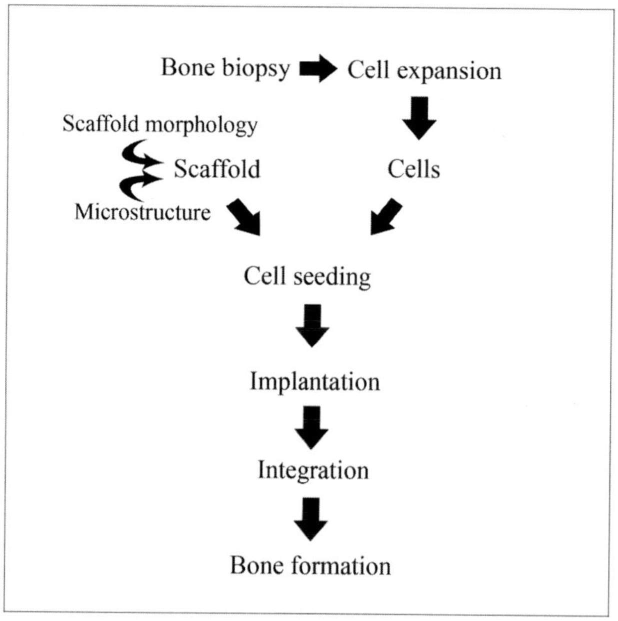

Figure 9.1. Schematic presentation of a tissue engineering approach for dental applications.

During the last two decades, treatment concepts have been developed to provide an alternative to autogenous bone grafts for maxillofacial reconstruction, and especially new ways of augmenting the maxillary sinus for placement of dental implants have been explored (Hollinger et al. 1996, Merkx et al. 2003, Vacanti and Bonassar 1999). First clinical trials have postulated that bone augmentation procedures of the maxilla before dental implant placement based on tissue-engineering concepts offer significant advantages compared with conventional allografts and autografts (Schmelzeisen et al. 2003).

The regeneration of the periodontal tissues depends on four basic components: the appropriate signals, cells, blood supply, and scaffold need to target the tissue defect. Each of these elements plays a fundamental role in the healing process in a simultaneous and temporal time frame and is interconnected into the generation of new tissues. Cells provide the machinery for new tissue growth and differentiation. Growth factors or morphogens modulate the cellular activity and provide stimuli to cells to differentiate and produce the matrix to develop tissue. New vascular networks promoted by angiogenic signals provide the nutritional base for tissue growth and homeostasis. Finally, scaffolds guide and create a template structure three-dimensionally to facilitate the above processes that are critical for tissue regeneration (Sampath and Reddi 1984).

Choosing the carrier material is a crucial step toward the development of a tissue-engineered transplantable bone construct. Over the past 30 years, an enormous array of biomaterials proposed as ideal scaffolds for cell growth have emerged, yet few have demonstrated clinical efficacy (El-Ghannam 2005). Scaffolds for engineering bone, regardless of whether they are permanent or biodegradable, naturally occurring or synthetic, should satisfy a number of criteria. Such matrices should be: (1) biocompatible, i.e., nonimmunogenic and nontoxic; (2) absorbable (with rates of resorption commensurate to those of bone formation); (3) preferably radiolucent (to allow the new bone to be distinguished radiographically from the implant); (4) osteoconductive; (5) easy to manufacture and sterilize; and (6) easy to handle in the surgery room, preferably without preparatory procedures (to limit the risk of infection) (Simon et al. 2002). These materials provide cell anchorage sites, mechanical stability, and structural guidance, and in vivo provide the interface to respond to physiologic and biologic changes as well as to remodel the extracellular matrix to integrate with the surrounding native tissue (Sampath and Reddi 1984).

A prevalent misconception in the literature is that craniofacial bones do not receive heavy loading and hence do not rely on functional strain for their maintenance. This idea arose from the fact that the skull does not support body weight (but it does support brain weight and monumental muscle forces), from incorrect assumptions about the strength of craniofacial elements (Hylander 1975), and from reports of low in vivo strains in skull bones (Rawlinson et al. 1995, Hillam 1996). As it turns out, in vivo studies show that most craniofacial bones are strained at levels comparable with those of limb bones (Herring and Ochareon 2005). Therefore, one unique feature that a suitable scaffold for the application in the maxillofacial region has to fulfil is the need for increased mechanical stability.

Hydroxyapatite (HA), $Ca_{10}(PO_4)_6(OH)_2$, is one of the most promising candidates as a suitable scaffold for bone tissue regeneration in the maxillofacial area due to its excellent biocompatibility and bioactivity. The crystallographic and chemical properties of HA closely resemble those of bones and the fact that HA is able to bond directly to tissues and promote tissue growth make it widely used in both orthopaedic and maxillofacial applications (Hench 1998, Bucholz 2002).

Maxilla Sinus Grafting with Marine Algae-derived Bone-forming Material

For the past 15 years, the authors used HA as an alternative graft material and followed up the input/output statistic of implants to evaluate whether this material provides results similar to the autogenous bone graft (Ewers 2005).

The natural macroporous HA ceramic is distributed worldwide as the Communauté Européenne-approved material AlgiPore® (Dentsply Friadent, Mannheim, Germany), as the US Food and Drug Administration-approved material C GRAFT™ (The Clinician Preference, LLC, Golden, CO, USA), and the Russian-approved material AlgOss® (Unexim Co., Moscow, Russia). AlgiPore®/C GRAFT™/AlgOss® (ACA) is a natural product synthesized out of two renewable marine red algae, *Corallina officinalis* and *Amphiroa ephredra*. The algae material is deproteinized by pyrolysis, during which the algae bushel (stems) fall into granules and the organic material is changed from calcium carbonate into HA (Simons et al. 1987, Spassova-Tzekova et al. 2004).

This material combines the desired properties for a bone graft substitute in a favorable way. ACA has a honeycomb-like interconnecting porosity that provides efficient osteoconduction and fast, new bone formation. The high absorptive pore structure of ACA guarantees moldability, ease of handling, and stability within the site. (See Figures 9.2A–C.)

Histological studies of ACA report almost total resorption of the material with simultaneously substitution by new bone in two to three years (Ewers et al. 1987,

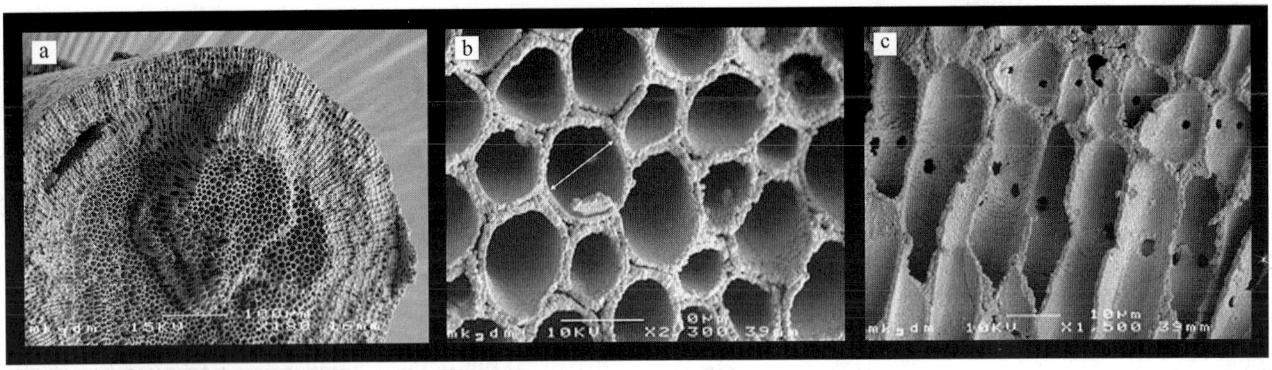

Figure 9.2. **A.** The unique three-dimensional (3D) morphologic structure of the calcite skeleton of the raw algae is maintained from the beginning through the production of the final material (magnification × 190; white bar = 100 μm). **B.** Cross section (magnification × 2,300; white bar = 10 μm). **C.** Longitudinal section. The particles of the biomaterial contain a regular arranged pore system (mean diameter of pores, 10 μm) that is periodically septated (mean length interval, 50 to 100 μm) and interconnected microperforated. Mean diameter of perforations, 1 to 3 μm (magnification × 1,500; white bar = 10 μm).

Ewers and Schumann 1994, Schopper et al. 2003). This process is commonly known as *creeping substitution*.

Previous studies have shown that this material has biocompatible properties as a bone graft substitute in vivo (Hench 1998, Bucholz 2002, Ewers et al., 2004). In vitro studies showed that this material supports the proliferation and differentiation of human osteoblast-like cells on its surface when grown in monolayer (Turhani et al. 2003, Turhani et al. 2005a, Turhani et al. 2005b) and in cell-seeded 3-D bone composites (Turhani et al. 2005c, Petite et al. 2000).

From September 5, 1990, to September 1, 2004, a total of 209 sinus grafts with ACA were performed on 118 patients who presented with a severely resorbed maxillary alveolar process with 1 mm to 5 mm (mean, 3.6 mm) of remaining bone. The available bone was a little less than Class C, according to the site classification proposed by Jensen (1994), comparable with Class D presented by Simion and others (2004). Implants were placed after six months, and six months later the implants were loaded. The longest observation period of loaded implants was 156 months (13 years). Implant loss was 27 out of 614 loaded implants (4.4%), showing a survival rate of 95.6%. Smokers and women over 50 are included. Although ACA undergoes a resorption process, we found only 14% volume loss after 6.4 months, compared with 49.5% after six months when autogenous bone was used. Our experience shows once again that the sinus lift procedure with grafting of the sinus floor and subsequent implant placement is a proven method.

Sinus Lift Operating Method

All 209 sinus grafts were augmented with a mixture of about 90% ACA and 10% autogenous collector bone gained from the bone trap and mixed either with venous blood or platelet-rich plasma (PRP). In a second-stage operation, after six months of primary healing, 614 implants were placed in 209 sinus-grafted sites on these 118 patients. Six months later the implants were again loaded by means of different prosthetic appliances. The patients underwent a very precise follow-up with a six-month recall interval. The postoperative and later complications were recorded and an input/output implant loss statistic was produced.

All patients received both clinical and radiographic examinations. Panoramic X-rays, lateral cephalograms, and dental computed tomographies were taken. All patients were treated under general anaesthesia. In this group all patients presented with a severely resorbed maxillary alveolar process with 1 mm to 5 mm (mean, 3.6 mm) of remaining bone. The operative approach is via an entrance to the piriform recess as described by Boyne and James (1980), Tatum (1986), and Loukota and others (1992).

According to the anatomic investigation of Solar and others (1999), we attempted to preserve the superior posterior alveolar artery by preparing a trough, starting posterior to the canine apex and continuing back to the area of the tuberosity. To achieve this we prepared a trough with the drill or the Piezo surgery instrument according to Vercellotti (2001).

Elevating the sinus mucosa was performed using either the sinus lift instruments designed by Dr. Kirsch from the Dentsply Friadent Company or the Piezo surgery unit from the Mectron Medical Technology Company (Carasco, Italy).

The authors believe that the elevated bone beneath the sinus mucosa is not needed as a protecting shield. Rather, the drilled bone was collected in the bone trap and this autogenous material was used as part of the graft material.

The authors always suture the perforated mucosa membrane with a 7-0 resorbable suture material and apply a small piece of collagen membrane (Reguarde, The Clinician's Preference, LLC) to cover the site. When the perforation is larger and more than three sutures are used, the sutures and the collagen membrane are sealed with fibrin glue (Baxter, Deerfield, IL, USA) according to the suggestion by Sullivan and others (1997).

The longest observation period of loaded implants on 614 implants placed in 209 sinus-grafted sites on 118 patients was 156 months (13 years). The authors used IMZ, Frialit II, and Xive implants (Dentsply Friadent). Implant loss was 27 out of 614 loaded implants (4.4%), showing a survival rate of 95.6%. This retrospective study over 14 years shows once again that the sinus lift procedure with grafting of the sinus floor and subsequent implant placement is a proven method. The good implant survival rate of 95.6% with a follow-up time of up to 13 years in this study proves that sinus floor grafting after sinus lift is an adequate method to solve the problems of the atrophied posterior part of the maxilla allowing dental implants with a fixed prosthetic.

Additionally, this 14-year longitudinal study shows that the marine-derived HA material ACA, in a mixture with approximately 10% of autogenous collector bone and blood, is able to enhance enough new bone in six months to allow implant osseointegration after six more months.

Maxilla Sinus Grafting with Autologous Cells Successful implantation of autologous cells augmented the maxillary sinus prior to the placement of dental implants in three patients.

The group of three patients consisted of one male (aged 55) and two females (aged 58 and 60) with the diagnosis of severe atrophy of the maxilla. Four weeks before the augmentation of the maxillary sinus, small periost biopsies were taken from the molar region. These biopsies were used to establish autologous cell cultures that were expanded under good laboratory practice (GLP) guidelines. (See Figure 9.3A.) For isolation of periosteal cells, an enzymatic digestion method was used as previously described (Spitzer et al. 2002). Briefly, after purification the biopsies were digested over three hours with collagenase CLS II (315 U/milliliter [mL]; Biochrom AG, Germany) in DMEM/Ham's F12 medium 1:1 (Glutamax II, Gibco) supplemented with 10% autologous serum, 100 IU/mL benzylpenicillin (G), 100 µmL streptomycin sulphate, and 1 µmL amphotericin (B).

Confluence was reached after approximately 10 days of cultivation under standard cell culture conditions. After approximately three weeks of culture, approximately 40 million of the cells could be harvested and were collected in three aliquots containing cells and 1 mL of culture medium, as shown in Figure 9.3B.

The graft material composed of AlgiPore®/C GRAFT™/AlgOss®, the harvested autologous cells, and fibrin glue (Baxter Deerfield, IL, USA) was applied to the graft site of the maxillary sinus. Figure 9.4 shows the

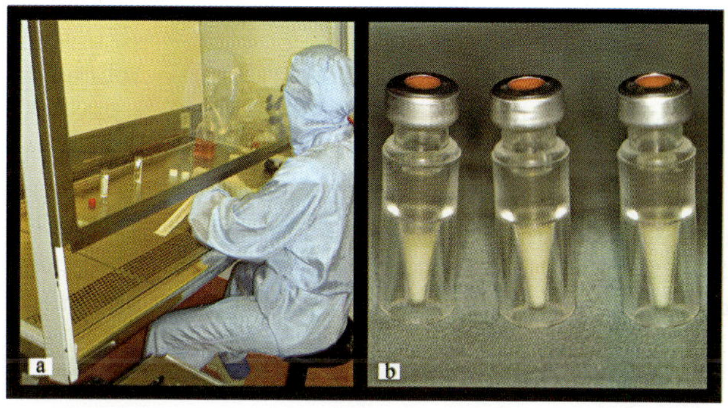

Figure 9.3. **A.** Establishment of autologous cell cultures under good laboratory practice (GLP) conditions. **B.** Harvested cells after expansion under GLP conditions.

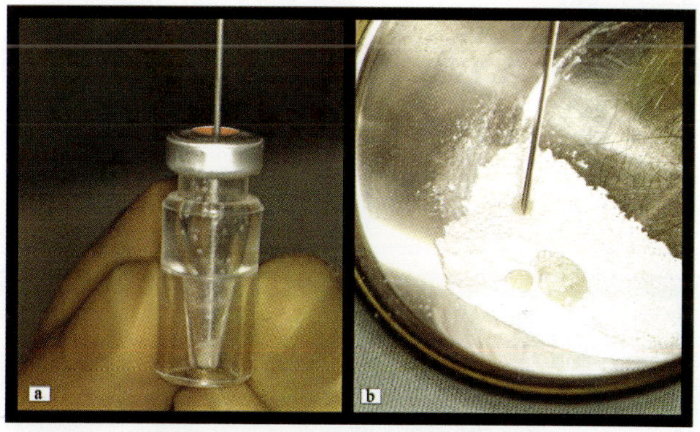

Figure 9.4. **A.** Harvested cells are collected from the vials. **B.** The collected cell suspension is carefully mixed with the AlgiPore®/C GRAFT™/AlgOss® particles.

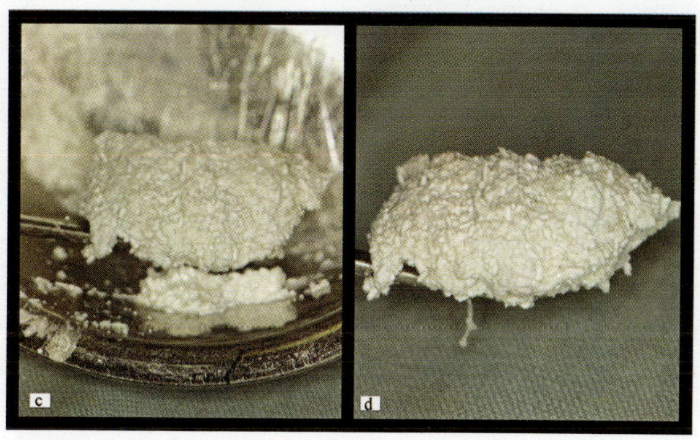

Figure 9.4. **C.** Fibrin glue is added to this mixture. **D.** The resulting polymerized mixture ready for implantation in the sinus recess.

preparation of this mixture directly before implantation. The maxillary sinus makes a good graft recipient for augmentation material because the quality of the surrounding bone is good and no mechanical stress is placed on the graft site. After filling the sinus recess with the mixture, as shown in Figures 9.5A–B, a titanium membrane was placed and fixed with titanium tacks to prevent the augmentation material from dislocating, as shown in Figure 9.5C.

The patients underwent a very precise follow-up with a six-month recall interval. All patients received both clinical and radiographic examinations. Panoramic X-rays, lateral cephalograms, and dental computed tomographies were taken. Figures 9.6A–B shows pictures of panoramic X-rays and computed tomographies before sinus grafting and six months after primary healing, prior to the placement of dental implants.

Six months after the sinus-grafting procedure, the amount of newly formed bone was sufficient to place dental implants. Six months after the implants were placed, they were loaded by means of different prosthetic appliances according to the individual needs of the patient. The patients had no complications caused by local infections or severe pain during the period of primary healing.

In conclusion, our results suggest that periosteum-derived osteoblasts on a suitable matrix can form lamellar bone within three to five months after transplantation and provide a reliable basis for simultaneous or secondary insertion of dental implants. Although long-term results are not yet available, the method of augmenting

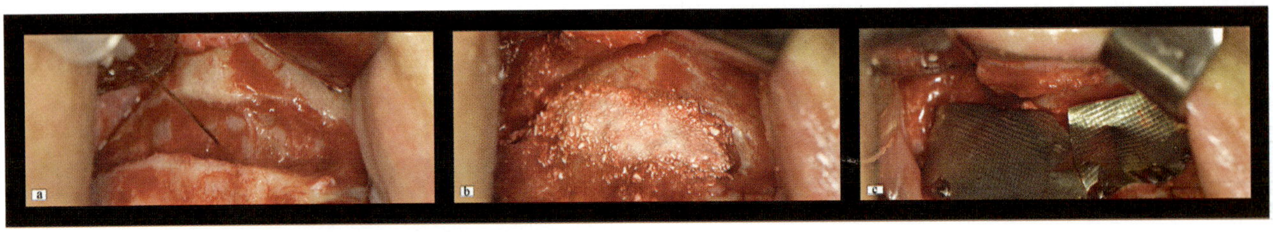

Figure 9.5. **A.** Sinus grafting procedure. Preparation of the graft site. **B.** Grafting site filled with augmentation material. **C.** Fixation of the grafting material with a titanium membrane to prevent dislocation.

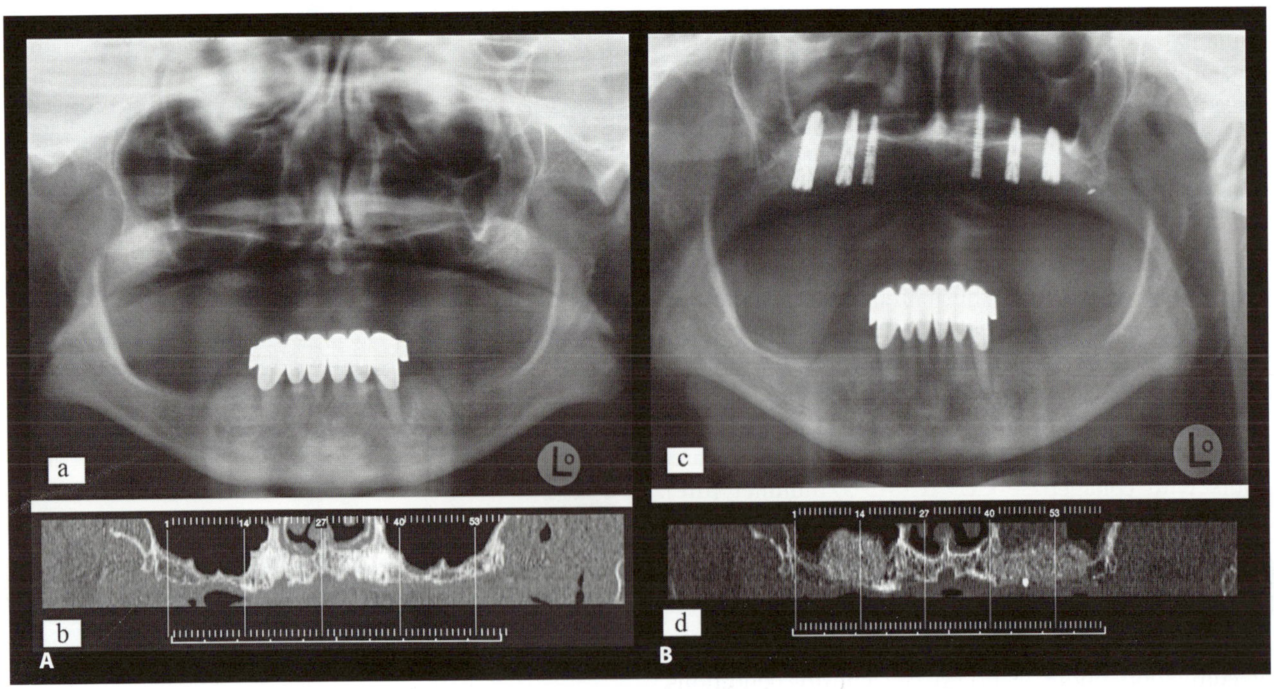

Figure 9.6. **A.** Picture taken before the sinus augmentation showing the severely atrophied condition of the maxilla. **B.** Condition 6 months after the sinus augmentation and the placement of dental implants.

the atrophic maxillary alveolus using tissue-engineered bone offers great potential for craniomaxillofacial surgery and bone reconstruction procedures in other parts of the skeleton.

Future research must address the mechanical stability of engineered bone, its possible resorption, and its application in less-vascularized environments.

References

Ahsan, T., and R.M. Nerem. 2005. Bioengineered tissues: the science, the technology, and the industry. *Orthod Craniofac Res.* 8, pp. 134–140.

Albandar, J.M., and A. Kingman. 1999. Gingival recession, gingival bleeding, and dental calculus in adults 30 years of age and older in the United States, 1988–1994. *J Periodontol*, 70, pp. 30–43.

Asahina, I., M. Seto, E. Oda, A.M. Marukawa, S. Imranul, and S. Enomoto. 1999. *Bone Engineering, 1st edition*, Em squared, Toronto, p. 526.

Bell, E., P. Ehflich, D.J. Buttle, and T. Nakatsuji. 1981. Living tissue formed in vitro and accepted as skin-equivalent of full thickness. *Science*, 221, pp. 1052–1054.

Bisceglie, V. 1933. Ueber die antineoplastische Immunnitaet; heterologe Einpflanzung von Tumoren in Huehnerembryonen. *ZtschrfKrebsforsch*, 40, pp. 122–140.

Boyne, P.J., and R.A. James. 1980. Grafting of the maxillary sinus floor with autogenous marrow and bone. *J Oral Surg*, 38, pp. 613–616.

Bucholz, R.W. 2002. Nonallograft osteoconductive bone graft substitutes. *Clin Orthop Relat Res*, 395, pp. 44–52.

Burke, J.F., I.V. Yannas, W.C. Quimby, C.C. Bondoc, and W.K. Jung. 1981. Successful use of a physiologically acceptable artificial skin in the treatment of extensive burn injury. *Ann Surg*, 194, pp. 413–448.

Chick, W.L., A.A. Like, and V. Lauris. 1975. Beta cell culture on synthetic capillaries: an artificial endocrine pancreas. *Science*, 187, pp. 847–848.

El-Ghannam, A. 2005. Bone reconstruction: from bioceramics to tissue engineering. *Expert Rev Med Devices*, 2, pp. 87–101.

Ewers, R., C. Kasperk, and B. Simons. 1987. Biologisches Knochenimplantat aus Meeresalgen. *Zahnärztliche Praxis*; 38, pp. 318–320.

Ewers, R., and B. Schumann. 1994. Experimental and Clinical Applications of Algipore, a Phycogenic Hydroxylapatite. *J Craniomaxillofac Surg*, 22, p. 92.

Ewers, R., W. Goriwoda, C. Schopper, D. Moser, E. Spassova. 2004. Histologic findings at augmented bone areas supplied with two different bone substitute materials combined with sinus floor lifting. Report of one case. *Clin Oral Impl Res*, 15, pp. 96–100.

Ewers, R. 2005. Maxilla Sinus Grafting With Marine Algae Derived Bone Forming Material: A Clinical Report of Long-Term Results. *J Oral Maxillofac Surg*, 63, pp. 1712–1723.

Griffith, L.G., and G. Naughton. 2002. Tissue engineering: current challenges and expanding opportunities. *Science*, 295, pp. 1009–1014.

Hench, L.L. 1998. Bioceramics. *J Am Ceram Soc*, 81, pp. 1705–1728.

Herring, S.W., and P. Ochareon. 2005. Bone—special problems of the craniofacial region. *Orthod Craniofac Res*, 8, pp. 174–182.

Hillam, R. 1996. Response of bone to mechanical load and alterations in circulating hormones, PhD Thesis. Bristol, UK: University of Bristol. Cited by J.D. Currey. How well are bones designed to resist fracture? *J Bone Min Res*, 18, pp. 591–598.

Hollinger, J.O., J. Brekke, E. Gruskin, and D. Lee. 1996. Role of bone substitutes. *Clin Orthop*, 324, pp. 55–65.

Hylander, W.L. 1975. The human mandible: lever or link? *Am J Phys Anthrop*, 43, pp. 227–242.

Jensen, O.T. 1994. Guided bone graft augmentation. In: D. Buser, C. Dahlin, and R.K. Schenk, Editors, *Guided Bone Regeneration in Implant Dentistry*, Quintessence, Chicago, IL, p. 235.

Jin, Q.M., H. Takita, T. Kohgo, K. Atsumi, H. Itoh, and Y. Kuboki. 2000. Effects of geometry of hydroxyapatite as a cell substratum in BMP-induced ectopic bone formation, *J Biomed Mater Res*, 51, pp. 491–499.

Kuboki, Y., H. Takita, D. Kobayashi, E. Tsuruga, M. Inoue, M. Murata, N. Nagai, Y. Dohi, and H. Ohgushi. 1998. BMP-induced osteogenesis on the surface of hydroxyapatite with geometrically feasible and nonfeasible structures: topology of osteogenesis, *J Biomed Mater Res*, 39, pp. 190–199.

Langer, R., and J.P. Vacanti. 1993. Tissue engineering. *Science*, 260, pp. 920–926.

Logeart-Avramoglou, D., F. Anagnostou, R. Bizios, and H. Petite. 2005. Engineering bone: challenges and obstacles. *J Cell Mol Med*. 9, pp. 72–84.

Loukota, R.A., S.G. Isaksson, E.L. Linner, and J.E. Blomqvist. 1992. A technique for inserting endosseous implants in the atrophic maxilla in a single stage procedure. *Br J Oral Maxillofac Surg*, 30, pp. 46–49.

MEDLINE. 1960. MeSH Browser. Bethesda, MD. National Library of Medicine, USA. http://pubmed.gov/. Accessed March 2005.

Merkx, M.A.W., J.C. Maltha, and P.J.W. Stoelinga. 2003. Assessment of the value of anorganic bone additives in sinus floor augmentation: a review of clinical reports. *Int J Oral Maxillofac Surg*, 32, pp. 1–6.

Petite, H., V. Viateau, W. Bensaid, A. Meunier, C. de Pollak, M. Bourguignon, K. Oudina, L. Sedel, and G. Guillemin. 2000. Tissue-engineered bone regeneration. *Nat Biotechnol*. 18, pp. 959–963.

Rawlinson, S.C.F., J.R. Mosley, R.F.L. Suswillo, A.A. Pitsillides, and L.E. Lanyon. 1995. Calvarial and limb bone cells in organ and monolayer culture do not show the same early responses to dynamic mechanical strain. *J Bone Min Res*, 10, pp. 1225–1232.

Ripamonti, U., S. Ma, and A.H. Reddi. 1992. The critical role of geometry of porous hydroxyapatite delivery system in induction of bone by osteogenin, a bone morphogenetic protein, *Matrix*, 12, pp. 202–212.

Rodan, G.A. 1992. Introduction to bone biology. *Bone*, 13, pp. 3–6.

Rose, F.R., and R.O. Oreffo. 2002. Bone tissue engineering: hope vs. hype. *Biochem Biophys Res Commun*. 292, pp. 1–7.

Salgado, A.J., O.P. Coutinho, and R.L. Reis. 2004. Bone tissue engineering: state of the art and future trends. *Macromol Bioscience*, 4, pp. 743–765.

Sampath, T.K., and A.H. Reddi. 1984. Importance of geometry of the extracellular matrix in endochondral bone differentiation, *J Cell Biol*, 98, pp. 2192–2197.

Schmelzeisen, R., R. Schimming, and M. Sittinger. 2003. Making bone: implant insertion into tissue-engineered bone for maxillary sinus floor augmentation. *J Cranio Maxillofac Surg*, 31, pp. 34–39.

Schopper, C., D. Moser, A. Sabbas, G. Lagogiannis, E. Spassova, F. Konig, K. Donath, and R. Ewers. 2003. The fluorohydroxyapatite (FHA) FRIOS$^-$ Algipore$^-$ is a suitable biomaterial for the reconstruction of severely atrophic human maxillae. *Clin Oral Impl Res*, 6, pp. 743 –749.

Simion, M., F. Fontana, G. Rasperini, and C. Maiorana. 2004. Long-term evaluation of osseo integrated implants placed in sites augmented with sinus floor elevation associated with vertical ridge augmentation. A retrospective study of 38 consecutive implants with 1- to 7-year follow-up, *Int J Periodont Restor Dent*, 24, pp. 208–221.

Simon, G.C., C.A. Khatri, S.A. Wight, and F.W. Wang. 2002. Preliminary report on the biocompatibility of a moldable, resorbable, composite bone graft consisting of calcium phosphate cement and poly(lactide-co-glycolide) microspheres. *J Orthop Res*, 20, pp. 473–482.

Simons, B., C. Kasperk, and R. Ewers. 1987. Ein neues phycogenes Hydroxylapatit-Implantatmaterial. Fortschritte der Mineralogie. Europäische Zeitschrift für Mineralogie, Kristallographie, Petrologie, Geochemie und Lagerstättenkunde, 65, p. 174.

Solar, P., U. Geyerhofer, H. Traxler, A. Windisch, C. Ulm, and G. Watzek. 1999. Blood supply to the maxillary sinus relevant to sinus floor elevation procedures. *Clin Oral Implant Res*, 10, pp. 34–44.

Sommerfeldt, D.W., and C.T. Rubin. 2001. Biology of bone and how it orchestrates the form and function of the skeleton. *Eur Spine J*. 10, pp. 86–95.

Spassova-Tzekova, E., Y. Dimitriev, B. Jilov, C. Schopper, D. Moser, E. Halwax, and R. Ewers. 2004. Bioactive Glass Ceramic Composites containing Phosphate Glasses and Phycogenic Apatite. Proceedings: XX Int. Congress on Glass. Kyoto, Japan.

Spitzer, R.S., C. Perka, K. Lindenhayn, and H. Zippel. 2002. Matrix engineering for osteogenic differentiation of rabbit periosteal cells using alpha-tricalcium phosphate particles in a three-dimensional fibrin culture. *J Biomed Mater Res*, 59, pp. 690–696.

Sullivan, S.M., R.A. Bulard, R. Meaders, and M.K. Patterson. 1997. The use of fibrin adhesive in sinus lift procedures, *Oral Surg Oral Med Oral Pathol Oral Radiol Endod*, 84, pp. 616–619.

Taba, M., Q. Jin, J.V. Sugai, and W.V. Giannobile. 2005. Current concepts in periodontal bioengineering. *Orthod Craniofac Res*, 8, pp. 292–302.

Tatum, O.H. 1986. Maxillary and sinus implant reconstructions. *Dent Clin North Am*, 30, pp. 207–229.

Tissue Engineering. 1995. 1, Vol. 1.

Turhani, D., C.B. Item, D. Thurnher, D. Kapral, B. Cvikl, M. Weiβenböck, K. Yerit, B. Erovic, D. Moser, F. Watzinger, R. Ewers, and G. Lauer. 2003. Osteocalcinexpression in biocomposits with osteoblast-like cells harvested from mandibula using RT-PCR and SDS—Page Western blotting. *Mund Kiefer Gesichtschir*, 5, pp. 294–300.

Turhani, D., B. Cvikl, E. Watzinger, M. Weiβenböck, K. Yerit, D. Thurnher, G. Lauer, and R. Ewers. 2005a. In vitro Growth and Differentiation of Osteoblast-like Cells on Hydroxyapatite Ceramic Granule Calcified from Red Algae. *J Oral Maxillofac Surg*, 63, pp. 793–799.

Turhani, D., M. Weiβenböck, E. Watzinger, K. Yerit, B. Cvikl, R. Ewers, and D. Thurnher. 2005b. In Vitro Study of Adherent Mandibular Osteoblast-Like Cells on Carrier Materials. *Int J Oral Maxillofac Surg*, 34, pp. 543–550.

Turhani, D., E. Watzinger, M. Weissenbock, B. Cvikl, D. Thurnher, G. Wittwer, K. Yerit, and R. Ewers. 2005c. Analysis of Cell-seeded Three-dimensional Bone Constructs Manufactured in vitro with Hydroxyapatite Ceramic Granulae obtained from Red Algae. *J Oral Maxillofac Surg*, 63, pp. 673–681.

Vacanti, C.A., and L.J. Bonassar. 1999. An overview of tissue engineered bone. *Clin Orthop Rel Res*, 7, pp. 375–379.

Vacanti, J.P., and R. Langer. 1999. Tissue engineering: the design and fabrication of living replacement devices for surgical reconstruction and transplantation. *Lancet*. 354, Suppl 1, pp. 32–34.

Vercellotti, T. 2001. The piezoelectric bony window osteotomy and sinus membrane elevation, Introduction of a new technique for simplification of the sinus augmentation procedure. *Int J Periodont Restor Dent*, 21, pp. 561–567.

Yaszemski, M.J., J.B. Oldham, L. Lu, and B.L. Currier. 1994. *Bone Engineering, 1st edition*, Em squared, Toronto, p. 541.

Chapter 10

Prosthetic Technologies and Techniques Beyond the Mere Fixture

Peter Gehrke

An accurate and systematic approach is required to evaluate, diagnose, and resolve esthetic problems predictably. Tooth color is obviously essential for the final result, but esthetic treatment planning should never be focused on shade improvements alone. The ultimate goal is achieving a pleasing smile architecture considering the proper proportion and relation according to established principles (Chiche and Pinault 1994, Magne and Belser 2002, Salama et al. 2002, Garber and Salama 2000).

Predictable osseointegration has taken implant dentistry beyond the mere restoration of function for the compromised edentulous case to esthetic single-tooth implant-supported restorations in the anterior region. Today, implants are a viable treatment option for partial edentulism. Consequently, sacrificing sound tooth structures for fixed bridgework can be prevented, and specific problems related to removable partial dentures can be eliminated.

However, to be the preferred treatment choice, implant-supported restoration should, cosmetically, be equal to or surpass that of conventional fixed prosthesis. This necessitates developing an implant recipient site in both hard and soft tissue for optimal placement of the implant and emergence of the restoration. Implants should not be limited by the osseous topography, which can compromise the final restoration, but implant placement should rather be restoration driven (Garber 1996). In addition, all restorative techniques available and adjunctive periodontal soft tissue procedures need to be applied to compensate for anatomical irregularities at the site and of the adjacent teeth. This allows for an implant restoration that mimics that of a natural tooth.

The increasing predictability and longevity of porcelain laminate veneers offer a beneficial asset to the esthetic modification of implant-adjacent teeth (Garber and Adar 1997, Fradeani et al. 2005). They allow for alteration of shade and tooth shape and convey the illusion of changes in tooth position. Smile design, restoration durability, and color conformity of natural and replaced teeth are prerequisites for a highly esthetic restoration. Although metal implant abutments have inherent esthetic disadvantages, they are most widely considered to be a standard treatment option for implant-supported restorations. The art of looking natural, however, has been perfected by ceramics. Their application in prosthodontics has opened up a new era in esthetic tooth replacement.

Zirconium Dioxide

Improved material characteristics, complying with clinicians' and patients' increased demands for highly esthetic results, have contributed significantly to the development of a new generation of implant abutments made from zirconium. These abutments are noted for their tooth-like color, high load strength, tissue tolerability, and intrasulcular design enhancement (Filser et al. 2001, Tinschert et al. 2001, Ichigawa et al. 1992, Yildirim et al. 2000, Yildirim et al. 2003, Sadoun and Perelmuter 1997, Brodbeck 2003). The phenomenon of transformation toughening of zirconium dioxide results in extremely high component strength and extraordinary bending capability and tensile strength, as well as fracture and chemical resistance (Gehrke and Kielhorn 2004, Gehrke et al. 2006). Oxide ceramics are equal to metals from a mechanical standpoint, but they are biologically stronger (Covacci et al. 1999, Ferraris et al. 2000).

Zirconium was introduced to material science in 1975 (Garvie et al. 1975), followed by its medical application in total hip replacements in the mid-1980s (Christel 1989). The use of zirconium dioxide for implant abutments has been introduced recently due to its high fracture resistance shown when comparing zirconium dioxide to aluminum oxide and other dental ceramics (Tinschert et al. 2001, Ichigawa et al. 1992, Yildirim et al. 2000, Yildirim et al. 2003, Gehrke and Kielhorn 2004, Gehrke et al. 2006). So far, only little data are available on the survival rate and average life times of zirconium implant restorations (Döring et al. 2004).

The word "zirconium," as used in our habitual language, represents a simple form of the chemically correct name "zirconium dioxide." The German chemist M.H. Klaproth discovered zirconium dioxide in 1789 by heating zirconium rocks (Hoppe et al. 1987). The name zircon is derived from the Persian word *zargon*, which means "gold color." The main material used for the extraction of zirconium dioxide is the mineral zircon ($ZrSiO_4$), which is found in volcanic rocks (granites, syenites, and gneisses). The majority of zircon is mined in Australia, the United States, India, and South Africa. Zirconium oxide is gained by melting coke with lime and zircon. A highly purified raw product must be used to develop high-performance ceramics. For this reason, a special synthesis method was developed to obtain highly pure zirconium oxide. (See Figures 10.1A–N.)

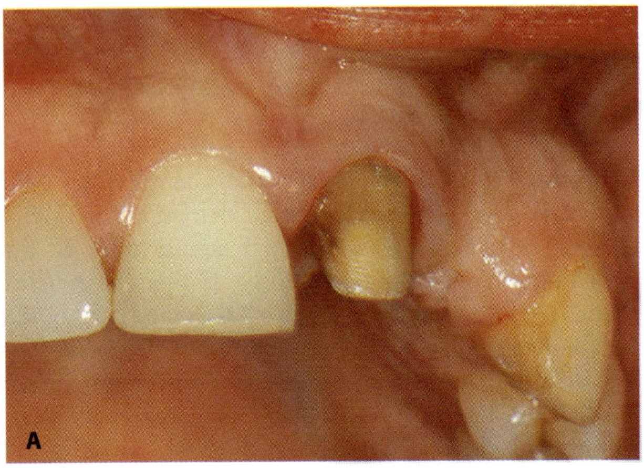

Figure 10.1A. Preoperative labial view after continuous decementation of fixed restoration with distal cantilever.

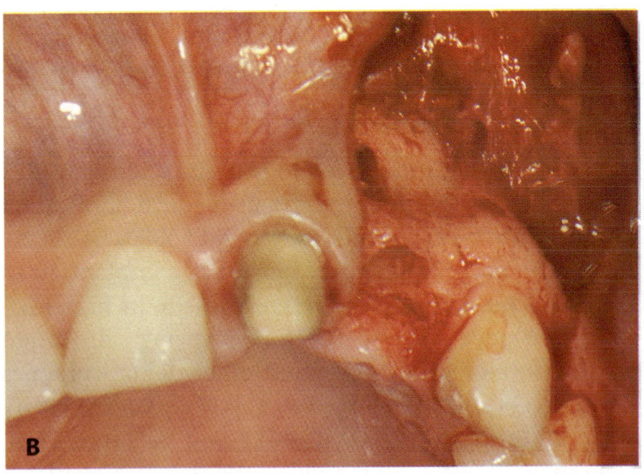

Figure 10.1B. Incision and elevation of mucoperiosteal flap. Note labial bone depression and fenestration. (Surgery: Dr. Orcan Yüksel).

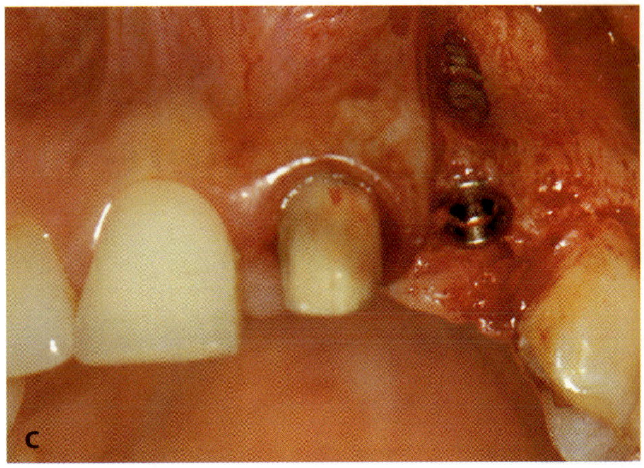

Figure 10.1C. XiVE Implant (DENTSPLY Friadent, Mannheim, Germany), 3.8 mm in diameter and 11 mm in length. Additional augmentation with FRIOS Algipore (Friadent, Mannheim, Germany) and Bio-Gide Membrane (Geistlich Pharma AG, Wolhusen, Switzerland).

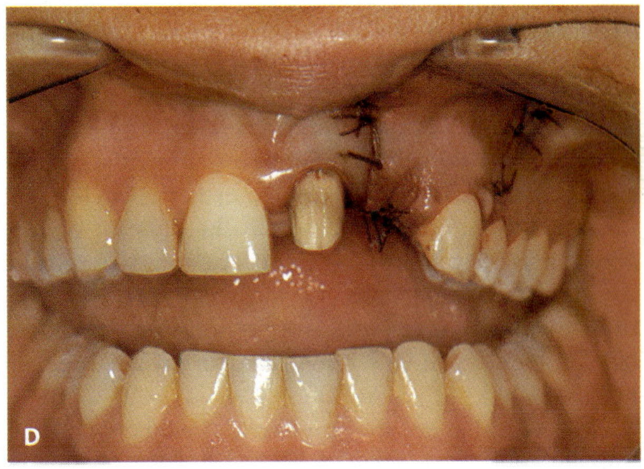

Figure 10.1D. Labial view immediately after implant placement, augmentation, and flap closure.

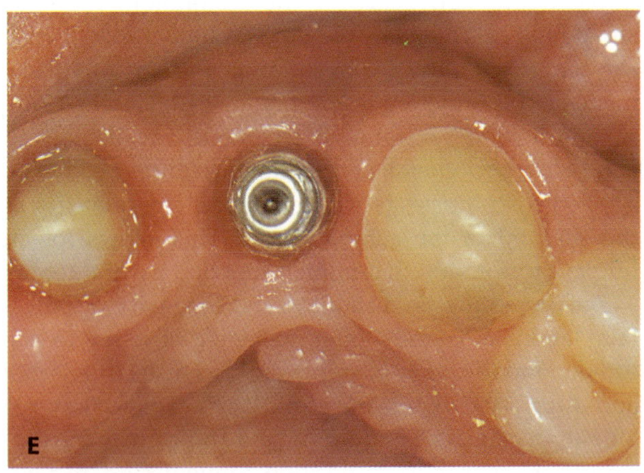

Figure 10.1E. Occlusal view 6 months after implant placement. Preparation of left canine for porcelain laminate veneer.

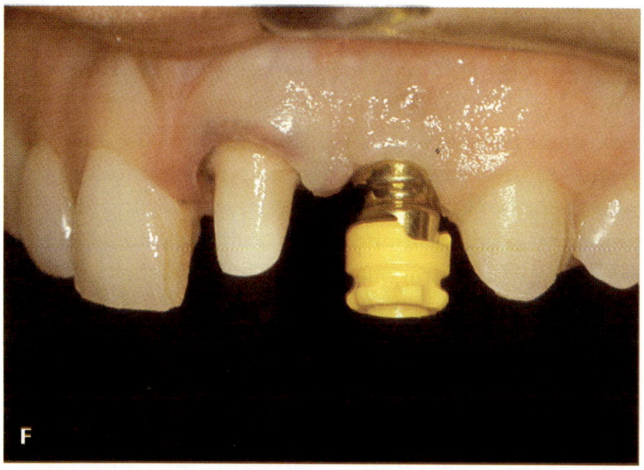

Figure 10.1F. Labial view after insertion of implant transfer coping with Transfer Cap and placement of retraction cord around central incisor for impression taking.

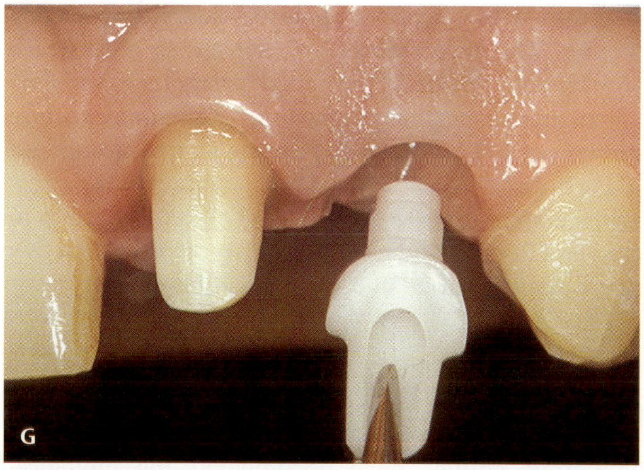

Figure 10.1G. Try-in of customized CERCON® zirconium abutment with hexagonal connection.

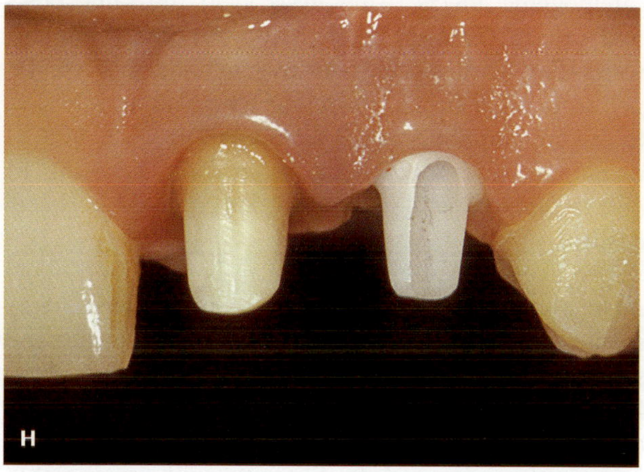

Figure 10.1H. Labial view of inserted zirconium abutment in situ.

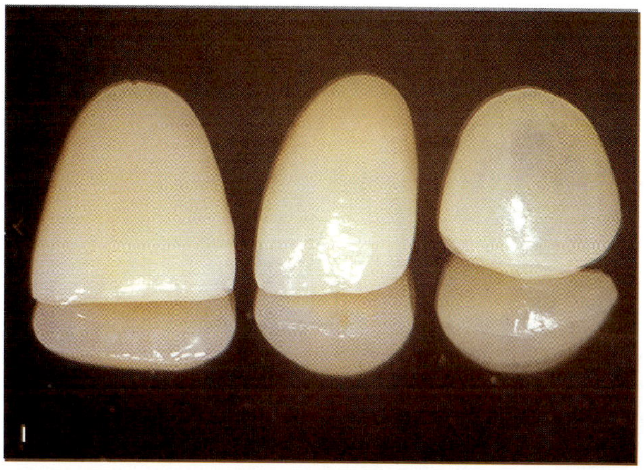

Figure 10.1I. Laboratory: Porcelain laminate veneer for canine. Full-ceramic crowns for central incisor and implant abutment.

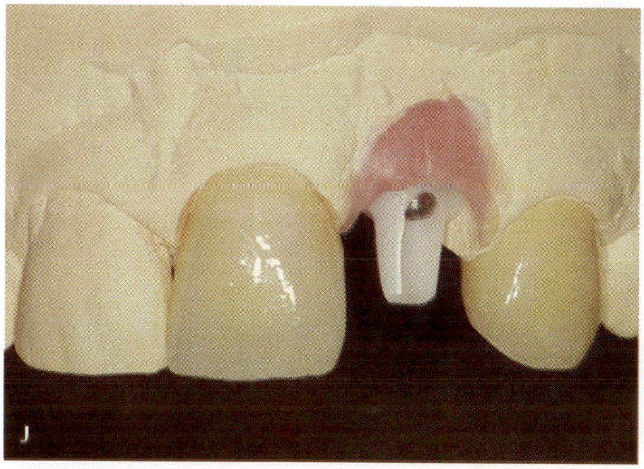

Figure 10.1J. Full-ceramic restorations and porcelain laminate veneer on master cast.

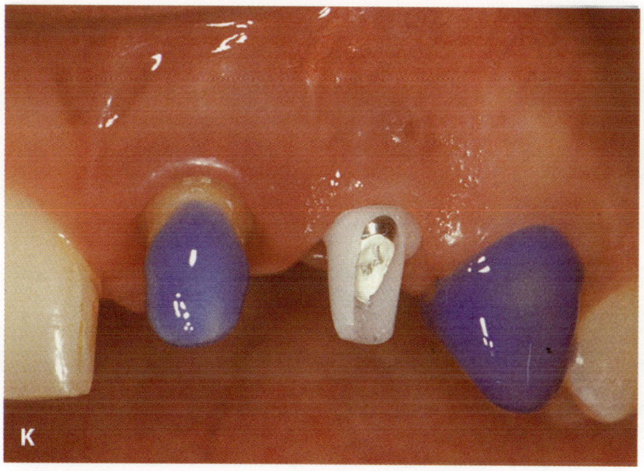

Figure 10.1K. Conditioning of left central incisor and canine for bonding of ceramic restorations.

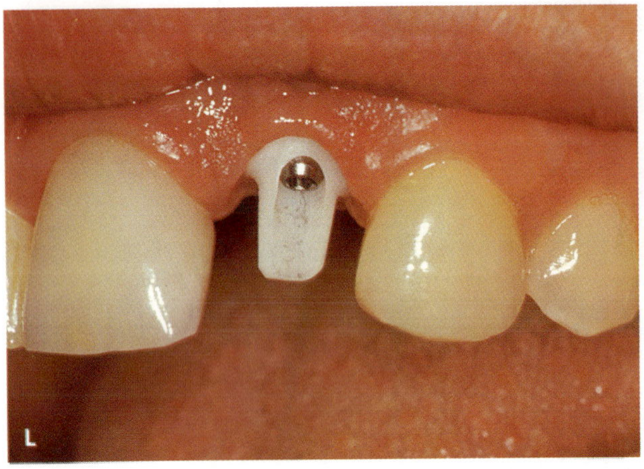

Figure 10.1L. Labial view after bonding of ceramic restorations to implant-adjacent teeth.

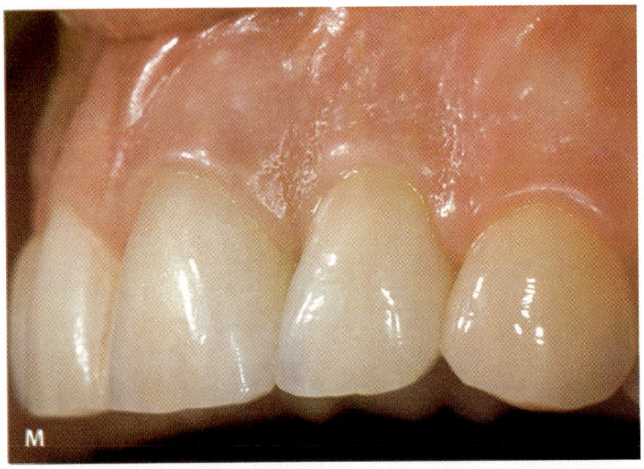

Figure 10.1M. Pleasing smile architecture with proper relation of implant restoration to adjacent teeth. Labial view of final restoration. (In collaboration with Dr. Orcan Yüksel)

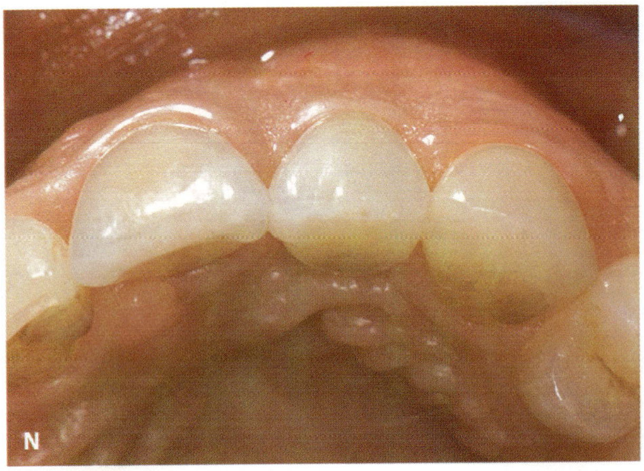

Figure 10.1N. Occlusal view of final restoration displaying compensated irregularities of buccal contour and overlying tissue.

Transformation Toughening

Zirconium dioxide has "self-repairing" properties, preventing crack propagation (Gehrke and Kielhorn 2004). It exists in three crystal conditions, even if the chemical composition is identical. This material characteristic is called *polymorphism*. At temperatures exceeding 2300°C, zirconium oxide is found in the cubic crystal phase; it changes into a tetragonal crystal phase when it cools down. Zirconium oxide transforms into a monoclinic phase at temperatures below 1200°C. The transformation from tetragonal to monoclinic is completed with a volume increase of approximately 3–5%.

These volume changes lead to very high inner-structure tensions and component fracture. For this reason, oxide additives (e.g., magnesium oxide, calcium oxide, or yttrium oxide) are necessary to completely or partially stabilize the high-temperature phases (cubic or tetragonal) down to room temperature. This reduces compression stress within the structure to a controlled level and prevents component destruction while cooling. The phenomenon of preventing microcrack propagation resulting from high material tension is called "transformation toughening." Maximum fracture strength of 672 Newtons (N) during static loading and 403 N during cyclic loading has been reported for zirconium ceramic abutments (Gehrke et al. 2006). Further in vitro and in vivo studies are necessary to prove that this claim can is accurate in clinical situations. (See Figures 10.2A–Z.)

Biocompatibility

Numerous studies have documented the biological safety of zirconium dioxide (Covacci et al. 1999, Ferraris et al. 2000). No toxic effects occurred at the interface of zirconium dioxide with bone or soft tissue. Tests of the mutagenic effects (chromosome aberration test) and carcinogenic effects (Ames test) yield the same positive results (Ferraris et al. 2000). An intact implant restoration requires the effective maintenance of the peri-implant margins, including low plaque adhesion to the implant abutment. Inadequate soft tissue attachment may lead to bacterial penetration, resulting in peri-implantitis and progressive loss of hard and soft tissues.

The degree of adhesion between bacteria and abutment depends on the abutment's and bacteria's free surface energy, the roughness of the surface, and the saliva's ionic conductivity (Quirynen and Bollen 1995). Recent studies by Scarano and others (2004) confirmed a 40% reduction in bacterial adhesion on zirconium oxide compared to titanium with comparable roughness.

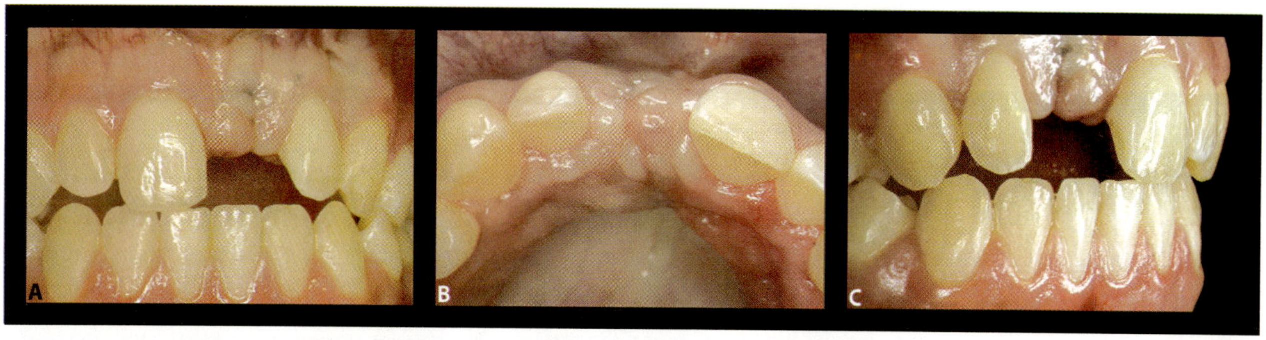

Figure 10.2. **A.** Tissue healing in region of left central incisor 8 months' post implant placement and guided tissue regeneration/membrane. Note unfavorable scar tissue and exposure of membrane tack. **B.** Occlusal view of soft tissue conditions in region of left central incisor. **C.** Labial view of soft tissue conditions in region of left central incisor.

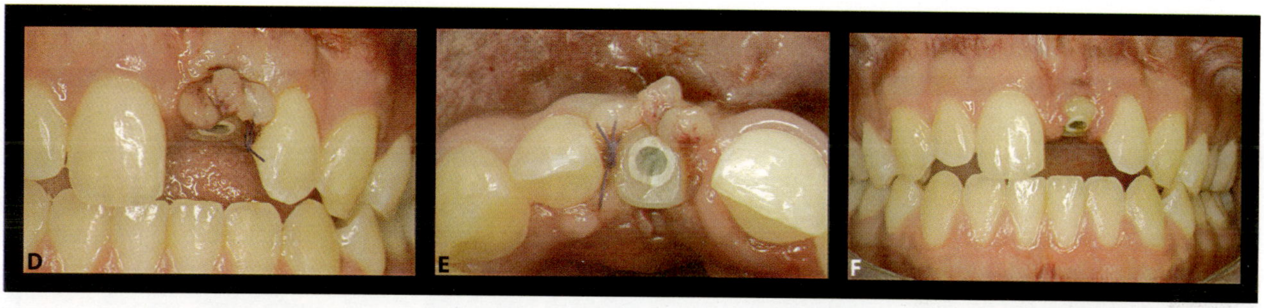

Figure 10.2. **D.** Labial view after pedicle soft tissue graft. (Surgery Prof. Dr. Günter Dhom). **E.** Occlusal view of pedicle soft tissue graft around acrylic anatomically contoured gingival former (FRIADENT, EsthetiCap). **F.** Situation 10 days after implant recovery and guided soft tissue management.

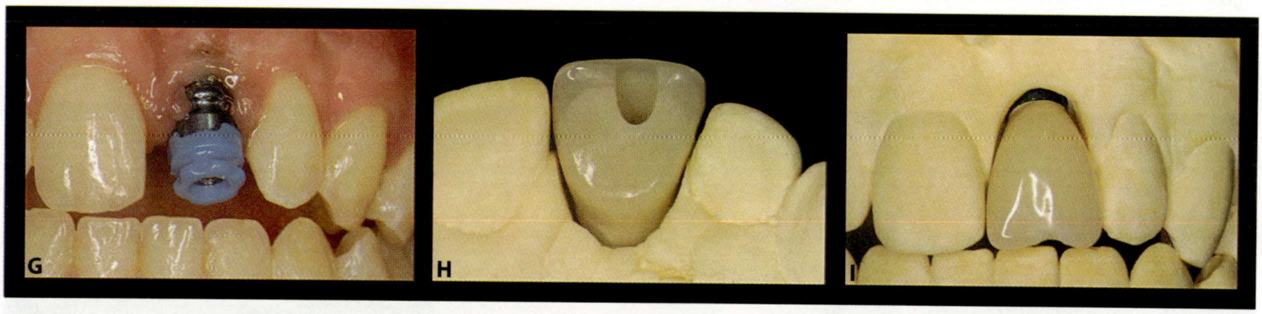

Figure 10.2. **G.** Impression taken with transfer coping and cap for fabrication of long-term provisional restoration. **H.** Incisally screw-retained provisional crown on acrylic abutment (FRIADENT, ProTect). **I.** Labial view of provisional acrylic crown on master cast prior to delivery.

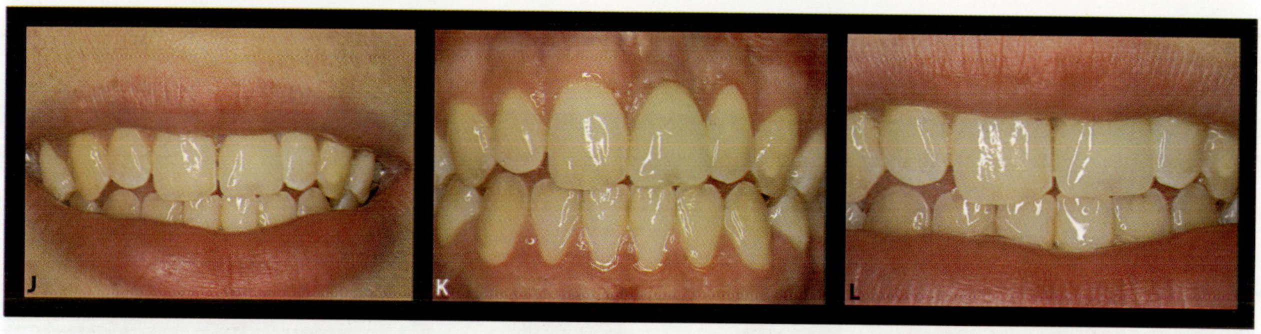

Figure 10.2. **J.** Smile line after delivery of provisional single restoration for left central incisor. **K.** Intraoral view of screw-retained provisional after closing of incisal access hole with acrylic. **L.** Close-up of smile line with provisional acrylic restoration.

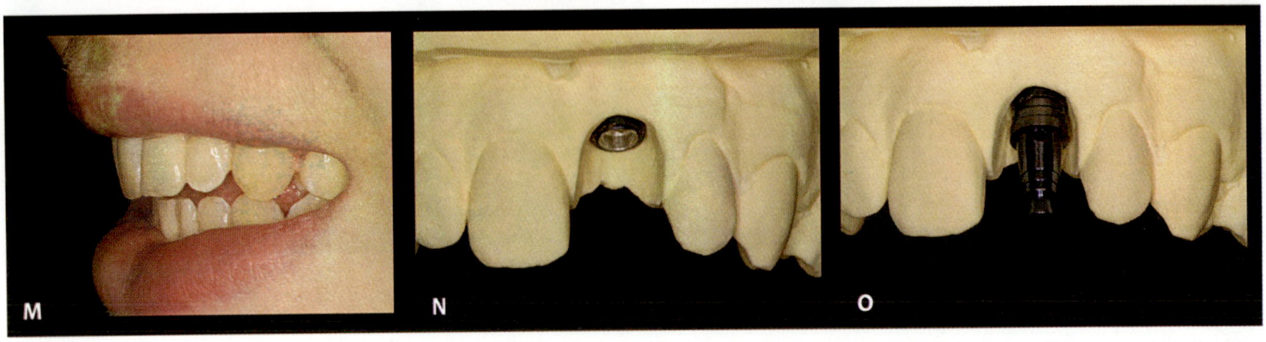

Figure 10.2. **M.** Lateral view of smile line in temporary stage. **N.** The gingival profile is checked and gingival height with select abutment on master cast. **O.** Selection of the abutment size & height.

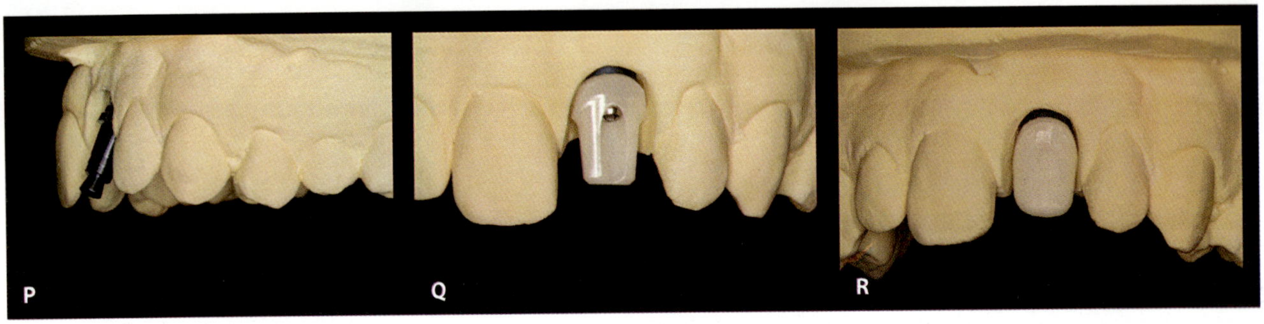

Figure 10.2. **P.** Selection of the abutment angulation. **Q.** CAD/CAM fabricated Zirconium abutment in place. **R.** CAD/CAM fabricated zirconium copings in place.

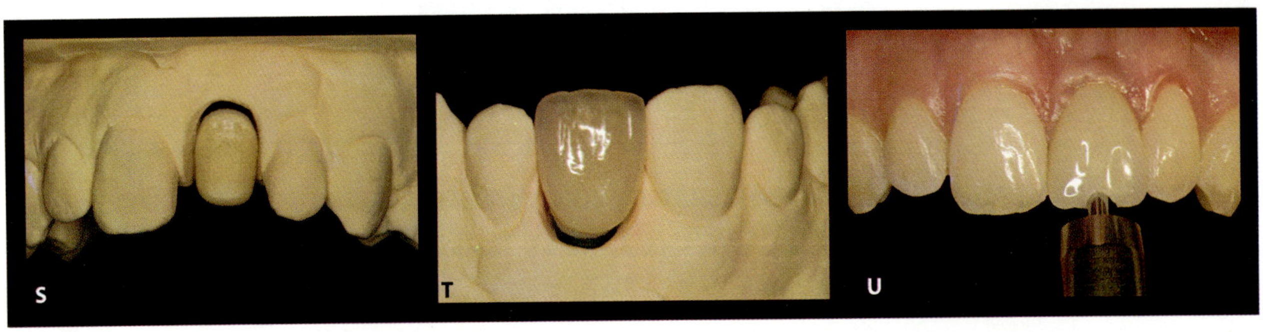

Figure 10.2. **S.** Zirconium copings after customization. **T.** Final full ceramic crown prior to delivery. **U.** Removal of provisional screw-retained crown.

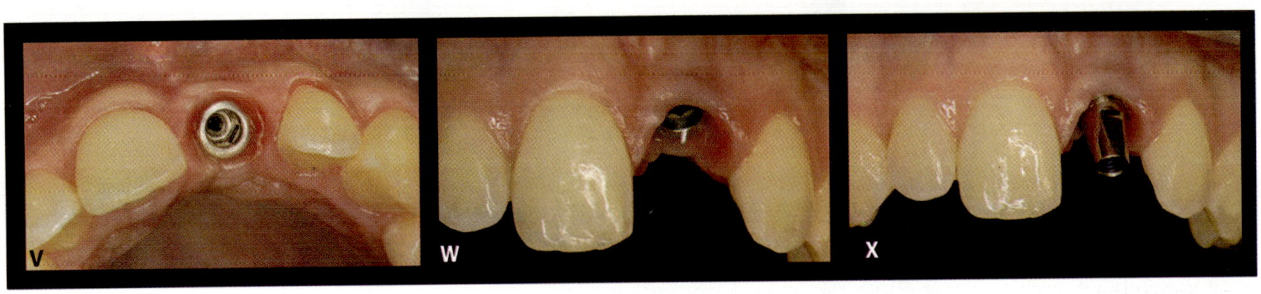

Figure 10.2. **V.** Incisal view if the Soft tissue condition. **W.** Labial view of the emergence profile 3 months after implant recovery. **X.** Clinical try-in with titanium abutment that shows the difference from the zirconium abutment.

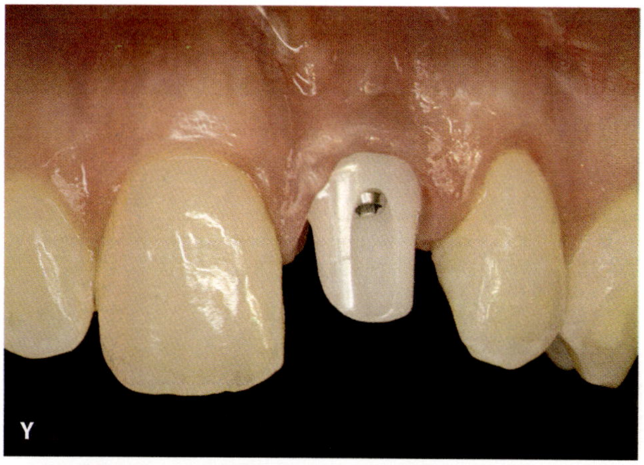

Figure 10.2Y. The zirconium abutment intra-orally.

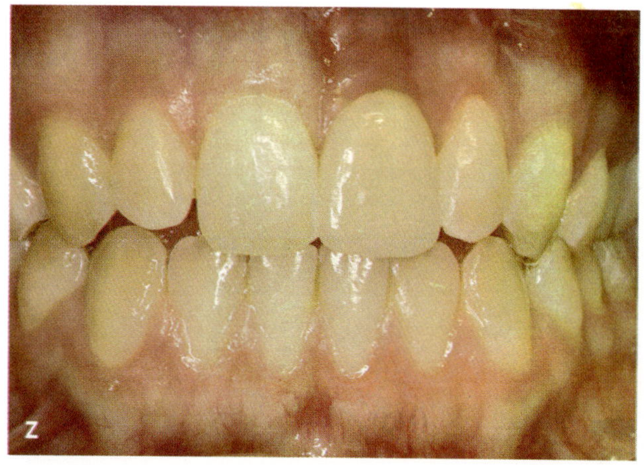

Figure 10.2Z. Intraoral view of final full ceramic restoration in situ.

Most infections in the oral cavity are due to the initial adhesion of bacterial colonization. These start on surface irregularities, such as grooves or abrasive defects, and extend gradually over the entire abutment. Bacteria are inaccessible to mechanical removal in the subperi-implant region, which allows bacteria to attach strongly to the abutment. The adhesion of bacteria directly correlates to the roughness and the number of surface defects. Abutments with low roughness values show a significant reduction in plaque adhesion and plaque growth. Poortinga and others (2001) demonstrated the significant influence of energy on bacterial adhesion, besides surface roughness. Bacteria absorbing and passing electrons from the fluid substrate adhere in stronger and greater numbers compared to bacteria only receiving electrons. These results prove that the electron transfer between bacteria and their substrate also influences the adhesion and thus plaque formation.

A comparative immunohistochemical evaluation of vascular growth factor, inflammatory infiltrate, proliferative activity expression, and microvessel density in the peri-implant soft tissues surrounding titanium and zirconium dioxide healing caps revealed statistically decreased values for zirconium dioxide (Degidi et al. 2006). Consequently, zirconium actively contributes to peri-implant tissue protection. The ideal synergy of mechanical, functional, biological, and esthetic features contributes significantly to the esthetic result of a full-ceramic implant restoration. Conventional titanium abutments can produce a bluish, metal shimmer at the restoration margin, especially in cases of thin soft tissue. This results in a significant loss of esthetic quality and may contribute to an unsatisfactory treatment outcome, particularly for patients with a high smile line. Zirconium ceramics appear to be an alternative abutment material for these cases.

Restorations in the esthetically demanding anterior region present significant challenges in both the surgical and prosthetic stages of implant dentistry. Titanium has been established as the material of choice for endosseous implants, resulting in a high degree of predictability. Zirconium dioxide appears to be a suitable material for manufacturing implant abutments with a high fracture strength and low bacterial colonization potential. Ceramic abutments also minimize the gray color associated with metal components shining through the peri-implant tissues. Their durability and color conformity are prerequisites for highly esthetic implant restorations.

Using Prefabricated Zirconium Copings on Corresponding Implant Abutments

New implant restorative treatment protocols aim for an effective and shortened treatment concept, both in the laboratory and chairside. The following clinical case summarizes a systematic restorative approach using a novel premanufactured zirconium abutment/coping system in partially edentulous patients. The prosthetic and laboratory procedures for an implant-supported single-tooth replacement in the esthetic region are addressed and illustrated in a step-by-step approach.

After osseointegration and stage-two soft tissue healing, a zirconium dioxide abutment (CERCON®, DENTSPLY Friadent, Mannheim, Germany) was attached to an implant (XiVE®, DENTSPLY Friadent, Mannheim, Germany) replacing the right lateral incisor. (See Figures 10.3A–N.) After placing the abutment, a

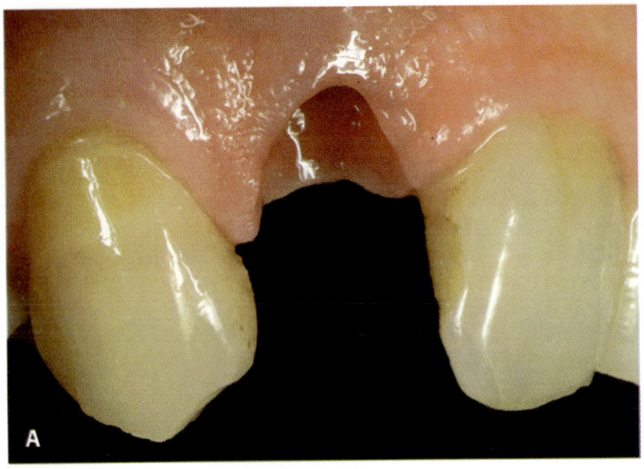

Figure 10.3A. Labial view after implant osseointegration (right lateral incisor) and stage two soft tissue healing.

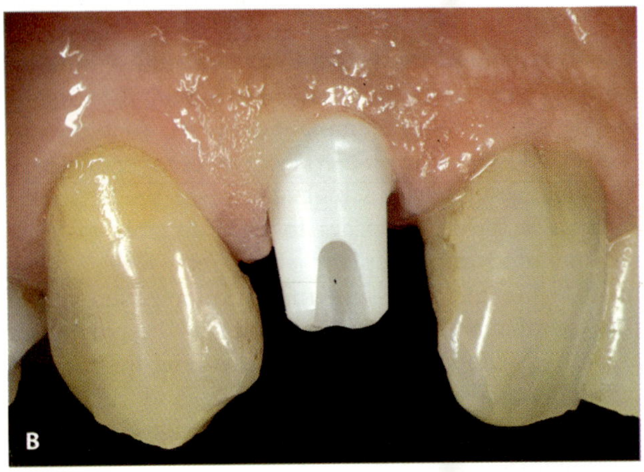

Figure 10.3B. Try-in of zirconium ceramic abutment (CERCON® neutral/dentin).

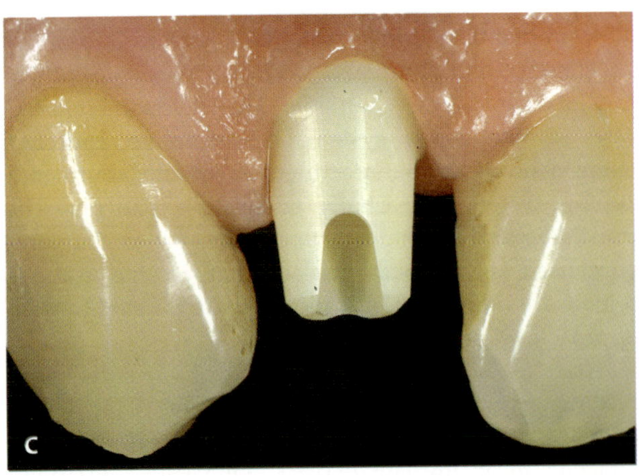

Figure 10.3C. Try in of another shade of the zirconium abutment (CERCON® neutral/dentin).

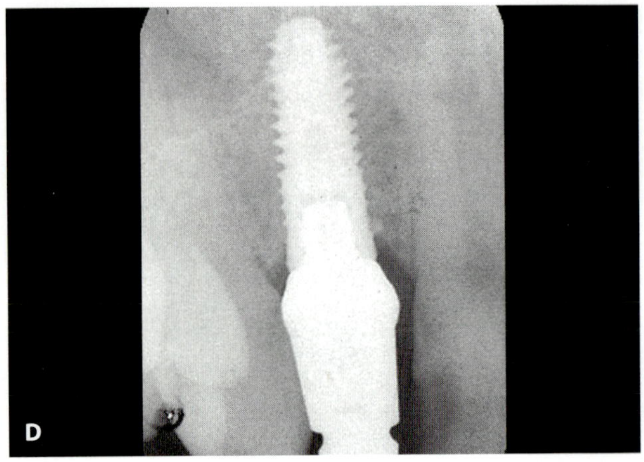

Figure 10.3D. Seating of premanufactured zirconium cap for impression taking.

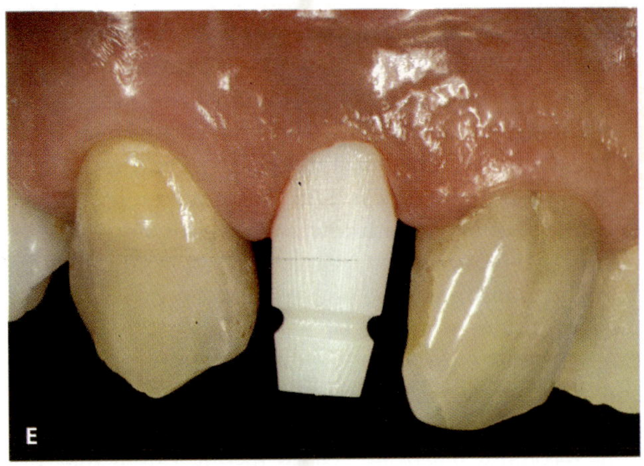

Figure 10.3E. Cap fully seated.

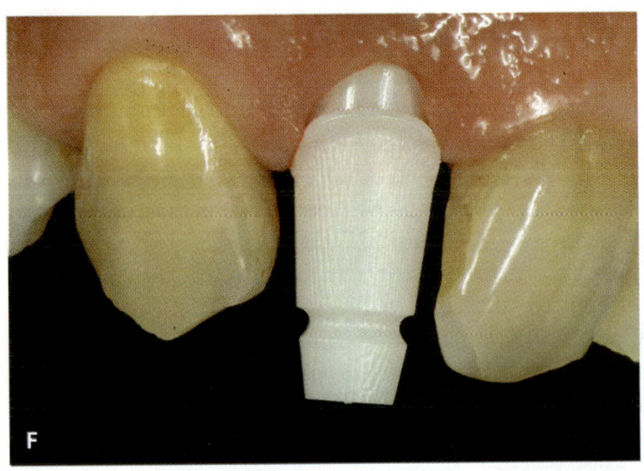

Figure 10.3F. Periapical X-ray of ZrO2-abutment/cap unit on implant.

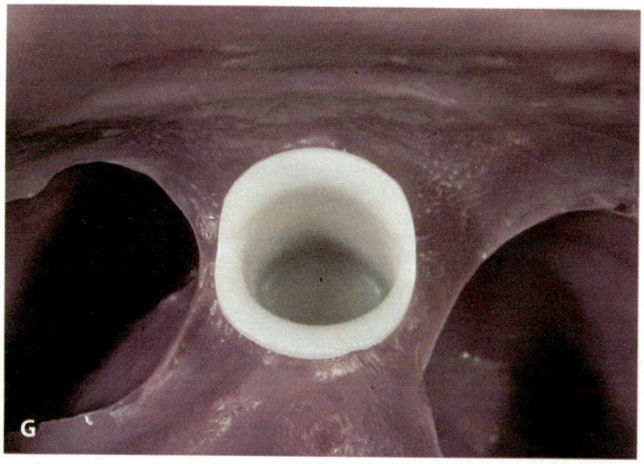

Figure 10.3G. Impression with polyether material and picked-up cap.

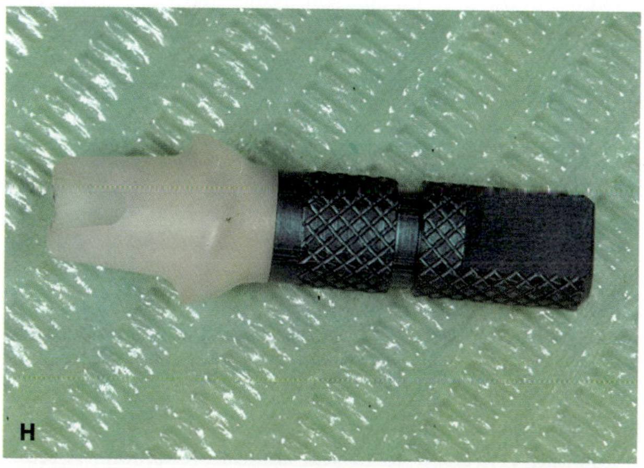

Figure 10.3H. Zirconium abutment connected to an implant analogue.

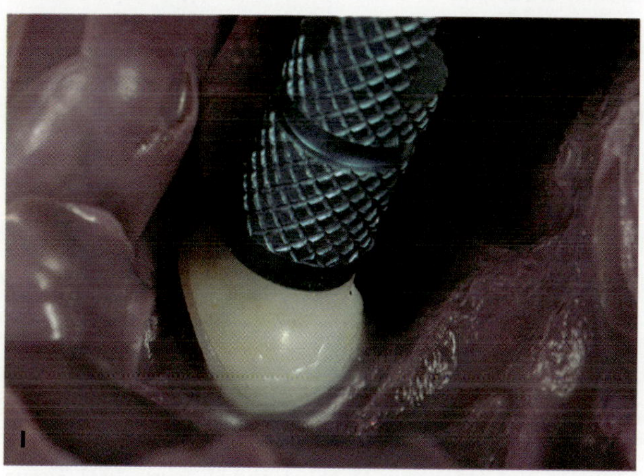

Figure 10.3I. Reseating of implant analogue/abutment unit into impression.

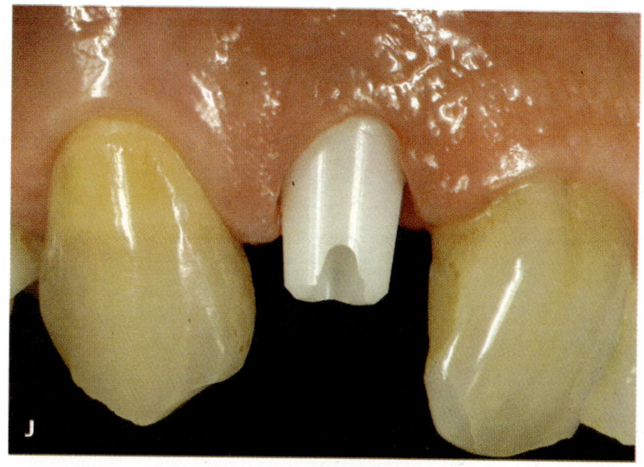

Figure 10.3J. Finalized full-ceramic restoration in the laboratory. Premanufactured coping serves as foundation for porcelain crown.

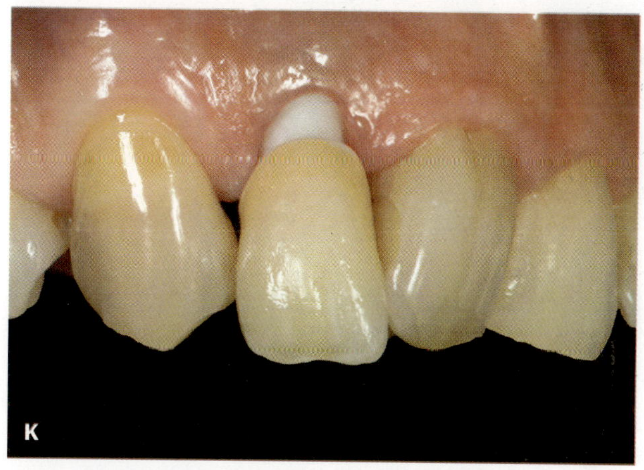

Figure 10.3K. Seating of zirconium ceramic abutment.

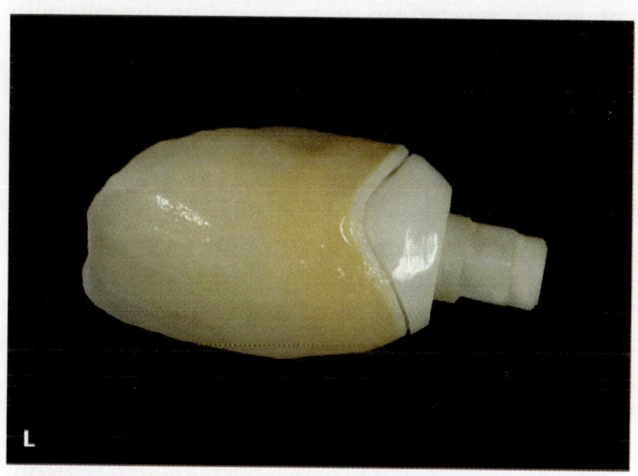

Figure 10.3L. Try-in of full ceramic crown.

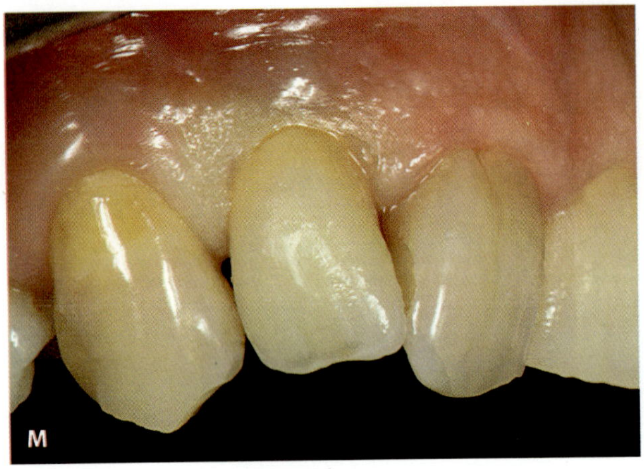

Figure 10.3M. Crown in situ immediately after cementation.

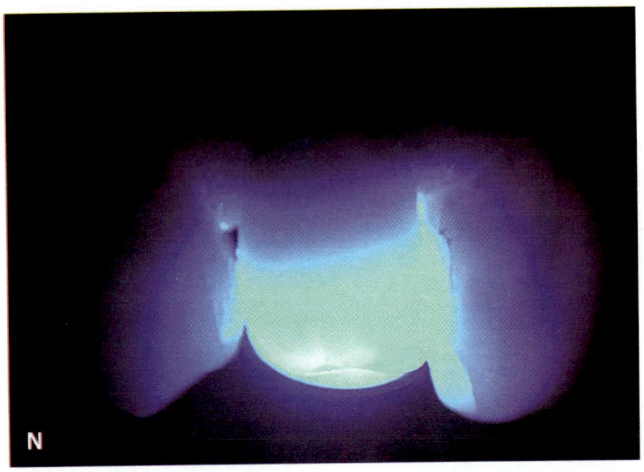

Figure 10.3N. Labial view of full ceramic implant restoration with polymerization light.

premanufactured corresponding zirconium coping was seated and an impression was taken for the fabrication of a master cast. The ceramic coping served as an impression transfer cap, to be picked up directly with the impression. Before pouring the cast, the zirconium abutment was connected to an implant analogue and securely reseated into the cap. No additional modifications were required, and porcelain was applied directly to the ceramic coping to complete a full-ceramic crown. The coping served as the foundation for the porcelain applied by the laboratory to create the final restoration. No additional ceramic crown or wax-up was necessary. The full ceramic crown, based on the zirconium cap was delivered and subsequently luted with resin cement. The clinical results indicate that the investigated zirconium restorative system allows an expedited and systematic treatment to resolve esthetic challenges with a premanufactured ceramic abutment/coping system in partially edentulous patients.

References

Brodbeck, U. 2003. The ZiReal post: A new ceramic implant abutment. *J Esthet Restor Dent*, 15, (1), pp. 10–24.

Chiche, G.J., and A. Pinault. 1994. *Esthetics of anterior fixed prosthodontics*. Textbook, Quintessence Publishing Co, Inc., Chicago, pp. 13–31.

Christel, P.S. 1989. Zirconia: the second generation of ceramics for total hip replacement. *Bull Hosp Jt Dis Orthop Inst.*, 49, (2), pp. 170–177.

Covacci, V., N. Bruzzese, G. Maccauro, C. Andreassi, G.A. Ricci, C. Piconi, E. Marmo, W. Burger, and A. Cittadini. 1999. In vitro evaluation of the mutagenic and carcinogenic power of high purity zirconia ceramic. *Biomaterials*, 20, (4), pp. 371–376.

Degidi, M., L. Artese, V. Pernotti, P. Gehrke, and A. Piattelli. 2006. Inflammatory infiltrate, microvessel density (MVD), nitric oxide synthase (NOS) expression, vascular endothelial growth factor (VEGF) expression, and proliferative activity (Ki-67) in the peri-implant soft tissues around titanium and zirconium oxide healing caps. *J Periodontol*, 77, pp. 73–80.

Döring, K., E. Eisenmann, and M. Stiller. 2004. Functional and esthetic considerations for single-tooth ANKYLOS implant-crowns: 8 years of clinical performance. *J Oral Implantol*, 30, pp. 198–209.

Ferraris, M, E. Verne, P. Appendino, C. Moisescu, A. Krajewski, A. Ravaglioli, and A. Piancastelli. 2000. Coatings on zirconia for medical applications. *Biomaterials*, 21, (8), pp. 765–773.

Filser, F., P. Kocher, F. Weibel, H. Lüthy, P Schärer, and L.J. Gauckler. 2001. Reliability and strength of all-ceramic dental restorations fabricated by direct ceramic machining (DCM). *Int J Comput Dent*, 4, (2), pp. 89–106.

Fradeani, M., M. Redemagni, and M. Corrado. 2005. Porcelain laminate veneers: 6- to 12-year clinical evaluation—A retrospective study. *Int J Periodontics Restorative Dent.*, Feb, 25, (1), pp. 9–17.

Garber, D.A. 1996. The esthetic dental implant: letting restoration be the guide. *J Oral Implantol.*, 22, (1), pp. 45–50.

Garber, D.A., and P. Adar. 1997. Securing the position of ceramic veneers in dentistry, *Summer*, 4, (2), pp. 2–4.

Garber, D.A., and M. Salama. 2000. The Aesthetic Smile: Diagnosis and Treatment. *Periodontology*, 1996, 11, pp. 18–28.

Garvie, R.C., R.H. Hannink, and R.T. Pascoe. 1975. Ceramic steel. Nature, 258, (5537), pp. 703–704.

Gehrke, P., and J. Kielhorn. 2004. CERCON~ implant abutments: Beauty follows function. *International Magazine Oral Implantol*, 5, (3), pp. 6–13.

Gehrke, P., G. Dhom, J. Brunner, D. Wolf, M. Degidi, and A. Piattelli. 2006. *Zirconium Implant Abutments: Fracture Strength and Influence of Cyclic Loading on Retaining-Screw Loosening.* Quintessence Int, 37, pp. 19–26.

Hoppe, G., F. Damaschun, and G. Wappler. 1987. An appreciation of Martin Heinrich Klaproth as a mineral chemist. (Article in German). *Pharmazie.*, Apr, 42, (4), pp. 266–267.

Ichigawa, Y., Y. Akagawa, H. Nikai, and H. Tsuru. 1992. Tissue compatibility and stability of a new zirconia ceramic in vivo. *J Prosthet Dent*, 68, pp. 322–326.

Magne, P., and U. Belser. 2002. *Bonded porcelain restorations*. Textbook, Quintessence Publishing Co, Inc., Berlin, pp. 58–96.

Poortinga, A.T., R. Bos, and H.J. Busscher. 2001. Charge transfer during staphylococcal adhesion to TiNoX coatings with different specific resistivity. *Biophys Cem*, 91, (3), pp. 273–279.

Quirynen, M., and C.M.L. Bollen. 1995. The influence of surface roughness and surface-free energy on supra- and subgingival plaque formation in man. A review of the literature. *J Clin Periodontol*, 22, (1), 1–14.

Sadoun, M., and S. Perelmuter. 1997. Alumina-zirconia machinable abutments for implant-supported single-tooth anterior crowns. *Pract Periodontics Aesthet Dent*, 9, (9), pp. 1047–1054.

Salama, M., H. Salama, and D.A. Garber. 2002. Guidelines for Aesthetic Restorative Options and Implant Site Enhancement. *Pract Proced Aesthet Dent*, (14), 2, pp. 125–130.

Scarano, A., M. Piattelli, S. Caputi, G.A. Favero, and A. Piattelli. 2004. Bacterial adhesion on commercially pure titanium and zirconium oxide disks: An in vivo human study *J Periodontol*, 75, (2), pp. 292–296.

Tinschert, J., G. Natt, W. Mautsch, M. Augthun, and H. Spiekermann. 2001. Fracture resistance of lithium disilicate-, alumina-, and zirconia-based three-unit fixed partial dentures: A laboratory study. *Int J Prosthodont*, 14, (3), pp. 231–238.

Yildirim, M., D. Edelhoff, O. Hanisch, and H. Spiekermann. 2000. Ceramic abutments—A new era in achieving optimal esthetics in implant dentistry. *Int J Periodontics Restorative Dent.*, Feb, 20, (1), pp. 81–91.

Yildirim, M., H. Fischer, R. Marx, and D. Edelhoff. 2003. In vivo fracture resistance of implant-supported all-ceramic restorations. *J Prosthet Dent*, 90, (4), pp. 325–331.

Chapter 11

The Art and Science of Shade Matching in Esthetic Implant Dentistry

Stephen Chu, Jonathan Zamzok, and Adam Mieleszko

Introduction

The importance of color matching in implant dentistry cannot be overemphasized. Implant dentistry is a painstaking, methodical, and highly scientific discipline. Dental implants serve as the solid, unwavering foundation for the teeth that are placed upon them. Furthermore, they are placed with the intention of providing the patient with a lifetime of worry-free dentition. But equally as important as the functionality of implants are their form, beauty, and outward appearance. They must mimic the function of the natural teeth they are there to replace, and they also must be undetectable to the casual observer, blending in side-by-side with the patient's natural dentition so perfectly that no one but the patient and their dentist know the "secret" the patient wishes to keep to himself.

Color Theory

Although there are solid scientific principles regarding the physics of color, due to innumerable differences in perception from one person to another, color is best described as an abstract science, as shown in Figure 11.1. That is because color has emotive properties; it appeals to the visceral and emotional senses, and can also be highly subjective. Each individual views the same object differently. The way in which we perceive color is influenced by many factors, both environmental (physical surroundings) and viewer-centric (physiological), including lighting conditions, background effects, color blindness, binocular differences, eye fatigue, age, and other physiological factors. But even in the absence of these physical considerations, each observer interprets color differently, based on their experiences with color. For example, most people would say the color of a McIntosh apple is simply red. Others might describe it as ruby or scarlet red. No matter what descriptive terms are used, everyone believes their assessment is most accurate (X-Rite 2002, Hunter and Harold 1987, Judd and Wyszecki 1975, Kuehni and Marcus 1979, Chu 2002a, Berns 2000, Commission Internationale de l'Eclairage 1971, Miller 1987, Wyszecki and Stiles 1982).

Visible Light and Color

Most of us have contemplated the answer to the riddle "If a tree falls in the woods and no one is around to hear it, does it make a sound?" Applied to color theory, that question becomes "If the petals of a rose are pink, and there is no one there to view them, are they actually pink?" According to color theorists, the answer is a resounding "no." In order for color to exist, three elements must be present: light, an object, and a viewer. (See Figure 11.2.) Without the simultaneous interaction of all three, color does not exist.

Importance of Color in Dentistry

The study of color is an integral part of esthetic dentistry. If the color of a restoration is off, even slightly, the mistake can be glaringly evident. It looks false, and the patient is unhappy. However, luckily for us, there is a true science behind the art of understanding and communicating color effectively. Once the processes of color perception and reproduction are well understood, they can be applied to dentistry, specifically to shade-matching techniques. The important concepts include pigment colors and the dimensions of color that must be considered when matching shades.

Science of Color—The Constituents of White Light

Visible light is light that can be perceived by the human eye. The visible light of the sun is referred to as "white" light. White light is not the light of a single color or frequency. In fact, it is composed of a combination of many color frequencies. Case in point: when sunlight passes through a glass of water and the light travels through the glass and onto a nearby wall, we see a rainbow of colors on the wall. This happens because white light is a mixture of all of the colors of the visible spectrum. The water acts as a filter to separate the white light into all

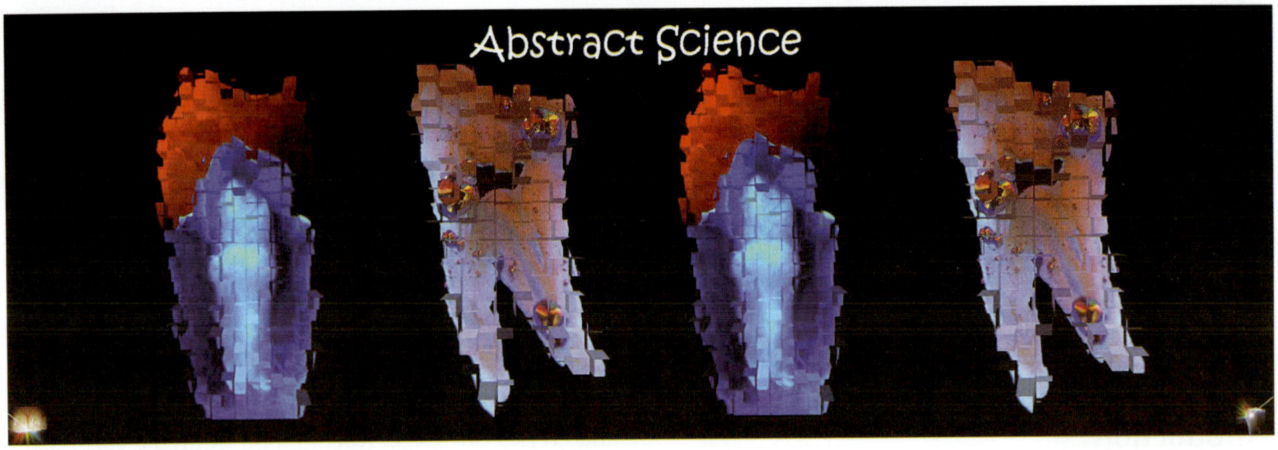

Figure 11.1. Color is best described as an abstract science, appealing to the visceral and emotional senses. The abstract part of the science of color has to do with individual perception. Each observer interprets color differently based on a number of physiological, psychological, and environmental factors. The scientific component is evidenced by the fact that each tooth has a specific numerical value associated within color space. Reproduced by permission of Quintessence Publishing, copyright Quintessence.

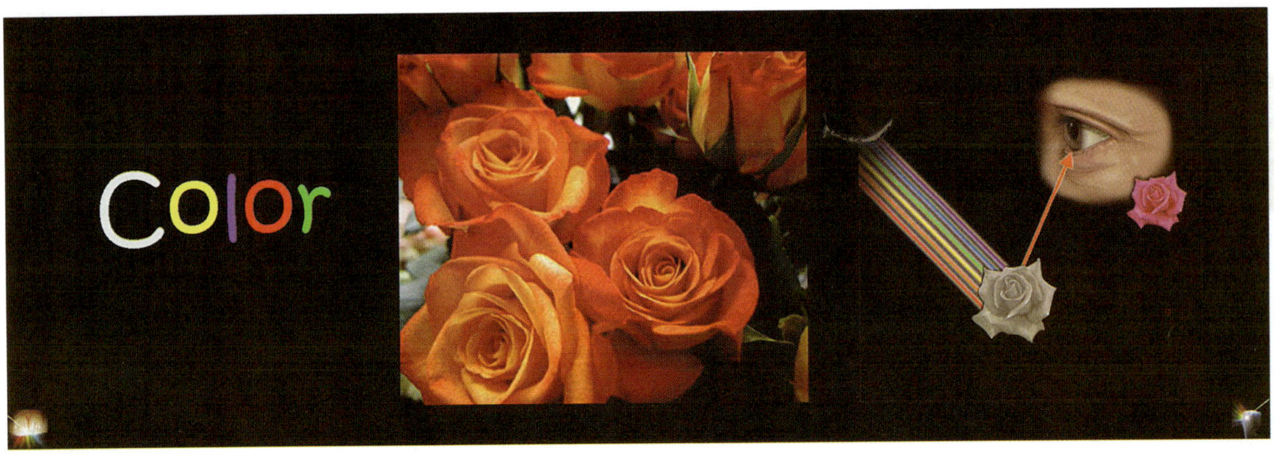

Figure 11.2. The wavelengths of visible light reflect off the object (a rose), resulting in the perception of color by the viewer. Without the simultaneous interaction of light, an object, and a viewer, color does not exist. Reproduced by permission of Quintessence Publishing, copyright Quintessence.

of its visible components. Isaac Newton was the first person to demonstrate this by passing sunlight through a glass prism to separate wavelengths into the colors of the rainbow spectrum, as shown in Figure 11.3.

Newton described the resulting continuous series of colors as a spectrum, and named these colors in the following order: red, orange, yellow, green, blue, indigo, and violet, as represented by the commonly used mnemonic association Roy G. Biv. These wavelengths are perceived by the three types of color receptors (called *cones*) in the human eye as variations of red, green, and blue light. The human eye can perceive only these wavelengths of light (Roy G. Biv), hence the term *visible light spectrum*. In physical terms, the wavelengths of visible light range from approximately 400 to 700 µm. Each hue is accurately defined by its wavelength or frequency (X-Rite 2002), as shown in Table 11.1.

Newton's significant breakthrough in the study of color science shifted attention to the light source (Chu et al. 2004, Bunting 2003). His observation was simple: White light contains all colors. If an object appears to be a particular color, this means that the light reaching our eyes when viewing that object has somehow been changed by the object. In other words, it is the interaction of the light with the object that allows perception of color. Therefore, without light, there would be no color. The basic process of color perception can be described as follows:

> Light is emitted from a light source. This light may reach the eye directly, or it may either strike or pass through an object. If the light interacts with an object, in some cases all light is either reflected or transmitted through the object, but more often some of the light is absorbed by

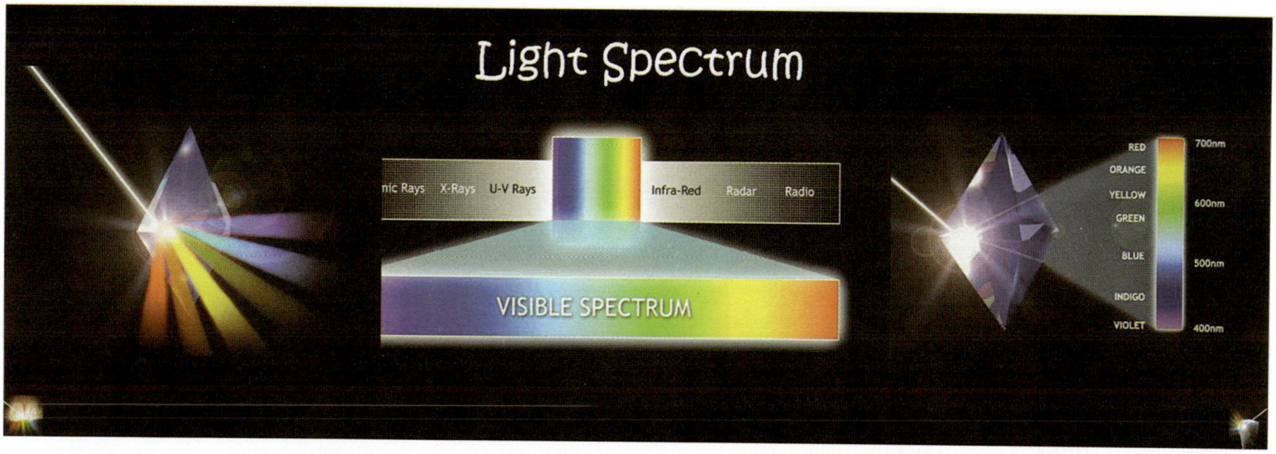

Figure 11.3. Dispersion of light through a prism breaks the light up into its component color frequencies, which are called wavelengths. For visible white light, the range of this spectrum is 400–800 nm. Reproduced by permission of Quintessence Publishing, copyright Quintessence.

Table 11.1 Wavelengths of light.

White Light	Wavelength (0.000001 mm = 1 nanometer)
Red	800–650
Orange	640–590
Yellow	580–550
Green	530–490
Blue	480–460
Indigo	450–440
Violet	430–390

the object. The wavelengths that are not absorbed (i.e., those that are reflected, transmitted, or emitted directly to the eye) are perceived by receptor cells in the eye (rods and cones) and recognized by the brain as a specific color.

Emission

Emission of light from a source occurs through a chemical or physical process. Every process releases more light at certain wavelengths than at others. To create perfectly white light, a light source would have to emit exactly the same amounts of each wavelength. In some cases, emissive objects are intended to produce specific colors. These objects, such as computer monitors, produce color by emitting light with distinct wavelength compositions of red, green, and blue light.

Transmission

When light passes through a transparent or translucent material, such as a slide or film, this is an example of light transmission. If light encounters molecules or larger particles in the material, some wavelengths of light are absorbed by these artifacts. The number of light rays and the specific wavelengths, or colors, that are absorbed are determined by the density and makeup of the material the light travels through (referred to as *spectral data*); the wavelengths that are transmitted compose the color that is perceived. If a material is completely translucent, all light is absorbed and/or transmitted, and the color black is perceived. If the material is completely opaque, all light is reflected, and the color white is perceived. In most cases, however, some of the wavelengths (colors) are absorbed and others transmitted. If this occurs, the color that is perceived corresponds to the wavelengths that are transmitted. For example, if a material absorbs red wavelengths and transmits green and blue wavelengths, a combination of green and blue (referred to as *cyan*) is the resultant color.

Reflection

Reflection occurs when rays of light strike a solid object and then bounce off of it. Depending on the spectral data (molecular structure or density) of the object or medium, certain wavelengths (colors) may be absorbed rather than reflected. The wavelengths that are reflected compose the color that is perceived. An object that reflects all light is perceived as white. An object that absorbs all light is perceived as black. In most cases, however, the object absorbs some wavelengths (colors) and reflects others. If this occurs, the object is perceived to be the color of the wavelengths that are reflected. For example, an object that absorbs green wavelengths but reflects red and blue wavelengths is perceived as a combination of red and blue (referred to as magenta).

Perception: The Eyes Have It

The wavelengths that reach the eye, whether by emission, transmission, or reflection, are received by the sensory cells on the retina—the rods and cones, as shown in Figure 11.4. Rods perceive the brightness of the

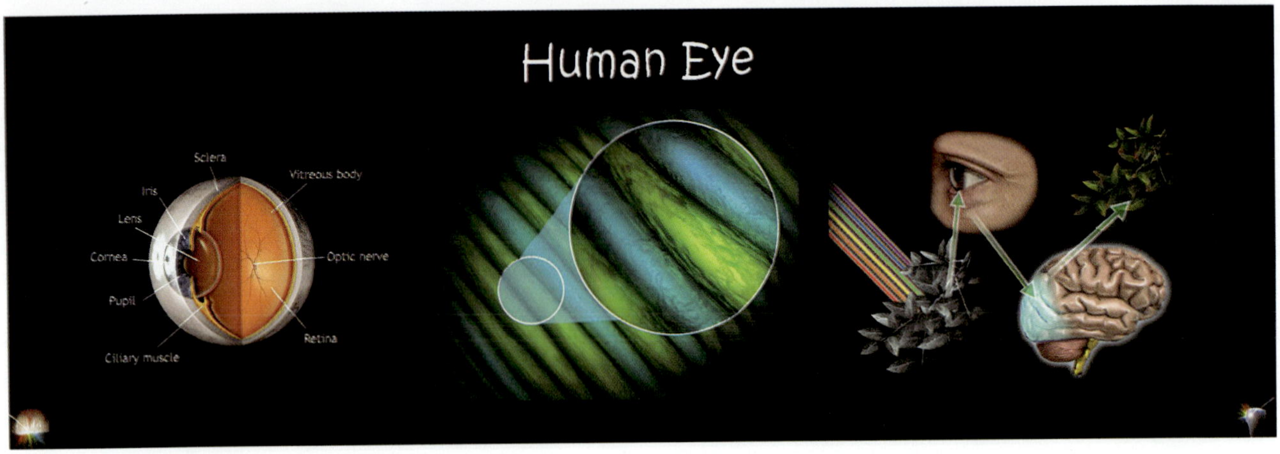

Figure 11.4. The retina of the eye contains three types of cone cells (represented as aqua color) responsible for color perception, as well as rod cells (represented as green color), which are responsible for perception of lightness and darkness. These cells send signals to the brain, resulting in color perception. Physiologically, the human eye possesses more rods cells than cones cells; therefore, we are able to perceive lightness/darkness greater than color. Reproduced by permission of Quintessence Publishing, copyright Quintessence.

color, or the intensity of the light rays reaching the eye. The cones perceive the hue, which is also known as the color tone. As discussed previously, the human eye contains three different types of cones, each one responsive to wavelengths approximating the colors red, green, and blue. Variations of these wavelengths stimulate each cone at different intensities. The cone cells then send signals to the brain, which translates the signals into colors.

Color Reproduction

Color is reproduced by means of 3-D color models that are based on the same mechanism by which color is perceived by the human eye (referred to as *tristimulus data*) as well as the emission, reflection, or transmission of light, depending on the medium. Colors may appear to be different depending on how they are reproduced. Tristimulus data are properties that describe how the color of an object appears to the observer or how the color data would be reproduced on a specific device such as a computer monitor or printer in terms of values.

Emissive Media: RGB Color Model

Electronic media such as computer monitors and television sets create color by emitting wavelengths that are mixtures of red, green, and blue (RGB) light to stimulate the cones in the human eye. Such media therefore can produce a color spectrum that includes nearly all of the colors in the visible spectrum. Theoretically, if the RGB wavelengths were to be combined, white light would result. For this reason, red, green, and blue are referred to as the additive primary colors. We start with black and color is created by adding certain amounts of RGB wavelengths of light. The process by which images are captured to be reproduced on emissive media, such as a digital camera, is similar to the process that occurs when the human eye perceives color. A digital camera picks up tiny pixels (picture elements) of red, green, and blue light and blends them together in varying intensities to create different colors. With that said, it is important to note that a digital camera carries the same subjective values as the human eye, and might not always be an accurate means to assess a patient's shade.

Reflective and Transmissive Media: CMY(K) Color Model

Media such as printed materials and photographs are considered reflective, and media such as slides and transparencies are considered transmissive, because they are visualized through the reflection of light off of their surfaces and the transmission of light through their surfaces, respectively. Color reproduction in reflective and transmissive media is based on the color-absorbing qualities of materials such as ink or dyes. These materials are formulated to absorb some wavelengths and reflect/transmit others to create specific colors.

The primary colors in these color systems are those created by the absorption of one of the RGB wavelengths and the reflection/transmission of the others. They are referred to as cyan, magenta, and yellow (CMY). Cyan is produced when red is absorbed and green and blue are reflected/transmitted; magenta is produced when green is absorbed and red and blue are reflected/transmitted; and yellow is produced when blue is absorbed and red and green are reflected/transmitted.

The absence (or subtraction) of these three colors would mean that no wavelengths could be absorbed, and therefore all wavelengths would be reflected/transmitted, resulting in the color white. For this reason, cyan, magenta, and yellow are referred to as the subtractive primary colors: Color is created by subtracting (absorbing) certain numbers of RGB wavelengths. Conversely, the presence of all three colors (CMY) should result in all wavelengths being absorbed and none reflected/transmitted (i.e., the color black).

Although this is true for CMY dyes used in photography, use of all three colors of printing ink actually results in a muddy brown because of inherent imperfections in the ink. Therefore, black (indicated by K in order to differentiate it from blue [B]) ink is usually added to improve the appearance of darker colors and to create better shadow density, which is why "CMYK" and "four-color processing" are the terms usually associated with full-color printing (Miller and Zaucha 1992).

Pigment Colors

Pigment colors contribute to the hues of an object. Because these colors are perceived through either transmission or reflection of light, they are essentially the same as the subtractive colors used in color reproduction for reflective and transmissive media, as discussed above. It is imperative to understand pigment colors in dentistry, especially because they are inherent in restorative materials such as ceramics, composites, and acrylic resins. Moreover, understanding primary, secondary, and complementary colors is critical to achieving accurate, esthetic shades.

The Primary Colors: Red, Yellow, Blue

The primary pigment colors are the same as the subtractive primaries, but they are referred to as red, yellow, and blue (instead of magenta, yellow, and cyan, respectively). Like the subtractive primaries, these are the colors that are perceived when one of the RGB wavelengths is absorbed. Red is perceived when green is absorbed; yellow is perceived when blue is absorbed; and blue is perceived when red is absorbed.

Secondary Colors: Orange, Green, Violet

The secondary colors are formed by combining two of the primary colors. For example, red and yellow create orange; yellow and blue create green; and blue and red create violet.

Complementary Colors

Complementary colors are so named because they "go well" together; these are the colors often seen paired in advertising. Complementary colors are those that, when combined in equal proportions, form a dull gray that absorbs and reflects/transmits all wavelengths in equal amounts, as shown in Figure 11.5. For example, orange and blue are complementary colors because orange is a combination of red and yellow, which absorb green and blue, respectively, while blue absorbs red. Other pairs of complementary colors include red/green and yellow/violet.

Dimensions of Color

Like the teeth and restorations we try to match, color is truly multidimensional. At the beginning of the twentieth century, Professor Albert H. Munsell (1969) noted that each color has a logical relationship to all other colors. He brought clarity to color communication by establishing an orderly system for accurately identifying every color. This "color wheel" includes the dimensions of hue, value, and chroma, as shown in Figure 11.6. To

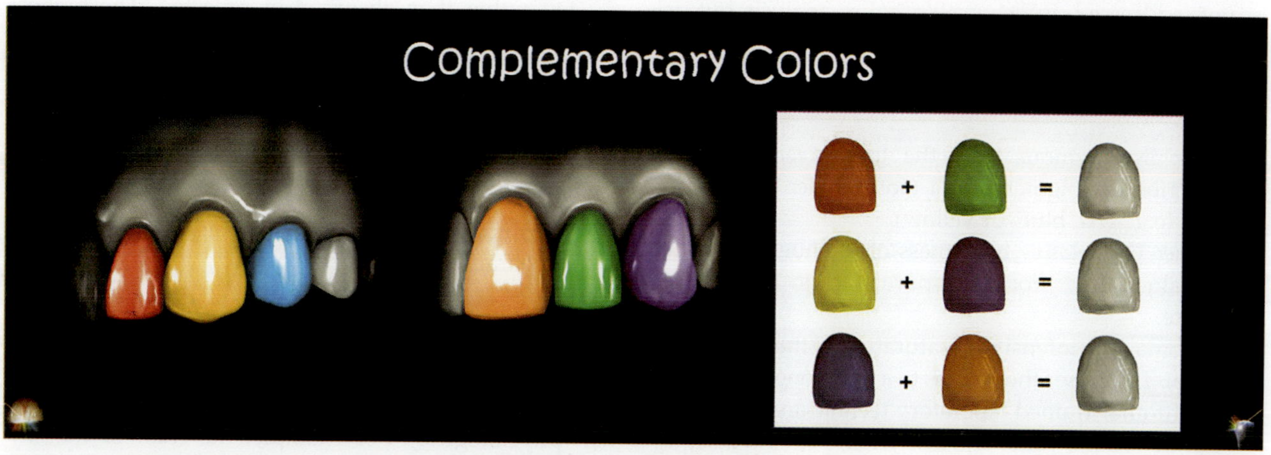

Figure 11.5. The primary pigment colors are referred to as red, yellow, and blue. The secondary pigment colors—orange, green, and violet—are formed when two primary colors are added together. When complementary colors are added together, they neutralize each other and form gray. This is clinically significant because complementary colors can be combined to lower the value of excessively bright restorations. Reproduced by permission of Quintessence Publishing, copyright Quintessence.

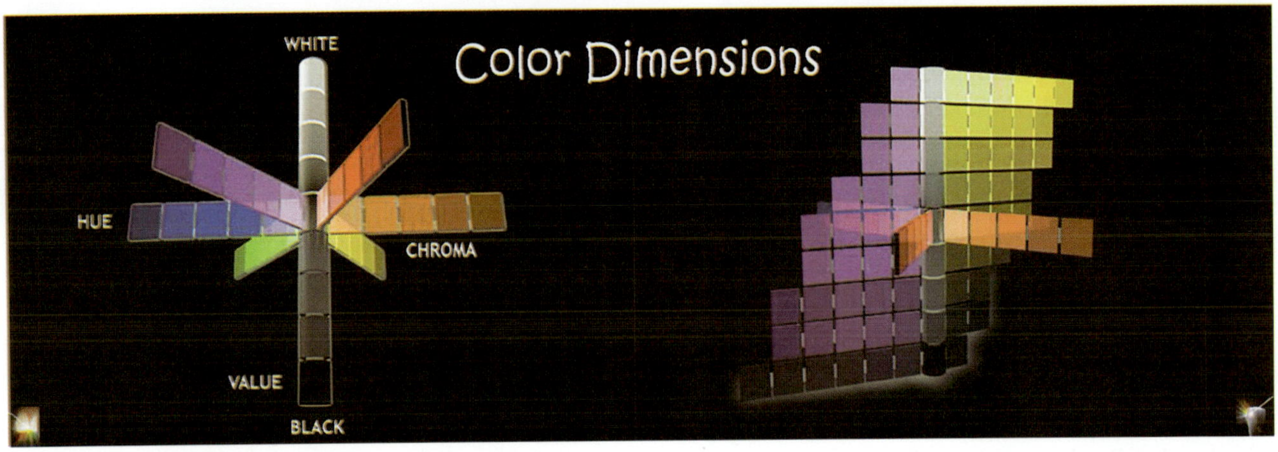

Figure 11.6. In Munsell's color wheel, color is described in terms of hue, chroma, and value. Reproduced by permission of Quintessence Publishing, copyright Quintessence.

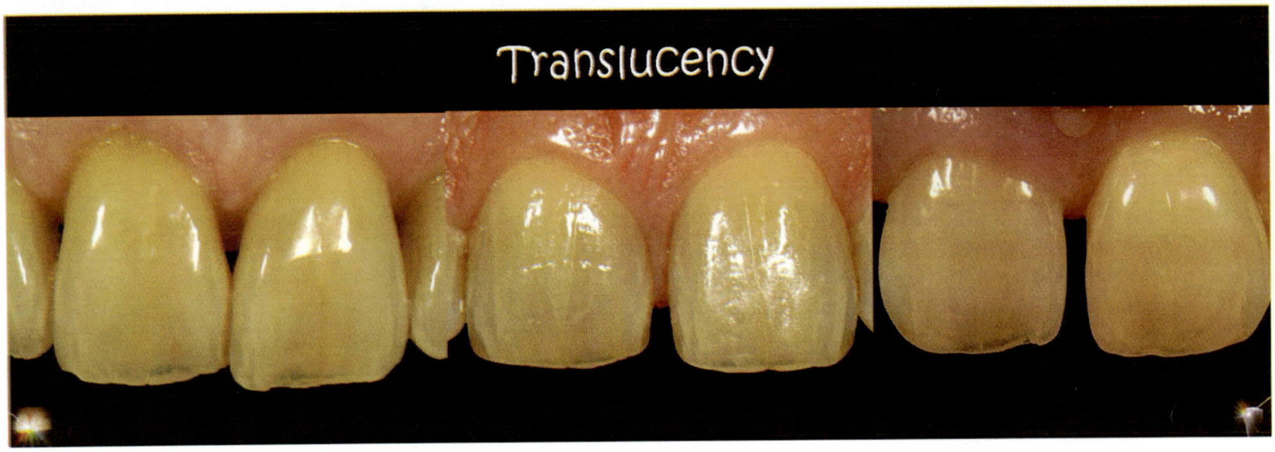

Figure 11.7. Various levels of translucency are exhibited by the natural dentition. Translucency is defined as the amount of transmitted light that passes through an object. The perception and quantification of translucency still remains elusive in dentistry. Reproduced by permission of Quintessence Publishing, copyright Quintessence.

these dimensions should be added translucency, which is not addressed in Munsell's color analysis but is perhaps the most critical factor in the quest for an esthetic restoration.

The four dimensions of color are defined as follows:

1. Hue: Synonymous with the term *color*. Used to describe the pigments of a tooth or dental restoration (e.g., red, blue, or yellow).
2. Value: The relative brightness of the hue. The scale of value ranges from 0 for pure black to 10 for pure white.
3. Chroma: The intensity or saturation of the color tone (hue). The closer the color is to a gray tone, the lower its chroma. Trained laboratory technicians generally can determine value and hue when presented separately. However, difficulties arise when value and chroma are coupled, and inconsistencies often occur when value determinations are made for dental restorations (Chu 2002b).
4. Translucency: The degree to which light is transmitted rather than absorbed or reflected. The highest translucency is defined as transparency (i.e., all light is transmitted), while the lowest is opacity (i.e., all light is reflected or absorbed). The incisal edges of natural teeth are translucent, and accurate translucency determination is vital to a restoration's esthetic success. (See Figure 11.7.) A mistake in translucency greatly compromises the natural appearance of a restoration.

Elements Affecting Color

There are many variables that affect how a color is perceived. These can be external (environmental) or internal (physiological). For example, the color of the sky cannot carry a blanket description of blue. The sky appears to be a different color in the morning than it does at midday or evening, with varying hues at different levels of relative lightness and brightness. The surrounding scenery, such as buildings, mountains, and vegetation, can create contrasts that affect the perceived color of the sky, particularly at the horizon. Moreover, different viewers may perceive the sky as being different colors even when viewing it under the same conditions. The same rules apply in the dental operatory during shade-matching procedures. The lighting conditions, the environment, and the viewer all play vital roles in color perception and evaluation (Sim et al. 2001).

Let There Be Light—The Right Light!

Without proper illumination, color can be neither accurately perceived nor correctly evaluated. (See Figure 11.8.) It is crucial to have sufficient lighting available to evaluate color properly, and it is also essential to achieve the proper quality of lighting in order to do so. This is accomplished by using the correct light intensity and the proper illuminants. However, even when these variables are well controlled, there are certain clinical challenges associated with lighting and shade matching that must be considered (i.e., light intensity, illuminants [light sources], metamerism, and environmental and human predispositions regarding perception).

Light Intensity

The intensity of light is the most common regulator of pupil diameter, which is a crucial factor in accurate shade matching (Carsten 2003). The accurate identification of color is only determined at the center of the visual field (i.e., what is perceived by the fovea). The fovea is located in the center of the retina and contains a high concentration of cone cells, which provide the greatest visual acuity and most accurate color perception. Much of the rest is "synthesized" by the visual cortex of the brain (Lamb and Bourriau 1995). Therefore, the most accurate color reading is obtained by the human eye when the pupil is opened just enough to fully expose the cones in the fovea. This is achieved by maintaining a lighting intensity of 150 to 200 foot-candles, as verified by a light meter.

Standard Illuminants (Light Sources)

The type of illuminant used can significantly impact the perception of color. A system created in 1931 by the Commission Internationale de l'Èclairage (CIE, which translates to International Commission on Illumination) categorized illuminants based on their effect on color perception (CIE 1971). This system was created to allow manufacturers of products such as paints and inks to specify and communicate the colors of their products. In their report, the CIE designated three standard illuminants, A, B, and C, to which they later added a series of D illuminants, a hypothetical E illuminant, and, unofficially, a series of fluorescents designated by the letter "F."

Clinical Challenges: Operatory Lighting

Dental professionals have long relied on so-called "color-corrected" lighting when evaluating tooth shade, yet using lights with that particular designation does not ensure accurate color matching (Carsten 2003). The reason for this is two-fold: conflicts in lighting and metamerism. The dental operatory has many sources of direct and indirect lighting to take into consideration. Light that streams in through a window mixes with the fluorescent light emanating from the hallway and the color-corrected lighting in the dental operatory. Amidst these various lighting conflicts, it is the job of the clinician to analyze the opposing teeth and determine an accurate shade match. The tips (Chu 2003) in the following sections aid in that process.

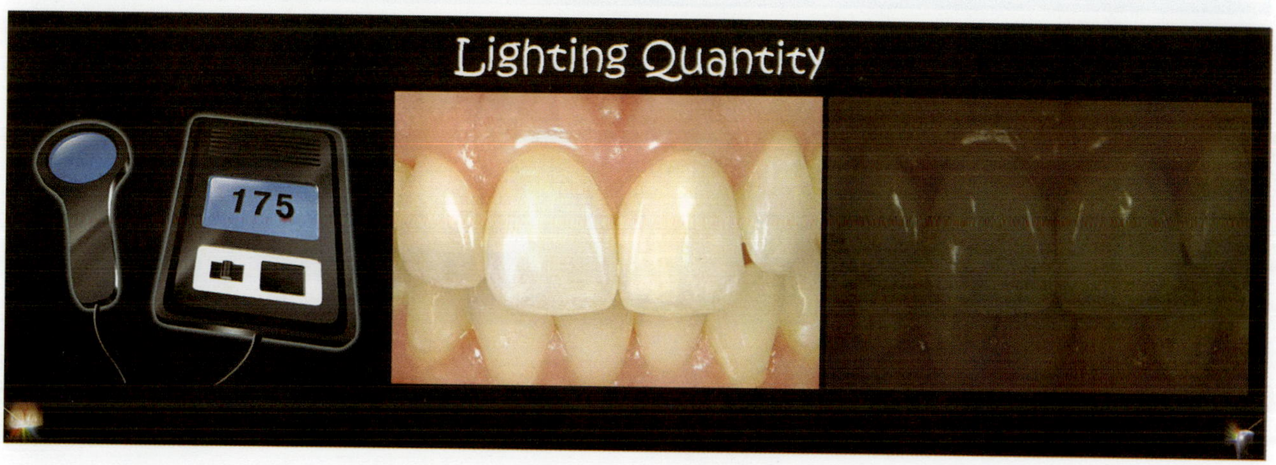

Figure 11.8. A light meter can be used to assess the proper quantity of light (150 to 200 foot-candles) in the dental operatory. Too much illumination obliterates detail necessary for accurate shade matching. Conversely, insufficient illumination makes it difficult to discern tooth shades as well. Reproduced by permission of Quintessence Publishing, copyright Quintessence.

Environmental Effects on the Perception of Color

Metamerism

Color-corrected lighting is designed to match the wavelengths and relative quantity of visible light coming from the sun; however, a person's smile will be viewed under any number of different lighting conditions, causing restorations to appear completely different in terms of hue, value, and chroma, as shown in Figures 11.9A–B. Like the restorations themselves, traditional shade tabs will appear different when viewed under various lighting conditions, creating difficulties in shade matching.

The phenomenon of two objects appearing to match in color in one setting, place, or environment, but showing apparent differences in others, is termed *metamerism*. This is known in some circles as the "jacket and pants problem." What can appear to be a perfectly matched pair under the fluorescent lighting of a clothing store can look significantly different in natural light. The two objects are referred to as a *metameric pair*.

In dental terms, metamerism occurs when a restoration is matched to the natural dentition under incandescent light, but, when viewed under color-corrected or fluorescent light, appears different in color when compared to the natural teeth. This can occur frequently, and mistakes can often be glaring, resulting in a return visit, an unhappy patient, and unproductive chair time. The only sure way to avoid metamerism is to achieve a spectral curve match. Pairs of colored objects that have the same spectral curve always match, regardless of the light in which they are viewed. Advanced technology in dentistry has greatly increased the chances of achieving a spectral curve match. Pairs of colored objects that do not have the same spectral components may or may not match under different lighting conditions.

Although some manufacturers have tried to combat metamerism by developing materials that exhibit a chameleon effect by taking on the color of their surroundings, metamerism continues to be a problem in the dental operatory. (See Figure 11.10.) Metamerism complicates shade selection and, on the whole, can only be

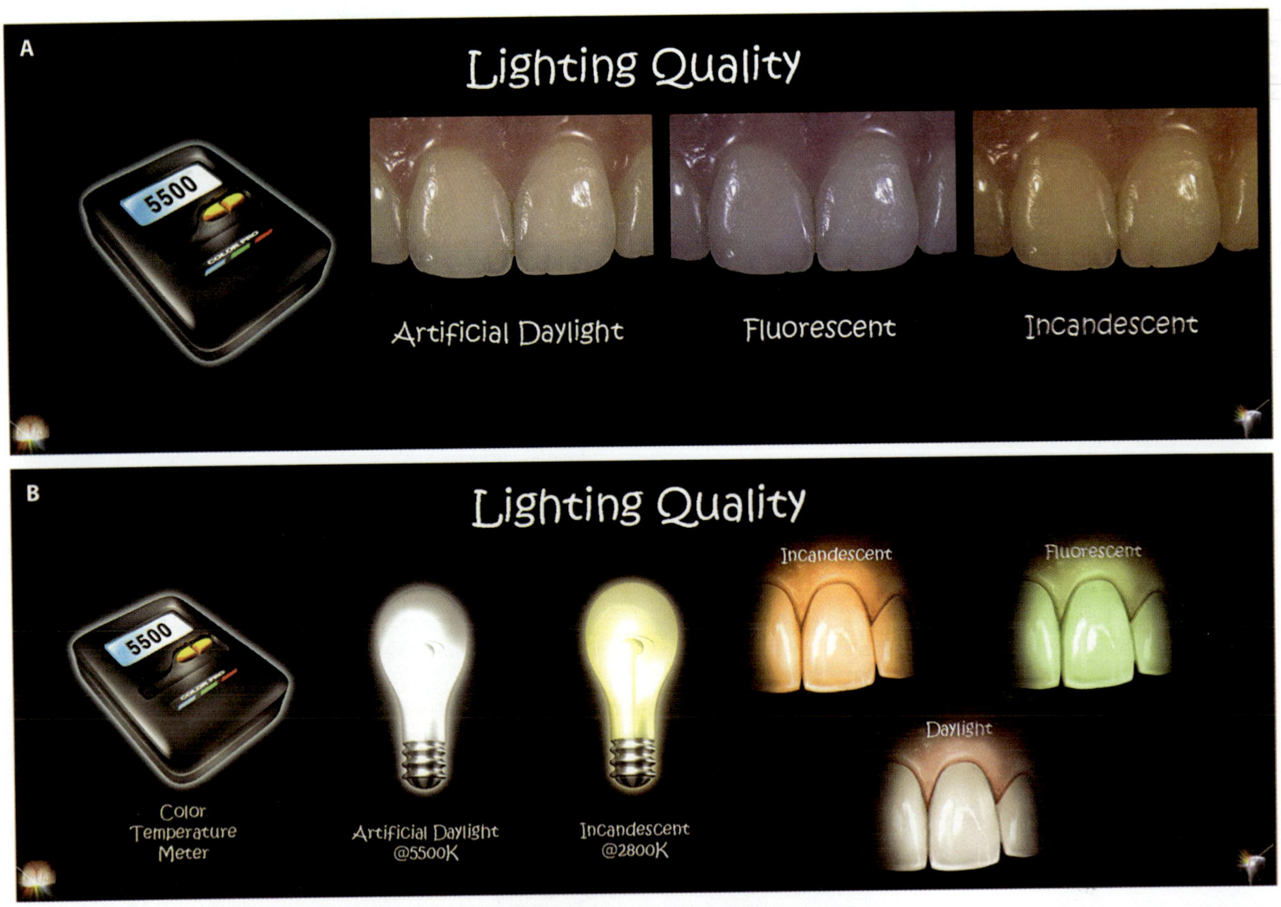

Figure 11.9A, B. A color temperature meter measures the quality of lighting. The proper color temperature for the dental operatory is about 5,500°K. Here we see the same two maxillary anterior central incisors viewed under artificial daylight, fluorescent light, and incandescent light, respectively, demonstrating that operatory lighting conditions have a big impact on tooth shade and color perception. Reproduced by permission of Quintessence Publishing, copyright Quintessence.

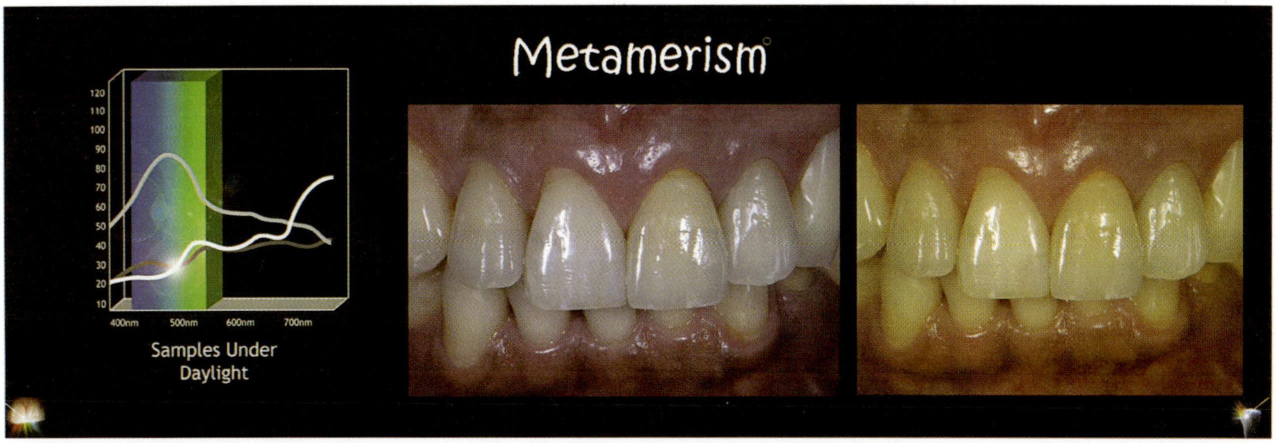

Figure 11.10. Metamerism in action: The graph shows spectral curves for light source approximating daylight conditions (gray line) and two gray objects (white and black lines). Note that the objects appear to match under these lighting conditions where the lines intersect in the graph at 500 nm. The crown on the left side photo shown under fluorescent lighting appears to match very well. However, the same crown shown in the right side photo under incandescent lighting least appears to match under this common household lighting. Reproduced by permission of Quintessence Publishing, copyright Quintessence.

Table 11.2 Clinical significance of contrast effects.

Contrast Effect	Clinical Effect	Clinical Application
Value	Correlated to surrounding environment; i.e., skin tone, hair color, eye color, and the value of the adjacent dentition and periodontium. A darker environment imparts the perception of object lightness.	Select brighter shades for light-toned patients; darker shades for pigment-toned individuals since the tendency is for the opposite contrast to occur (teeth will appear darker for lighter patients and vice versa). Error toward the value tendency of the surrounding is dentition (i.e., low value if dentition is dark; high value if dentition light).
Hue	The complementary color of the surrounding background or environment is more apparent.	Use a light blue or neutral gray (18%) when selecting shades to eliminate surrounding distractions as well as precondition the eyes for improved perception of color (complementary) tones.
Areal	Size does matter: larger teeth will tend to look brighter; bright teeth will appear to look larger; dark teeth will appear smaller.	Consider decreasing the value and/or increasing the chroma of the restoration by half a shade.
Spatial	Tooth position will affect the perception of brightness/darkness. More recessed teeth will appear darker; more protruding teeth will appear brighter.	Recessed teeth can be made brighter; protruding teeth can be made darker. Consider orthodontic therapeutic correction, bleaching, or conservative esthetic restoration.

recognized and explained. With all variables being equal, there is often no solution to it. Therefore, clinicians must explain to patients that in some situations a restoration may not match as well as in others and that this is an occurrence, not a fault (Sproull 1973).

Proper Shade Selection: It's Actually a Matter of Contrast

Understanding how color perception can potentially deviate due to various contrast effects allows the dentist to select a shade more effectively. With a working knowledge of how opposing and adjacent colors can play tricks on the interpreter, the chances for an accurate shade match can be dramatically improved. (See Table 11.2.)

Simultaneous Contrast

Simultaneous contrast occurs when two objects are observed at the same time. When perceiving more than one color at once, the brain attempts to achieve a harmonic balance of the colors. Perception of the color therefore is affected by two factors: (1) its surrounding relative lightness, making the color appear to be darker or lighter; and (2) its surrounding color, making the color appear to have shifted toward its surrounding color's complement. Identical colors will appear to be different when framed by different backgrounds or patterns in reference to brightness and color.

Value Contrast

Visual judgment of brightness is not dependable, primarily because the relative brightness of an object is affected by the brightness of the contrasting background or surroundings. For example, if the surrounding background is dark, an object will appear light. However, if the same object is placed against a lighter background, it is perceived as darker. (See Figure 11.11.)

This illustrates that the perceived brightness can vary, even though the reflectivity of the object is constant. This is because the retina is very sensitive to light. It expands and contracts in response to varying light intensities as they are interpreted by the brain. If the background is darker than the object, the retina must adapt to the relatively brighter object, causing the brain to perceive it as brighter than it would be if the object were viewed by itself. If the background is lighter than the object, the opposite effect results. However, because the eye adapts much more quickly from dark to light than from light to dark, the effect of a darker object on a lighter background is always more pronounced.

A practical dental example of this phenomenon is when a restoration is viewed adjacent to inflamed gingival tissues. (See Figure 11.12.) The redness (darkness) of the gums (background) distorts color perception, making the restoration (object) appear brighter. As a result, a crown that is too low in value (dark) may be chosen. The mistake becomes apparent when the tissues heal and the crown appears too dark because the shade was selected falsely dark under those pretenses and poor shade selection conditions.

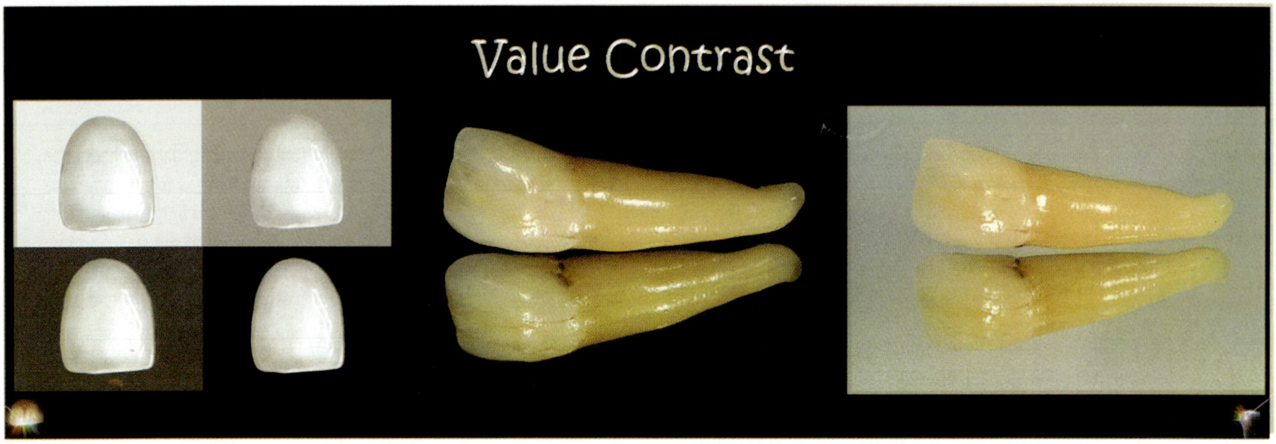

Figure 11.11. The value contrast effect makes the same tooth appear increasingly lighter as the background becomes darker. Reproduced by permission of Quintessence Publishing, copyright Quintessence.

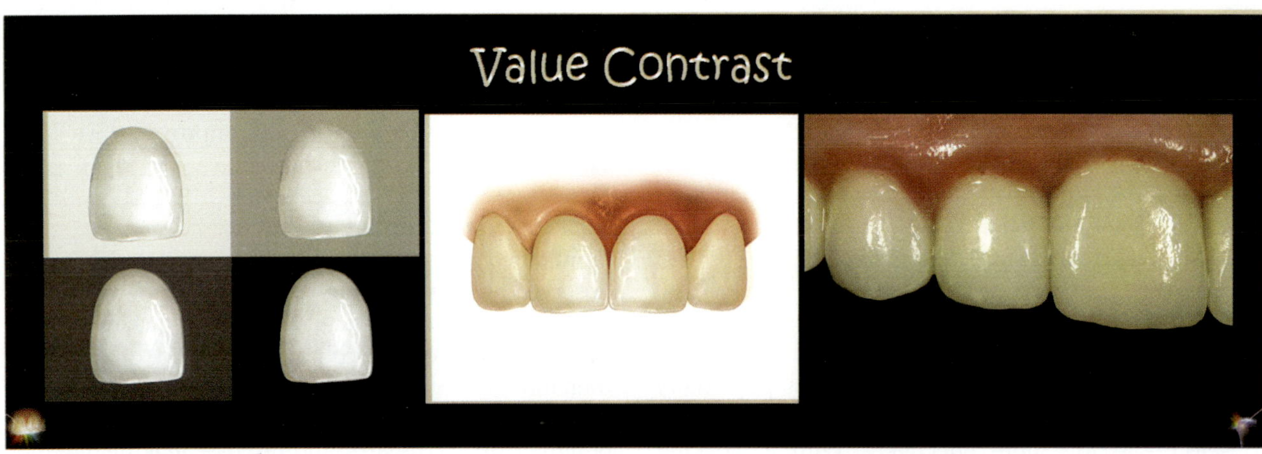

Figure 11.12. Value contrast effects have clinical significance when dealing with excessively inflamed gingival tissues. The dark value of the inflamed gums will trick the eyes into perceiving the tooth shade as being lighter than it actually is. As a result, the fabricated restoration will appear too dark once the tissues have healed. Reproduced by permission of Quintessence Publishing, copyright Quintessence.

Hue Contrast

A color will be perceived differently when viewed in conjunction with various background or adjacent colors with contrasting hues. For example, a tooth or restoration appears bluish against an orange background and purplish if the background is yellow. (See Figure 11.13.) When a color is viewed simultaneously with another color, the perceived hue of the first color appears more similar to the complementary color of the second color. Using this contrast effect, dental professionals can precondition their eyes when taking shades by first looking at a complementary color, then looking at the tooth shades. This allows the clinician to see the color of the tooth shades more effectively.

Chroma Contrast

This contrast follows the same effect as the value and hue contrasts. An image appears darker against a light background, which is low in chroma (light), and brighter against a more chromatic background, which is high in chroma (dark). However, there is a variation to the theme: the closer the tooth is to the hue and chroma of the surrounding background, the less visible it becomes, and therefore it is difficult to distinguish the shade of the tooth. (See Figure 11.14.)

Areal Contrast

The size of the object can also influence visual color perception. For instance, a larger object appears brighter than a smaller object of the same color. Likewise, a brighter object appears to be larger than a darker object of the same size, as shown in Figure 11.15. This type of contrast accounts for the fact that darker clothes have a tendency to make an individual look smaller and thinner, while whiter clothes tend to make the individual appear larger and heavier.

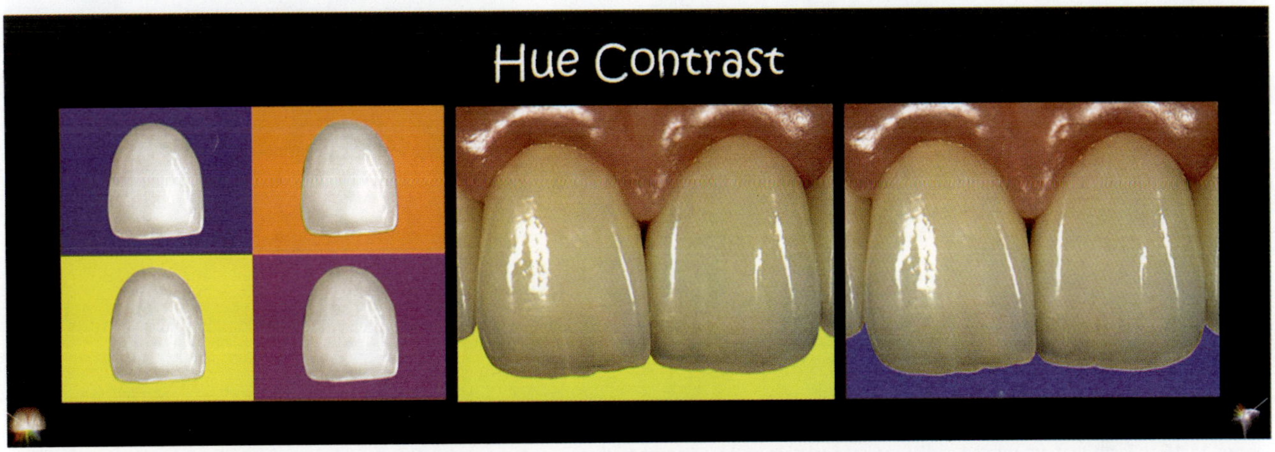

Figure 11.13. When viewed against different background colors, the teeth appear to take on the hue of the background's complementary color. The yellow background causes the ceramic veneer to take on a purple case, and the same veneers appear orange in hue against a blue background. Reproduced by permission of Quintessence Publishing, copyright Quintessence.

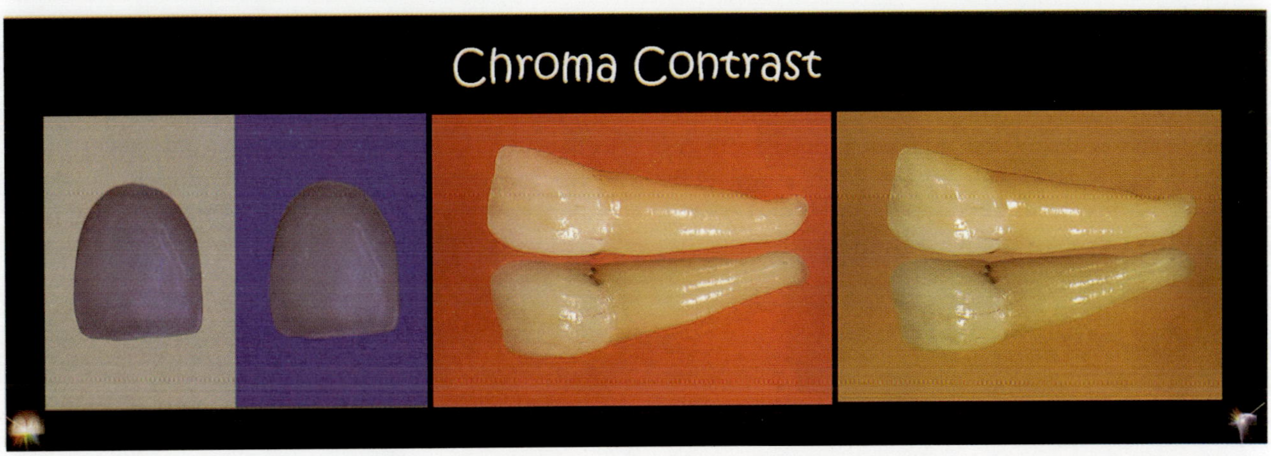

Figure 11.14. Against a background that is low in chroma, the tooth appears much more vibrant when compared to the same tooth against a background that closely matches the chroma of the tooth. The ceramic tooth against the orange background is not as visible because the orange is a similar chroma. The ceramic tooth against the yellow-orange background is even less visible because the background very closely approximates the tooth's chroma. Reproduced by permission of Quintessence Publishing, copyright Quintessence.

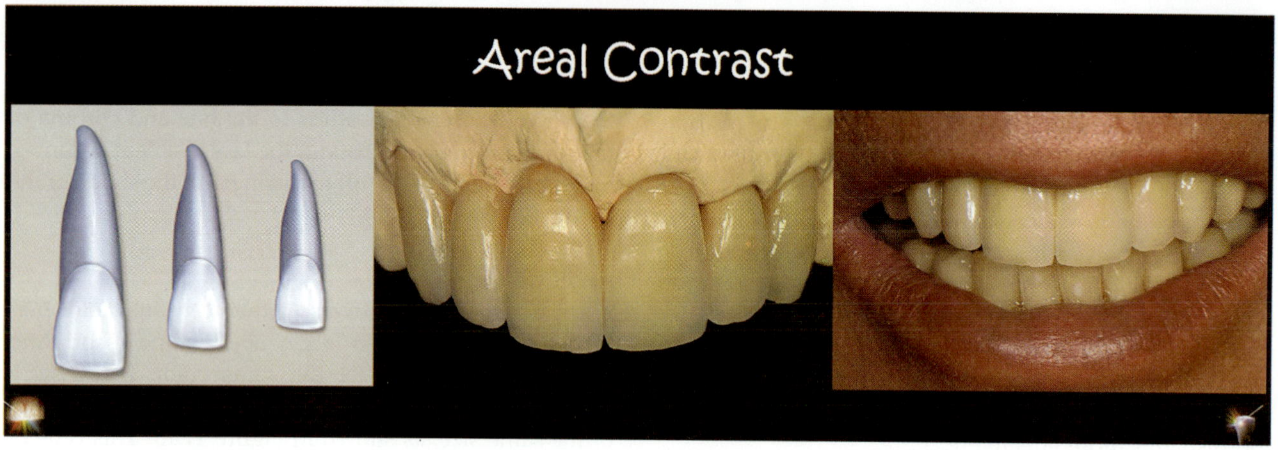

Figure 11.15. A large image appears lighter since the surface area is greater and reflects more light back to the observer. Even though all of the teeth in this clinical case of very large maxillary incisors (as part of a fixed prosthesis) are the same shade (Vita A3), the central incisors appear lighter because of areal contrast effects. Reproduced by permission of Quintessence Publishing, copyright Quintessence.

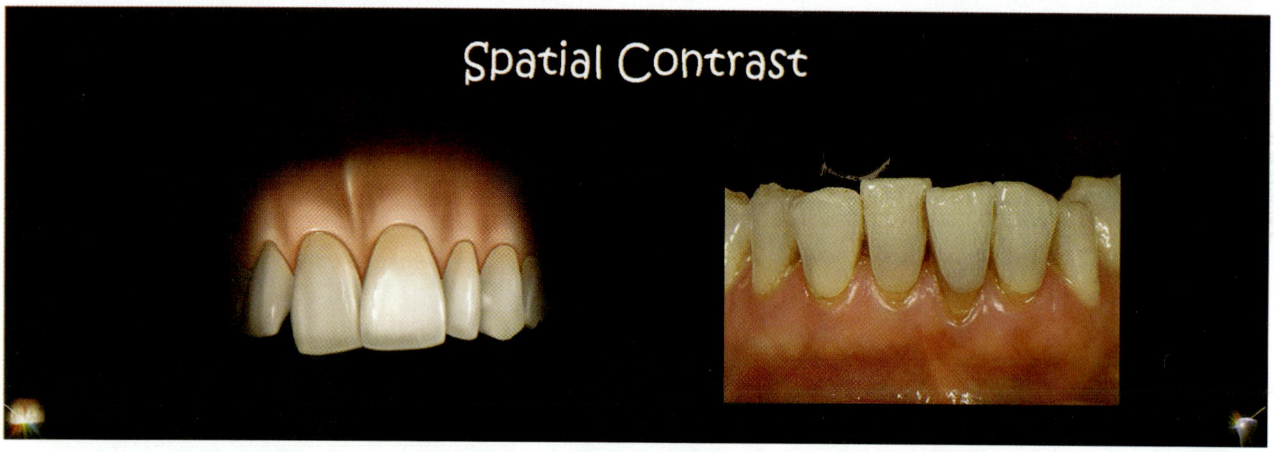

Figure 11.16. Teeth that are rotated and/or recessed relative to the adjacent teeth appear to be darker. The clinical example on the right shows a mandibular right central incisor that appears darker than the other teeth because of its recessed position. Reproduced by permission of Quintessence Publishing, copyright Quintessence.

Spatial Contrast

An object closer to the observer appears larger and brighter, whereas a more recessed object appears to be smaller and not as bright. This phenomenon is frequently seen with rotated and overlapped teeth, as shown in Figure 11.16. The recessed teeth appear to be darker. Posterior teeth also appear to be darker, and the shadows in the mouth further contribute to this appearance.

Successive Contrast

Successive contrast occurs when one color is viewed following the observation of another color. The visual perception remains after the eye has left the object. Afterimages are categorized as positive (similar) or negative (different). Positive afterimages have the same color as the original perception; negative afterimages have the opposite or complementary color to the original perception. Positive afterimages occur following a short visual interaction, while negative afterimages occur after long visual contact with an object. The physiochemical effect is that the neurotransmitter "rodopsin" in the cones of the retina are quickly depleted during prolonged staring. Therefore, the ability to see that color is no longer a physical reality.

Physiological (Viewer-Dependent) Effects

Color Blindness

A person with color blindness has trouble seeing red, green, blue, or mixtures of these colors. The term "color vision problem" is often used instead of color blindness because most people with color blindness can see some color. Although the condition might be perceived as rare,

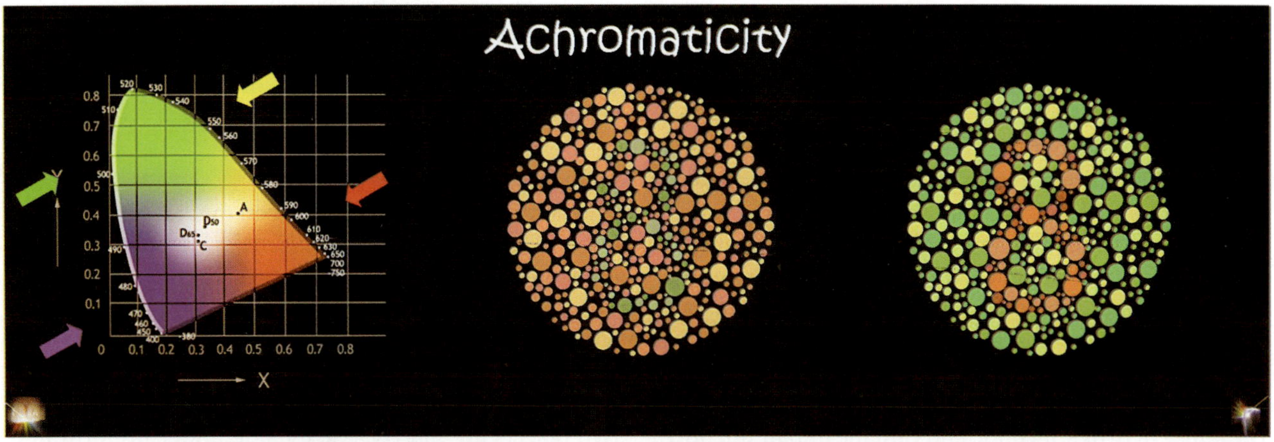

Figure 11.17. The chromaticity diagram shows the distribution of color that the cones of the human eye can perceive. The cones are most sensitive to reds and purples (wider area of the graph) than they are to greens and yellows (narrower area of the graph). Therefore, is more difficult to see the yellow-green number 8 in the middle image than it is to see the red-purple number 8 in the far right image because of the physiologic limitations of the human eye as it relates to color perception. Reproduced by permission of Quintessence Publishing, copyright Quintessence.

approximately 10% of U.S. males (but only 0.3% of U.S. females) are affected by color blindness (Chu et al. 2004, p. 31). Most optical exams include tests for color blindness, as shown in Figure 11.17. Color blindness is caused by a deficiency in or absence of one or more of the three types of photosensitive pigments able to detect red, green, and blue. The essential effect of color blindness is that hues that appear different to most people look the same to those with color blindness. This is a serious problem for a clinician performing shade matching, since determining the hue, value, and chroma of a restoration is critical to the natural appearance of the restoration.

Age

Aging is detrimental to color-matching abilities because the cornea and lens of the eye become yellowed with age, imparting a yellow-brown bias and causing the differentiation between white and yellow to become increasingly difficult. This process begins at age 30, becomes more noticeable after age 50, and has clinical significance after 60 years of age. After age 60, many people have significant difficulties in perceiving blues and purples (Wasson and Schuman 1992, Quackenbush 1997, Rosenthal and Phillips 1997).

Fatigue

Tired eyes cannot perceive colors as accurately as alert eyes. Compromised visual perception is the consequence of systemic, local, and/or mental fatigue. The inability to accurately determine hue and chroma is most evident during times of fatigue; in addition, color may be perceived as faded or blurry. Successive shade observations (i.e., a lot of patients requiring shade assessment during a typical work day) can be one of the primary causes of fatigue. Fatigue is the most common cause for an inaccurate shade match.

Nutrition

An individual's eating habits play an important role in the health of the eye. Some scientists have suggested that there is an association between macular degeneration (a physical disturbance of the center of the retina, called the macula, which causes gradual loss of vision) and a large intake of substances high in saturated fat (The Schepens Eye Research Institute 2003). There is also evidence that eating fresh fruits and dark green, leafy vegetables may delay or reduce the severity of macular degeneration. Additionally, supplementation with antioxidants such as vitamins C and E has been shown to have positive effects in slowing the progression of the disease in some cases. Other trace minerals and nutrients such as zinc and lutein are also important for the health of the eyes (Age-Related Eye Disease Study Research Group 2001). An individual's nutrition is an essential factor in the overall health of the body, and the eye is certainly no exception.

Emotions

Color can function as a language. For example, in many places throughout the world, red suggests anger or passion, yellow represents joy, and blue is associated with sadness. Without delving into the complexity of the human emotional tie to color, it is worthwhile to note the following scientific evidence, which is significant to the dental professional.

It is generally known that emotion can affect pupillary diameter, causing dilation or constriction, and, as stated in the previous discussions about light intensity and light/dark contrast, pupillary diameter has a direct effect on color discrimination. Additionally, it has been shown that in the practice of meditation, a subject can be trained to control brain wave patterns to favor delta waves. When in meditation, people report the appearance of colored halos around objects, as well as other alterations of visual perception. It is therefore clear that regardless of how a color may affect a person's mood, the initial mood or mental state of the observer can be a critical factor in color determination (Gimbel 1994).

Medications

The abuse of drugs, alcohol, and caffeine impair not only judgment, but also color perception. In addition, many prescription and even over-the-counter medications are associated with visual side effects. Medications can act on any part of the visual system, from the visual cortex to the retina. Like all drug side effects, they vary from person to person. Some side effects are neither predictable nor apparent to the individual taking the medication. It is safe to assume that most dentists will take some medication in their lives, and the older people get the more likely they are to take multiple medications. Viagra, a drug used to treat erectile dysfunction, is notorious for causing vision to have a blue tint, which makes it difficult to distinguish between blue and green. As a result of these findings, the Federal Aviation Administration (FAA) now requires all commercial airline pilots to refrain from the consumption of Viagra 12 hours prior to flight time (Carsten 2003). Of special concern for dentists, particularly female practitioners, are the side effects caused by oral contraceptives (i.e., red-green or yellow-blue discrimination defects). They also can cause a blue tinge, and there are several studies that indicate that long-term use of oral contraceptives causes a decrease in color perception of blues and yellows (Fraunfelder 1996).

Binocular Difference

The perception difference between the right eye and the left eye is called *binocular difference*. It often becomes evident during an eye exam when a person can see the vision chart better with one eye than the other. While color disparity between a person's eyes is relatively minor, one should be aware of it and, if necessary, compensate for it. To check for binocular color difference, two objects are placed side by side under uniform illumination, as shown in Figure 11.18. They may appear different (e.g., the one on the right may seem slightly lighter than the one on the left). A binocular color difference exists if the object on the right still appears lighter when the placement is reversed. (It is not uncommon during a routine eye examination that color blindness tests are conducted to establish the patient's deficiencies between each eye).

Materials Selection: The "Optical Triad"

The choice of material is extremely important to determine the accuracy of a shade. The relative translucency of the tooth to be matched and the material selected must coincide. Bleached teeth can be especially problematic to match. This is because color is achromatic; hue is white, chroma is low (little saturation of hue), and value is high (bright). Value is the only tangible parameter that can be addressed, but it relates to opacity and translucency. Therefore, material selection is signifi-

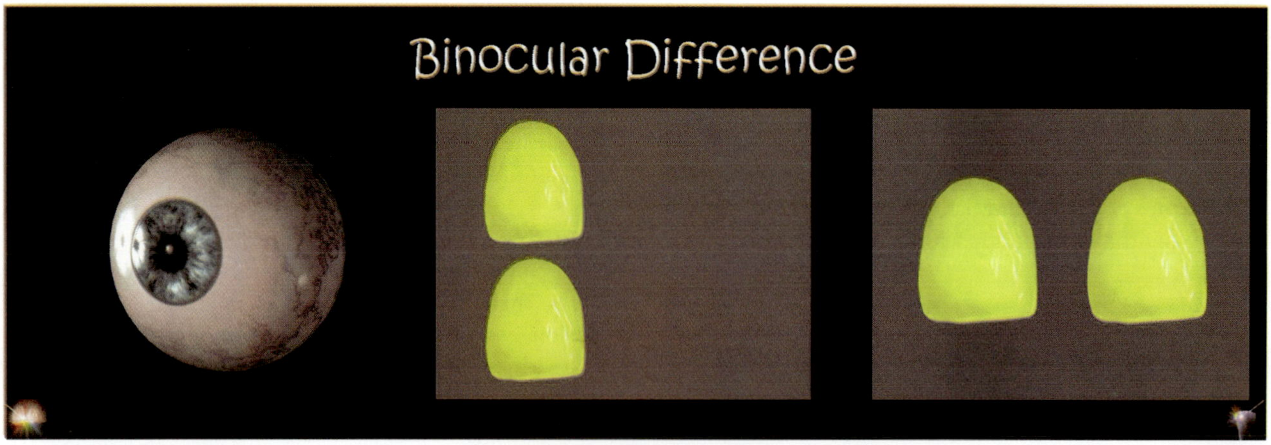

Figure 11.18. When two objects of the same shape and color are arranged side by side, they may appear to be different. For example, one may seem to be slightly lighter than the other. However, if the two objects are placed on the same side, the effect is not evident. That is because the left and right eyes do not see color and brightness the same. Reproduced by permission of Quintessence Publishing, copyright Quintessence.

cantly more important. Certain materials are higher in translucency (synthetic ceramics) while others are higher in opacity (zirconia and alumina); therefore, identification of the material's inherent qualities is imperative when quantifying shade. These qualities, fluorescence, opalescence, and translucency, make up the "optical triad," and it is the job of the dentist-technician team to recognize and account for those variances.

Fluorescence and Opalescence

For clinicians who practice esthetic restorative dentistry, particularly in the field of ceramics, fluorescence is an important physical property. By their very nature, teeth and more specifically, dentine, are fluorescent because they emit visible light when exposed to ultraviolet light. Fluorescence adds to the natural look of a restoration and minimizes the metameric effect. When creating a restoration, the porcelain consists of agents that cause the restoration to react and become fluorescent. On the other hand, opalescence is the ability of a translucent material to appear blue in reflected light and red-orange in transmitted light. Fluorescence and opalescence both contribute to the vitality of a restoration (Leinfelder 2000, Chu et al. 2004).

Fluorescence, opalescence, and translucency are responsible for the vivacity of natural teeth and dental porcelain. The opalescent effect is based on the behavior of translucency of natural teeth. Under direct illumination, the shorter wavelengths of the visible spectrum (blue = 400 nanometer [nm]) are reflected from the fine particle size of natural enamel and dental porcelain giving the white tooth color a bluish appearance while the longer wavelengths (red-orange = 700 nm) are absorbed. In transillumination, however, light penetrating through a natural tooth appears orange because the longer wavelengths are reflected at the surface and, conversely, the shorter blue wavelengths are absorbed. This effect, known in optical physics as the "Tyndall Effect," is called opalescence of natural teeth. Both opalescence and fluorescence are responsible for the intrinsic brilliance of natural teeth that we try to imitate when fabricating artificial restorations made of dental porcelains while depth of vitality is conveyed through translucency. (See Figure 11.19.)

Bleaching

What are white teeth? Essentially the color white is a contradiction. It is scientifically described as being completely reflective of all visible wavelengths of light (Roy G. Biv). White is not a color; all it describes is the level of brightness or translucency of a tooth or restoration. When you bleach teeth, you're increasing the relative lightness (value) of the teeth, making them appear whiter. Therefore, bleaching teeth is associated with a loss of colored pigments in the tooth structure. Bleaching does not necessarily imply that the teeth are becoming more opaque and reflective. It means that intrinsic colored pigments are removed and a tooth can become whiter yet can remain highly translucent.

Usually, bleaching is performed through the application of a gel containing oxidants (i.e., carbamide-peroxide). Oxygen radicals released from the gel penetrate the enamel and oxidize many of the dark colorants in the dentine layer that may be of intrinsic or extrinsic origin. The structure of the teeth remains the same, yet the value of the teeth increases. A myriad of factors can influence the dental professional's color assessment. When using

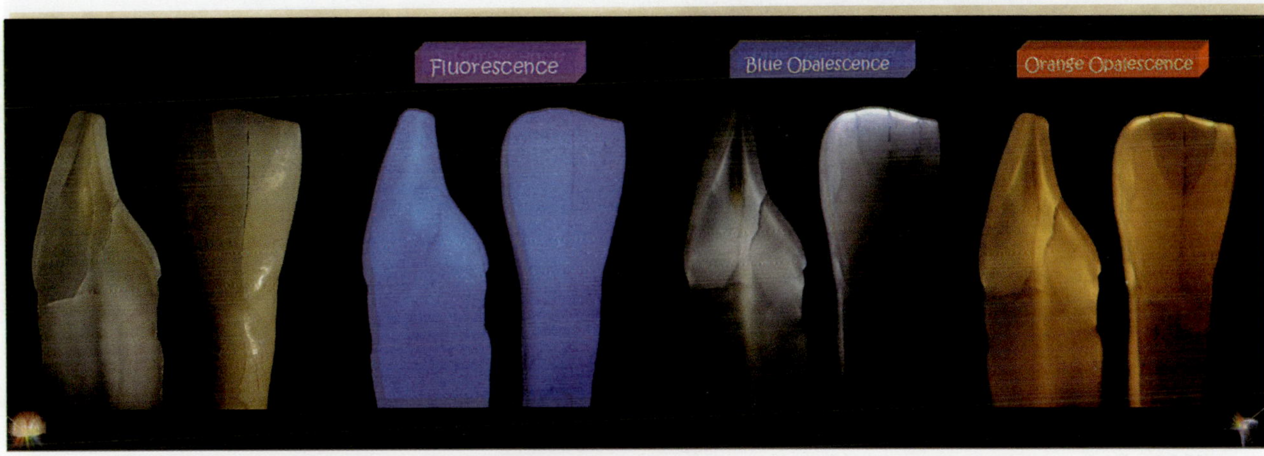

Figure 11.19. On the far left are extracted teeth under natural daylight conditions. The same teeth under ultraviolet light show a greater fluorescence of the dentinal layer compared with the enamel layer. A blue opalescent effect is caused by the reflection and transmission of the shorter blue wavelengths of light, and an orange opalescent effect is caused by the transmission and reflection of the longer red-yellow (orange) wavelengths and the absorption of blue wavelengths. Reproduced by permission of Quintessence Publishing, copyright Quintessence.

traditional shade-matching techniques, the dental professional should consider several variables. For example, changes in operatory lighting, fatigued eyes, and various contrast effects can create optical illusions. Additionally, the side effects associated with the use of oral contraceptives are a problem primarily for female practitioners, and the high incidence of color blindness among U.S. males is of equal concern. Although no dental practitioner can read color perfectly, and no dental operatory is free from problems, a thorough understanding of the potential factors affecting color perception allows the dental professional to compensate for them as required to achieve the most accurate shade matching possible.

Steps to Predictable Shade Matching and Color Communication: 7-Step Approach to Successful Shade Matching

The seven steps to successful shade matching are:

1. Patient/Tooth Evaluation
2. Image Capture/Shade Analysis
3. Communication
4. Interpretation
5. Fabrication
6. Verification
7. Placement of Restoration.

Shade matching is a critical final step in implant dentistry because implants require indirect restorations. By now you should understand the complexity involved in matching a shade. The variables in the dental treatment room and human error are recognized obstacles. Color is both a science and an art, and can often be difficult to measure. Historically, conventional shade methods and technology by themselves have limitations, since technicians require more "visual" information to interpret shade information (Quintessence Publishing 2004).

Advances in technology have greatly elevated the likelihood of a clinically acceptable shade match through accurate shade analysis, if properly performed. After much research and clinical evaluation, this segment of the chapter addresses a culmination of knowledge that embodies how the authors perceive predictable shade matching. A step-by-step protocol to shade matching is comprehensively outlined through a case study using a combination of the technology-based instrumentation, conventional techniques (i.e., shade tabs), and reference photography, a wonderful way for predictable shade-matching limiting remakes.

Predictable Shade-matching Protocol

Step 1: Evaluation This phase of treatment may be the most clinically significant because proper shade matching depends directly upon the tooth type (i.e., whether the tooth is high or low in translucency). (See Figure 11.20.)

This affects material selection, since the choices of materials that can be used for the definitive restoration (i.e., ceramometal, as shown in Figures 11.21 and 11.22) or high strength computer-aided design/computer-aided manufacturing (CAD/CAM)-based ceramics (such as alumina or zirconia, as shown in Figure 11.23) will ultimately dictate the tooth/abutment preparation

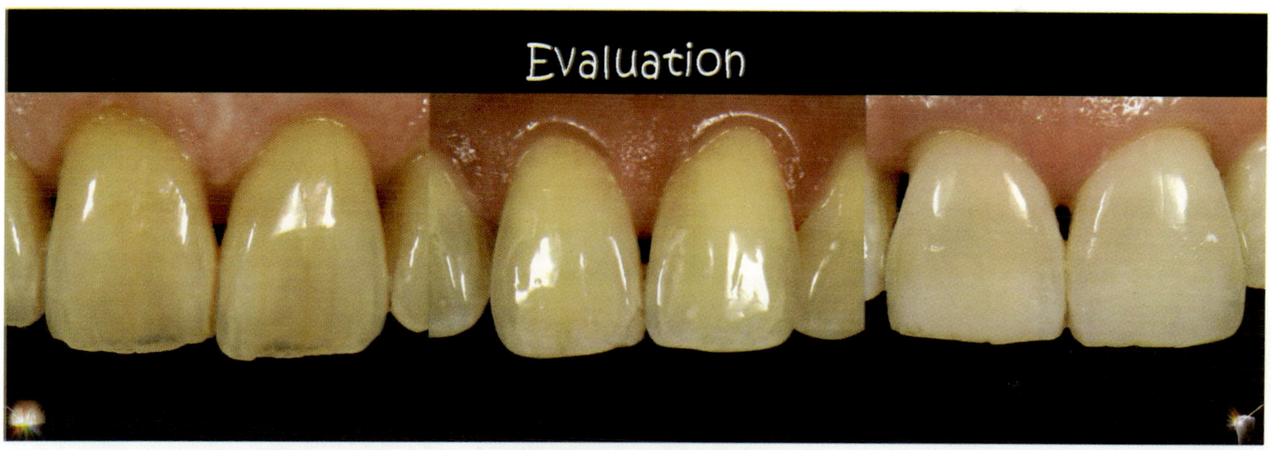

Figure 11.20. The central incisor teeth represented in this photograph on the far left are high in translucency. Note the orange amber opalescence through the middle-incisal third of the teeth and the blue opalescence/translucency at the incisal edge. Materials selection for these teeth, if they should ever require treatment, may comprise the following list: all-ceramic feldspathic bonded restorations, leucite reinforced pressable ceramics, porcelain butt margin CAD/CAM-based ceramics such as zirconia or alumina. The central incisor teeth represented on the far right are low in translucency, or high in opacity. Matching these teeth, if necessary, would be serviced nicely with ceramometal restorations. Reproduced by permission of Quintessence Publishing, copyright Quintessence.

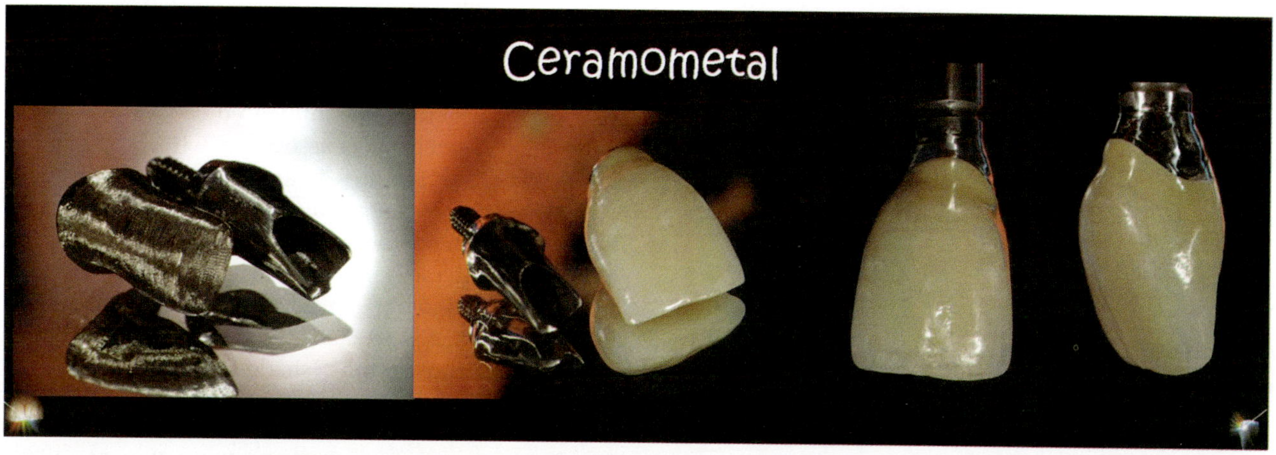

Figure 11.21. A 135-degree angular shoulder (45-degree beveled shoulder) preparation can be used for the custom implant abutment, which requires a slight metal collar for the cement-retained final restoration. Reproduced by permission of Quintessence Publishing, copyright Quintessence.

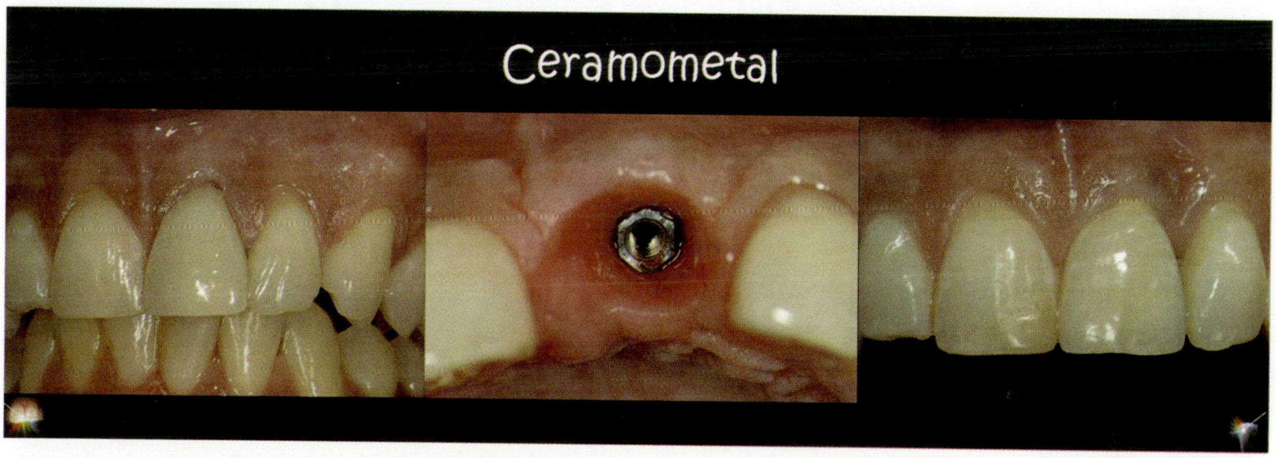

Figure 11.22. The definitive implant restoration replacing tooth No. 9 with a cement-retained ceramometal restoration matching tooth No. 8, which has low translucency/high opacity. Reproduced by permission of Quintessence Publishing, copyright Quintessence.

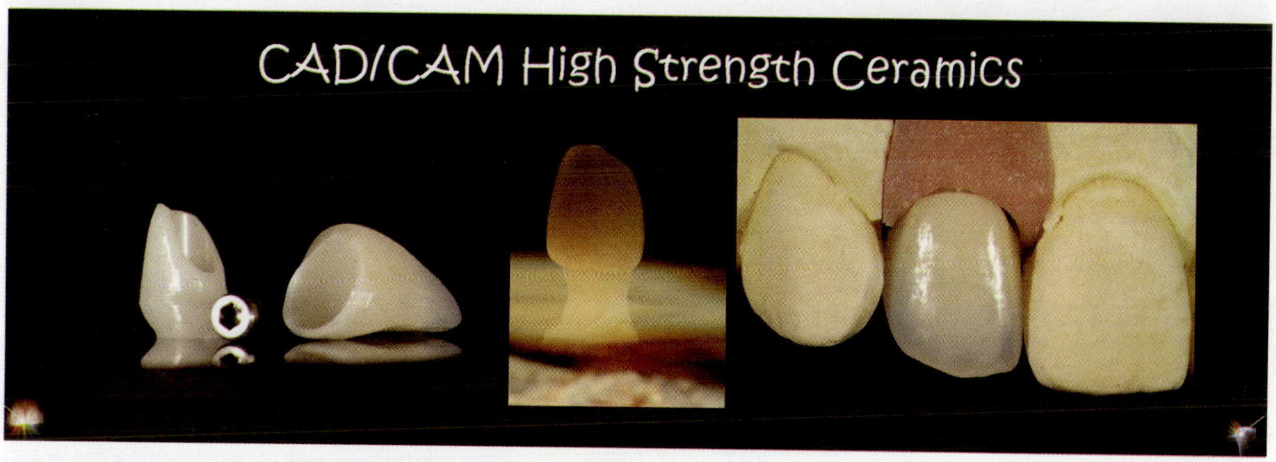

Figure 11.23. High strength CAD/CAM materials are available in various types of ceramic (i.e., alumina and zirconia) to satisfy the strength and esthetic requirements anywhere in the mouth. They possess light transmission qualities greater than that of ceramometal restorations. However, optical properties vary; familiarity with these materials is a must as CAD/CAM has become increasingly popular and widely accepted among dentists and laboratory technicians alike. Reproduced by permission of Quintessence Publishing, copyright Quintessence.

design. (See Figure 11.24.) Questions to consider during the preoperative patient evaluation include:

- Is there a significant variance in the shade of the gingival, body, and incisal?
- Are there any special characterizations or effects in the tooth?
- Can the patient's teeth be categorized as high in translucency or high in opacity?
- Can materials selection affect the final esthetic outcome of the restoration?

After those questions have been addressed, a treatment plan can be developed and the clinician can determine the ideal material selection and preparation for the restoration.

Step 2: Image Capture/Shade Analysis The best way to analyze the shade is to use technology (SpectroShade Micro, MHT S.P.A., Milan, Italy), as shown in Figure 11.25, since it is the least influenced by contrast effects and visual discrepancies associated with proper lighting. Technology requires image capture, as shown in Figure 11.26, or image acquisition. Once the images are brought into the database and stored, they can then be analyzed for shade, as shown in Figures 11.27 and 11.28.

Today's technology streamlines shade analysis by indicating which shade tabs the clinician should select for reference photography (shade communication).

Step 3: Transferring the Information into a Visual Format (Shade Communication) High-quality digital photo-

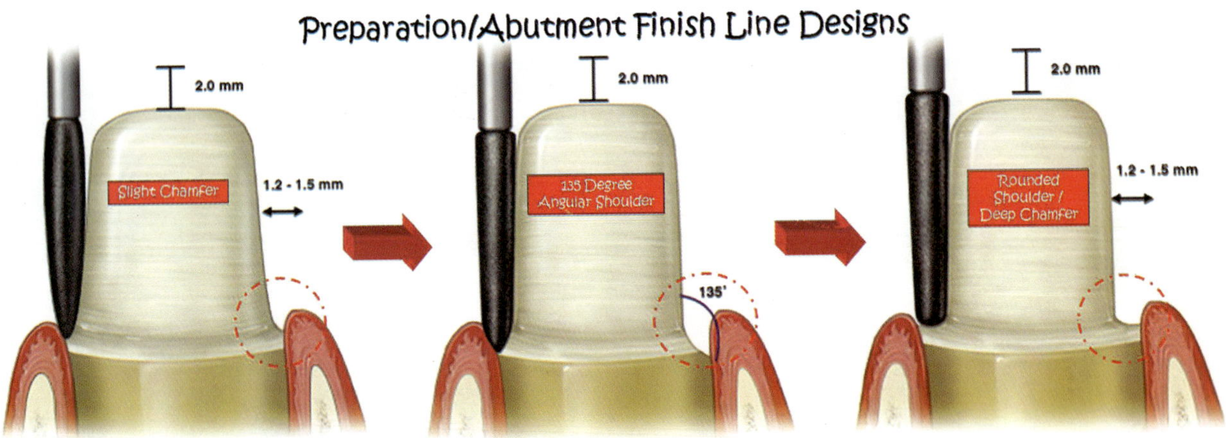

Figure 11.24. Tooth preparation/abutment design may take many forms and is primarily dependent on the material chosen and collar design for the final restoration. The shade/material of the implant abutment (i.e., metal versus Ceramic) must be taken into consideration as it may influence the value of the material/final restoration placed on top of it. Reproduced by permission of Quintessence Publishing, copyright Quintessence.

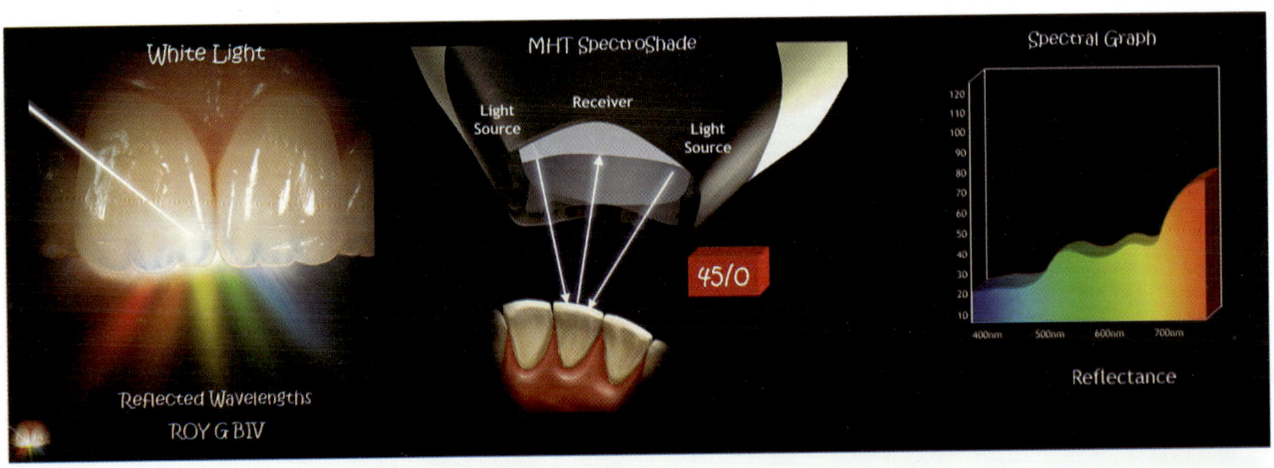

Figure 11.25. Digital spectrophotometers measure and record the amount of visible radiant energy reflected by the teeth one wavelength at a time for each hue, value, and chroma present in the entire visible spectrum. Present spectrophotometers used illuminate the teeth at a 45-degree angle of incidence to the object to eliminate reflectance glare and distortion of the data and captures the image at a zero-degree angle. A specific and unique fingerprint of the image (far right image) is recorded at intervals of 10 nm without the whole visible light spectrum (400–800 nm). Reproduced by permission of Quintessence Publishing, copyright Quintessence.

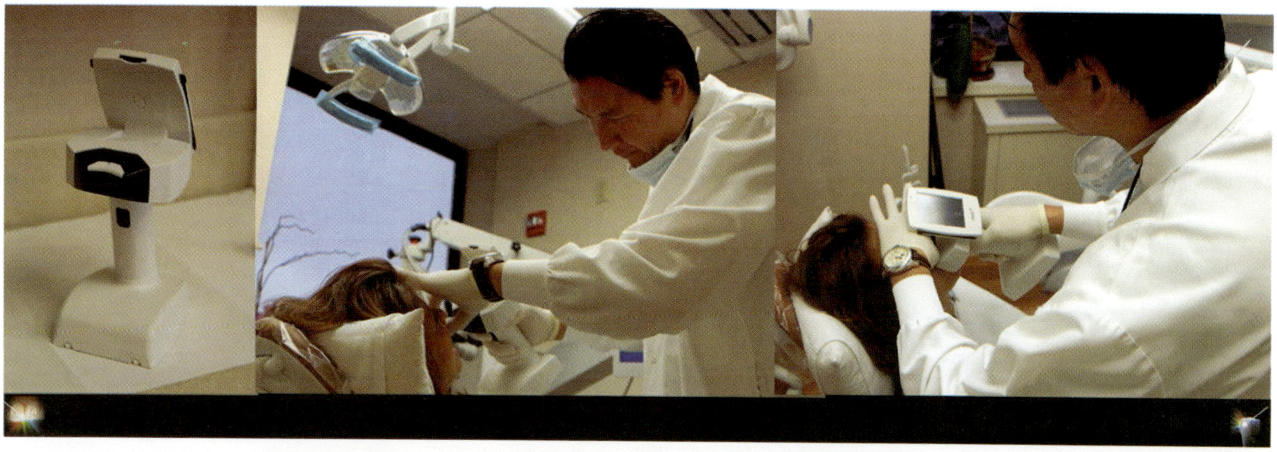

Figure 11.26. Portable handheld spectrophotometers such as the SpectroShade Micro System from MHT uses dual digital cameras and LED light technology to measure the color of teeth and allows readings of its reflectivity and interpreted inferred translucency. A "pop up" color PDA screen allows easy image visualization during image capture. Reproduced by permission of Quintessence Publishing, copyright Quintessence.

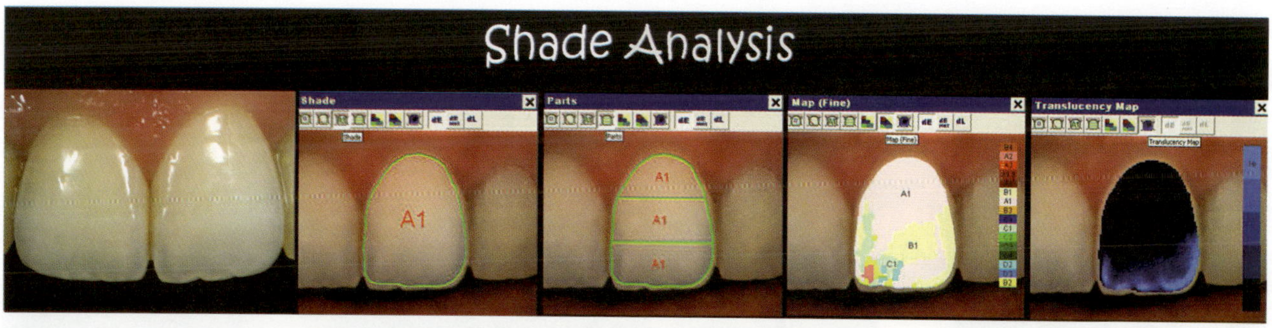

Figure 11.27. Once the image is acquired, the teeth are analyzed for overall or basic shade and the gingival/body/incisal (GBI) shade. A fine shade map, and inferred translucency map are also displayed. Reproduced by permission of Quintessence Publishing, copyright Quintessence.

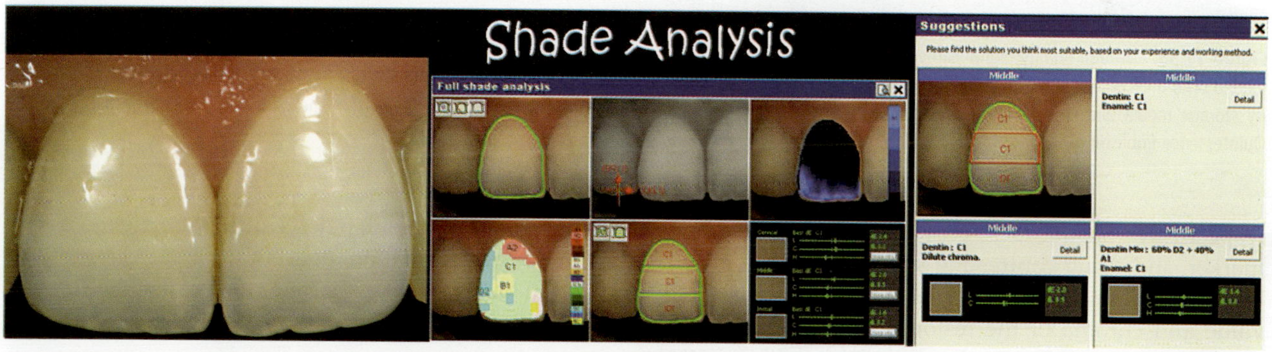

Figure 11.28. Besides giving a GBI map of the tooth, delta E values can be generated and quantified (far right image). This is unique to spectrophotometers since they have true numerical values associated with the tooth shade and these numbers can be mathematically compared to the values of shade tabs. The change in E (delta E) can then be calculated. A delta E of 0 is a perfect match. The human eye is sensitive to a delta E of 2; therefore, any number greater than 2 will be noticeable and not a clinically acceptable match. Reproduced by permission of Quintessence Publishing, copyright Quintessence.

graphs are the best means to communicate shade. With digital photography, images can be immediately evaluated and assessed for quality. With cost-efficient storage media devices, there is no penalty for taking a poor image since it can be erased. Special effects and characterizations can be best visualized by altering the object's exposure to brightness, viewing angle, and flash orientation, as shown in Figure 11.29. Shade tabs and reference photography, as shown in Figure 11.30, should be employed to gather and communicate the precise shade,

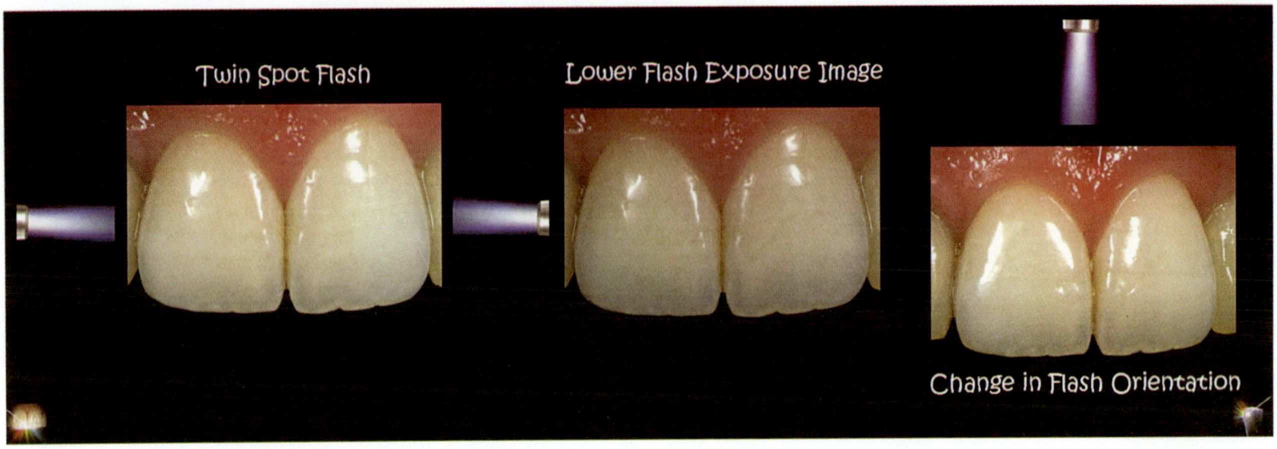

Figure 11.29. Photographs of these central incisors with lighting from a twin spot (both sides) flash, light emanating from below, as well as from the top, allows nuances in tooth shade and characterization to be clearly visualized. Also, a lower exposure image should be provided to the technician thereby allowing visualization of special effects and characterizations in the tooth shade (middle image). Reproduced by permission of Quintessence Publishing, copyright Quintessence.

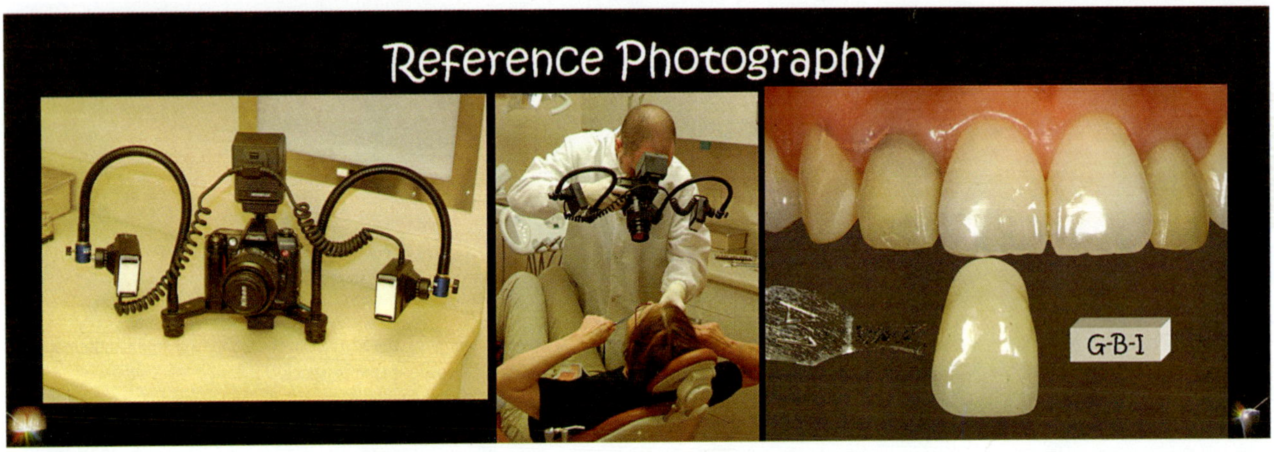

Figure 11.30. A high quality digital camera system is recommended for use since it produces quality images for shade interpretation. Images can be downloaded onto a CF II/III or SD card. There is no penalty for a poor image taken since they can be evaluated immediately and erased if necessary. Also, high capacity storage media allows literally hundreds of images to be taken prior to formatting and eliminating them from the card. Reproduced by permission of Quintessence Publishing, copyright Quintessence.

respectively. Shade tabs provide a visual reference marker, and using contrasting shade tabs that are both bright and dark allows clinicians to better determine the value and chroma of the restoration. Taking reference photographs provides the lab technician with a better understanding of how the shade tabs compare to the shade of the surrounding dentition and the value changes of the tooth to be matched, as shown in Figure 11.31. As an adjunct, black and white photographs are helpful in determining the shade value, which is the most significant variable, as shown in Figure 11.32.

After the shade information is gathered by the clinician, it must be delivered to the lab. This can be accomplished in two ways: (1) sent as a hard copy stored on a CD, or (2) sent via e-mail. (See Figure 11.33.) Reference photography and written descriptions are the most critical pieces of information for accurate shade communication that must be sent to the laboratory. All of the analysis information can now be delivered electronically.

Step 4: Interpreting the Shade Information (Interpretation)
When the laboratory technician receives the shade information, they must interpret all of the pieces. A color map report alone is insufficient; all materials should be taken into account when interpreting the shade. (See Figures 11.34, 11.35, and 11.36.) The reference photography is tantamount to the lab technician to better understanding the shade tab selection and the variance in value and chroma. The digital color map provides a close-to-accurate depiction of the shade reading (shade analysis).

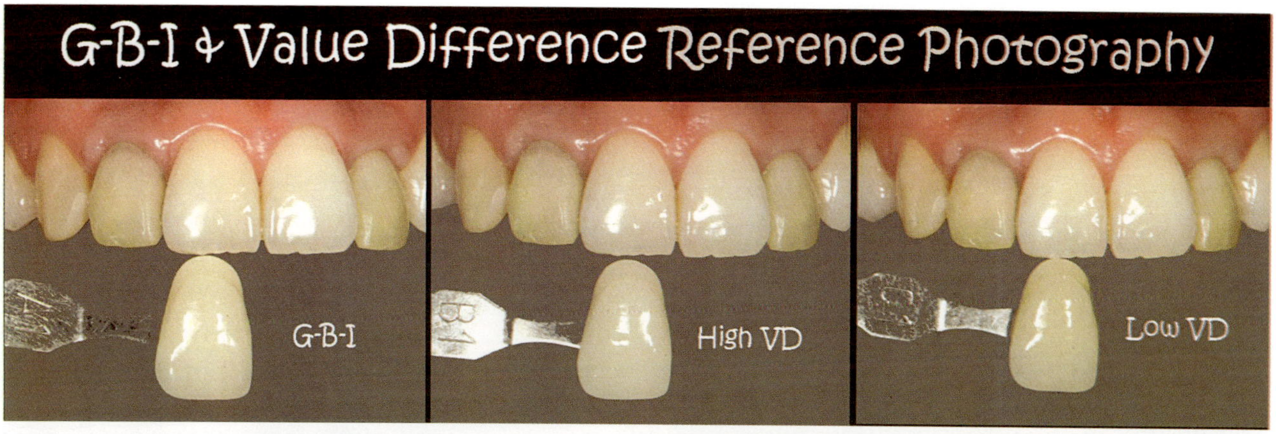

Figure 11.31. Reference photographs using contrasting shade tabs that are both bright and dark, as well as the actual matched GIB tab, will provide a better overall picture of surrounding dentition as well as the tooth to be matched. An 18% gray background eliminates visual distractions that can lead to poor shade perception. Reproduced by permission of Quintessence Publishing, copyright Quintessence.

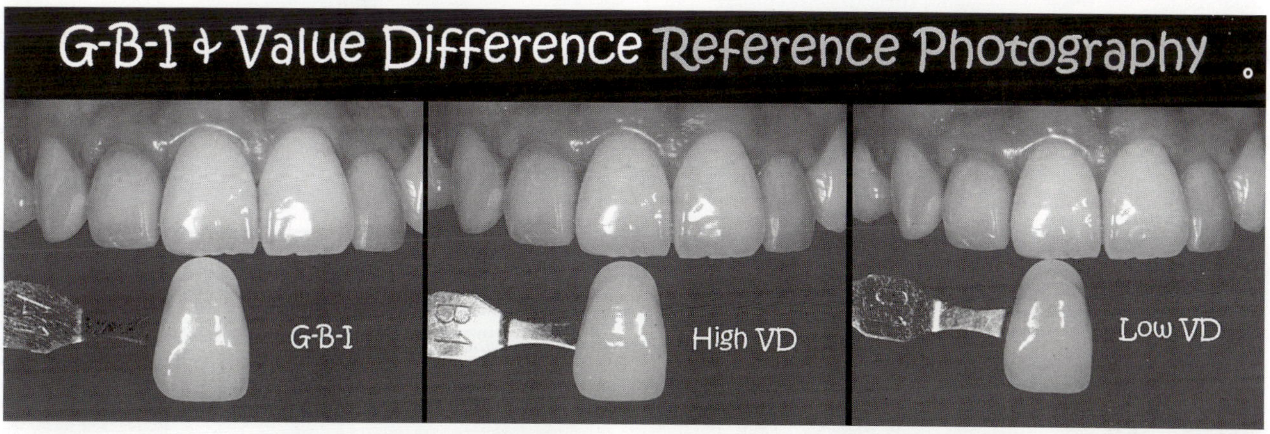

Figure 11.32. Taking and/or converting the same three photographs in a black and white format are helpful to determine which value shade tab is the most significant variable. Reproduced by permission of Quintessence Publishing, copyright Quintessence.

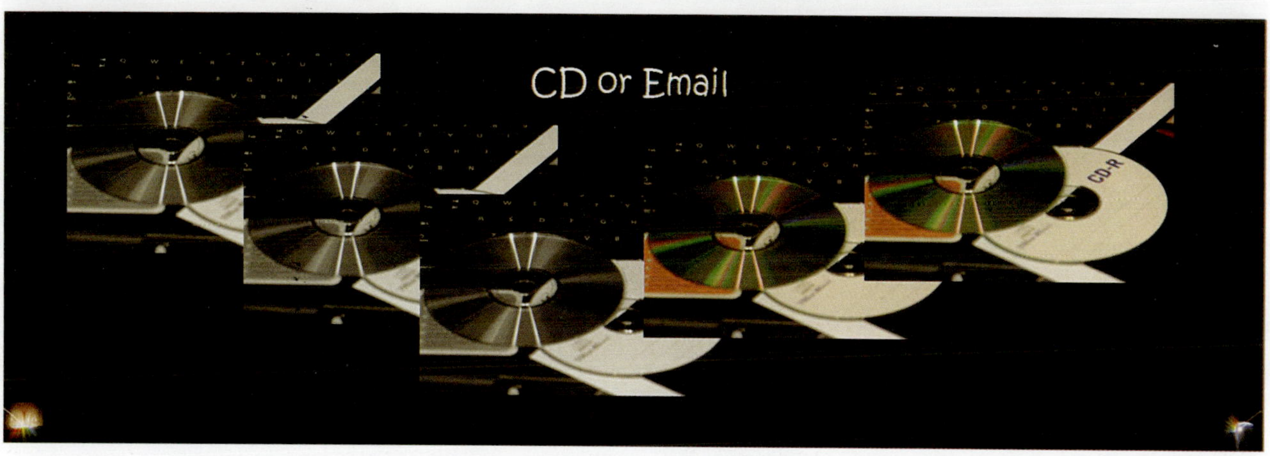

Figure 11.33. E-mail allows for "instant" transferal of shade information to and from the lab provided the server allows high capacity Internet file transfer. Also, the shade data may be mailed to the lab on a CD along with the actual case. Reproduced by permission of Quintessence Publishing, copyright Quintessence.

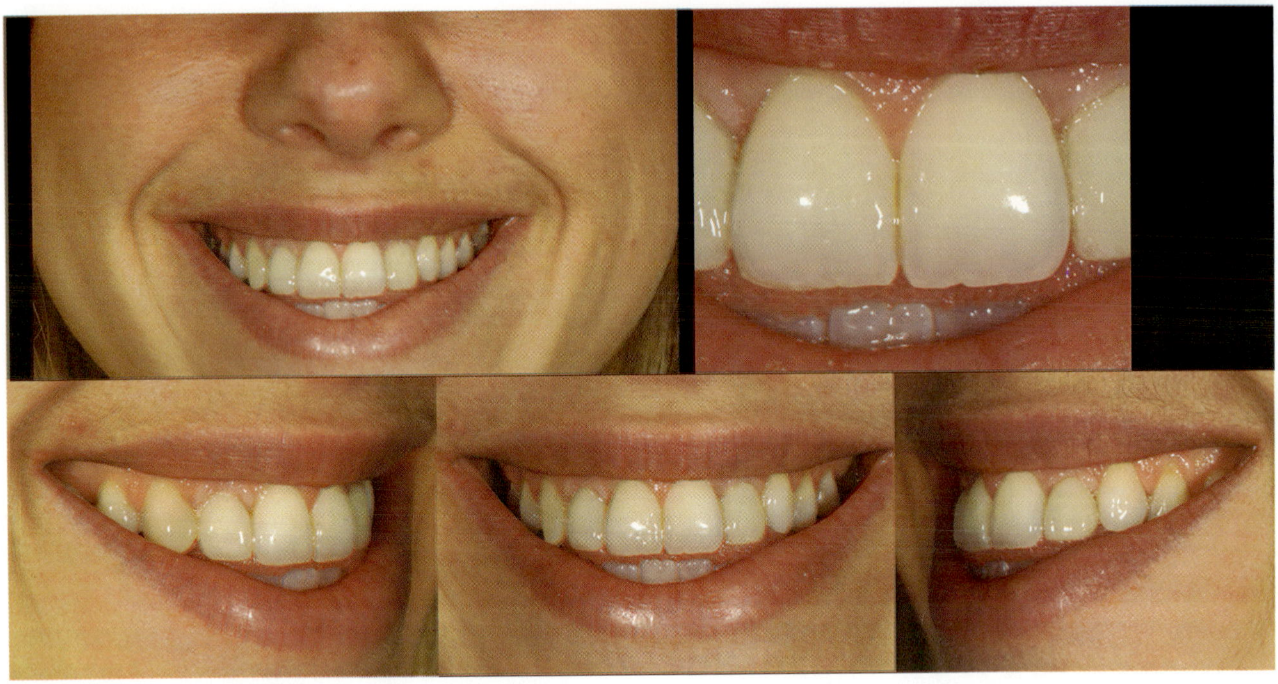

Figure 11.34. Composite photographs allows the technician to evaluate the "smile design" of the case and different angles to the subject gives a "feel" for overall tooth size and proportion. Reproduced by permission of Quintessence Publishing, copyright Quintessence.

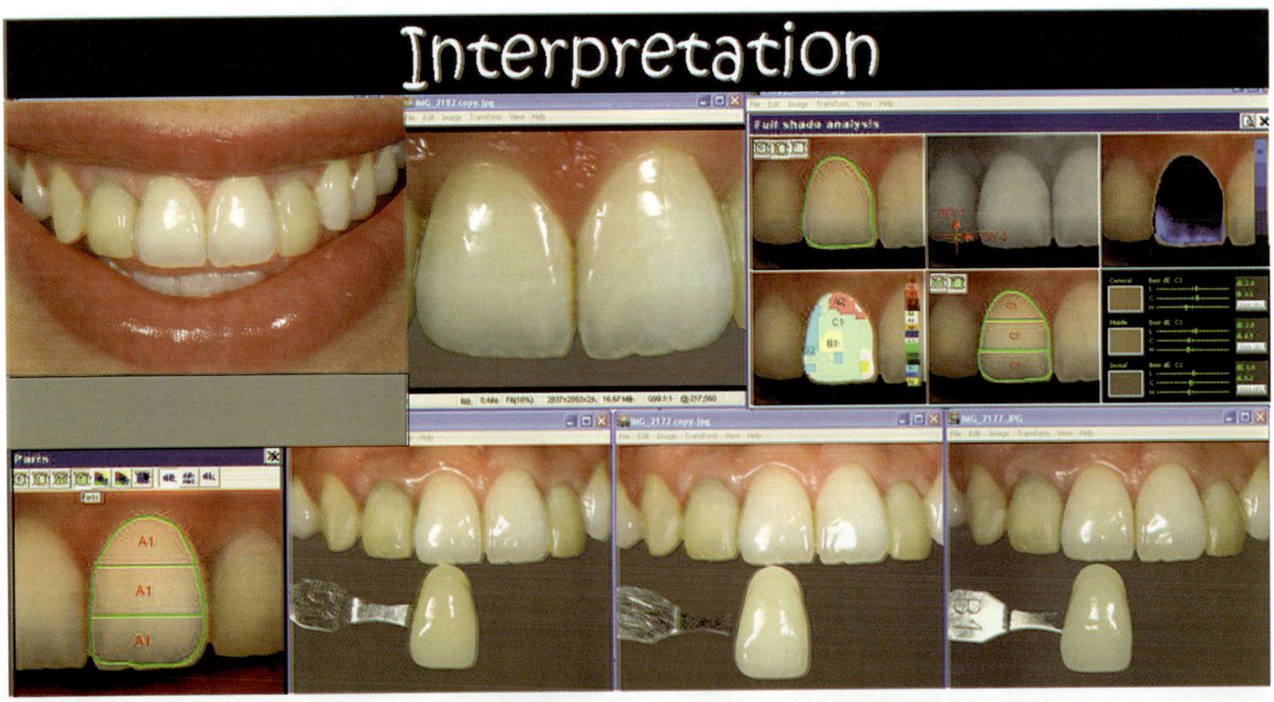

Figure 11.35. Photographs of the tooth to be matched, digital shade reports, and reference photographs can be compiled as a composite collage to allow easy and simple shade interpretation and understanding of color. Interpretation of shade information can be termed "visual understanding of the color." Reproduced by permission of Quintessence Publishing, copyright Quintessence.

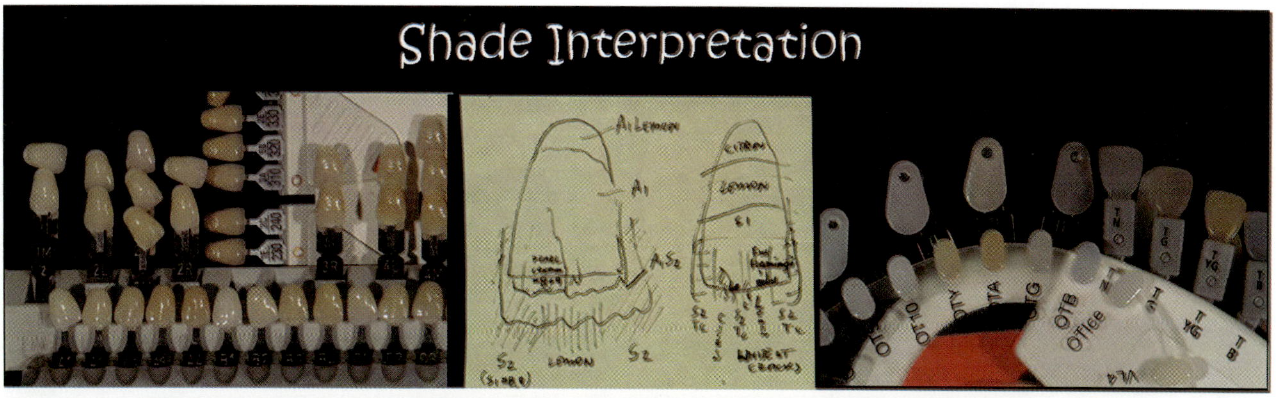

Figure 11.36. With all the shade information at hand, the lab technician translates this information into the language of the ceramic system to be used. Reproduced by permission of Quintessence Publishing, copyright Quintessence.

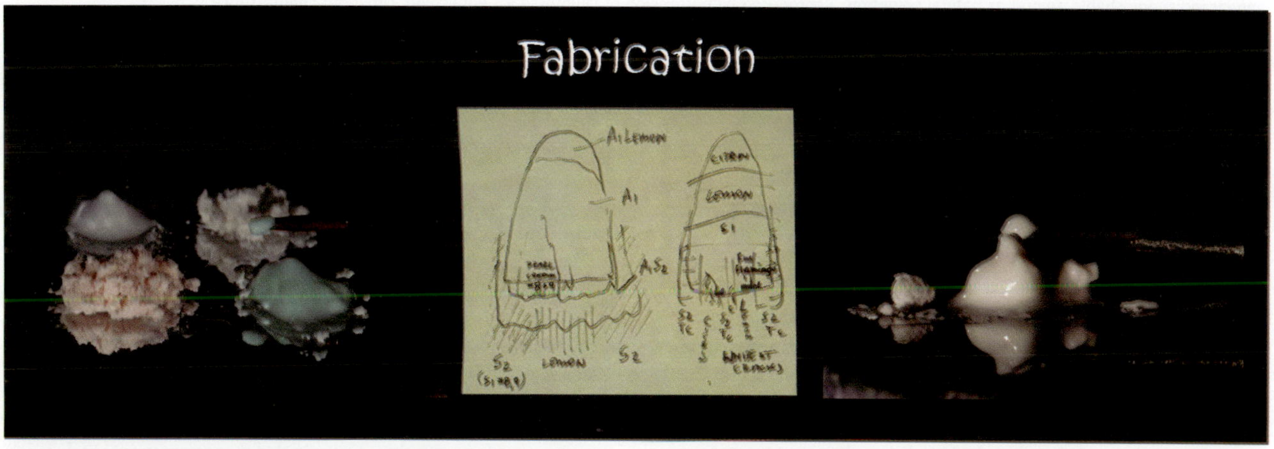

Figure 11.37. The ceramist creates detailed tooth maps defining where the system's special effects powders should be used to achieve the desired nuances in shade. Reproduced by permission of Quintessence Publishing, copyright Quintessence.

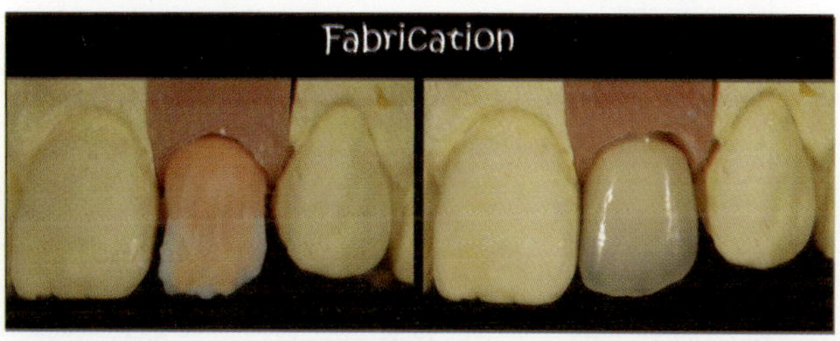

Figure 11.38. Ceramic powders and internal colors are layered and stacked to proper shape, size, and contour to impart the correct visual effect upon firing. Extrinsic glazes are added to finalize the color effects of the final restoration. Reproduced by permission of Quintessence Publishing, copyright Quintessence.

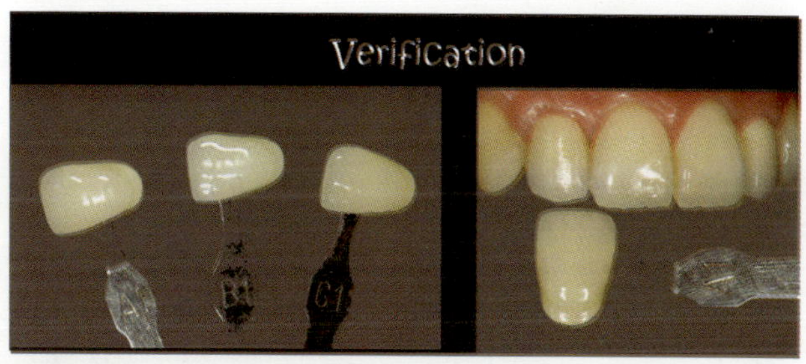

Figure 11.39. Shade verification should always be done in the laboratory with an 18% gray card prior to the restoration being returned to the clinician. The reference photographs should be compared to the completed restoration and the shade tab against an 18% gray card. Reproduced by permission of Quintessence Publishing, copyright Quintessence.

Step 5: Fabricating the Restoration (Fabrication) After assessing the shade and determining what material works best given the particular clinical application, the lab technician uses a chart similar to that shown in Figure 11.37 to fabricate the restoration and add the necessary details in the staining and glazing stage to match the opposing dentition, as shown in Figure 11.38.

Step 6: Verifying the Accuracy of the Shade Match (Verification) Shade verification is one of the most critical phases of treatment. This should always be performed in the laboratory by the technician prior to it being returned to the clinician for try-in and/or insertion. (See Figure 11.39.) The simplest means of shade verification is through the use of shade tabs. Using an 18% gray card

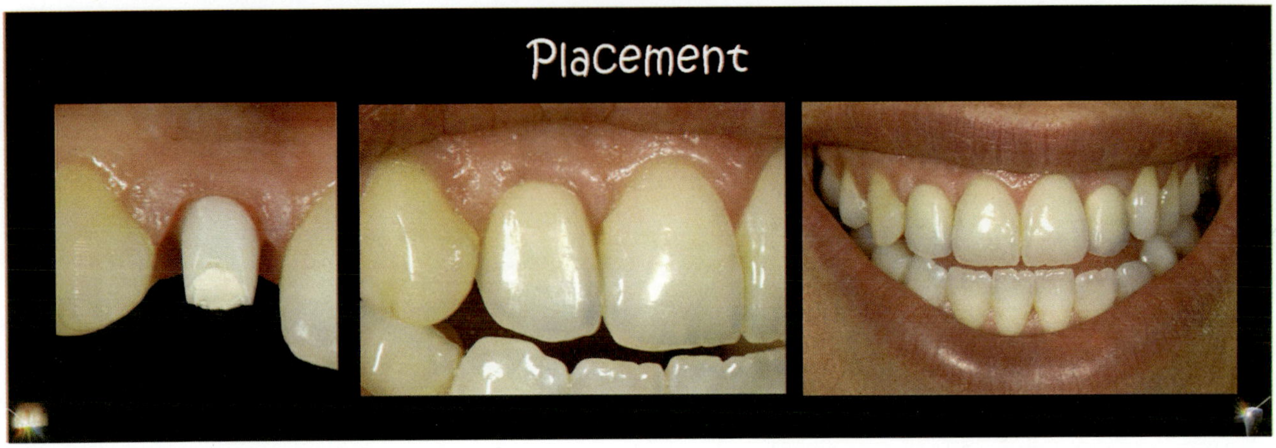

Figure 11.40. Any discrepancies in the final restoration will be immediately evident upon placement by the clinician. Likewise, a "perfect" restoration will appear indistinguishable among its natural neighbors. Reproduced by permission of Quintessence Publishing, copyright Quintessence.

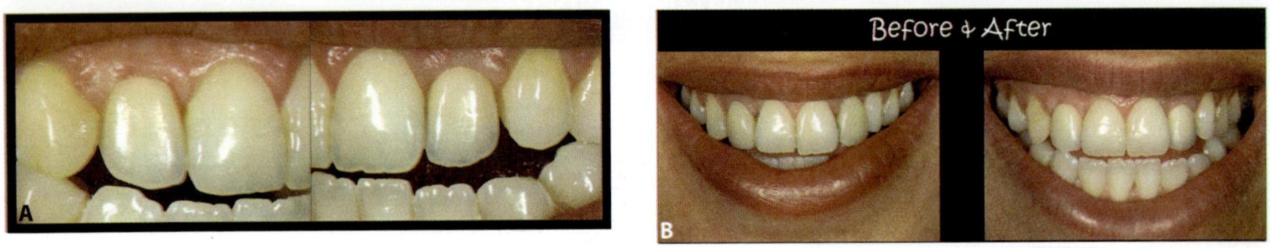

Figure 11.41. 11.41A. Using the 7-step shade-taking and communication protocol, challenging anterior restorations can be matched confidently and predictably, and repeatedly, case after case. Reproduced by permission of Quintessence Publishing, copyright Quintessence.

as a background is also helpful to eliminate any surrounding distractions that could cause poor shade perception.

Step 7: Placement (Clinical Insertion/Cementation) The ultimate verification of the restoration's accuracy happens when the clinician fits the restoration. (See Figures 11.40, 11.41A–B.) Does it match or doesn't it? If the restoration does not match, it should be a glaring problem. However, by using this protocol, remakes should be significantly minimized. If the restoration does not match, steps 2–6 should be repeated. The reference photographs should be taken with the new restoration in place and referred to accordingly.

Summary

The highlights to remember for shade matching are:

- The best way to analyze shade objectively is to use technology-based systems. However, shade tabs can be used judiciously.
- Details added by the lab technician in the fabrication process often can increase the natural appearance of a shade. This is best communicated with digital images/reference photography and an 18% gray card as the background to eliminate contrasting effects.
- Successful shade taking involves a combination of technology-based systems, shade tabs, and reference photography.

References

Age-Related Eye Disease Study Research Group. 2001. A randomized placebo-controlled clinical trial of high-dose supplementation with Vitamins C and E beta carotene and zinc for age-related macular degeneration and vision loss. *AREDS Report No. 8. Archives of Ophthalmology*, Oct., 119, (10), pp. 1417–1436.

Berns, R.F. 2000. *Billmeyer and Saltzman's principles of color technology*. 3rd Ed. New York: Wiley, pp. 75–104.

Bunting, F. 2003. *The ColorShop Color Primer*. Available at: www.xrite.com/documents/mktg/ColorPrimer.pdf. Accessed 18 September.

Carsten, D. 2003. Successful shade matching—What does it take? *Compend Contin Educ Dent*, 24, pp. 175–178, 180, 182.

Chu, S.J. 2002a. The science of color and shade selection in aesthetic dentistry. *Dent Today*, 21, (9), pp. 86–89.

Chu, S.J. 2002b. Precision shade technology: Contemporary strategies in shade selection. *Pract Proced Aesthet Dent*, 14, 79–83.

Chu, S.J. 2003. *Science and Art of Porcelain Veneers*: Color (Chapter 5). Chicago, IL: Quintessence Publishing, pp. 157–206.

Chu, S.J, A. Devigus, and A. Mieleszko. 2004. *Fundamentals of Color: Shade Matching and Communication in Esthetic Dentistry*. Quintessence Publishing Co, Inc., Chicago, IL, pp. 4, 31.

Commission Internationale de l'Èclairage. 1971. *Colorimetry, official recommendations of the International Commission on Illumination*. Publication CIE No. 15 (E–1.3.1). Paris: Bureau Central de la CIE.

Fraunfelder, F.T. 1996. *Drug-Induced Ocular Side Effects*. Philadelphia: Williams & Wilkins.

Gimbel, T. 1994. *Healing with Color and Light*. New York: Simon and Schuster.

Hunter, R.S., and R.W. Harold. 1987. *The measurement of appearance*. New York: Wiley, pp. 3–68.

Judd, D.B., and G. Wyszecki. 1975. *Color in business, science and industry*. 3rd Ed. New York.

Kuehni, R.G., and R.T. Marcus. 1979. An experiment in visual scaling of small color differences. *Color Res Appl*, 4, pp. 83–91.

Lamb, T., and J. Bourriau, Eds. 1995. *Colour: Art and Science*. Cambridge, UK: Cambridge University Press.

Leinfelder, K. 2000. Porcelain Aesthetics for the 21st Century. *JADA*, Vol. 131, June.

Miller, L. 1987. Organizing color in dentistry. *J Am Dent Assoc*, (Spec Iss), 26E–40E.

Miller, M.D., and R. Zaucha. 1992. Color and tones. In: *The Color Mac: Design Production Techniques*. Carmel, IN: Hayden, pp. 23–39.

Munsell, A.H. 1969. *A Grammar of Color*. New York: Van Nostrand Dreinhold.

Quackenbush, T.R. 1997. *Relearning to See*. Berkeley, CA: North Atlantic Books.

Quintessence Publishing. 2004. *The Fundamentals of Color*. Carol Stream, IL.

Rosenthal, O., and R. Phillips. 1997. *Coping with Color-Blindness*. New York: Avery.

The Schepens Eye Research Institute. 2003. www.eri.harvard.edu *Macular Degeneration*. Accessed October 6.

Sim, C.P., A.U. Yap, and J. Teo. 2001. Color perception among different dental personnel. *Oper Dent*. Sep–Oct, 26, (5), pp. 435–439.

Sproull, R.C. 1973. Color matching in dentistry, part I. The three-dimensional nature of color. *J Prosthet Dent*, 29, pp. 416–424.

Wasson, W., and N. Schuman. 1992. *Color vision and dentistry*. Quintessence Int. May 23, (5), pp. 349–353.

Wyszecki, G., and W.S. Stiles. 1982. *Color science concepts and methods, quantitative data and formulae*. 2nd Ed. New York: Wiley, pp. 83–116.

X-Rite. 2002. *A Guide to Understanding Color Communication*. Grandville, MI.

Chapter 12

Treatment Complications in the Esthetic Zone

Abd El Salam El Askary

Implant failure is defined as the total failure of the implant to fulfill its purpose (functional, esthetic, or phonetic) due to mechanical or biological reasons (El Askary et al. 1999a). On the other hand, treatment complications may occur for the same reasons, but they might be reversible (El Askary et al. 1999b). Treatment complications can range from fracture of the prosthetic components to a transient inflammatory condition; however, this chapter addresses the possible complications in the esthetic zone, which involves the possibility of failure due to esthetic reasons.

An implant with successful osseointegration might still be considered a failure if the final prosthesis does not provide the optimal required esthetics. Such a failure could be due to several reasons, some of which are untreatable. The esthetic outcome of an implant-supported restoration is affected by four main factors: (1) implant placement, (2) soft tissue condition, (3) osseous condition, and (4) prosthetic condition (El Askary and Meffert 1999).

The failure to replicate the patient's natural dentition in the final implant-supported prosthesis may result in a disturbing appearance that is considered an absolute failure. The accurate identification of any potential esthetic complications prior to implant installation permits alternative planning and eliminates the need for more complex treatment or retreatment at a later date (Balshi 1998). In addition, fabrication of a preoperative prototype is necessary because it provides helpful information about the final prosthesis and facilitates proper implant positioning.

The possible treatment complications in the esthetic zone can be divided according to the reason of the occurrence:

1. Etiological, which is concerned with the etiological factors that lead to implant failures or complications. This type of failure can be divided into host factors, surgical placement, implant selection, and/or restorative problems. Among the main etiological factors that lead to implant failure are (a) implant misplacement errors (e.g., placement of the implant in an infected socket, pathological lesion, or immature bone previously augmented, or placement of a contaminated implant in the osteotomy) or lack of primary stabilization of the implant; (b) intraoral infection or soft tissue complications; (c) lack of biocompatibility of the implant material or inserting the implant in poor-quality bone (immature grafted bone or D4 bone that leads to an insufficient bone contact surface area; (d) excessive surgical trauma; and/or (e) faulty loading or excessive torque during abutment connection.
2. Biological, which involves the bacterial invasion of the peri-implant tissues that results in soft tissue inflammatory changes and rapid bone loss. This condition was termed *peri-implantitis* and was defined by Meffert (1992) as the progressive loss of peri-implant bone as well as soft tissue inflammatory changes. This definition implies that bone loss and soft tissue inflammation occur together as a result of bacterial invasion. On the other hand, Tonetti and Schmid (1994) divided the host's reaction to bacterial invasion into two groups: peri-implant mucositis, which implies that the inflammatory changes are localized only to the surrounding soft tissue, and peri-implantitis, in which the reaction affects the deeper soft tissues and surrounding bone. The latter explanation may be based on the concept that the tissues surrounding a functioning oral implant can be divided into two distinct anatomical compartments, both with different functions. These are the soft tissues, which can seal the implant from aggression of exogenous bacteria, and bone, which plays the supporting role for the implant (Esposito et al. 1998).
3. Personal factors, because the overall clinical success of the dental implant relies on close cooperation among a dental team that involves the patient as well. Each member has his own role in certain stages of treatment. The poor clinical skills of the clinician might lead to the failure to obtain a reasonable esthetic result. On the other hand, the well-trained

laboratory technician greatly contributes to the long-term success of dental implant therapy, both esthetically and functionally.

4. Defective tissues. Krekeler and others (1985) suggested a relationship between implant failure and the absence of an adequate band of keratinized mucosa surrounding the abutment. This was based on the ability of the keratinized mucosa to withstand bacterial insult and ingression. Tonetti and Schmid (1994), in supporting this concept, stated that the late failures that occur as a result of peri-implantitis (infectious etiology) occur because of a defective function of the soft tissues. Therefore, the marginal periabutment tissues should constitute a functional barrier between the oral environment and the host bone by sealing off the osseous fixture site from noxious agents and thermal and mechanical trauma (Adell et al. 1981). Gingival loss might lead to continuous recession around the implant with subsequent bone loss. This leads to a soft tissue type of failure. On the contrary, Strub and others (1991) stated that the keratinized mucosa or dental plaque does not seem to be related to implant failure but that its presence might facilitate the patient's hygienic procedures.However, in the esthetic zone, the relationship between the available keratinized mucosa and the overall success of the implant-supported prosthesis becomes very valuable. On the other hand, the loss of the supporting alveolar bone leads to serious treatment complications.

Adell and others (1981) stated that marginal bone height depends on both proper marginal stress distribution and adequate function of the marginal soft tissue. They also listed several factors that contribute to marginal bone loss, including (1) surgical trauma, such as detachment of the periosteum and damage caused during drilling, (2) improper stress distribution caused by defective prosthetic design and occlusal trauma, (3) physiological ridge resorption, and (4) gingivitis, which, if allowed to progress, will lead to the ingression of bacteria and their toxins to the underlying osseous structure.

Implant Positioning Complications

Incorrect implant position in the alveolar ridge may occur due to many factors such as the imprecise fabrication of surgical template, the lack of control during the drilling procedure, poor presurgical planning, poor armamentarium, and the lack of knowledge or experience. The minor deviation from the standard known clinical guidelines for esthetic implant positioning in any dimension will surely result in esthetic fallout. Some can be treated, while for others, implant removal will be the only possible option. As is the case of any positioning error, there is always a consequence or repercussion. Therefore, all efforts should be made to avoid any misplacement errors. It is also essential that the clinician be familiar with the various unfortunate clinical situations that may arise due to misplacement and the ways to solve any associated problems.

The axial misplacement of the dental implant within its housing can be damaging to the overall health of the soft and hard tissues surrounding the implant. A deep gingival sulcus with long junctional epithelium can be a serious consequence due to the further deep positioning of the implant. This creates a favorable environment for several types of bacteria, including anaerobic bacteria, to colonize and populate (Misch 1995).

Logically speaking, the deeper an implant is inserted into the bone, the more bone will be resorbed around the implant following the second-stage surgery with abutment connection. This bone resorption is not a pathological condition but a physiological reaction to the implant misplacement. (See Figure 12.1.) Inflammation and gingival bleeding usually occur as a result of the inaccessibility for hygiene measures from one side and the bacterial endotoxins from another side. The problem begins at the time of the insertion, when it becomes difficult to seat the protheses. (See Figures 12.2A–B.) These symptoms are common clinical events that often occur when placement is too far apical. Likewise the prosthetic margins of a deeply seated implant also become inaccessible at the time of insertion, especially when the restora-

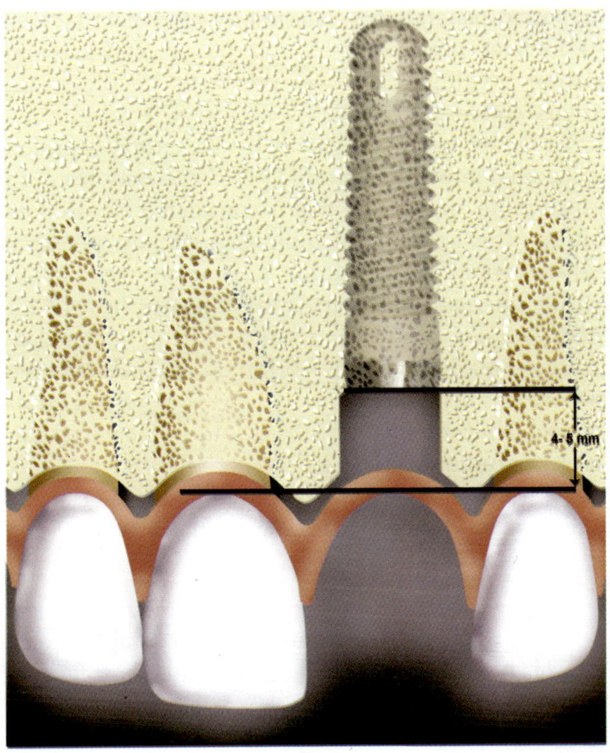

Figure 12.1. Too deep placement of an implant fixture; showing a resultant increased pocket depth.

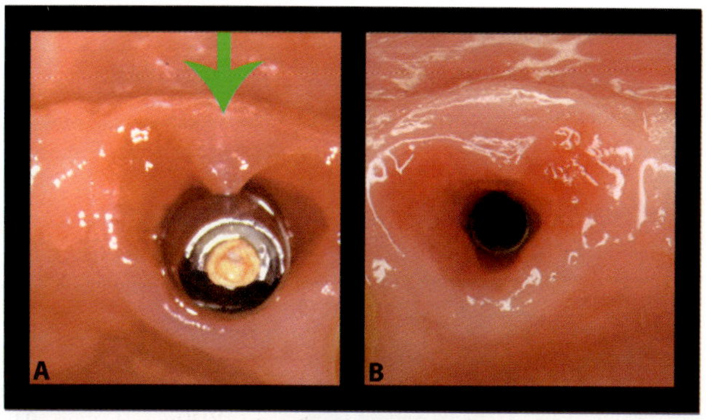

Figure 12.2. **A.** A deeply seated implant revealing severe gingival inflammation, the green arrow points at gingival hyperplasia. **B.** The gingival condition post crown removal, note the collapsed gingival collar.

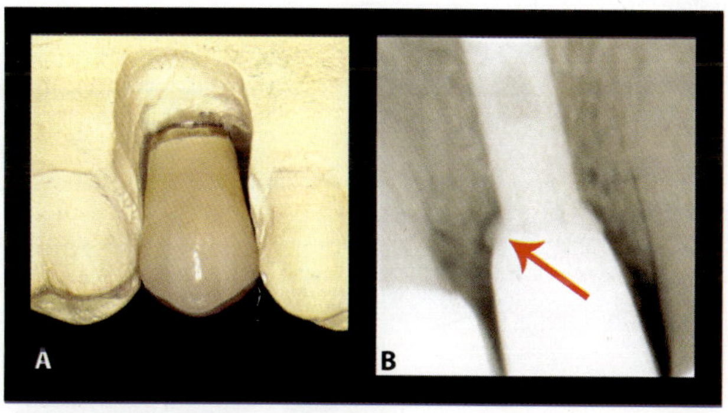

Figure 12.3. **A.** A deeply seated implant on the cast reveals a long crown margin that is impossible to be accessed for cleaning. **B.** A radiographic view shows the red arrow points at the excess luting cement being retained in the sulcus due to the difficulty to remove it.

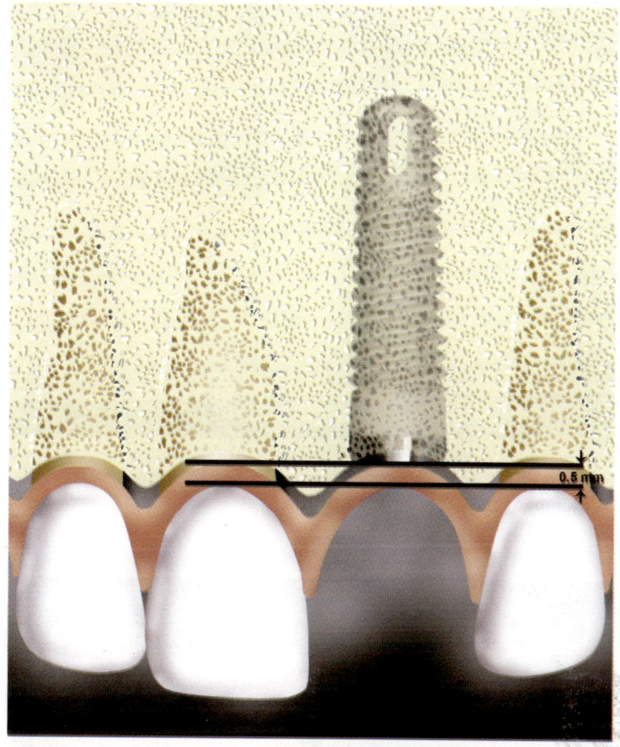

Figure 12.4. Insufficient depth positioning of an implant fixture.

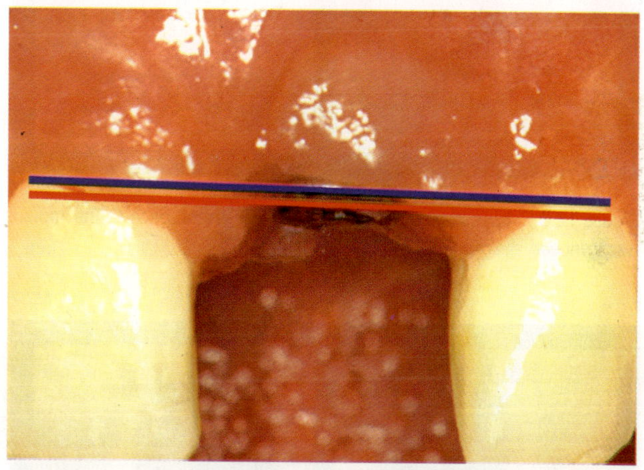

Figure 12.5. The implant head is placed shallow leaving no running room. The red line represents the implant head location and the blue line represents the gingival zenith, not the decreased space between them.

tion is cemented. It is extremely important to ensure the complete removal of the excess luting cement from the interface between the abutment and the restoration. The correction of this clinical dilemma is almost impossible (Agar et al. 1997). (See Figures 12.3A–B.)

The failure to position the implant in its optimal depth—for instance, if it is placed too shallow—often results in a short crown with constricted margins due to the absence of "running room." This places the prosthetic components in a supragingival location, and this clinical predicament is impossible to amend or rectify. The difficulty remains in handling the margins of the final prosthesis and hiding the abutment collar sublingually. (See Figures 12.4 and 12.5.) In this particular condition, it may be necessary to remove the implant. The improper mesiodistal positioning of the implant might lead to the total absence of restorative possibilities. If the implant is placed in the interdental papilla space, as shown in Figures 12.6A–C, or is placed too mesially or with zero or minimal space left for restoration, the case becomes impossible to restore. (See Figures 12.7A–B.)

Violating the labial plate of bone or the labial soft tissues might constitute a major clinical dilemma that is impossible to correct, even with the use of the angulated abutments, as shown in Figure 12.8. Violating the labial plate integrity extends beyond the teeth, and affects to the lip support—it might impinge on the lip harmony.

Placing the implant angulation too far lingually might result in tongue crowding, impinging on the tongue space, which can significantly compromise speech and mastication. The chances of restoring a misplaced implant with an acceptable esthetic result are minimal. This is especially the case if the implant has been positioned too far labially or incisally, as seen in Figure 12.9.

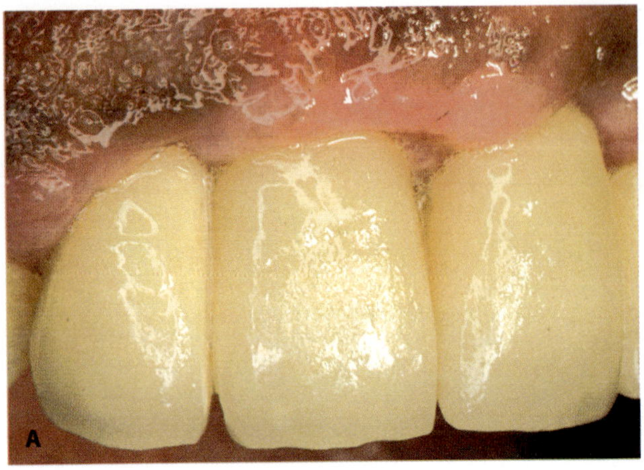

Figure 12.6A. Missing inter-implant papilla due to improper mesio-distal implant positioning.

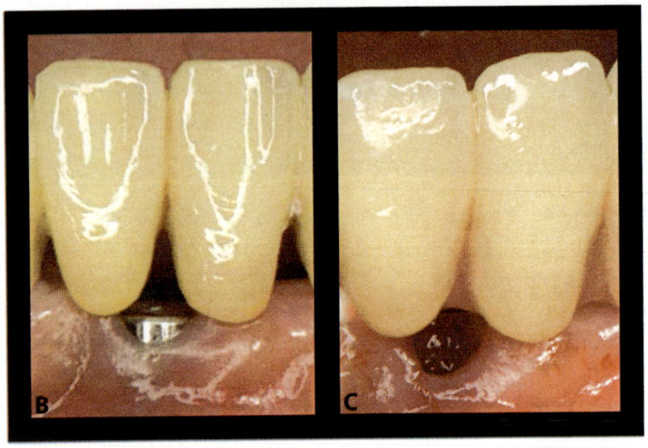

Figure 12.6. B. An implant is placed in the inter-dental space. **C.** The implant was removed.

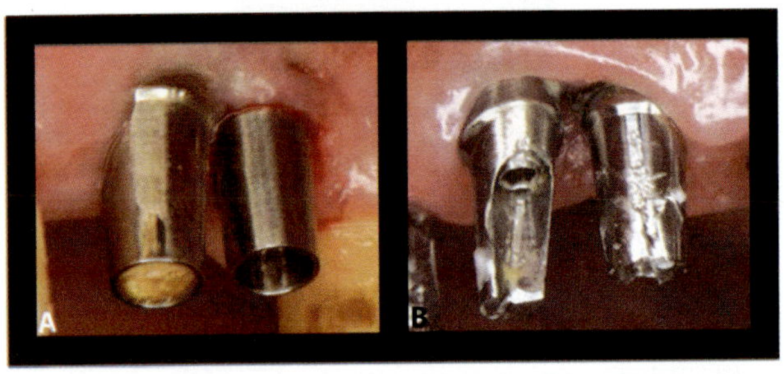

Figure 12.7. A. Implants are misplaced leaving no embrasure space. **B.** The use of angulated abutments was not able to solve the misplacement.

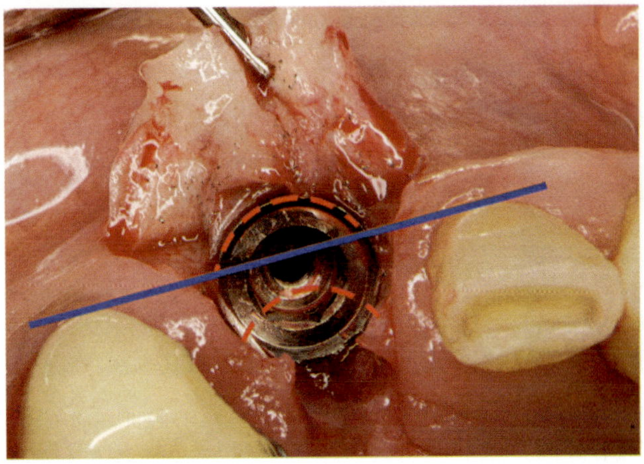

Figure 12.8. An implant is placed too far labillay that is impossible to restore.

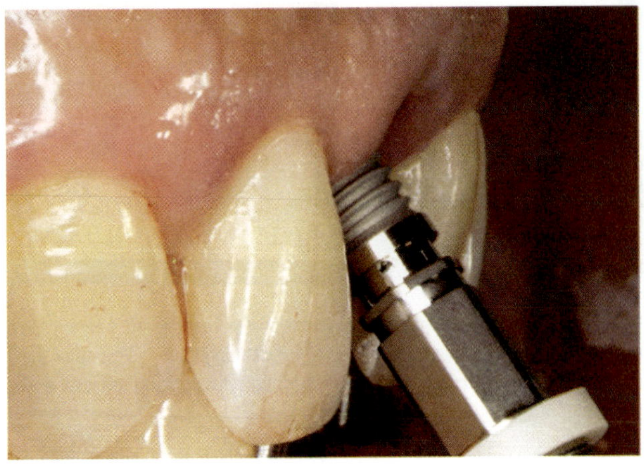

Figure 12.9. Improper violation of the labial plate via improper implant angulation.

Fair numbers of clinical approaches have been described for resolving misaligned and malpositioned dental implants. If unfavorable inclination of the implant fixture is the only problem, angulated abutments can often improve the prosthetic results of an implant-supported restoration. Using the preangulated abutments in cases in which the implant has been placed too far labially is not effective in most clinical situations because the preangled abutment usually requires a larger restorative dimension than other types. In addition, the gingival collar of the preangled abutment might encroach upon the peri-implant soft tissue and violate its natural contours.

Interestingly, Nishimura and others (1999) have described an alternative approach for patients with misplaced dental implants that are difficult to restore with the regular commercially available abutments. This approach suggests using a custom-fabricated abutment that is specially designed to meet the esthetic and functional needs of each particular patient; however, this approach does not solve many misplaced implant cases. Other attempts have been made to correct implant misplacement by performing an osteotomy around the osseous housing of the implant fixture, moving the

segment to the required correct position and stabilizing it with microplates and screws. The possibility of using segmental maxillary or mandibular osteotomies to reposition an alveolar segment with its implants may be an effective method to treat misplacements.

The procedure requires delicate surgery with minimal stripping of the periosteum to ensure uninterrupted blood supply to the segment, promote faster healing, and avoid necrosis. The segments are minimally stripped to enhance vascularization, and surgery is performed under copious irrigation to avoid bone overheating. The titanium micro plate used for rigid fixation is microsized and placed strategically in a position that does not require postsurgical removal. A longer period of immobilization is indicated, and the occlusion should be checked to eliminate any premature contacts. A restoration on a straight abutment of an ideal shape, length, and inclination is fabricated by measuring the same tooth on the other side if possible. A surgical guide is made and osteotomy is carried out accordingly. The segment is then placed in the ideal position (Warden 2000, Guerrero et al. 1999).

This procedure can eliminate the need for several surgical procedures to remove and replace the misplaced implant, which involves longer treatment time. However, the limited space between the existing natural root and the implant fixture sometimes makes the osteotomy clinically inapplicable. Additional limitations may include insufficient keratinized tissues to cover the surgical site, any existing anatomical landmark, and risk of morbidity or other unforeseen surgical difficulties.

Another clinical suggestion for restoring a partially edentulous area in patients with compromised oral hygiene or unfavorably positioned implants is the use of an implant-supported milled metal bar with acrylic resin partial overdenture (Asvanund and Morgano 2004). When dental implants were poorly positioned, ZAAG (Zest Anchors, Inc., Escondido, CA, USA) attachments were used with a milled bar to restore the partially edentulous area with a parallel-sided milled bar to prevent the prosthesis from rotating labiolingually. The method improved the patient's speech, function, and esthetics.

Peri-implant Soft Tissue Complications

Postoperative soft tissue complications can be devastating to the implant's overall success. Unfortunately, the factors that influence soft tissue healing are numerous and can be either local or systemic. However, the clinician should be able to avoid these possible complications and deal with them if they occur. Thin scalloped tissue biotypes are more liable to have postoperative rescission, because tissue instability is a common characteristic among such patients. The possible soft tissue complications follow.

Marginal Soft Tissue Recession

Stable peri-implant soft tissue contours are vital for the long-term stability of the esthetic outcome of dental implants. Implants should not only be well integrated within the bone to maintain function, but they should also meet long-term esthetic demands. Following implant restoration therapy, soft tissue margins may move in an apical direction early on, with the potential for exposing the titanium collar and creating an unfavorable esthetic situation. It is possible that these early changes may be associated with the remodeling of the underlying bone following functional loading and the re-establishment of the biological width. Marginal soft tissue status around the labial surface of implant-supported restorations might be influenced by many factors, such as:

1. The biocompatibility of the transmucosal components, because the adhesion of the junctional epithelium and connective tissue is possible only on highly biocompatible materials. If the transmucosal components are not biocompatible, the soft tissue migrates apically. The best materials are probably zirconium and titanium, and the least favorable materials are gold and acrylic resin.

   A study by Abrahamsson and others (1998) evaluated the response of the soft tissue to the different types of abutment materials and found that the material used in the abutment portion of an implant system influenced the quality of the mucosal barrier that formed following implant installation. Five beagle dogs were included in the study. The mandibular premolars and the first, second, and third maxillary premolars were extracted. Three fixtures of the Branemark system were installed in each mandibular quadrant (a total of six fixtures per animal). Abutment connection was performed after three months of healing. In each dog the following types of abutments were used: two "control abutments" (commercially pure [CP] titanium), two "ceramic abutments" (highly sintered aluminum oxide [Al2O3]), one "gold abutment," and one "short titanium abutment." The short titanium abutment was provided with an outer structure made of dental porcelain fused to gold. Following abutment, connection to a plaque control program was initiated and maintained for six months. Semithin sections representing the mesial, distal, buccal, and lingual aspects of the peri-implant tissues were produced and subjected to histological examination.

The findings from the analysis demonstrated that the material used in the abutment portion of the implant influenced the location and the quality of the attachment that occurred between the peri-implant mucosa and the implant. Abutments made of CP titanium or ceramic allowed the formation of a mucosal attachment, which included one epithelial and one connective tissue portion that were about 2 mm and 1–1.5 mm high, respectively. At sites where abutments made of gold alloy or dental porcelain were used, no proper attachment formed at the abutment level, but the soft tissue margin receded and bone resorption occurred. The abutment fixture junction was hereby occasionally exposed and the mucosal barrier became established to the fixture portion of the implant.

2. Repeated removal and placement of the abutment, which leads to cell tear and biological width disruption, because the repeated unscrewing of the abutment mechanically disrupts the cellular attachment mechanism and might lead to apical migration of the attachment apparatus.
3. Loosening of the implant interface connection, which forms a gap that harbors bacteria that can invade the surrounding tissues. The further long-term screw loosening activates bone loss and apical soft tissue migration.
4. A muscle pull on the implant site, which might lead to a continuous steady gingival recession around natural teeth.
5. The location of the implant-abutment connection in relation to the osseous crest.
6. Shear loading beyond reasonable limits, which can induce screw loosening and destroy the marginal bone crest and lead to subsequent gingival recession.
7. The location of the smooth collar of the implant in relation to the bone level, which might induce bone resorption due to the lack of bone affinity to smooth surfaces, which could further lead to the possible migration of the attachment levels.
8. The continuous pressure induced from a removable prosthesis or faulty prosthetic margins might lead to gingival recession.
9. Premature delivery of the final prosthesis (minimum of two months), which has proven to lead to postinsertion gingival recession because the soft tissue should reach a stable status prior to final crown insertion.
10. Osseous contouring in the second-stage surgery, which might stimulate further bone resorption that initiates gingival recession.
11. The geometry of the implant diameter in relation to the size of the abutment used, which might influence bone levels via platform switching, as shown in Figure 12.10.
12. The use of alcohol disinfectants for the healing abutments, which might lead to cell death of the peri-implant tissues and further recession. (See Figures 12.11A–C.)

A study by Oates et al. (2002) assessed the long-term changes of the facial soft tissue when a one-stage implant system was used. A total of 106 one-stage implants (ITI, Straumann, Switzerland) were evaluated in 39 patients. Implants were placed in maxillary and mandibular anterior regions. Clinical assessment of the soft tissues on the midfacial aspect of the implants was performed over a two-year period, at three- and six-month intervals, following placement of the final restoration.

The overall soft tissue rescission on the facial aspect of 61% of the 106 implants was 1 mm or more, whereas 19% of the implants showed 1 mm or more gain in soft tissue height. There was a significantly ($P < 0.01$) greater number of implants showing a gain in soft tissue levels in the mandibular implants compared with the maxillary implants. The study concluded that there was a significant decrease in the mean levels of tissue height of 0.6 mm within the first six months; however, in evaluating only patients showing a loss in tissue height around one or more implants, the mean loss in tissue height was 1.6 mm after 24 months.

These results suggested that the potential for significant changes in soft tissue levels after completion of restorative therapy need to be considered for implant therapy in esthetic areas. Despite the fact that the study did not state the postabutment connection provisionalization time for the implants used within the study, a conclusion can be drawn that the soft tissue around

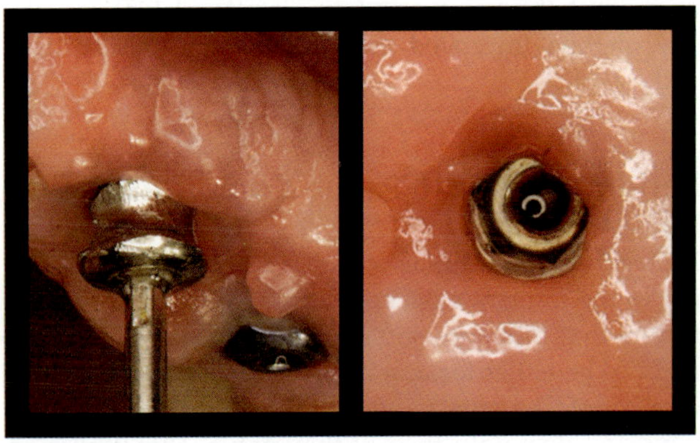

Figure 12.10. The O-ring effect of the platform switching.

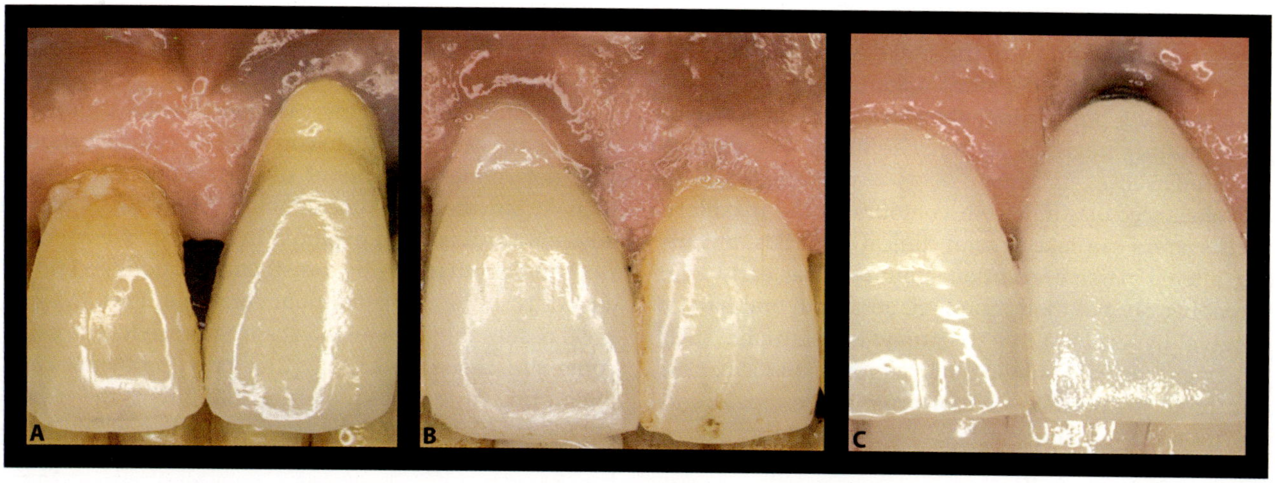

Figure 12.11A, B, C. Variable degrees of soft tissue recession around dental implants.

dental implants attains a certain behavior pattern that could be dealt with or avoided by using long-term provisionalization until soft tissue margins reach a stable situation. The position of the soft tissue is primarily related to the position of the marginal bone, especially in thin scalloped tissue biotypes.

Another study by Small and Tarnow (2000) evaluated the soft tissue behavior around dental implants following surgery to determine whether a predictable pattern of soft tissue changes could be identified. This study evaluated 63 implants in 11 patients. Subsequent measurements were recorded at one week, one month, three months, six months, nine months, and one year after baseline measurements. The majority of the recession occurred within the first three months, and 80% of all sites exhibited recession on the buccal surface. It is therefore recommended that a waiting period of three months be allowed for the tissue to stabilize before selecting a final abutment or making a final impression.

Some studies evaluated the soft tissue behavior around dental implants on a long-term basis. Apse and others (1991) evaluated the peri-implant tissues over four to nine years. The study examined plaque, keratinized mucosa, gingival indices, probing depth, and the height of the abutment above the peri-implant mucosa. The authors reported a decrease in probing depth, from 4.27 mm in the first year to 2.51 mm in the ninth year. Approximately 1.75 mm of tissue shrinkage occurred around dental implants over the nine years.

Bengazi and others (1996) evaluated peri-implant tissues longitudinally for two years following implant-supported prosthesis placement. They measured plaque, gingival inflammation, probing depth, bleeding upon probing, marginal soft tissue level, width of masticatory mucosa, and marginal soft tissue mobility. Though they did not publish an overall mean value for the recession, it appeared to be approximately 0.5 mm. All of the recession occurred within the first six months after prosthesis placement, and mandibular lingual sites showed the greatest tendency toward recession.

Recently, an interesting study by Meijndert et al. (2004) has led to the standardized assessment of the soft and hard peri-implant tissue levels. The study aimed to fabricate a simple acrylic device using standardized color slides and standardized dental X-rays so the changes in both the soft and hard tissue around implant-supported crowns can be evaluated. The reproducibility of the technique was tested on color slides as well as on dental X-rays in a series of implant-supported crowns and their neighboring teeth. The method showed a very minimal error of 0.14 ± 0.02 mm in soft tissue measurement. As a result, the future assessment of soft tissue marginal status around dental implants can be more precise and predictable.

When gingival asymmetry around natural teeth is to be corrected, the amount of free gingiva can be determined by probing through the connective tissue at the base of the sulcus after anesthesia has been administered. Measuring more than 2 mm beyond the base of the sulcus indicates a long junctional or connective tissue attachment that can be rectified by simple gingivectomy or flap procedure without osseous resection. Otherwise, bone must be resected as is needed for crown elongation to preserve normal "biologic width." When soft tissue recession occurs around dental implants, the treatment options are not versatile. A connective tissue graft might be used to mask the exposed metal collar. In the case of muscle pull, a vestibuloplasty might be performed, and in the case of a reduced amount of keratinized tissue, an onlay soft tissue graft might be used to prevent further recession. Severe gingival recession around dental implants is probably due to severe bone loss; therefore, the overall grafting that includes hard and soft tissues might be used to improve the situation. Sometimes gingival recession around dental implants can be a result of poor implant positioning; therefore, implant removal with grafting might be the only solution. (See Figures 12.12A–D.)

Unbalanced natural teeth contours in the maxillary incisor areas can take several clinical scenarios, including altered passive eruption; trauma at an early age, impeding normal tooth eruption; abnormal oral habits; gingival hyperplasia due to chronic local irritants such as cement retained subgingivally on orthodontic bands; and tooth malposition or root prominence (Spear and Townsend 1991). The selection of appropriate corrective procedures for gingival asymmetries depends on several factors: adequacy of attached gingiva, localized excessive exposure of tooth root structure, the necessity for apically positioning existing bands of keratinized tissue, the nature of the gingival attachment and position of the cemento-enamel junction, the type of planned restoration, and root angulation (Maynard and Wilson 1979).

Asymmetrical margins around dental implants usually are very tedious to correct. The clinician should first determine the amount of correction needed and then locate the cementoenamel junction (CEJ) of the adjacent teeth with an explorer. In the case of asymmetrical implant margins, the prosthetic solutions should be a priority. If the first attempt at correction fails, the gingival tissues might require a grafting procedure to overcome the tissue deficiency. The only problem when attempting to treat asymmetrical margins is the resultant long pocket around the abutment collar, which complicates the long-term health of the area. An implant repositioning protocol could be a valid solution to move the osseous levels to appropriate levels to avoid violating the biological width and forming a long pocket. (See Figures 12.13A–F.)

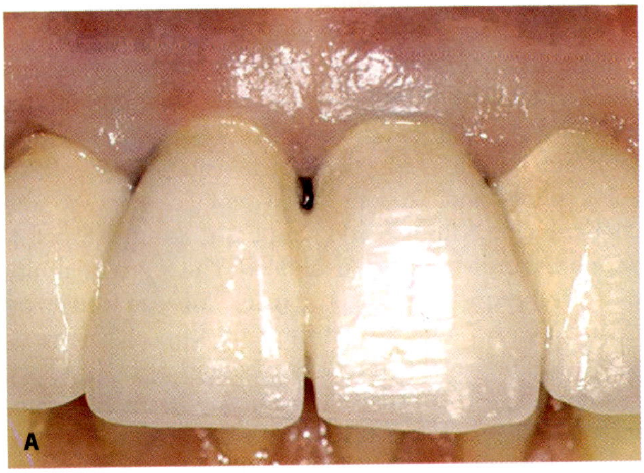

Figure 12.12A. Implant supported prosthesis replacing the upper four maxillary incisors, note the excellent marginal condition of the gingiva.

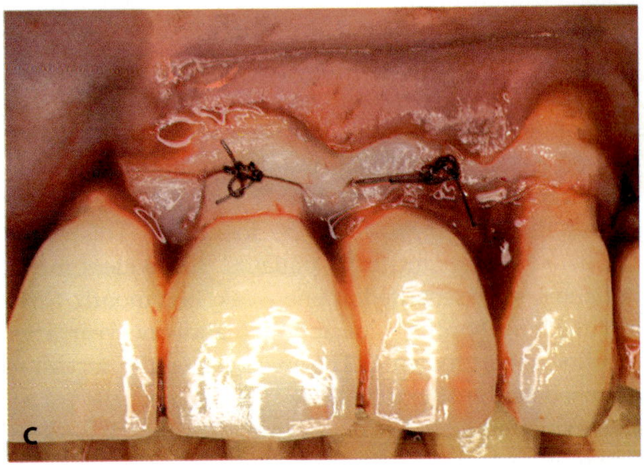

Figure 12.12C. A connective tissue graft is being used to mask the metal show.

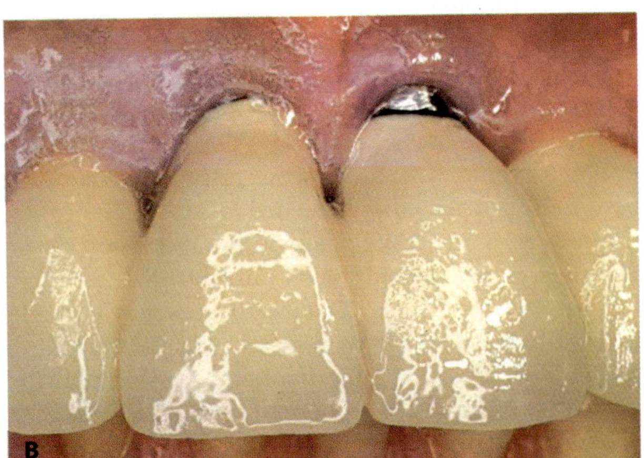

Figure 12.12B. One year post restorative gingival recession.

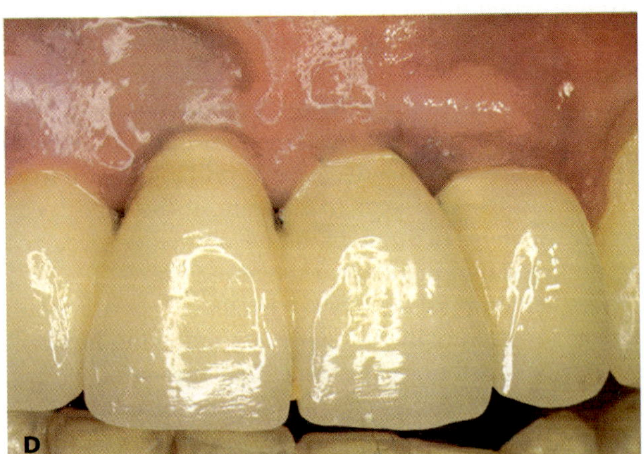

Figure 12.12D. The post healing clinical result.

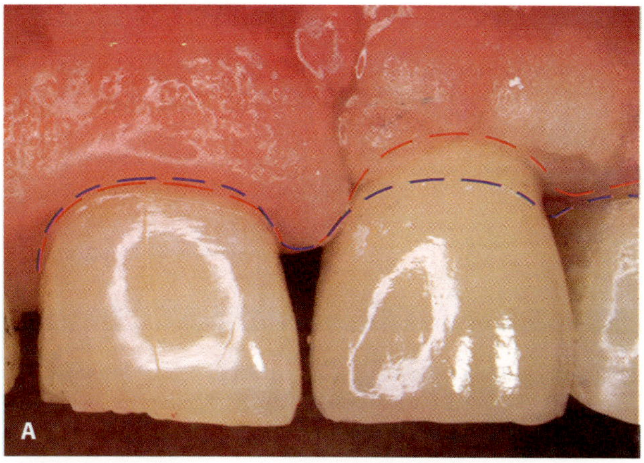

Figure 12.13A. Asymmetrical implant supported prothesis contour.

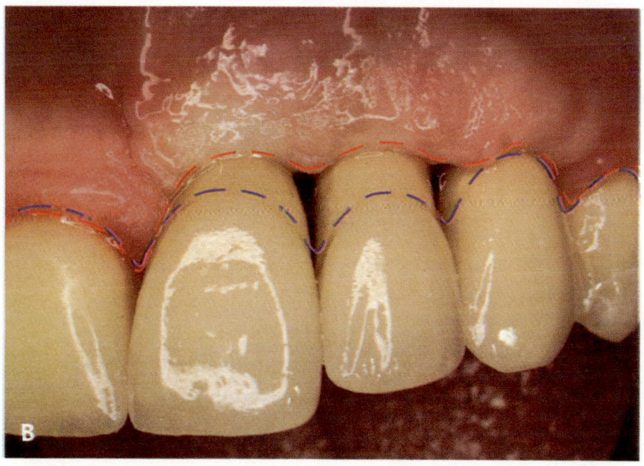

Figure 12.13B. Tissue deficiency that lead to an asymmetrical prosthetic contour.

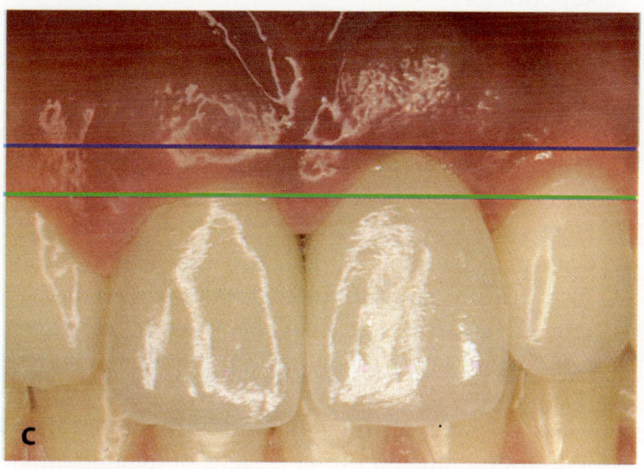

Figure 12.13C. Asymmetrical implant supported prosthetic contour related to the place of the maxillary left central incisor.

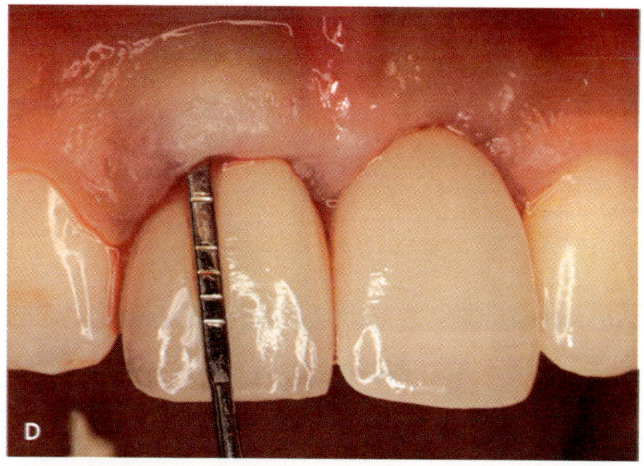

Figure 12.13D. A deep pocket around the adjacent natural central right incisor that mandates reduction.

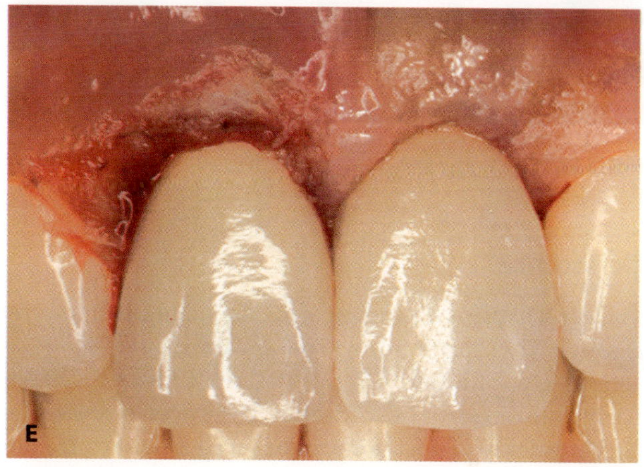

Figure 12.13E. Gingival excision and recountouring was performed in order to allow hygienic pocket depth and solve the asymmetrical problem.

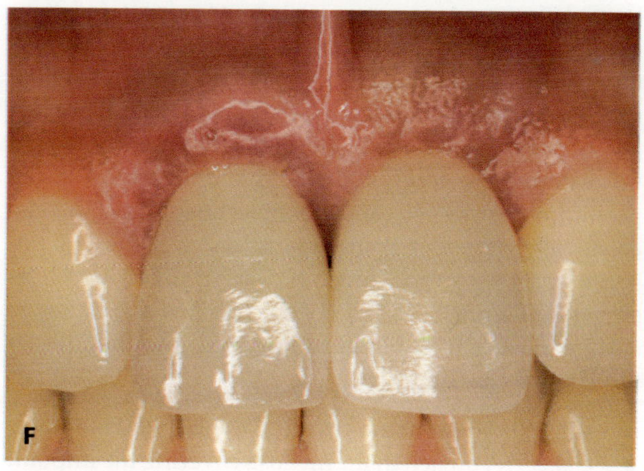

Figure 12.13F. The case shows three months post soft tissue healing a more satisfactory appearance and almost symmetrical contours.

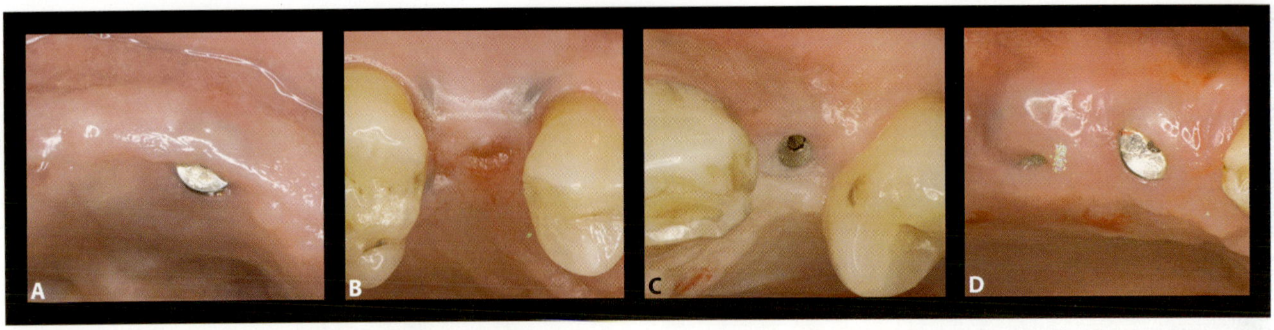

Figure 12.14. **A.** Class E Gingival dehiscence over an implant fixture (Barboza classification). **B.** Class A Gingival dehiscence over an implant fixture(Barboza classification). **C.** Class B Gingival dehiscence over an implant fixture. (Barboza classification). **D.** Class A & E Gingival dehiscence over an implant fixture (Barboza classification).

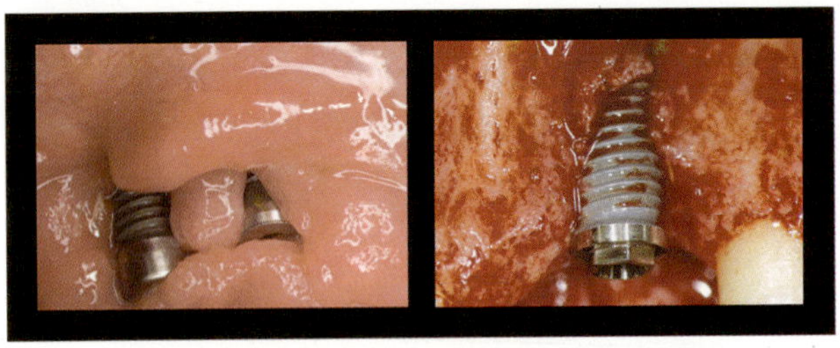

Figure 12.15. Osseous breakdown of the bone-implant interface due to soft tissue dehiscence.

Dehiscence

The early exposure of a part of the dental implant fixture through the surrounding soft tissue may lead to a serious complication during the initial healing phase. Early full or partial exposure of the cover screws can be considered a foci for plaque accumulation. If left untreated, this may result in inflammation, damage to the peri-implant mucosa, and possible bone loss (Barboza and Caula 2002). (See Figures 12.14A–D.)

Dehiscence might occur from over-tightened sutures, flap closure under tension, a decreased amount of keratinized tissues, torn wound edges or a lacerated flap, muscle pull along the wound edges, and/or oral habits (i.e., smoking, alcohol). The potential threat of dehiscence is bacterial colonization that could occur between the implant surface and the oral environment. If left untreated, there could be inflammation, damage to the peri-implant mucosa, and possible bone loss (Toljanic et al. 1999). Thus, it is important to detect these exposures early to avoid more serious complications, as shown in Figure 12.15. Tal (1999) classified spontaneous early exposure of submerged implants into the following clinical classes:

- Class 0: The mucosa covering the implant is intact.
- Class 1: A breach in the mucosa covering the implant is observed. The cover screw can be detected by a periodontal probe.
- Class 2: The mucosa above the cover screw is fenestrated. The cover screw is visible. The borders of the perforation's aperture do not reach or overlap the borders of the cover screw at any point.
- Class 3: The cover screw is visible. In some parts, the borders of the perforation's aperture overlap the borders of the cover screw.
- Class 4: The cover screw is completely exposed.

(See Figure 12.16A–E.)

Barboza and Caula (2002) described another detailed division for implant exposure, as well as clinical recommendations for the treatment:

- Class I: Cover screw spontaneous early partial exposure—a communication between the cover screw and oral cavity, with a fenestrated mucosa still partially covering the cover screw.
- Class II: Cover screw spontaneous early total exposure—the fenestration reveals the cover screw completely. Subdivisions are proposed based on clinical signs of healthy, inflammation, and suppuration.
- Class A: No signs of inflammation. Mucosa texture, volume, and color are within the normal limits of health. No purulent exudate is observed.
- Class B: No signs of inflammation with suppuration. Mucosa texture, volume, and color are within the normal limits of health; however, purulent exudate is present.
- Class C: The signs of inflammation and the mucosal texture and/or color are altered, edematous mucosa and/or pain may be present. However, visually or upon palpation, no purulent exudate is observed.
- Class D: Signs of inflammation with suppuration, fenestrated mucosa presents signs of inflammation, and, visually or upon palpation, purulent exudate is observed.

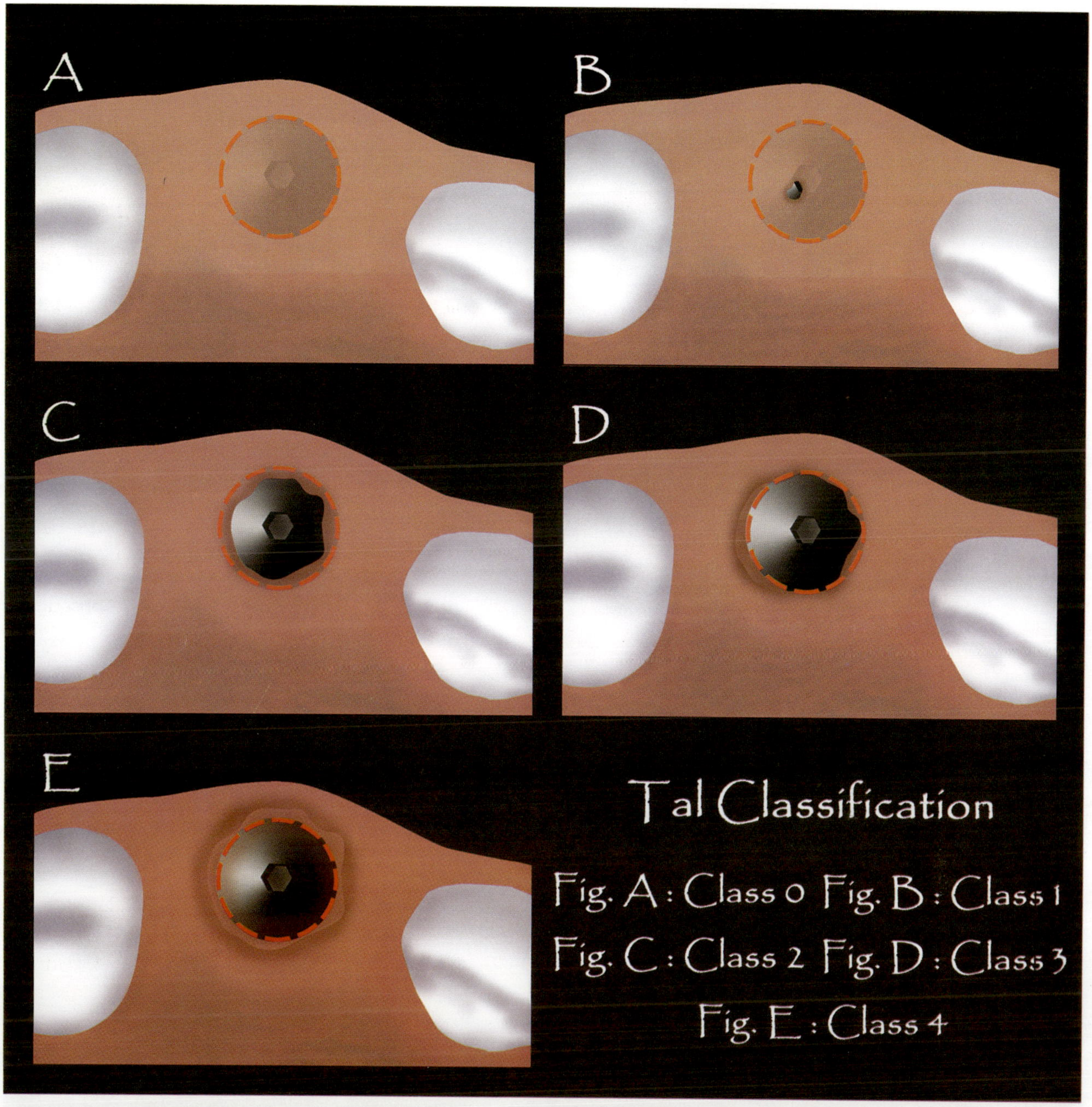

Figure 12.16. **A.** Tal classification for gingival exposure on top of an implant site. Class 0: The mucosa covering the implant is intact. **B.** Class 1: A breach in the mucosa covering the implant is observed. Cover screw can be detected by a periodontal probe. **C.** Class 2: The mucosa above the cover screw is fenestrated. Cover screw is visible. The borders of the perforation's aperture do not reach or overlap the borders of the cover screw at any point. **D.** Class 3: Cover screw is visible. In some parts, the borders of the perforation's aperture overlap the borders of the cover screw. **E.** Class 4: Cover screw is completely exposed.

(See Figure 12.17A–F.)

Dealing with implant dehiscence can vary according to its category. Barboza and Caula (2002) introduced four distinctive treatment modalities for implant dehiscence:

- Treatment modality No. 1 includes professional cleaning of the cover screw if plaque or calculus is detected. The cover screw should be mechanically cleaned using specific curettes, abrasive air, rubber cup, polishing paste, oral hygiene instructions reinforcement, and rinses with chlorhexidine digluconate 0.12%. Shortened recall periods are called for if inflammation signs are present. Radiographs are indicated to evaluate peri-implant bone morphology.

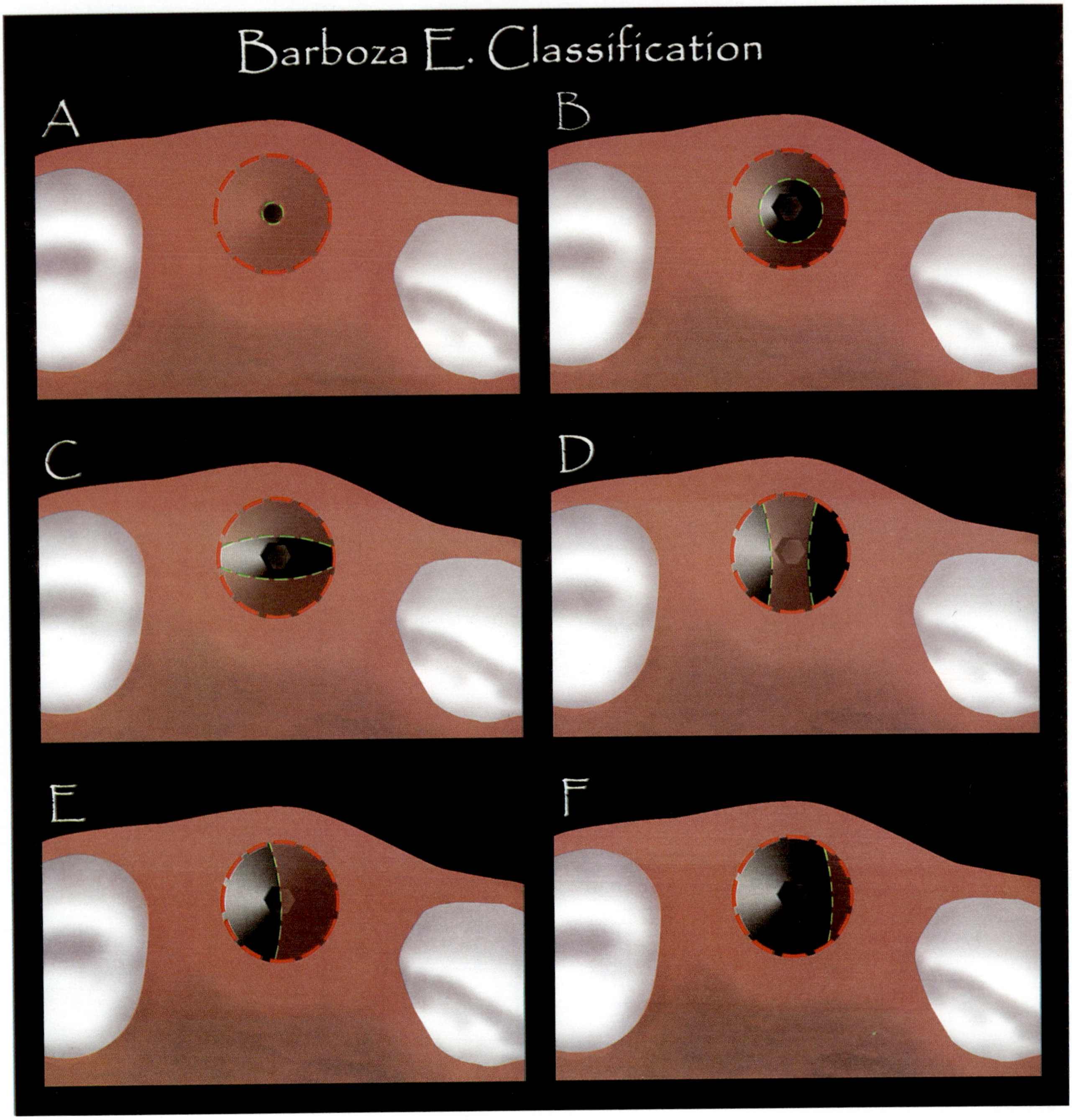

Figure 12.17A–F. Barboza classification for gingival exposure on top of an implant site.

- Treatment modality No. 2 includes the identification of microorganisms and antibiotic therapy. In the presence of purulent exudates, specific microbial information is indispensable. Microbiological samples must be collected to identify the putative pathogens. If the patient presents a localized peri-implant problem, a topical antibiotic therapy can be considered. If other areas of peri-implant or periodontal disease are present, a systemic antibiotic should be administered.
- Treatment modality No. 3 includes surgical exposure of the cover screw and adaptation of a healing abutment to avoid the mucosa regrowth and facilitate patient oral hygiene.
- Treatment modality No. 4 includes typical peri-implantitis treatment. If bone destruction is radiographically detected, surgical intervention is necessary to correct tissue morphology or to apply guided bone regeneration techniques. Another treatment protocol (Nemcovsky and Artzi 2002) was pro-

posed to treat the dehiscence with the bone regenerative therapy in treating buccal type dehiscent defects around 102 dental implants (42 microtextured, 56 titanium-plasma-sprayed, and 4 hydroxyapatite-coated). Dental implants were placed according to the surgical techniques outlined by the implant system being used. Following implant stabilization, the distance from the most apical aspect of the buccal crest to the fixture platform was recorded as the defect height. The widest mesiodistal dimension of the bony defect was recorded as the defect width. After grafting and barrier membrane application, the implants were allowed to heal for six to eight months. At second-stage surgery, defect height and width were again recorded. Resolution of defect height and width was reported as the millimeter linear change between stage one and two surgeries. The percentage area of defect fill at stage two was also reported. Early bone loss is linked to the exposure of an implant between stage one and stage two implant surgery (Toljanic et al. 1999). Bone levels were measured during placement of 275 implants in the maxillae of 50 subjects. Repeated bone height measurements were obtained at implant uncovering. Fourteen implants in seven patients were exposed to the oral cavity through the mucosa at the second-stage surgery. Patients with one or more exposed sites demonstrated a likelihood of bone loss 3.9 times greater than patients with nonexposed sites. These results suggested that the exposure of an implant during the healing period might serve as a potential indicator of the occurrence of early bone loss (Guerrero et al. 1999). An inverse relationship was noted between the incidence of unanticipated surgical events and the level of crestal bone loss. The nature of the event and the surgical response at the time of implantation may account for this finding. However, the study did not distinguish whether thin scalloped or thick flat tissue biotypes were tested.

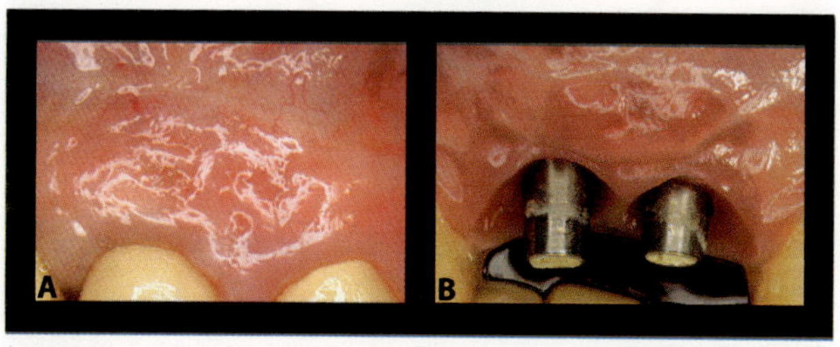

Figure 12.18. **A.** Post surgical scar tissue formation. **B.** Another example of deeper scar tissue.

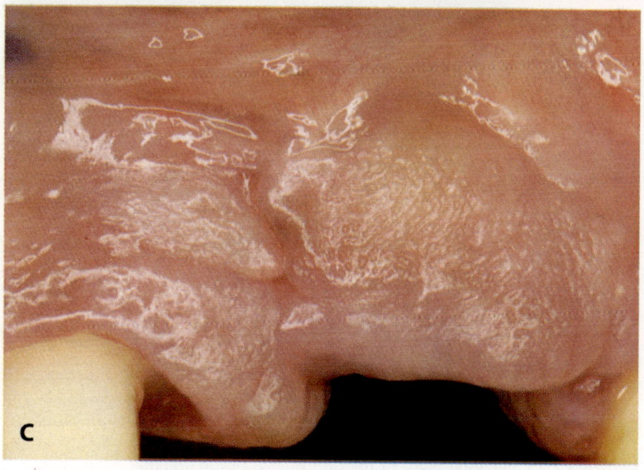

Figure 12.18C. Post surgical scar tissue formation.

Postsurgical Scar Formation

As a result of multiple surgeries, improper approximation of flap edges, improper flap design, or nonmeticulous tissue manipulation, scar tissue or a soft tissue callus may form. Usually soft tissue scars are not esthetically determinant if not shown while smiling; in other words, when the patient possesses a high smile line, scars become an esthetically compromising factor. Scar tissues can be dealt with either by laser resurfacing or excision and onlay soft tissue grafting, as shown in Figures 12.18A–F.

Missing Papilla

The preservation of the interimplant or the interdental papilla is an important issue to the overall treatment success, because the missing peri-implant papilla or the interimplant papilla might lead to serious esthetic concerns, such as a blunted papilla between two adjacent implants or a black triangle-like appearance between teeth. All efforts should be made to preserve or spare the papilla during the treatment, and in case the papilla is

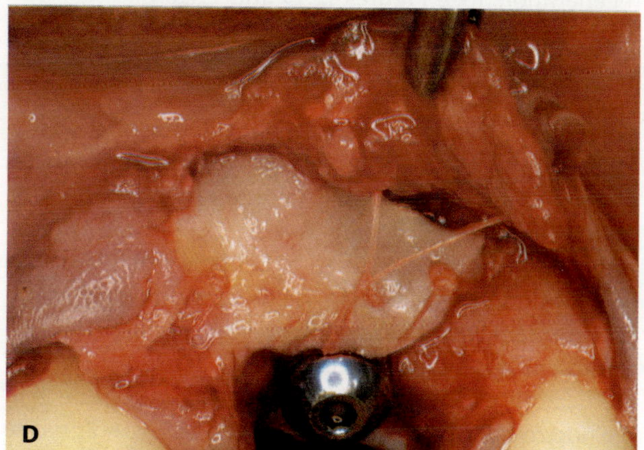

Figure 12.18D. The scar tissue is excised and a connective tissue graft is placed underneath the defect in order to provide a better tissue profile.

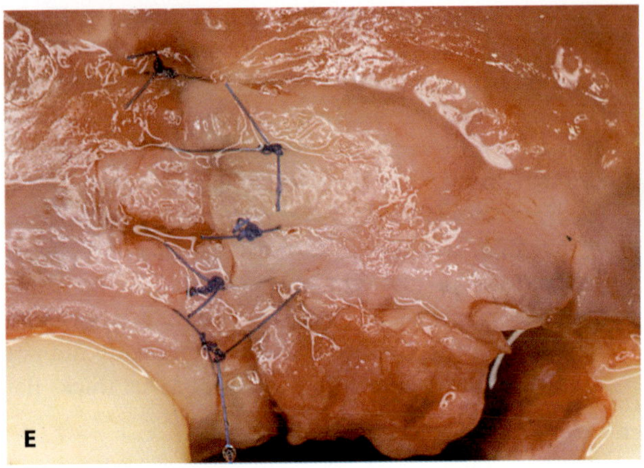

Figure 12.18E. Soft tissue closure suing ultra fine cosmetic sutures.

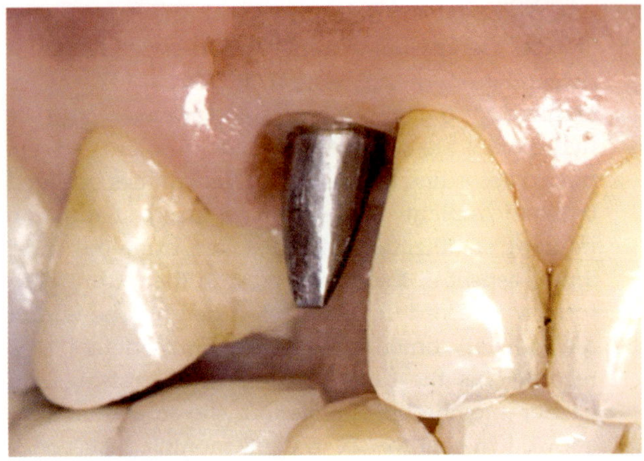

Figure 12.19. Missing peri-implant papilla.

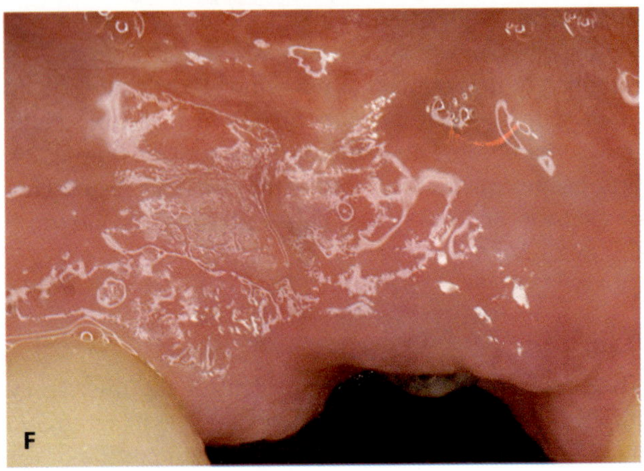

Figure 12.18F. The final healing showing the eliminated scar tissues.

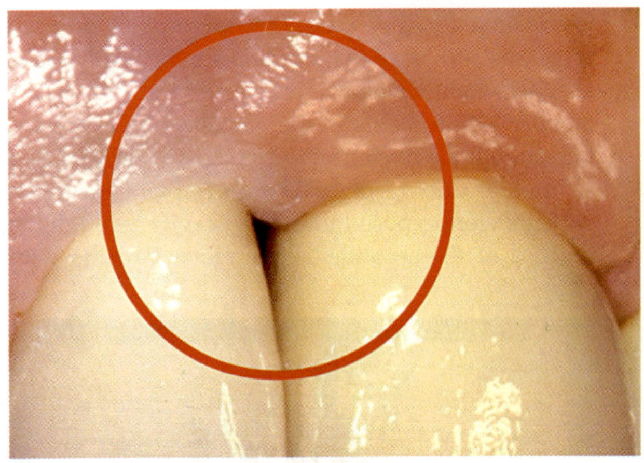

Figure 12.20. The red circle shows the black triangle between two implant supported restorations.

lost, all efforts should be made to achieve predictable regeneration. (See Figures 12.19 and 12.20.)

Missing Buccal Tissue Volume

Missing buccal tissue volume can result due to poor surgical manipulations, either when the implant fixture is inserted in insufficient tissue volume, or when soft tissue sloughing occurred during healing. The overall buccal soft tissue volume is reduced either horizontally or vertically, and this reduction in the tissue volume can influence implant esthetics and the overall prosthetic profile. Treatment options to regain the lost tissue volume are predictable, especially if the missing tissue volume is in the horizontal dimension, because connective soft tissue grafts can be used routinely to regain the missing bulk. (See Figures 12.21 and 2.22.)

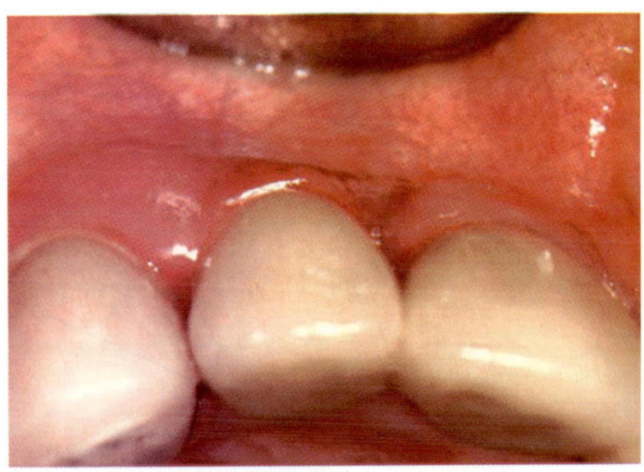

Figure 12.21. Labial view of missing buccal tissue volume.

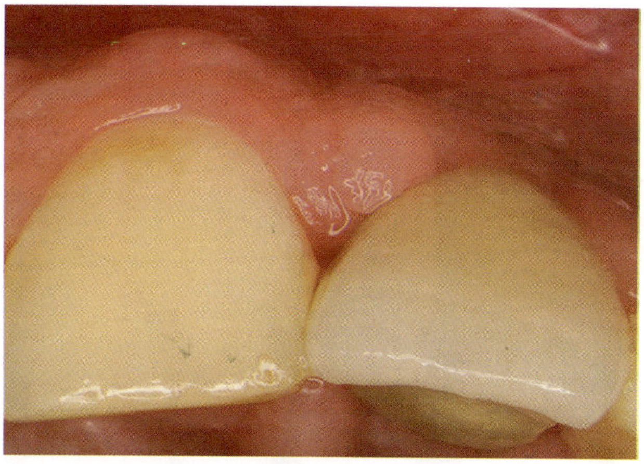

Figure 12.22. Another labial deficiency.

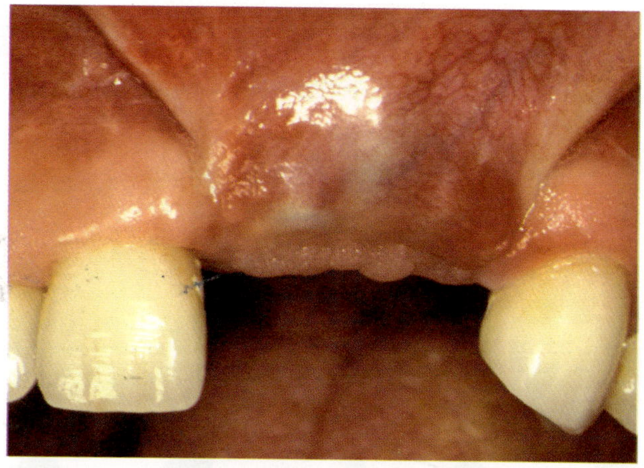

Figure 12.23. Keratinized tissue loss post surgical intervention.

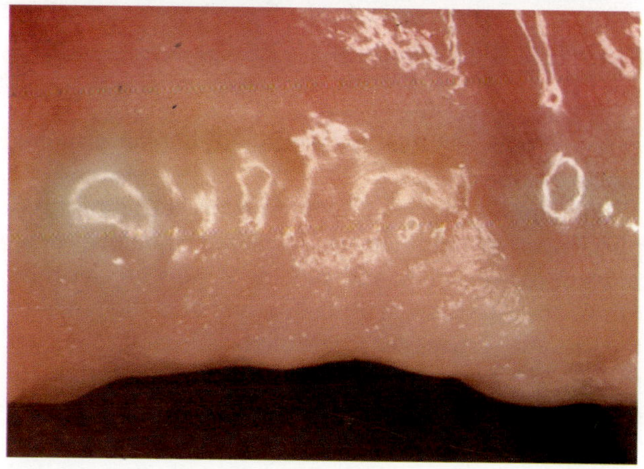

Figure 12.24. Keratinized tissue loss opposite to two dental implants.

Loss of Keratinized Tissue

As a result of successful tissue healing or a bone-grafting procedure, a possible reduction of the amount of keratinized mucosa sometimes occurs. A significant tissue reduction may be due to the coronal displacement of the labial tissues to close the tissues without tension. The resultant reduction in the keratinized tissues might require an onlay-grafting procedure to regain the tissue band continuity or an apical repositioning flap. A vestibuloplasty can be performed after the onlay graft is completed. A connective tissue graft also may be used to enhance the tissue quality either at the first- or second-stage surgery. (See Figures 12.23 and 12.24.)

Incision Line Opening

The incision line opening is a very common event that occurs during the healing phase. There are several contributing factors, both systemic or local. The incision line opening can lead to the rapid breakdown of the bone graft or the bone-implant interface. The reasons for the opening should be identified in the case of an incision line opening that exposes the underlying graft or the implant fixture. Most of the incision line opening usually is due to flap closure under tension, local irritation from an existing prosthesis, or uncontrolled systematic conditions, such as diabetes mellitus. The opened flap edges should be resutured and approximated. If the opening exposes mature bone, healing by secondary intention may occur eventually. In this case, a periodontal wound pack may be applied to the area and the area is monitored to ensure satisfactory closure. (See Figures 12.25A–C.)

Soft Tissue Inflammation

Bacterial invasion of the peri-implant tissues may result in soft tissue inflammatory changes and rapid bone loss. This condition was termed peri-implantitis and was defined by Meffert (1992) as the progressive loss of peri-implant bone as well as soft tissue inflammatory changes. This definition implies that bone loss and soft tissue inflammation occur together as a result of bacterial invasion. As previously noted, Tonetti and Schmid (1994) also divided the host's reaction to bacterial invasion into two groups: peri-implant mucositis and peri-implantitis. Mombelli and others (1987) have shown that gram-negative rods, including *bacteroides* and *fusobacterium* ssp., are consistent with failing implants. Rosenberg and others (1991) later suggested the association between the presence of spirochetes and motile rods (which, on average, made up 42% of the total morphotypes in the subgingival microflora, with a predominance of *Peptostreptococcus micros, Fusbacterium* species, and

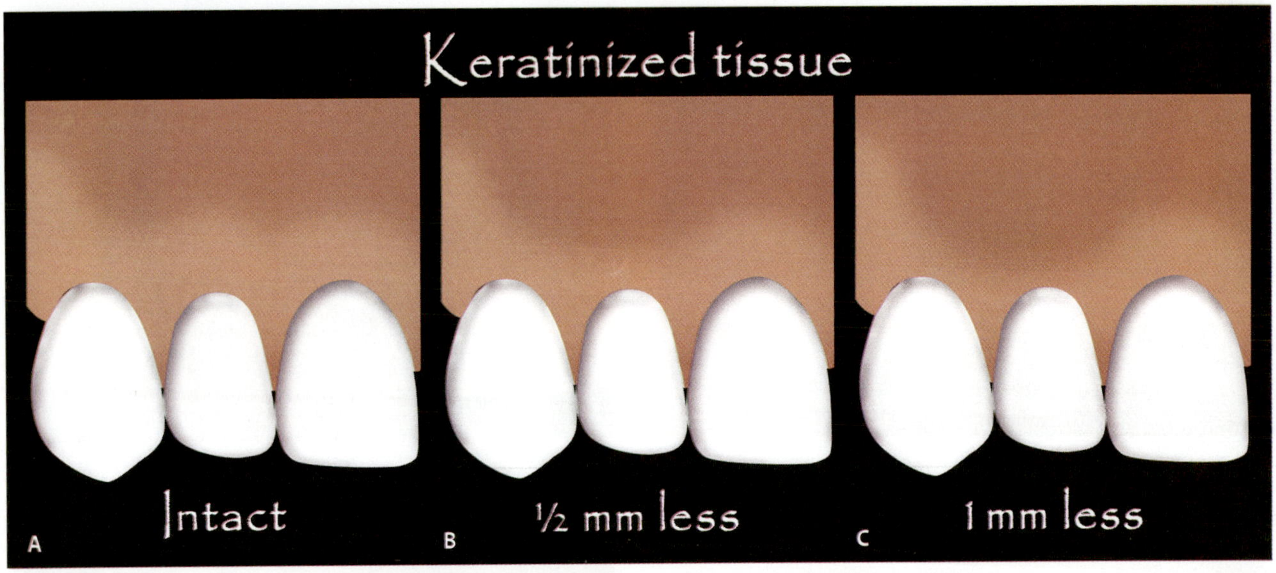

Figure 12.25A, B, C. Different clinical situations for incision line opening.

enteric gram-negative rods) around implants failing because of infection.

The clinical signs of inflammation, bleeding, and purulence, in addition to increased mobility, peri-implant radiolucency, and probing depths greater than 6 mm, are associated with failing implants. Removal of the irritating cause is of prime importance. The clinician should select the proper antibiotics type and dosage to overcome the condition. (See Figure 12.26.)

A study by Powell et al. (2005) evaluated a sample comprised of 395 patients, including 1,053 fully documented surgical procedures. Surgical techniques included several periodontal, implantology, grafting clinical procedures. Infection was defined as increasing and progressive swelling with the presence of suppuration. The impact of various treatment variables was examined, including postsurgical antibacterial rinses, systemic antibiotics, and dressings. Results were analyzed using Fisher's exact test and Pearson's chi-square test. Of the 1,053 surgical procedures evaluated, there were 22 infections for an overall prevalence of 2.09%. Patients who received antibiotics as part of the surgical protocol (pre- and/ or postsurgically) developed 8 infections in 281 procedures (2.85%) compared to 14 infections in 772 procedures (1.81%) in which antibiotics were not used. Procedures in which chlorhexidine was used during postsurgical care had a lower infection rate (17 infections in 900 procedures, 1.89%) compared to procedures in which chlorhexidine was not used (5 infections in 153 procedures, 3.27%). Surprisingly, the use of a postsurgical dressing demonstrated a slightly higher rate of infection (8 infections in 300 procedures, 2.67%) than nonuse of a dressing (14 infections in 753 procedures, 1.86%).

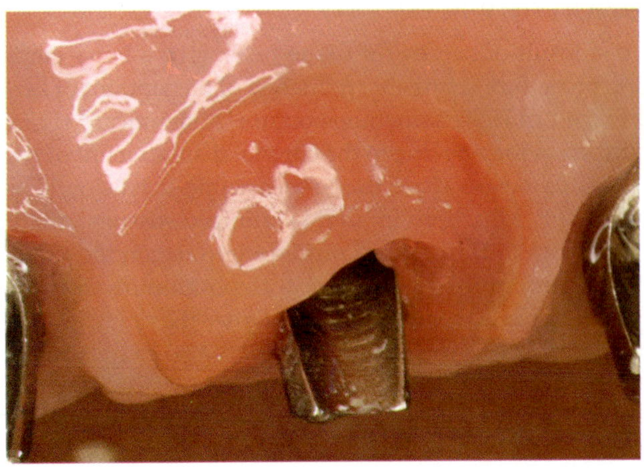

Figure 12.26. Soft tissue inflammation due to the intrusion of local irritating factor.

Despite these trends, no statistically significant relationship was found between postsurgical infection and any of the treatment variables examined, including the use of preoperative antibiotics. The study stated that although preoperative antibiotics are commonly used when performing certain regenerative and implant surgical procedures, data from this and other studies suggest that there may be no benefit in using antibiotics for the sole purpose of preventing postsurgical infections. Further large-scale, controlled clinical studies are warranted to determine the role of preoperative antibiotics in the prevention of periodontal postsurgical infections. In general, purulent areas respond to home irrigation devices. In the event of abscess formation, amoxicillin with clavulanate potassium (Augmentin,

SmithKline Beecham, Pittsburgh, PA, USA), 250 milligrams (mg), three times daily for 10 days, is prescribed. Augmentin has been suggested for treatment of abscessed sites because the clavulanate potassium portion of this drug renders the beta-lactamase enzyme produced by penicillin-resistant microflora inactive. The beta-lactamase enzyme destroys the beta-lactam ring in penicillin, rendering penicillin inactive.

In conclusion, the role of infection in the etiology of dental implant failure is evident, as previously suggested and from the results of Boutros and others (1996). Therefore, careful attention should be taken when placing implants in a partially edentulous periodontally involved mouth. In addition, complete periodontal therapy should be attempted before implant placement to avoid unnecessary complications.

Peri-implant Hard Tissue Complications

Numerous bone-grafting methods have been introduced to restore maxillary and mandibular osseous defects. However, postoperative and intraoperative treatment complications have been recorded, these have been due to the failure to detect hidden systemic issues, improper conceptual decisions by the clinician, or a combination of biological or technical reasons.

The use of allogenic and alloplastic bone-grafting materials as an alterative to autogenous grafts has been documented extensively in the literature (Jovanovic and Nevins 1995, Tolman 1995, Burchardt 1987, Friedlander 1987, Schwartz et al. 1996). Their advantages include the elimination of donor site entry. However, the clinical predictability is still in question. It has been shown that the amount of healed bone following guided bone regeneration (GBR) with demineralized freeze-dried bone allograft (DFDBA) and a bioabsorbable membrane is significantly less than the initial quantity.

Recently, a study by Zubillaga and others (2003) was designed to determine if the amount of GBR would be affected by using an osteoinductive DFDBA and bioabsorbable membrane and membrane stabilization. Eleven extraction sites (10 patients) were treated with DFDBA and bioabsorbable membrane before placing endosseous implants. Standardized alveolar height and width measurements were taken after extraction, following GBR, and four months postoperatively, at predetermined measurement points (sites midpoint and 3 mm mesial and distal from the midpoint) and classified as augmented (<1 mm increase of GBR height or width) or grafted (>1 mm increase). Five membranes were stabilized.

Results showed that 3 mm from the crest, augmented points exhibited a complete loss of augmented width. There was also some loss of pre-GBR bone width (ranging from 4.7% to 20%) at augmented and grafted points. Augmented points lost 83.3% to 92.3% of augmented width 4 mm from the crest, and grafted points lost 12.9% to 18% of pre-GBR width. Loss of augmented height ranged from 93.5% to 100%. Augmented (except distal) and grafted measurement points lost 2.1% to 12% of pre-GBR height. Comparing tacked and nontacked sites, the former manifested better augmented bone width, while the latter better augmented bone height. The study recommended meticulous membrane handling as well as stabilization to attain better clinical results. (See Figures 12.27A–C.)

Other disadvantages of allografts include the risk of rejection, high rate of infection, nonunion, risk of rapid resorption, and problems related to the considerable technical precision required to pack and hold the graft in place in bleeding sites (Lane 1995, Tatum 1996, Barboza et al. 1999, Wang et al. 1990, Toriumi et al. 1991). The main complication in regenerating bone defects using nonresorbable membranes that use expanded polytetrafluoroethylene (ePTFE; W.L. Gore and Associates, Flagstaff, AZ, USA) is the membrane exposure rates that reached up to 31% (Lang et al. 1994) caused by flap

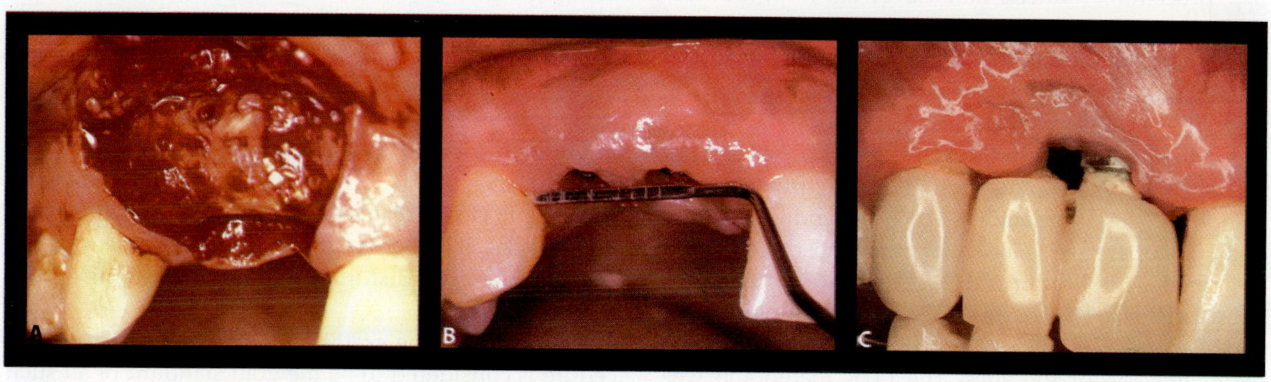

Figure 12.27. **A.** Vertical osseous defect that has been augmented via titanium mesh. **B.** The soft tissue profile pre-abutment connection. **C.** Two year's post-restorative; one implant was lost and bone resorption occurred. (Failed bone grafting procedure)

sloughing or incision-line opening. These complications have led to further postsurgical complications and failures. Membrane exposure provided a channel of communication between the oral environment and newly forming tissues, increasing the chance for infection and decreasing bone regeneration potential.

Guided tissue regeneration (GTR) procedures using resorbable or nonresorbable membranes have caused a small portion of the coronal aspect of the membrane to be exposed, usually near a crestal incision site or adjacent to a proximal tooth surface and a space lateral to where the e-PTFE barrier is created. This space, sometimes called a "pseudopocket," represents a potential site for bacterial colonization (Selvig et al. 1990, Schallhorn and McClain 1988), which leads to a rapid breakdown of the grafted material underneath the membrane. Cocci and nonmotile rods, constituting 46.2% and 49.1% of the flora, respectively have been found. Spirochetes (1.7%) and motile rods (2.9%) were found. Streptococcus and Actinomyces species were also found (Murphy 1995, pp. 363–375).

The exposure of the membrane subsequently alters the normal healing response of the surrounding tissues. Unlike resorbable membranes, nonresorbable membranes seem to block the blood supply to the underlying mucoperiosteal flap. This prevents the establishment of the collateral microvasculature anastomoses necessary for gingival flap survival (Selliseth and Selvig 1994).

The frequency of this complication ranges from 4% to 41% of sites treated and depends heavily on the surgical experience of the clinician (Buser et al. 1990, Lang et al. 1994). The chance of soft tissue dehiscence might increase when GBR is performed in conjunction with immediate implant placement in extraction sockets. Sloughing or necrosis of a portion of the flap could be frequent due to blood perfusion. Studies have demonstrated that blood flow to the coronal edges of the mucosal flap is significantly decreased after a GTR procedure, compared to the blood flow allowed by a regular flap procedure (Zanetta-Barbosa et al. 1993, Gottlow et al. 1986). GTR complications usually are accompanied by clinical manifestations such as purulence exudate, tissue sloughing, swelling, pain, and membrane piercing through the mucosa.

A retrospective study (Murphy 1995, pp. 549–561) of 102 sites in 62 patients examined the frequency of complications associated with GTR and concluded that postoperative pain was the most frequently described complication (16%). Purulence occurred in approximately 11% of the sites. Swelling, sloughing, and the presence of exophytic tissue occurred in approximately 7% of the sites. The GTR membrane was exposed in 87% of the sites. The average time to exposure was between two and three weeks (16.2 days) postoperatively.

Swelling exerts a tensile force on the coronal edge of the healing gingival flap. Purulence occurs only at sites that demonstrate material exposure. However, in many sites that demonstrated purulence, associated gingival tissues present with only mild gingival inflammation. Because only sites that demonstrate material exposure display purulence, the presence of purulence appears to depend on the development of the pseudopocket or gingival space. Prevention of purulence is related to timely removal of the material within four to six weeks (Murphy 1995, pp. 549–561).

Antibiotic administration had no significant effect on the flora, when given after four weeks of GTR placement (Demolon et al. 1993). However, antibiotics were associated with a significant decrease in the clinical signs of inflammation. Ciancio and others (1990) have demonstrated that systemic doxycycline improves the immediate postoperative health of the gingival tissues and decreases swelling in a GTR procedures. It has also been proposed that applying a metronidazole gel locally at the time of surgery decreases the amount of microorganisms present during early healing of GTR procedures; this was only limited to 2 weeks time (Sander et al. 1994). The treatment of the purulence depends on whether or not the membrane is removed. However, premature removal of the membrane results in significantly decreased regeneration (Lekholm et al. 1993). It has been suggested that the maintenance of the exposed membrane should take six to eight weeks, along with strict oral hygiene procedures (Buser et al. 1994). If the membrane is to remain, then local irrigation with chlorhexidine, mechanical oral hygiene procedures, and proper antibiotic therapy are administered.

Complications from GTR are associated with smoking, poor oral hygiene, and decrease in the vascular supply to the flap. Placement of the membrane in an apical direction, beveled flap edges, and remote incisions might help to reduce membrane exposure (Buser et al. 1994). It has been suggested to replace the membrane with another one if it becomes exposed, but the final regeneration predictability and soft tissue management is still questionable (Valentini et al. 1993).

Many clinicians tend not to pay attention to membrane displacement underneath the mucosa, which may lead to insufficient volume of regenerated bone. This might be attributed to wearing a partial denture postsurgery and the failure to stabilize the membrane, whether it is resorbable or nonresorbable, with membrane tacks. It is believed that micromovement of the membrane might disturb the callus formation underneath the wound.

Autogenous bone grafting in any reconstructive procedure is considered to be the gold standard of all such procedures because it provides proteins such as bone-enhancing substrates, minerals, and vital bone cells to the recipient site, resulting in high success rates

(Burchardt 1987, Schwartz et al. 1996). Experimental evidence indicates that grafts from membranous bone show less resorption than endochondral bone. This is due to early revascularization, better potential for incorporation in the maxillofacial region because of a biochemical similarity in the collagen content, and greater inductive capacity is because of a higher concentration of bone morphogenetic proteins and growth factors (Lu and Rabie 2003, Smith and Abramson 1974).

Trabecular grafts provide numerous osteogenic cells in their structure, while a cortical graft has fewer surviving osteogenic cells but provides the most bone morphogenetic protein (BMP), the essential agent for bone formation (Burchardt 1987). BMP differentiates host mesenchymal cells into osteoblasts (Friedlander 1987). In addition, BMP provides more resistance to the graft structure, which impedes soft tissue ingrowth, but also may prolong the time needed for blood vessels to infiltrate the graft (Friedlander 1987). Corticotrabecular grafts can be shaped and trimmed to fit the recipient bed, and the trabecular part is placed to face the recipient bed. The healing process follows one of three paths: (1) the graft becomes viable, gradually acquiring the characteristics of adjacent bone, (2) the graft resorbs partially or completely, resulting in instability, or (3) the graft becomes sequestrated and is treated by the host as a foreign body (Smith and Abramson 1974).

The dense structure of the cortical portion of the graft offers improved implant stability and stress transmission upon implant loading (Schwartz-Arad and Dori 2002). A study showed that an intraoral block bone graft was suitable for augmentation of short spans such as in a single tooth area, medium spans such as in a two- to three-tooth area from an adjacent donor area, and long spans up to complete jaw augmentation. Both vertical and horizontal addition can be achieved successfully (Schwartz-Arad et al. 2005). While Misch (1999) recommended that only short spans be augmented using intraoral block bone grafts that study showed the length of the recipient site did not influence the complication or failure rates.

However, the use of onlay autogenous grafts has shown that complications other than graft ununion and graft morbidity can be expected, such as extensive graft resorption, especially with iliac grafts, but less with mandibular grafts (because they are from the same embryonic origin as the recipient site). (See Figures 12.28A–I.) Complications might occur at the recipient

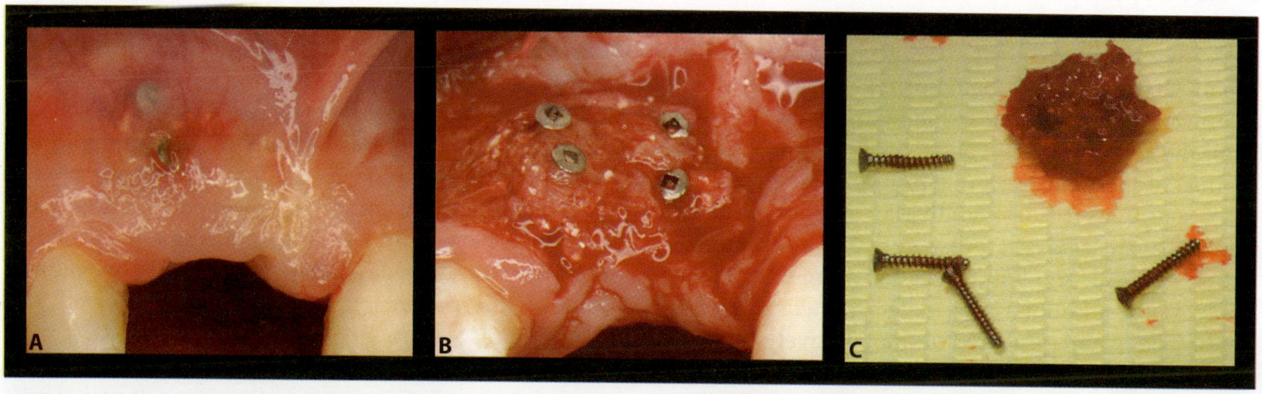

Figure 12.28. A. Exposed titanium screws due to thinning of the keratinized tissues and graft separation. B. The bone graft is exposed. C. The bone graft is being removed along with the screws and the area curetted.

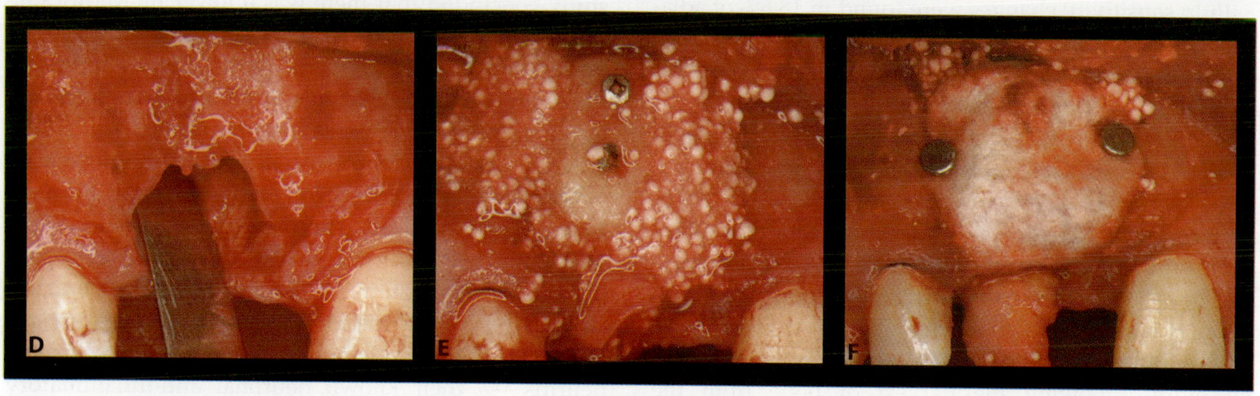

Figure 12.28. D. The underlying host bed is prepared. E. A new autogenous block graft stabilized and the spaces filled with particulate bone graft. F. Biomend membrane was stabilized with membrane taks.

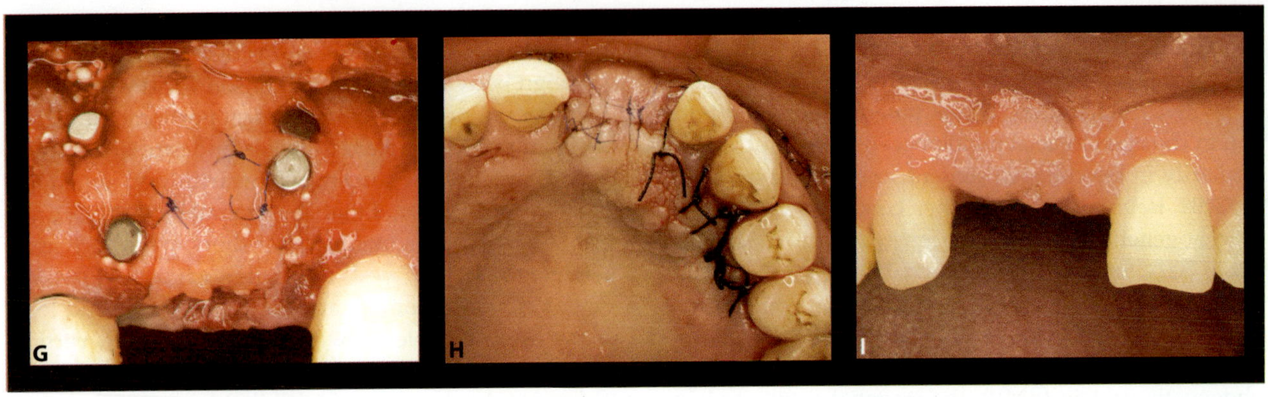

Figure 12.28. **G.** Pedicle connective tissue is laid on top to allow tissue bulking. **H.** The area sutured. **I.** Two months post healing showing favorable tissue condition and vertical tissue development.

site or the donor site. The possible complications or morbidity that might occur on the donor sites are numerous. A study by Joshi (2004) has evaluated the morbidity at the donor site following harvest of chin bone for intraoral augmentation. Thirty-three percent of the patients suffered postoperative morbidity, and 18.5% experienced woodiness/numbness of the lower anterior teeth at the first postoperative visit and at 12 months.

Intraoral neurosensory complications at the donor site also have been investigated. A study by von Arx and others (2005) analyzed the occurrence and resolution of neurosensory disturbances following bone harvesting from the symphysis. It evaluated 30 patients who complained of skin sensitivity of the chin/lower lip area and pulp sensitivity of all mandibular anterior teeth. The patients were assessed preoperatively, at the time of suture removal, and both at six and 12 months postoperatively. In addition, bone defect dimensions of the donor site were measured intraoperatively, and distances from defect margins to adjacent anatomical structures (such as root apices, mental foramen, and inferior border of mandible) were assessed postoperatively on a panoramic radiograph.

Pulp sensitivity changes were found in 18.6% of adjacent teeth at the time of suture removal. At the six-month follow-up, 8.1% of teeth, and at the 12-month reexamination, 0.6% of teeth, presented with altered sensitivity. This decrease over time of the number of affected teeth per patient with sensitivity changes was significant ($P = 2.35e - 007$). Radiographic measurements of distances between donor defect and adjacent anatomical structures only reached significant difference for one parameter in patients with sensitivity changes, compared with patients without sensitivity changes.

Nkenke et al. (2004) also assessed the extraoral morbidity following the harvest of bone from the anterior and posterior ilium in elective preprosthetic augmentations. They studied 50 consecutive healthy patients (30 female, 20 male, mean age 52.5 ± 9.3 years, age range 31 years to 65 years) who underwent augmentations of implant sites by iliac crest bone grafts. In 25 cases the bone harvest was from the anterior and in 25 cases it was from the posterior ilium. The superficial sensory function of the skin toward pain and thermal sensitivity was determined quantitatively preoperatively seven and 30 days after surgery. On the same occasions, subjective pain and gait disturbances were documented.

A significant impairment of the superficial sensory function could be found after one week and a significant tendency toward recovery was noted after one month. Gait disturbances were seen in seven patients after anterior bone harvest and in three patients after posterior bone harvest seven days after surgery. After one month, none of the patients from either group showed gait disturbances.

The maximum subjective pain level was found on the second postoperative day in both groups. It was significantly higher for the anterior approach. At days 7 and 30, the pain levels no longer differed significantly. The study concluded that there was a lower morbidity rate of bone harvest from the posterior ilium in the early postoperative phase compared to the anterior approach. Therefore, it seems that this approach should be preferred in elective augmentation procedures.

A minor nerve injury usually heals spontaneously within days or months. However, prolonged pressure from neuritis may lead to permanent degeneration of the affected nerve. Adjunct drugs such as clonazepam (Rivotril®, Hoffmann La Roche Ltd., Switzerland), carbamazepine (Tegretol®, Novartis Pharmaceutical, Inc., NJ, USA), or vitamin B-complex might alleviate neuritis via their known neuronal anti-inflammatory actions (Park and Wang 2005).

Systemic factors such as diabetes mellitus, poor oral measures, and smoking have proven to increase the risk for graft morbidity. Smoking impairs wound healing in various surgical operations. In orthopedic surgery, such as hip or knee arthroplasty, smoking is the single most important risk factor for the development of postoperative complications, particularly those relating to wound healing, cardiopulmonary complications, and postoperative intensive care (Esposito et al. 1998). One of the methods that has led the way to solve some clinical dilemmas of failed bone grafts, or sever osseous defects, is the use of sandwich osteotomy with an inlay autogenous bone graft or with interposition allograft blocks with sandwich techniques. (See Figures 12.29A–F.)

A study by Stellingsma and others (1998) evaluated 10 candidates ranging in age from 19 to 57 over a 31-month period. Several variables were measured, including condition of the peri-implant tissues, radiographic bone changes, and patient satisfaction. Results indicated that the technique offers a solid base for bone grafting in dental implantology. No implants were lost, bone loss was limited, and patients were satisfied. Another study by Satow and others (1997) evaluated the use of interposed bone grafts to accommodate endosteal implants

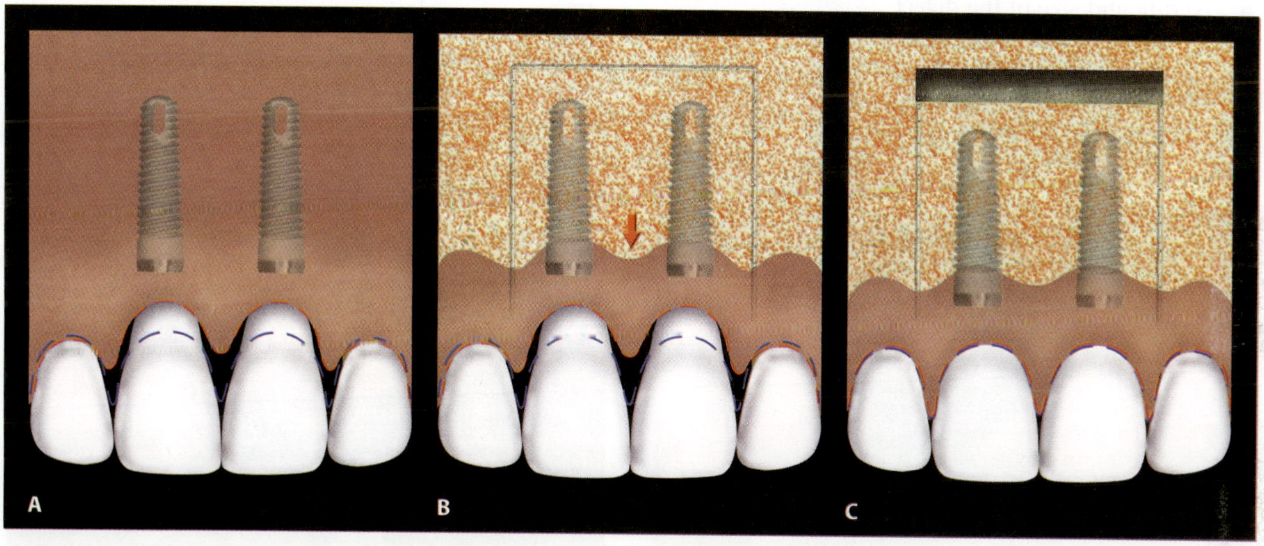

Figure 12.29. **A.** An illustration showing improper peri-implant soft tissue margin that indicates deficient bone support. The red line represents the actual gingival marginal condition and the blue line represents the optimal gingival level. **B.** The outline of the block osteotomy of the segment to move it in an incisal direction. **C.** The space developed after the segment is being moved.

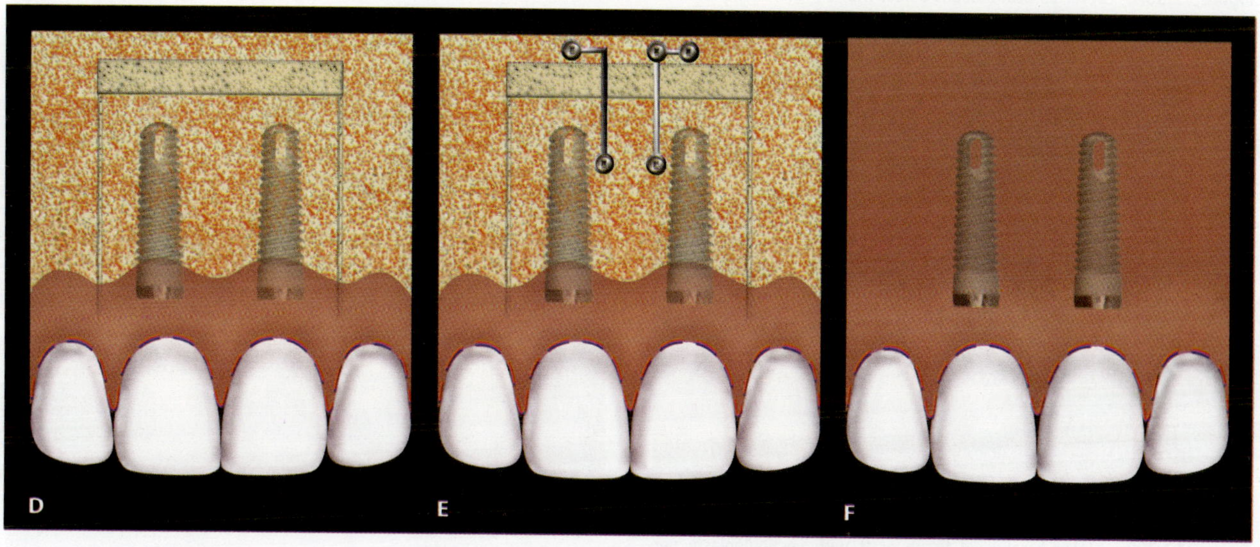

Figure 12.29. **D.** The interposition graft in place. **E.** The osseous segment is being stabilized to the basal bone. **F.** The case post healing.

for retaining mandibular over dentures. Results were reported in 34 edentulous patients who underwent interposed autogenous bone graft augmentation in the symphysis of the mandible, combined with onlay augmentation of the area posterior to the mental foramina. Two to four implants were placed in the grafted symphysis after 3–5 months. An over denture was constructed three months later. The follow-up period ranged from one to seven years. An average loss of mandibular bone height of 10–13% was observed. (See Figures 12.30A–G.)

The decision to use any particular grafting material or grafting technique should be based on the following:

- Nature and size of the defect
- Physical properties of the graft
- Chemical properties of the graft
- Mechanism(s) of action of the graft
- Assumed rehabilitation planning

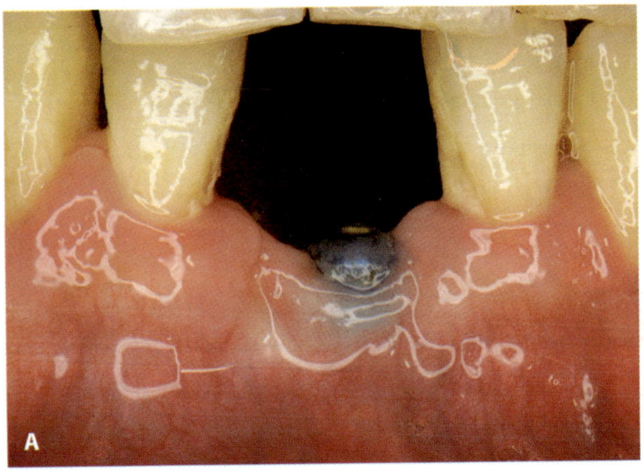

Figure 12.30A. Sever vertical osseous defect with un-retored implant.

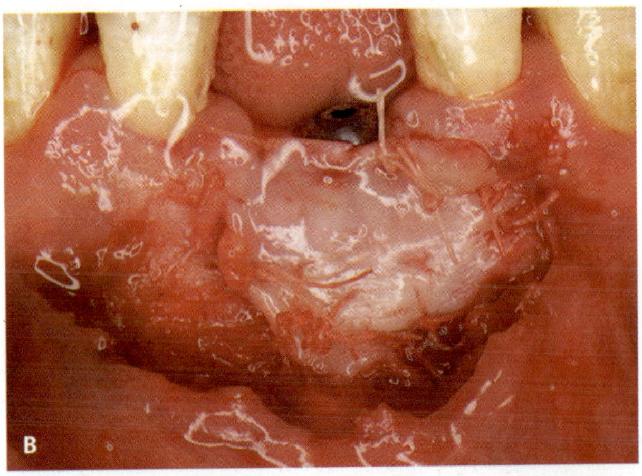

Figure 12.30B. Onlay keratinized tissue graft with vestibuloplasty performed in order to enhance the soft tissue at the site.

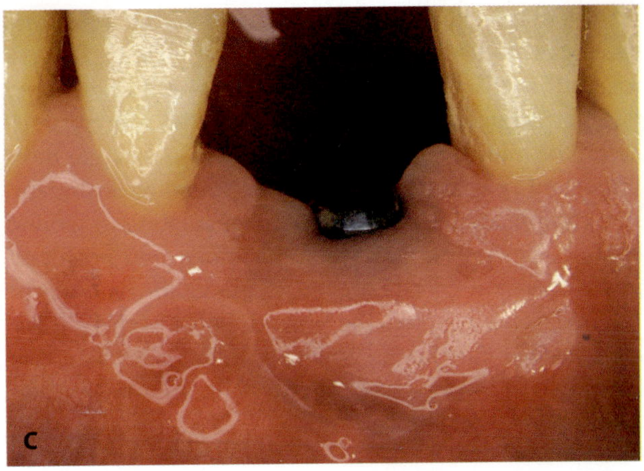

Figure 12.30C. Post operative view showing the improvement in the vestibular area as well as the quality and quantity of the keratinized mucosa.

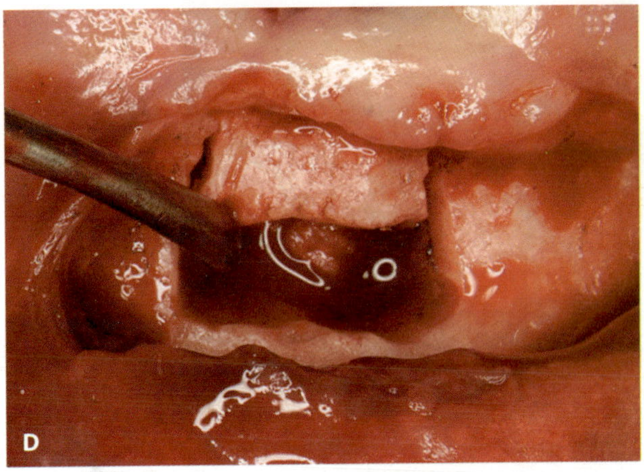

Figure 12.30D. The osseous segment is being displaced vertically.

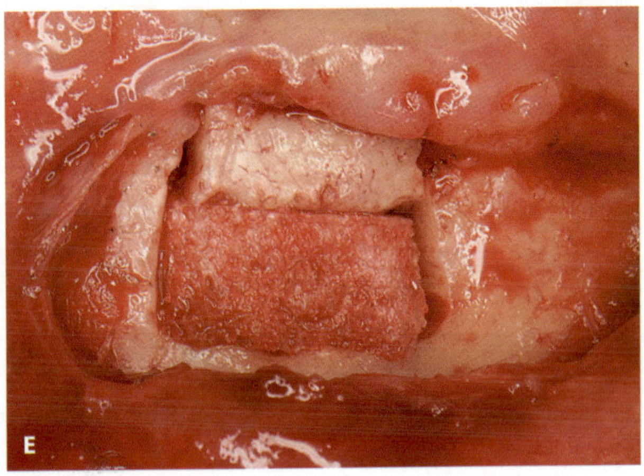

Figure 12.30E. The interposition graft is finally seated.

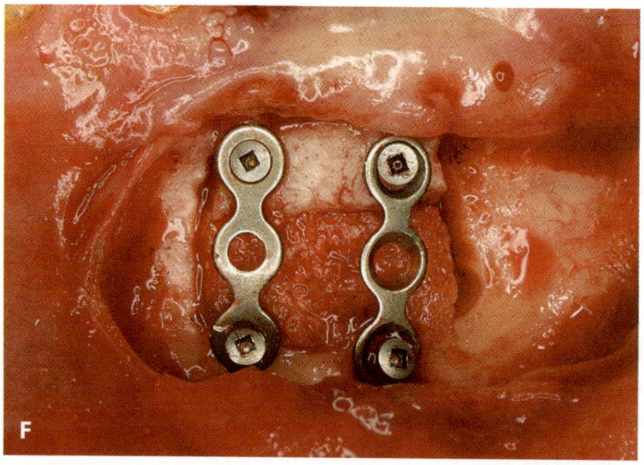

Figure 12.30F. Two micro-Ti-Plates are being used to stabilize the segment and the interposition graft to the basal bone of the mandible.

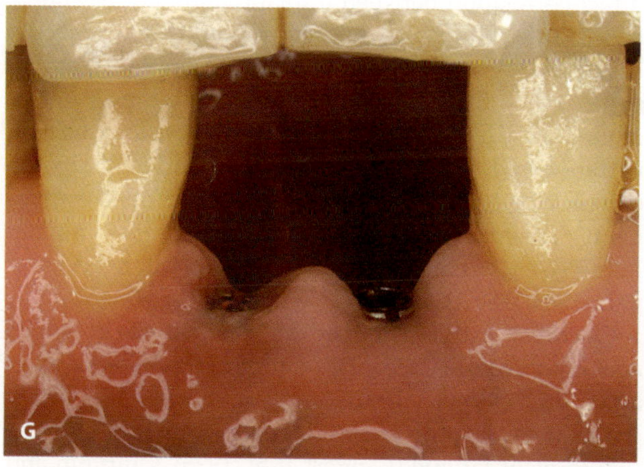

Figure 12.30G. Two month post operative healing showing an improvement of the vertical bone defect condition with the development of the inter-implant papilla due to the enhancement of the osseous support.

Today there is a wide array of grafting materials that can minimize the possibility of treatment complications. The use of modern materials has tremendously widened the scope and expectations for implant surgery. Research and clinical experience have shown that certain materials are better suited for specific applications than others and are much easier to handle than others. Keeping this in mind, the clinician must give priority to thorough presurgical planning and to considering less invasive procedures that attain predictable results. Selection of the appropriate grafting technique or grafting material influences the success and predictability of the final treatment outcome. Defect size and type and the patient's general health condition are some factors that influence the decision making in bone-grafting procedures.

Prosthetic and Biomechanical Complications

A recent consensus that provided a report on technical complications included implant fracture and connection-related and superastructure-related complications. Based on seven cohort studies with five years of follow-up and four studies with 10 years of follow-up, the incidence of implant fracture was 0.4% after five years and 1.8% after 10 years. The incidence of connection-related complications (screw loosening or fracture) was 7.3% (five years). The incidence of superastructure-related complications (veneer and framework fracture) was 14% after five years. Of the 7% of the restorations that were cemented, loss of retention of the restoration occurred in 2.9% within five years and 16.2% within 10 years. Regarding connecting natural teeth to dental implants in the same prostheses, the cumulative survival rate of implants used in implant-/tooth-supported fixed partial denture (FPD) was 90.1% after five years of function and 82.1% after 10 years of function. This evidence is derived from eight cohort studies with a mean follow-up of 5.7 years and four cohort studies with a mean 10-year follow-up period (Lang et al. 2004).

Proper patient selection and biomechanical prosthetic planning are the main components for achieving treatment success. Misch (1993b) stated that 10 prosthetic considerations should be evaluated before the final treatment plan is presented to the patient: (1) interarch space, (2) implant permucosal position, (3) existing occlusal plane, (4) arch relationship, (5) arch form, (6) existing occlusion, (7) existing prostheses, (8) number and location of missing teeth, (9) lip line, and (10) mandibular flexure. Any treatment plan aimed at success should include these 10 considerations in its prosthetic planning.

One of the most crucial factors is achieving passive fit during prosthesis insertion. This is considered to be one of the keys to success of dental implant-supported restorations in the esthetic and functional zones. Passive fit reduces long-term stresses along the implant superastructure or any related components, and protects bone adjacent to the implants (Jemt 1991). The failure to achieve passive fit may be manifested clinically by pain and discomfort in the short term, and loosening or fracture of implant components in the long term (Lekholm et al. 1985), because of excessive strains on the peri-implant bone (Scher 1991). According to Rangert and others (1989), the passive fit should exist at the 10-µm level and is required to achieve an optimum load distribution.

Millington and Leung (1995) found a positive correlation between the size of fit discrepancy and stress on the superastructure. Some of the factors that impair achievement of a passive fit are dimensional changes in ceramometal restorations during firing cycles, improper impression techniques, improper spacer application, and use of poor metal type for casting. A passive fit is considered to be an important factor in the success of dental implants. Many procedures have been applied to prevent nonpassivity, such as segmenting the metal try-in (in case of long-span restorations) and resoldering it properly to compensate for dimensional changes.

To evaluate whether the fabrication and retention methods have an influence on the passivity of superastructure fit, Karl and others (2004) conducted a study to quantify the strain development of various cemented and screw-retained FPDs. Forty samples of four different types of FPDs (10 of each type) were investigated. Each sample had three ITI implant abutments and two pontics. The three implants were anchored in a straight-line configuration in a measurement model simulating a real-life patient situation. Strain gauges were mounted close to the implants and on the pontics. The developing strains were recorded during cement setting and screw fixation. For statistical analysis, multivariate two-sample tests were performed, with the level of significance set at P = .1. All FPDs investigated revealed a considerable amount of strain, with no significant difference between cement and screw retention. Furthermore, no significant difference was found between the conventional fabrication modes for screw-retained FPDs. The lowest strains were found in prostheses that were intraorally bonded onto gold cylinders.

Because bonding of the superastructure in the oral cavity may compensate for impression and laboratory variables, restorations with the best possible passive fit can result from this retention technique. The study concluded that an absolute passive fit of superastructures is not possible using conventional clinical and laboratory procedures, and because clinical fit-evaluation methods often do not detect "hidden" inaccuracies, the more sensitive strain-gauge technique should be used for an objective accuracy test. Reference strain values from implant-supported prostheses that have served without complications could help define a "biologically acceptable fit." Another biomechanical critical factor that affects the long-term success of implant-supported restorations in the esthetic zone is the excessive application of cantilevers within any prosthetic design. For partially edentulous patients, this places offset loads to the most distal implant abutments and results in greater tensile and shear forces on cement or screw fixation, especially when the number of implants used for support is diminished. Many problems can be associated with cantilevers supported by dental implants. Such problems include fracture of the prosthesis (Rangert 1991), deintegration (Lekholm et al. 1985), and bone fatigue (Johns et al. 1992).

If any given three-unit prosthesis is supported by two implants and has a cantilevered tooth, the bending moment may be twice that of a prosthesis in which both ends are supported. With occlusal forces acting on the cantilever, the implant becomes a fulcrum and is subjected to axial, rotational, and torsional forces (English 1993). English also stated that distally extended cantilevers must be approached more cautiously because an increase of occlusal forces is encountered in the first and second molar areas. Fingerlike extensions to keep a maxillary second molar from extruding may be sufficient. Achieving a proper abutment-fixture interface fit is critical. It might lead to improper locking between the two parts of the antirotational implant device that leads to an increased strain on the implant components, with subsequent bone loss and rapid screw-joint failure. There is a direct correlation between implant-abutment rotational misfit and screw-joint failure (Binon 1996), probably because of micromovement between implant components. When there is no rotational misfit, the abutment immediately engages the external hexagon, and the load is transferred to the external hexagon and is dissipated by relieving compressive stresses in the clamped components. Therefore, the establishment of proper implant interface engagement with the superastructure becomes valuable to the long-term success of the treatment.

Overload can be defined as a situation in which occlusal forces on an implant-supported prosthesis exert a bending moment on the implant cross section at the crestal bone, leading to marginal bone loss and/or eventual implant fatigue (Rangert et al. 1995). Quirynin and others (1992) and Hoshaw and others (1994) have shown, both clinically and experimentally, that bone resorption around an implant may be caused by overload. This induces bending moments on the implant. In addition, analysis of clinically retrieved fractured implants and in vitro fatigue tests on implant components have demonstrated bending overload to be a causative factor in implant fracture (Rangert et al. 1995). Misch and others (2005) have investigated the literature to determine the relationship between occlusal overload and peri-implant bone loss via a Medline-assisted and hand search of peer-reviewed English literature. The search used a selective review of articles addressing biomechanical stress and bone loss in cellular biomechanics, engineering principles, mechanical properties of bone, animal studies, clinical reports, bone physiology, and implant design biomechanics. The results indicted a direct relationship between occlusal overload on implants and the incidence of marginal bone loss.

A retrospective clinical analysis by Rangert and others (1995) proposed three causative factors associated with bending of the implant: (1) in-line implants, (2) leverage, and (3) bruxism or heavy occlusal forces (Perel 1994). Misch (1993b) proposed a direct correlation between the bending force and the cube of the length of a fixed prosthesis, whereas Rangert and others (1989) proposed a proportional relationship between bending force and the distance from the occlusal contact to the crest of the supporting bone. It is important to properly manage the mechanical problems, as well as excessive bone resorption, with a proper response when they occur (Rangert et al. 1989).

The dentist should aim to reduce the amount of bending moments generated around an implant. This can be achieved if a careful treatment plan is made to select the appropriate location and number of implants to be placed. Avoiding or reducing cantilevers, narrowing the dimensions of the final restoration, and centering occlusal contacts are all clinical objectives. Loading of the implant too rapidly is considered to be one of the most common causes of prosthetic-related failure. In delayed loaded implant protocols, Branemark (1983) stated that strict protocol requires a stress-free healing period of three to six months for osseointegration to occur. Misch (1993c) stated that at 16 weeks, the surrounding bone is only 70% mineralized and still has woven bone as a component. The woven bone has an unorganized structure that cannot withstand full-scale stresses (Roberts et al. 1987). Also, Misch (1993c) has accordingly classified a specific healing period for each type of bone (from D1 to D4). Brunski (1993) stated that micromotion of more than 100 μm should be avoided; motion greater than this level causes the bone to undergo fibrous tissue repair rather than the desired osseous regeneration. But this is hard to apply practically. In fact, the precise level of micromotion that can be tolerated without being significantly inhibiting to bone formation is unknown (Esposito et al. 1998).

References

Abrahamsson, I., T. Berglundh, P.O. Glantz, et al. 1998. The mucosal attachment at different abutments. An experimental study in dogs. *J Clin Periodontol*, 25, (9), pp. 721–7.

Adell, R., U. Lekholm, and B. Rockler. 1981. A 15 year study of osseointegrated implants in the treatment of the edentulous jaws. *Int. J Oral Surg*, 10, pp. 387–416.

Agar, J., S. Cameron, J. Hughbanks, and M. Parker. 1997. Cement removal from restorations luted to titanium abutments with simulated subgingival margins. *J Prosthet Dent*, (78), pp. 43–47.

Apse, P., G.A. Zarb, A. Schmitt, and D.W. Lewis. 1991. The longitudinal effectiveness of osseointegrated dental implants. The Toronto study: Peri-implant mucosal response. *Int J Periodontics Restorative Dent*, 11, (2), pp. 94–111.

Asvanund, C.H., and S.M. Morgano. 2004. Restoration of unfavorably positioned implant for a partially edentulous patient by using an overdenture retained with a milled bar and attachments: A clinical report. *J Prosthet Dent*, 91, pp. 6–10.

Balshi, T.J. 1998. Preventing and resolving complications with osseointegrated Implants. *Dent Clin North Am.*, 33, pp. 821–868.

Barboza, E., and A. Caula. 2002. Diagnoses, Clinical Classification, and Proposed Treatment of Spontaneous Early Exposure of Submerged Implants. *Implant Dent*, 11, pp. 331–337.

Barboza, E., A. Caula, and F. Machado. 1999. Potential of recombinant human bone morphogenetic protein-2 in bone regeneration. *Implant Dent*, (4), pp. 360–366.

Bengazi, F., J.L. Wennstrom, and U. Lekholm. 1996. Recession of the soft tissue margin at oral implants. *Clin Oral Implant Res*, (7), pp. 303–310.

Binon, P.P. 1996. The effect of implant/abutment hexagonal misfit on screw joint stability. *Int J Prosthodont*, 9, pp. 149–160.

Boutros, S.M., B.S. Michalowicz, O.T. Smith, et al. 1996. Crevicular fluid enzymes from endosseous dental and natural teeth. *Int J Oral Maxillofac Implants*, 11, pp. 322–330.

Branemark, P.-I. 1983. Osseointegration and its experimental background. *J Prosthet Dent*, 50, pp. 399–440.

Brunski, J.B. 1993. Avoid pitfalls of overloading and micromotion of intraosseous implants [Interview]. *Dent Implantol Update*, 4, pp. 77–84.

Burchardt, H. 1987. Biology of bone transplantation. *Orthop Clin North Am*, 18, pp. 187–195.

Buser, D., U. Bragger, N.P. Lang, and S. Nyman. 1990. Regeneration and enlargement of jaw bone using guided tissue regeneration. *Clin Oral Implants Res*, 1, p. 22.

Buser, D., K. Dula, H.P. Hirt, and H. Berthold. 1994. Localized ridge augmentation using guided bone regeneration. In: Buser, D., Dahlin, C., Schenk, R., eds. *Guided Bone Regeneration in Implant Dentistry*. Chicago: Quintessence.

Ciancio, S., M. Mather, and M. Kazmierczak. 1990. Effectiveness of systemic antibiotics in a barrier method of periodontal regeneration. *J Dent Res*, 69, p. 165.

Demolon, I.A., G.R. Persson, B.J. Moncla, R.H. Johnson, and W.E. Ammons. 1993. Effects of antibiotic treatment on clinical conditions and bacterial growth with guided tissue regeneration. *J Periodontol*, 64, pp. 609–616.

El Askary, A.S., and R.M. Meffert. 1999. Aesthetic considerations in anterior single tooth replacement. *Implant Dent.*, 8, pp. 61–66.

El Askary, A.S., R.M. Meffert, and T. Griffin. 1999a. Why Do Dental Implants Fail, Part I. *Implant Dent*, 8, pp. 173–185.

El Askary, A.S., R.M. Meffert, and T. Griffin. 1999b. Why Do Dental Implants Fail, Part II. *Implant Dent*, 8, pp. 265–277

English, C.E. 1993. Biomechanical concerns with fixed partial dentures involving implants. *Implant Dent.*, 2, pp. 221–242.

Esposito, M., J.-M. Hirsch, U. Lekholm, et al. 1998. Biological factors contributing to failures of osseointegrated oral implants (II). Etiopathogenesis. *Eur J Oral Sci*, 106, pp. 721–764.

Friedlander, G. 1987. Current concepts review. Bone grafts: The basic science rationale for clinical applications. *J Bone Joint Surg*, 69, p. 786.

Gottlow, J., S. Nyman, J. Lindhe, T. Karring, and J. Wennstrom. 1986. New attachment formation in the human periodontium by guided tissue regeneration. *J Clin Periodontol*, 13, p. 604.

Guerrero, C., R. Laplana, N. Figueredo, et al. 1999. Surgical Implant Repositioning: A Clinical Report. *Int J Oral Maxillofac Implants*, 14, pp. 48–54.

Hoshaw, S., J. Brunski, and G. Cochran. 1994. Mechanical bending of Branemark implants affects interfacial bone modelling. *Int J Oral Maxillofac Implants*, 9, pp. 345–360.

Jemt, T. 1991. Failures and complications in 391 consecutively inserted fixed prostheses supported by Branemark implants in edentulous jaws: A study of treatment from the time of prosthesis placement to the first annual checkup. *Int J Oral Maxillofac Implants*, 6, pp. 270–275.

Johns, R.B., T. Jemt, M.R. Heath, et al. 1992. A multicenter study of overdentures supported by Branemark implants. *Int J Oral Maxillofac Implants*, 7, pp. 513–522.

Joshi, A. 2004. An investigation of post-operative morbidity following chin graft surgery. *Br Dent J.*, 196(4), pp. 215–218.

Jovanovic, S., and M. Nevins. 1995. Bone formation utilizing titanium-reinforced barrier membranes. *Int J Periodontics Restorative Dent*, 15, pp. 57–69.

Karl, M., W. Winter, T. Taylor, et al. 2004. In vitro study on passive fit in implant-supported 5 units fixed partial dentures, 19, pp. 30–37.

Krekeler, G., W. Schilli, and J. Diemer. 1985. Should the exit of the artificial abutment tooth be positioned in the region of the attached gingiva? *Int J Oral Surg*, 14, pp. 504–508.

Lane, J.M. 1995. Bone graft substitutes. *West J Med*, (163), pp. 565–567.

Lang, N.P., C.H. Hammede, U. Bragger, B. Lehman, and S.R. Nyman. 1994. Guided tissue regeneration in jawbone defects prior to implant placement. *Clin Oral Implant Res*, (5), pp. 92–97.

Lang, N., T. Berglundh, H. Mayfield, et al. 2004. Consensus Statements and Recommended Clinical Procedures Regarding Implant Survival and Complications. *J Prosthet Dent.*, 19, pp. 150–154.

Lekholm, U., R. Adell, and P.-I. Branemark. 1985. Complications. In: Branemark, P.-I., Zarb, G.A., Albrektsson, T., eds. Tissue-Integrated Prostheses: *Osseointegration in clinical dentistry*. Chicago: Quintessence Publishing Company, Inc., pp. 233–240.

Lekholm, U., W. Becker, C. Dahlin, B. Becker, K. Donath, and E. Morrison. 1993. The role of early versus late removal of GTAM membranes on bone formation at oral implants placed into immediate extraction sockets. An experimental study in dogs. *Clin Oral Implants Res*, 4, pp. 121–129.

Lu, M., and A.B. Rabie. 2003. Microarchitecture of rabbit mandibular defects grafted with intra-membranous or endochondral bone shown by micro-computed tomography. *Br J Oral Maxillofac Surg.*, 41, pp. 385–391.

Maynard, J.G., and R.D.K. Wilson. 1979. Physiologic dimensions of the periodontium significant to the restorative dentist. *J Periodontol*, 50, p. 170.

Meffert, R.M. 1992. Treatment of failing dental implants. *Curr Opin Dent*, 2, pp. 109–144.

Meijndert, L., H. Meijer, G. Raghoebar, et al. 2004. A Technique for Standardized Evaluation of Soft and Hard Peri-Implant Tissues in Partially Edentulous Patients. *J Periodontol*, 75, pp. 646–651.

Millington, N.D., and T. Leung. 1995. Inaccurate fit of implant superastructures. Part 1: Stresses generated on the superastructure relative to the size of fit discrepancy. *Int J Prosthodont*, 8, pp. 511–516.

Misch, C.E. 1993a. Prosthetic options in implant dentistry. In: Misch, C.E., ed. Contemporary implant Dentistry. St. Louis, MO: *Mosby Yearbook, Inc.*, pp. 43–50.

Misch, C.E. 1993b. Prosthodontic considerations. In: Misch, C.E., ed. Contemporary Implant Dentistry. St. Louis, MO: *Mosby Yearbook*, Inc., pp. 187–200.

Misch, C.E. 1993c. Progressive Bone Loading. In: Misch, C.E., ed. Contemporary Implant Dentistry. St. Louis, MO: *Mosby Yearbook*, Inc., 623–650.

Misch, C.E. 1995. The maxillary anterior single tooth implant aesthetic health compromise. *Int J Dent Symp*, (1), pp. 4–9.

Misch, C.E. 1999. The harvest of ramus bone in conjunction with third molar removal for onlay grafting before placement of dental implants. *J Oral Maxillofac Surg.*, 57, pp. 1376–1379.

Misch, C., J. Suzuki, F. Misch, et al. 2005. A Positive Correlation Between Occlusal Trauma and Peri-implant Bone Loss: Literature Support. *Implant Dent*, 14, pp. 108–116.

Mombelli, A., M.A.C. Van Oosten, E. Schurch, et al. 1987. The microbiota associated with successful or failing osseointegrated titanium implants. *Oral Microbiol Immunol*, 2, pp. 145–151.

Murphy, K.G. 1995. Incidence, characterization and effect of postoperative surgical complications using Gore-Tex periodontal material. Part II. Effect of complications on regeneration. *Int J Periodont Rest Dent*, 15, pp. 363–375, 549–561.

Nemcovsky, C., and Z. Artzi. 2002. Comparative Study of Buccal Dehiscence Defects in Immediate, Delayed, and Late Maxillary Implant Placement with Collagen Membranes: Clinical Healing Between Placement and Second Stage Surgery, *J Periodontol*, 73, pp. 754–761.

Nishimura, R.D., T.L. Chang, G.R. Perri, et al. 1999. Restoration of partially edentulous patients using customized implant abutments. *Pract Periodont Aesthet Dent*, (11), pp. 669– 676.

Nkenke, E., V. Weisbach, E. Winckler, et al. 2004. Morbidity of harvesting of bone grafts from the iliac crest for preprosthetic augmentation procedures: a prospective study. *Int J Oral Maxillofac Surg.*, 33, (2), pp. 157–63.

Oates, T., J. West, J. Jones, et al. 2002. Long-Term Changes in Soft Tissue Height on the Facial Surface of Dental Implants. *Implant Dent*, 11, pp. 272–279.

Park, S.H., and H.L. Wang. 2005. Implant Reversible Complications: *Classification and Treatments Implant Dent*, 14, pp. 211–220.

Perel, M.L. 1994. Parafunctional habits, night guards, and root form implants. *Implant Dent.*, 3, pp. 261–263.

Powell, C., B. Mealey, D. Deas, et al. 2005. Post-Surgical Infections: Prevalence Associated With Various Periodontal Surgical Procedures. *J Periodontol*, 76, pp. 329–333.

Quirynin, M., J. Naert, and D. Van Steenberghe. 1992. Fixture design and overload influence, marginal bone loss and implant success in the Branemark system. *Clin Oral Impl Res*, 3, pp. 104–111.

Rangert, B., T. Jemt, and L. Jorneus. 1989. Forces and moments on Branemark Implants. *Int J Oral Maxillofac Implants*, 4, pp. 241–247.

Rangert, B., J. Gunne, and D.Y. Sullivan. 1991. Mechanical aspects of a Branemark implant connect to a natural tooth: An in vitro study. *Int J Oral Maxillofac Implants*, 6, pp. 185–194.

Rangert, B., P.H.J. Krogh, B. Langer, et al. 1995. Bending overload and implant fracture: A retrospective clinical analysis. *Int J Oral Maxillofac Implants*, 10, pp. 326–334.

Roberts, W., P. Turley, N. Brezniak et al. 1987. Bone physiology and metabolism, *J Calif Dent Assoc*, 2, pp. 155–156.

Rosenberg, E.S., J.P. Torosian, and J. Slots. 1991. Microbial differences in two clinically distinct types of failures of osseointegrated implants. *Clin Oral Implants Res*, 2, pp. 134–144.

Sander, L., E.V.G. Frandsen, D. Arnbjerg, K. Warrer, and T. Karring. 1994. Effect of local metronidazole application on periodontal healing following guided tissue regeneration. Clinical findings. *J Periodontol*, 65, pp. 914–920.

Satow, S., A.P. Slagter, P.J. Stoelinga, et al. 1997. Interposed bone grafts to accommodate endosteal implants for retaining mandibular overdentures. A 1–7 year follow-up study. *Int J Oral Maxillofac Surg.*, 26, (5), pp. 358–64.

Schwartz, A., J. Melloing, D. Carnes, J. de la Fontaine, D. Cochran, D. Dean, and B. Boyan. 1996. Ability of commercial de-mineralized freeze-dried bone allograft to induce new bone formation. *J Periodontol*, 67, pp. 918–926.

Schallhorn, R.G., and P.R. McClain. 1988. Combined osseous composite grafting, root conditioning and guided tissue regeneration. *Int J Periodont Rest Dent*, 8, (4), pp. 9–31.

Scher, E.L. 1991. The use of osseointegrated implants in long span fixed partial prosthesis: A case report. *Int J Oral Maxillofac Implants*, 6, pp. 351–353.

Schwartz-Arad, D., and S. Dori. 2002. Intraoral autogenous onlay block bone grafting for implant dentistry. *Refuat Hapeh Vehashinayim*, 19, pp. 35–39.

Schwartz-Arad, D., L. Levin, and L. Sigal. 2005. Surgical Success of Intraoral Autogenous Block Onlay Bone Grafting for Alveolar Ridge Augmentation. *Implant Dent*, 14, pp. 131–138.

Selliseth, N.J., and K.A. Selvig. 1994. The vasculature of the periodontal ligament: A scanning electron microscopic study using corrosion casts in the rat. *J Periodontol*, 65, pp. 1079–1087.

Selvig, K., R. Nilveus, B. Kersten, and S. Khorsandi. 1990. Scanning electron microscopic observation of cell population and bacterial contamination of membranes used for guided tissue regeneration in humans. *J Periodontol*, 61, pp. 515–520.

Small, P.N., and D.P. Tarnow. 2000. Gingival recession around implants: A 1-year longitudinal prospective study. *Int J Oral Maxillofac Implants*, (15), pp. 527–532.

Smith, J.D., and M. Abramson. 1974. Membranous vs. endochondral bone autografts. *Arch Otolaryngol*, 99, pp. 203–205.

Spear, F., and C. Townsend. 1991. Esthetics: A multidisciplinary approach. Presented at the American Academy of Periodontology, 77th Annual Meeting, Vancouver, October 2.

Stellingsma, C., G.M. Raghoebar, H.J. Meijer, et al. 1998. Reconstruction of the extremely resorbed mandible with interposed bone grafts and placement of endosseous implants. A preliminary report on outcome of treatment and patients' satisfaction. *Br J Oral Maxillofac Surg.*, Aug, 36, (4), pp. 290–5.

Strub, J., T. Gaberthuel, and U. Grunder. 1991. The role of attached gingiva in the health of peri-implant tissue in dogs. Part I. Clinical findings. *Int J Periodontics Restorative Dent*, 11, pp. 317–333.

Tal, H. 1999. Spontaneous early exposure of submerged implants: 1. Classification and clinical observations. *J Periodontol*, 70, pp. 213–219.

Tatum, Jr., O.J. 1996. Osseous grafts in intra-oral sites. *J Oral Implant*, (22), pp. 51–52.

Toljanic, J.A., M.L. Banakis, L.A. Willes, et al. 1999. Soft tissue exposure of endosseous implants between stage I and II surgery as a potential indicator of early crestal bone loss. *Int J Oral Maxillofac Implants*, 14, pp. 436–441.

Tolman, D. 1995. Reconstructive procedures with endosseous implants in grafted bone: A review of the literature. *Int J Oral Maxillofac Implants*, 10, pp. 275–294.

Tonetti, M.S., and J. Schmid. 1994. Pathogenesis of implant failures. *Periodontol 2000*. 4, pp. 127–38.

Toriumi, D.M., H.S. Kotler, D.P. Luxenberg, et al. 1991. Mandibular reconstruction with a recombinant bone-inducing factor: Functional, histologic and biomechanical evaluation. *Aech Otolaryngol Head Neck Surg*, (17), pp. 1101–1112.

Valentini, P., D. Abensur, and P. Missika. 1993. Membrane exposure during bone regeneration before implant placement: Management and results. A report of two cases. *J Oral Implantol*, 19, pp. 364–368.

von Arx, T., J. Hafliger, and V. Chappuis. 2005. Neurosensory disturbances following bone harvesting in the symphysis: a prospective clinical study. *Clin Oral Implants Res*. Aug, 16, (4), pp. 432–9.

Wang, E.A., V. Rosen, J.S. D'Alessandro, et al. 1990. Recombinant human bone morphogenetic protein induces bone formation. *Proc Natl Acad Sci USA*, (87), pp. 2220–2224.

Warden, P.J. 2000. Surgical repositioning of a malposed, unserviceable implant: Case report. *Int J Oral Maxillofac Surg*, (58), pp. 433–435.

Zanetta-Barbosa, D., B. Klinge, and H. Svensson. 1993. Laser Doppler llowmetry of blood perfusion in mucoperiosteal flaps covering membranes in bone augmentation and implant procedures. A pilot study in dogs. *Clin Oral Implants Res*, 4, pp. 35–38.

Zubillaga, G., S. Von Hagen, B. Simon, et al. 2003. Changes in Alveolar Bone Height and Width Following Post-Extraction Ridge Augmentation Using a Fixed Bioabsorbable Membrane and Demineralized Freeze-Dried Bone Osteoinductive Graft. *J Periodontol*, 74, pp. 965–975.

Index